## Tenth Edition

Volume
3

*Competency Based*

**BD Chaurasia's**

# Human Anatomy

## Regional and Applied — Dissection and Clinical

As per the latest NMC Guidelines | Competency Based Medical Education (CBME) Curriculum under Graduate Medical Education Regulation

## Head and Neck

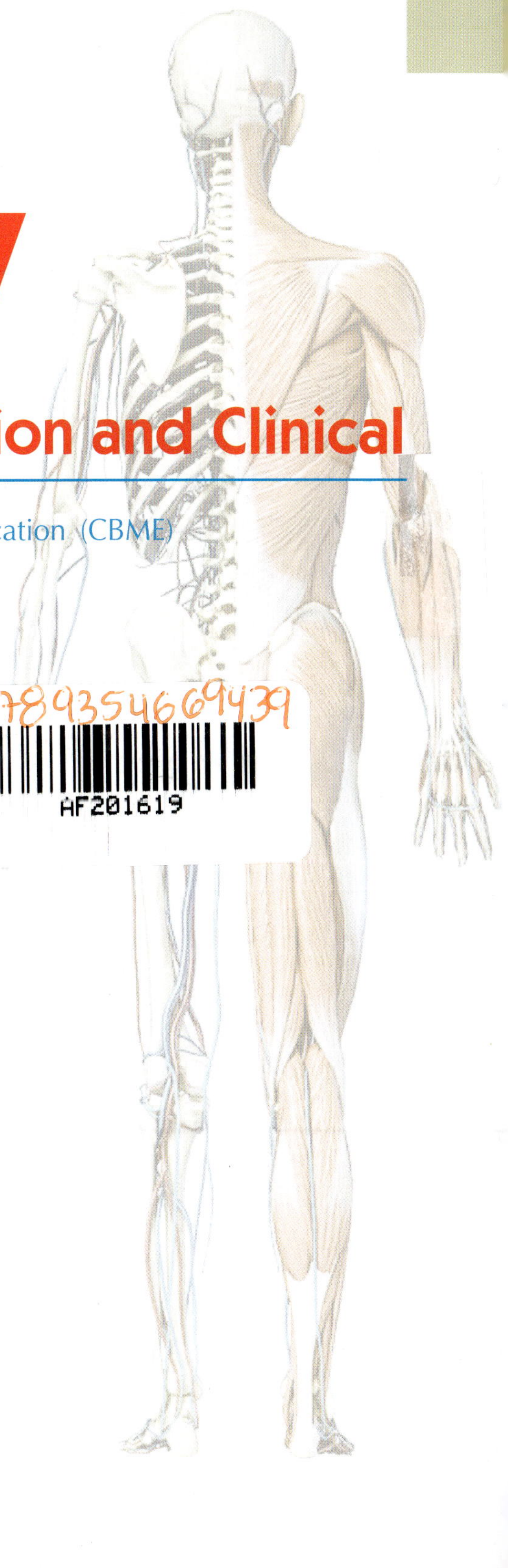

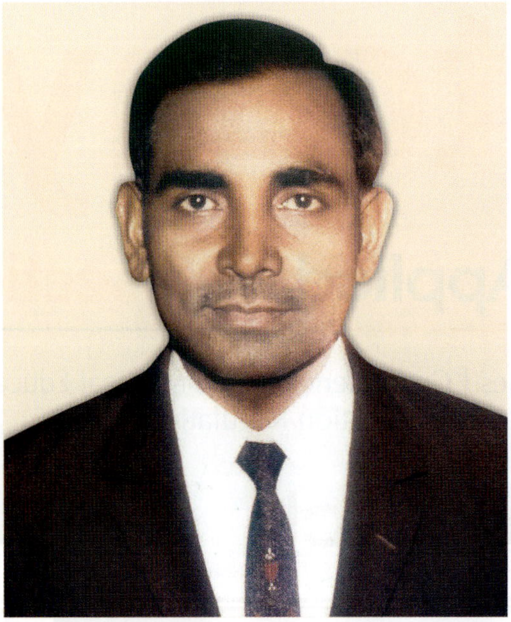

**Dr BD Chaurasia** (1937–1985)

was Reader in Anatomy at GR Medical College, Gwalior.
He received his MBBS in 1960, MS in 1965 and PhD in 1975.
He was elected fellow of National Academy of Medical Sciences (India) in 1982.
He was a member of the Advisory Board of the *Acta Anatomica* since 1981,
member of the editorial board of *Bionature*, and in addition
member of a number of scientific societies.
He had a large number of research papers to his credit.

**Tenth Edition**

**Volume 3**

*Competency Based*

**BD Chaurasia's**

# Human Anatomy

## Regional and Applied | Dissection and Clinical

As per the latest NMC Guidelines | Competency Based Medical Education (CBME) Curriculum under Graduate Medical Education Regulation

## Head and Neck

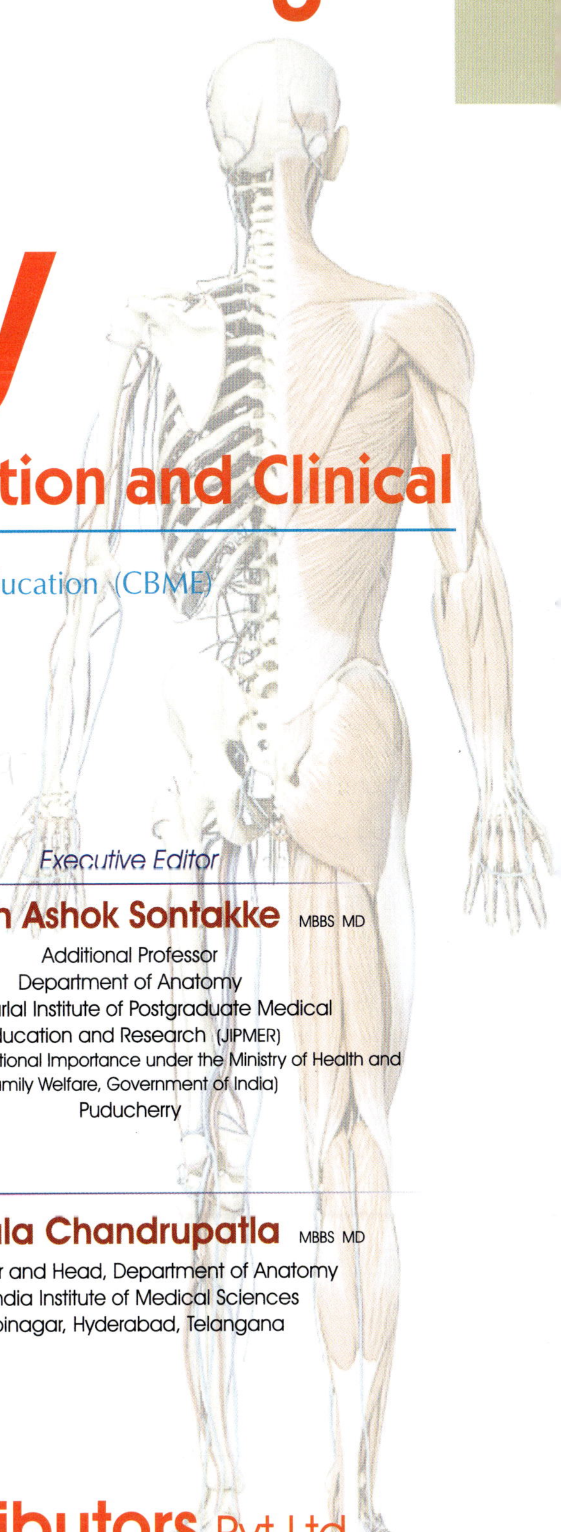


*Chief Editor*

**Krishna Garg**
MBBS MS PhD FIMSA FIAMS FAMS FASI
Legend of Anatomy; Nation's Who's Who
Fellow, Anatomical Society of India
Lifetime Achievement Awardee
DMA Distinguished Service Awardee
Ex-Professor and Head, Department of Anatomy
Lady Hardinge Medical College, New Delhi

*Executive Editor*

**Yogesh Ashok Sontakke** MBBS MD
Additional Professor
Department of Anatomy
Jawaharlal Institute of Postgraduate Medical Education and Research (JIPMER)
(An Institute of National Importance under the Ministry of Health and Family Welfare, Government of India)
Puducherry

*Editors*

**Pragati Sheel Mittal** MBBS MS
Professor, Department of Anatomy
Government Institute of Medical Sciences
Greater Noida, Uttar Pradesh

**Mrudula Chandrupatla** MBBS MD
Professor and Head, Department of Anatomy
All India Institute of Medical Sciences
Bibinagar, Hyderabad, Telangana



CBSPD

**CBS Publishers & Distributors** Pvt Ltd

New Delhi • Bengaluru • Chennai • Kochi • Kolkata • Lucknow • Mumbai
Gujarat • Hyderabad • Jharkhand • Nagpur • Patna • Pune • Uttarakhand

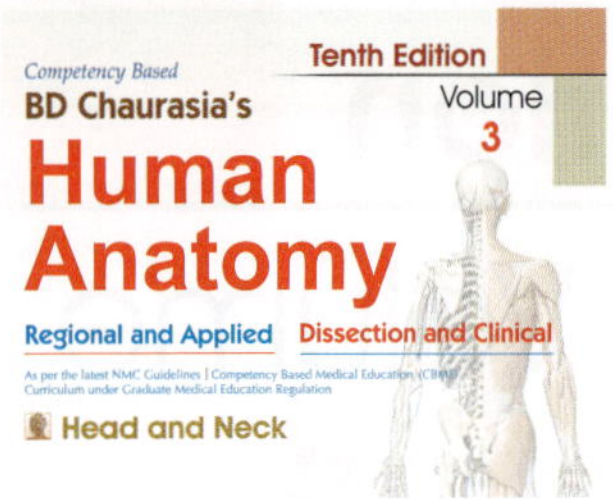




**ISBN:** 978-93-5466-943-9



**Tenth Edition: 2025**[1]
**Reprint: 2026**

First Edition: 1979
Reprint: 1980, 1981, 1982, 1983, 1984, 1985, 1986, 1987, 1988
Second Edition: 1989
Reprint: 1990, 1991, 1992, 1993, 1994
Third Edition: 1995
Reprint: 1996, 1997, 1998, 1999, 2000, 2001, 2002, 2003, 2004
Fourth Edition: 2004
Reprint: 2005, 2006, 2007, 2008, 2009
Fifth Edition: 2010
Reprint: 2011, 2012
Sixth Edition: 2013
Reprint: 2014, 2015
Seventh Edition: 2016
Reprint: 2017, 2018, 2019
Eighth Edition: 2020
Reprint: 2021, 2022
Ninth Edition: 2023
Reprint: 2024



Published by Satish Kumar Jain and produced by Varun Jain for

**CBS Publishers & Distributors** Pvt Ltd
4819/XI Prahlad Street, 24 Ansari Road, Daryaganj, New Delhi 110 002, India
Ph: 011-23289259, 23266838
Website: www.cbspd.com
e-mail: delhi@cbspd.com

*Corporate Office:* 204 FIE, Industrial Area, Patparganj, Delhi 110 092, India
Ph: 011-4934 4934 Fax: 011-4934 4935 e-mail: publishing@cbspd.com; publicity@cbspd.com

***Branches***

- **Bengaluru:** Seema House 2975, 17th Cross, K.R. Road, Banasankari 2nd Stage, Bengaluru 560 070, Karnataka, India
  Ph: +91-80-26771678/79 Fax: +91-80-26771680 e-mail: bangalore@cbspd.com
- **Chennai:** 18/8B, Subbarayan Street, Shenoy Nagar, Chennai 600 030, Tamil Nadu, India
  Ph: +91-44-42032115, 26681266 e-mail: chennai@cbspd.com
- **Kochi:** 42/1325, 1326, Power House Road, Opposite KSEB, Power House, Ernakulum 682 018, Kochi, Kerala, India
  Ph: +91-484-4059061–65, 67 Fax: +91-484-4059065 e-mail: kochi@cbspd.com
- **Kolkata:** 147, Hind Ceramics Compound, 1st Floor, Nilgunj Road, Belghoria, Kolkata 700 056, West Bengal, India
  Ph: +91-33-25633055/56 e-mail: kolkata@cbspd.com
- **Lucknow:** Basement, Khushnuma Complex, 7 Meerabai Marg (behind Jawahar Bhawan), Lucknow 226 001, UP, India
  Ph: +91-522-4000032 e-mail: tiwari.lucknow@cbspd.com
- **Mumbai:** PWD Shed, Gala No. 25/26, Ramchandra Bhatt Marg, Next JJ Hospital Gate No. 2, Opp. Union Bank of India, Noorbaug, Mumbai 400 009, Maharashtra, India
  Ph: +91-22-66661880/89 e-mail: mumbai@cbspd.com

***Representatives***

- **Gujarat** 0-9879558667
- **Hyderabad** 0-9885175004
- **Jharkhand** 0-9811541605
- **Nagpur** 0-8692091830
- **Patna** 0-9334159340
- **Pune** 0-9664372571
- **Uttarakhand** 0-9716462459

*Printed at:* Thomson Press (India) Ltd., Faridabad, Haryana, India

*to*

*my teacher*
*Shri Uma Shankar Nagayach*

— BD Chaurasia

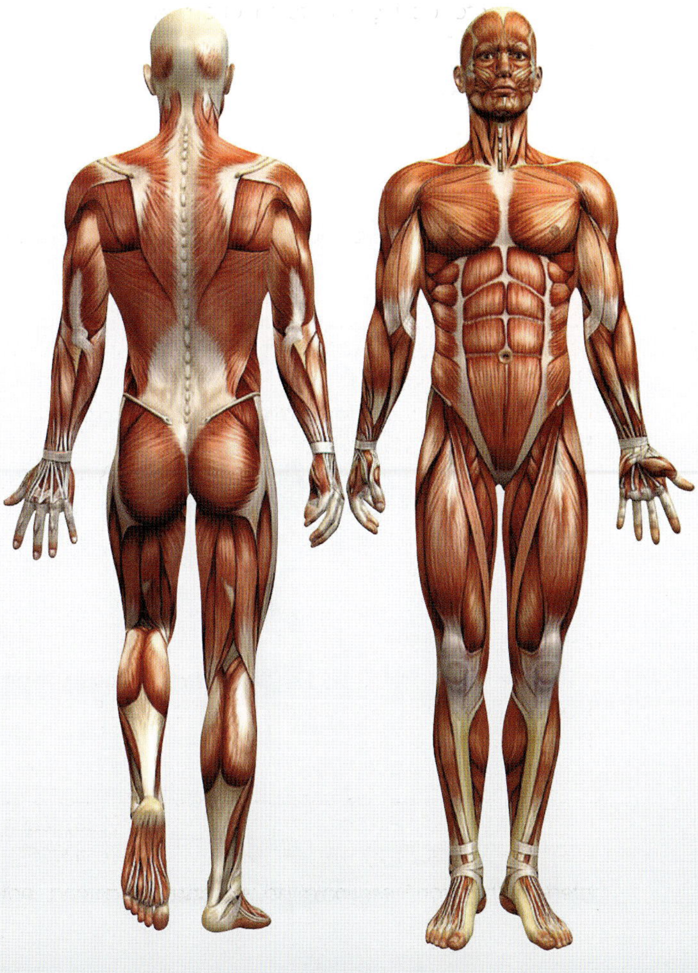

Volume 1 **UPPER LIMB and THORAX**

Volume 2 **LOWER LIMB, ABDOMEN and PELVIS**

Volume 3 **HEAD and NECK**

Volume 4 **BRAIN–NEUROANATOMY**

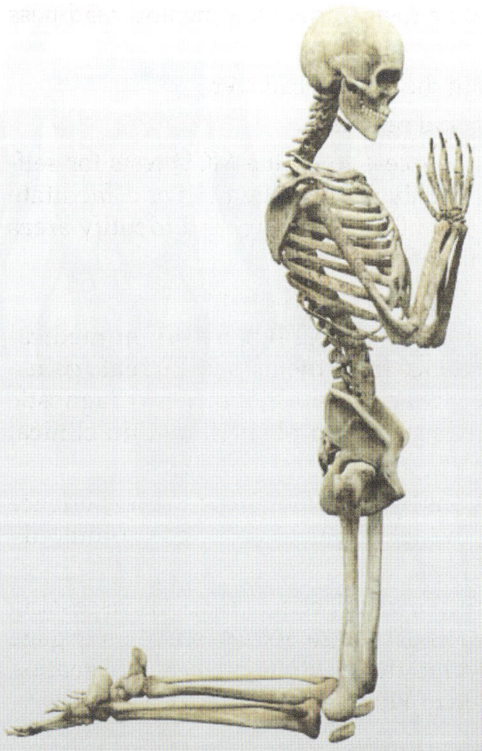

# Preface to the Tenth Edition

With the change in time, the needs of the students and curriculum are continuously changing. The science is continuously evolving. To integrate the solutions to common problems faced by the students and to follow the latest NMC guidelines for the CBME curriculum, the most widely accepted and read book has been revised thoroughly to maintain the standards of the last half-century. The primary goal of this book is to help the students for easy understanding and rapid grasping of knowledge for their higher academic achievements, to prepare them for all academic formative, summative and entrance examinations and to make it extremely student-friendly.

Anatomy forms the foundation of the clinical knowledge. This book has been made more clinically oriented with the following salient features:

- **Complete** and **time-tested textbook** boasting unparalleled **quality content** designed to enrich both fundamental and clinical understanding for students.
- **Simple text** is the main feature of the book. It will facilitate easier understanding for students. Small sentences minimize effort, enhancing readability and accessibility. This approach ensures clarity of information, aiding students in grasping complex concepts effortlessly.
- **Updated text and images:** The text and images updated as per the updates in the field of medicine, in the terms updates the facts and the data from the authenticated reference books. All the deviations from the traditional concepts, have been duly sourced and referenced to the standard international publications. It make the book suitable for all the academic university and entrance examinations need the updated information.
- **3D colour illustrated plates** will aid the students in comprehending anatomical structures and their relationships with clarity. These visual aids offer a dynamic perspective, enhancing spatial understanding and facilitating the identification of anatomical features.
- **Simple line diagrams** are incorporated. These diagrams will allow students to easily redraw them during examinations. These diagrams are designed for clarity and simplicity, ensuring that students can accurately reproduce anatomical structures in assessments and examinations efficiently.
- **Flowcharts** will facilitate rapid revision and memorizing of facts, alleviating students' concerns about time constraints during the subject review. These visuals will enhance comprehension and retention. Students can quickly navigate through key concepts, optimizing study time and effectively addressing time limitations in their revision process.
- **Clinical anatomy** sections are integrated at the end of each topic to maintain the purpose towards **early clinical exposure** (ECE). By seamlessly merging theoretical knowledge with practical application, this approach ensures students gain valuable insights into clinical contexts, enhancing their understanding and readiness for real-world clinical scenarios.
- **Dissection boxes** will guide the students in the step-wise dissection of the human cadaver.
- **Tables** are used to summarise essential facts for clear understanding and retention.
- *QR codes* for ***eSmartQuiz*** are embedded in the text, which will grant access to online MCQ tests for self-assessment at the end of each chapter. This interactive feature will enhance engagement and facilitate convenient self-evaluation. Students can assess their understanding, reinforce learning, and identify areas for improvement, facilitate a dynamic and effective learning experience.
- ***Free Workbook:*** The main textbook is supported with a workbook, which has the following:
  1. **Clinicoanatomical problems** emphasize early clinical exposure and vertical integration in medical education. By integrating anatomical knowledge with clinical practice from the outset, students gain a holistic understanding of medical concepts. This approach fosters practical skills, enhances diagnostic abilities, and promotes a deeper comprehension of the human body's complexities within clinical contexts.
  2. **Practice figures** aid in preparing students for academic examinations by providing hands-on experience with exam-style preparation. It will help to build confidence in tackling the challenges commonly encountered in academic assessments.
  3. **Multiple choice questions (MCQs)** will serve as potent tools for reinforcing learning, assessing comprehension, and enhancing attention and critical thinking skills. Through MCQs, students engage actively with the curriculum, consolidate understanding, and develop the ability to analyse information critically, ultimately fostering deeper comprehension and retention of knowledge.

4. **Spotters** and **question bank** introduce students to the examination system by familiarising them with the format and types of questions commonly encountered in assessments. These wide ranges of questions will aid the students in preparing for examinations and gaining confidence in tackling examination challenges effectively.

- ***Free MindMaps in Anatomy*:** A separate booklet of MindMaps in Anatomy is included with each volume. These MindMaps will help the students revise and memorise anatomy through visual impact in a precise manner.
- ***Free access to BDC's Anatomy eBook (digital content through CBSiCentral app)*:** It includes the following:
  a. Additional topics and clinical aspects
  b. *Viva voce* questions, and
  c. Topics for further reference and reading.

  This digital resource will enhance the book's utility, providing students with expanded knowledge and resources for comprehensive learning. Accessible supplementary materials will enhance understanding and facilitate deeper exploration, empowering students to excel in their studies and clinical practice.
- **Free Access to CBSiCentral App:** It includes videos of osteology and soft parts and chapter-wise self-assessment MCQ tests. The videos of the dissection will give three-dimensional image descriptions of tissues and organs, which get effectively registered in the brain for a longer time.
- **Wall charts:** Each volume is provided with meticulously crafted wall charts, elegantly designed and tailored to enhance students' comprehension of anatomy. These visually engaging aids can be easily affixed to walls to grasp the visual impressions of anatomy.

Always remember that success is achieved only through diligent effort and hard work.

*Chief Editor*
**Krishna Garg**

*Executive Editor*
**Yogesh Ashok Sontakke**

*Editors*
**Pragati Sheel Mittal**
**Mrudula Chandrupatla**

# Preface to the First Edition (excerpts)

The necessity of having a simple, systematized and complete book on anatomy has long been felt. The urgency for such a book has become all the more acute due to the shorter time now available for teaching anatomy, and also to the falling standards of English language in the majority of our students in India. The national symposium on 'Anatomy in Medical Education' held at Delhi in 1978 was a call to change the existing system of teaching the unnecessary minute details to the undergraduate students.

This attempt has been made with an object to meet the requirements of a common medical student. The text has been arranged in small classified parts to make it easier for the students to remember and recall it at will. It is adequately illustrated with simple line diagrams which can be reproduced without any difficulty, and which also help in understanding and memorizing the anatomical facts that appear to defy memory of a common student. The monotony of describing the individual muscles separately, one after the other, has been minimised by writing them out in tabular form, which makes the subject interesting for a lasting memory. The relevant radiological and surface anatomy have been treated in separate chapters. A sincere attempt has been made to deal, wherever required, the clinical applications of the subject. The entire approach is such as to attract and inspire the students for a deeper dive in the subject of anatomy.

The book has been intentionally split in three parts for convenience of handling. This also makes a provision for those who cannot afford to have the whole book at a time.

It is quite possible that there are errors of omission and commission in this mostly single-handed attempt. I would be grateful to the readers for their suggestions to improve the book from all angles.

I am very grateful to my teachers and the authors of numerous publications, whose knowledge has been freely utilised in the preparation of this book. I am equally grateful to my professor and colleagues for their encouragement and valuable help. My special thanks are due to my students who made me feel their difficulties, which was a great incentive for writing this book. I have derived maximum inspiration from Prof. Inderbir Singh (Rohtak), and learned the decency of work from Shri SC Gupta (Jiwaji University, Gwalior).

I am deeply indebted to Shri KM Singhal (National Book House, Gwalior) and Mr SK Jain (CBS Publishers & Distributors, Delhi), who have taken unusual pains to get the book printed in its present form. For giving it the desired get-up, Mr VK Jain and Raj Kamal Electric Press are gratefully acknowledged. The cover page was designed by Mr Vasant Paranjpe, the artist and photographer of our college; my sincere thanks are due to him. I acknowledge with affection the domestic assistance of Munne Miyan and the untiring company of my Rani, particularly during the odd hours of this work.

**BD Chaurasia**

# Acknowledgements

We have the blessings and good wishes of Prof NA Faruqi (Aligarh); Dr DC Naik (Rewa); Dr SD Joshi and Dr SS Joshi (Indore); Dr (Brig) Rakesh Gupta (Greater Noida); Dr DR Singh (Lucknow); Dr M Kaul; Dr C Anand and Dr I Bahl (Delhi); Dr Mohsin Azmi (Kanpur); Dr Medha Joshi (Ghaziabad); Dr Surbhi Gupta (Delhi); Dr Nitin Nagarkar (Raipur); Dr CK Shukla (Raipur); Dr Shakuntala Pai (Manipal); Dr Manik Chatterjee (Raipur) and Dr SN Kazi (Pune).

We are thankful to Dr Sangeeta Chouhan, Dr Seema Gupta (Jaipur); Dr Surjit Ghatak (Jodhpur); Dr Vinay Sharma (Muzzafarnagar); Dr Deepu Singh Kataria (UP); Dr Anup Singh Gurjar (Pali); Dr Jagmohan Sharma, Dr Deepak Sharma, Dr Rajesh Arora and Dr Sumit Gupta (Kota); Dr Gopal Sharma and Dr Manoj Sharma (Jhalawar); Dr Rekha Parashar (Dausa); Dr Santosh Kumar (Dholpur); Dr Isha Srivastav, Dr Aprajita Raizada, Dr Sajan Skaria, Dr Hitant Vohra, Dr Anjali Jain, Dr Kalpana Sharma, Dr Praveen Ojha, Dr Prakash KG, Dr Seema Prakash (Udaipur); for giving feedback for various sections of the volumes. We are greatful to Dr K Aravindhan, Dr V Gladwin, Dr Raveendranath V, Dr Suman Verma, Dr Sulochana Sakthivel, Dr Rajasekhar SSSN and Dr Vidhya G (Puducherry) for their support.

We are grateful to Dr Anupma Mahajan (Amritsar); Dr Vanita Gupta (Jammu); Dr Vikas Verma (Lucknow) and Dr Tripta Bhagat (Ghaziabad) for editing chapters to enhance the value of the volumes. We are grateful to Dr Sangeeta and Dr Nusrat Jabeen (Jammu); Dr Gurdeep Singh Kalyan (Gajrola); Dr Rajan Singla (Patiala); Dr Aprajita Sikka (Ludhiana); Dr Bashir (Srinagar) and Dr Ritu (Rajouri); Dr Mubeen (Kathua); Dr RK Srivastava (Kanpur); Dr Punita Manik (Lucknow); Dr Binod Kumar; Dr Sunita Nayak and Dr Shambhu Prasad (Patna); Dr AK Dubey (Ranchi); Dr Satyam Khare, Dr Shilpi Jain and Dr Alok Tripathi (Meerut), for promoting the volumes.

We have been getting constant encouragement and support from Dr Ranjana Verma, Dr Muthukrishnan P, Dr Yogesh Yadav, Dr Pullimi Vineel and Dr Nirupma Gupta (Greater Noida); Dr Nisha Kaul (Ghaziabad); Dr Vinay Singhal (Saharanpur); Dr RK Ashoka (Mathura); Dr Vineet Guhia (Khandwa); Dr Manisha Sinha (Raipur); Dr Jahan Shirin (Kanpur); Dr Damyanti (Manipur) and Dr MK Anand (Bhuj).

Our regards and affection to Dr Rewa Choudhry, Dr Shilpa Paul, Dr Smita Kakar, Dr Anita Tuli, Dr Gayatri Rath, Dr Shashi Raheja, Dr A Shariff, Dr SB Ray, Dr Vandana Mehta, Dr Sabita Mishra, Dr Renu Chauhan, Dr Jyoti Arora, Dr Sneh Agarwal, Dr TS Roy, Dr Ruchi Dhuria, Dr Shaifaly Madan Rustagi (Delhi) and Dr Anjoo Yadav for going through the volumes.

We would like to thank Dr Pritha Bhuiyan (Mumbai); Dr Brijendra Singh (Rishikesh); Retd (Brig) Dr Sushil Kumar (Faridabad); Dr AK Srivastava (Lucknow); Dr MK Pant (Dehradun); Dr Simmi Mehra (Rajkot); Dr Fatima M De Souza (Goa); Dr Mukesh Mittal (Shivpuri); Dr Priti Sinha (Saharanpur); Dr Rashmi Malhotra (Rishikesh); Dr Simmi Soni (Aziznagar); Dr Sunita Gupta (Ahmedabad); Dr Raghunandan Ramanathan (Chennai), Dr BK Aghera (Ahmedabad) and many-many other teachers all over the globe, for giving us good wishes.

We also acknowledge Drs Neetu Sivadasan, Rituraj Majumdar, Nandhini R, Nithya D, Kalaivani K, Jakkula Akhil, Ambiga R, S Nikilesh, Udit Narayan, Jayasree S, Bharathy Mohan P, Nandhini S, Aakriti Mehrotra, Sancy Charly, Madhusingh Thakur, Tarakeshwari RB, Dhivyaa Shree R, Thaiyal Nayagi and Prasanna Raj AV (Puducherry) for their support.

Videos of bones and soft parts of human body, prepared at Kathmandu University School of Medical Sciences, have now been added with the respective chapters and are available at our mobile App CBSiCentral. We are grateful to Dr R Koju, CEO of Kathmandu University School of Medical Sciences (KUSMS) and Dhulikhel Hospital, for his generosity.

The moral support of my (chief editor) family members, Late Dr DP Garg, Dr Suvira Gupta, Dr JP Gupta, Mr Manoj, Ms Rekha, Mr Sanjay, Ms Meenakshi, Dr Manish, Dr Shilpa Garg, Dr Naveen Garg, Dr Manoj, Dr Nalini Shukla, Dr Vikas Verma and Dr Swati Gupta, is appreciated.

The magnanimity shown by Mr SK Jain (Chairman) and Mr Varun Jain (Director), CBS Publishers & Distributors, has been always forthcoming. The unquestionable support of Mr YN Arjuna (Senior Vice President—Publishing, Editorial and Publicity) and his entire team comprising Ms Ritu Chawla (GM—Production), Mr Neeraj Prasad (Graphic Artist), Mr Binay Kumar (Editor) and Mr Vikrant Sharma (DTP operator) has made an excellent contribution to bring out this edition. We are really obliged to them and pray for their prosperity.

***Editors***

## Acknowledgements


We extend our heartfelt thanks to the following teachers of anatomy for their consistent academic support, encouragement, and well wishes.

- Dr AB Mishra (Mathura, UP)
- Dr A Hima Bindu (Visakhapatnam, AP)
- Dr Aaditya Madhusudan Tarnekar (Nagpur, Maharashtra)
- Dr Aarushi Jain (Kota, Rajasthan)
- Dr Abhijeet Joshi (Barmer, Rajasthan)
- Dr Abhilasha Priya (Jamshedpur, Jharkhand)
- Dr Abhinav Kumar Mishra (Sitapur, UP)
- Dr Abid Ali (Yenkapally, Telangana)
- Dr Abraham Joseph (Nandyal, AP)
- Dr Aditya Pratap Singh (Prayagraj, UP)
- Dr Ajay Kumar (Ludhiana, Punjab)
- Dr Ajay Nene (Alwar, Rajasthan)
- Dr Ajay Rathva (Vadodara, Gujarat)
- Dr AK Singh (Almora, Uttarakhand)
- Dr AK Srivastava (Lucknow, UP)
- Dr Akhilesh Trivedi (Gwalior, MP)
- Dr Alka Singh (Ayodhya, UP)
- Dr Alka Udainia (Surat, Gujarat)
- Dr Alka V Bhingardeo (Bibinagar, Hyderabad)
- Dr Alka (Kanpur, UP)
- Dr Alok Saxena (Dehradun, Uttarakhand)
- Dr Amar Jayanthi A (Idukki, Kerala)
- Dr Amarappa S Nagalikar (Belagavi, Karnataka)
- Dr Ambica Wadhwa (Jalandhar, Punjab)
- Dr Amit Kumar (Bilaspur, CG)
- Dr Amit Kumar Gupta (Jamshedpur, Jharkhand)
- Dr Amit Kumar Nayak (Varanasi, UP)
- Dr Amit Mehta (Chindwada, MP)
- Dr Amit Srivastava (Datia, MP)
- Dr Amol Durgkar (Chindwada, MP)
- Dr Amol Shinde (Pune, Maharashtra)
- Dr Amrita Kumari (Patna, Bihar)
- Dr Amrut Mahajan (Jalgaon, Maharashtra)
- Dr Amrutha Roopa Ramagalla (Siddipet, Telangana)
- Dr Amudha Mohan Ram (Chilakaluripet, Guntur, AP)
- Dr Anand Mishra (Basti, UP)
- Dr Anant Sachan (Orai, UP)
- Dr Angela A Viswasom (Kollam, Kerala)
- Dr Anil Agrawal (Bilaspur, CG)
- Dr Anil Kumar (Sangareddy, Telangana)
- Dr Anil Kumar Dwivedi (Srinagar, Uttarakhand)
- Dr Anil Rahule (Ramagundam, Telangana)
- Dr Anita (Bharatpur, Rajasthan)
- Dr Anita Fating (Amaravati, Maharashtra)
- Dr Anitha V (Kanyakumari, TN)
- Dr Anjali Aggarwal (Chandigarh)
- Dr Anjali Jain (Ludhiana, Punjab)
- Dr Anjali Jain (Udaipur, Rajasthan)
- Dr Anjali Prasad (Muzaffarpur, Bihar)
- Dr Anjali Sabnis (Navi Mumbai, Maharashtra)
- Dr Anju Partap (Shimla, HP)
- Dr Ankur Kumar (Karauli, Rajasthan)
- Dr Ankur Sharma (Greater Noida, UP)
- Dr Anne George (Kottayam, Kerala)
- Dr Annie Doley (Tezpur, Assam)
- Dr Anshu Gupta (Agra, UP)
- Dr Anshu Sharma (Chandigarh)
- Dr Anshu Soni (Ludhiana, Punjab)
- Dr Anterpreet Arora (Amritsar, Punjab)
- Dr Antima Gupta (Meerut, UP)
- Dr Anu Sharma (Ludhiana, Punjab)
- Dr Anuj Ram Sharma (Muzaffarnagar, UP)
- Dr Anup Singh Gurjar (Pali, Rajasthan)
- Dr Anupama Doddappaiah Panagar (Hosur, TN)
- Dr Anupama Mahajan (Amritsar, Punjab)
- Dr Anuradha (Amritsar, Punjab)
- Dr Anurag (Dehradun, Uttarakhand)
- Dr Anwar Unisa Sabry (Siricilla, Telangana)
- Dr Aparna (Vijayawada, AP)
- Dr Aparna Dixit (Unnao, UP)
- Dr Aparna K Vedapriya (Yadadri, Telangana)
- Dr Aparna Muraleedharan (Puducherry)
- Dr Aprajita Raizada (Udaipur, Rajasthan)
- Dr Aprajita Sikka (Ludhiana, Punjab)
- Dr APS Batra (Sonipat, Haryana)
- Dr Archana Rani (Lucknow, UP)
- Dr Archana Srivastava (Lucknow, UP)
- Dr Archana (Alzapur, Telangana)
- Dr Archana Goel (Shahbad, Haryana)
- Dr Archana Kalyankar (Aurangabad, Maharashtra)
- Dr Archana Kannamwar (Yavatmal, Maharashtra)
- Dr Arindam Banerjee (Durgapur, WB)
- Dr Arun Arya (Muzaffarnagar, UP)
- Dr Arun Kasote (Nagpur, Maharashtra)
- Dr Arun Prasad Singh (Patna, Bihar)
- Dr Arun Pundlikrao Kasote (Jalgaon, Maharashtra)
- Dr Arunabha Tapadar (Uluberia, WB)
- Dr Arvinder Pal Singh Batra (Sonipat, Haryana)
- Dr Arvind Kumar Pankaj (Lucknow, UP)
- Dr Asha Latha (Nellore, AP)
- Dr Ashfaq Ul Hasan (Srinagar, J&K)
- Dr Ashok Kumar Singh (Nalanda, Bihar)
- Dr Ashok Patil (Sangamner, Ahmednagar, Maharashtra)
- Dr Ashima (Nuh, Haryana)
- Dr Ashutosh Mangalagiri (Bhopal, MP)
- Dr Ashwani K Sharma (Jammu, J&K)
- Dr Ashwini Jadhav (Mumbai, Maharashtra)
- Dr AV Kulkarni (Dharwad, Karnataka)
- Dr Avanish Kumar (Patna, Bihar)
- Dr Avinash Abhaya (Chandigarh)
- Dr Avinash Rudrajwar (Durg, CG)
- Dr Azhar Ahmed Siddiqui (Badnapur, Jalna, Maharashtra)
- Dr Azmi Mohsin (Kanpur, UP)
- Dr B Naveen Kumar (Bachupally, Hyderabad, Telangana)
- Dr Babu Rao (Hyderabad, Telangana)
- Dr Badal Singh (Prayagraj, UP)
- Dr Banani Kundu (Uluberia, WB)
- Dr Bandi Sirisha (Telangana)
- Dr Bashir Ahmad Shah (Srinagar, J&K)
- Dr Beena Nambiar (Pariyaram, Kannur, Kerala)
- Dr Berjina Naqshi (Baramulla, J&K)
- Dr Bertha AD Rathinam (Bhopal, MP)
- Dr Bhagyashree (Bilaspur, HP)
- Dr Bharat Patel (Ahmedabad, Gujarat)
- Dr Bhaskar Pal (Haldia, WB)
- Dr Bhaudas Khanderao Jadhav (Mumbai, Maharashtra)
- Dr Bhavana Junagade (Mumbai, Maharashtra)
- Dr Bhavik Doshi (Ahmedabad, Gujarat)
- Dr Bindu Singh (Gorakhpur, UP)
- Dr Binod Kumar (Muzzafarpur, Bihar)
- Dr Bipinchandra Khade (Bhopal, MP)
- Dr Biswabina Ray (Kalyani, WB)
- Dr Bonita Gupte (Jammu)
- Dr Brajesh Ranjan (Banda, UP)
- Dr BR Singh (Nagpur, Maharashtra)
- Dr Brijendra Singh (Rishikesh, Uttarakhand)
- Dr BS Lala (Indore, MP)
- Dr BS Patil (Vijayapura, Karnataka)
- Dr C Kishan Reddy (Karimnagar, Telangana)
- Dr C Lalitha (Bengaluru, Karnataka)
- Dr Chandan Kumar Yadav (Lucknow, UP)
- Dr Charulata A Satpute (Nagpur, Maharashtra)
- Dr Chetan Sahni (Varanasi, UP)
- Dr Chetna Thakur (Agra, UP)
- Dr Chitti Narasamma (Kurnool, AP)
- Dr D Asha Latha (Machlipatnam, AP)
- Dr D Sudhakar Babu (Nizamabad, Telangana)
- Dr Daizy Singh (Ludhiana, Punjab)
- Dr Dalbir Kaur (Agroha, Haryana)
- Dr DAVS Sesi (Kakinada, AP)
- Dr Debjani Roy (Midinapore, WB)
- Dr Deepa Bently (Coimbatore, TN)
- Dr Deepa Deopa (Haldwani, Uttarakhand)
- Dr Deepa Devadas (Varanasi, UP)
- Dr Deepak Joshi (Mumbai, Maharashtra)
- Dr Deepak Sharma (Jaipur, Rajasthan)
- Dr Deepali G Vidhale (Amaravati, Maharashtra)
- Dr Deepali Onkar (Nagpur, Maharashtra)
- Dr Deepanshu Shukla (Lucknow, UP)
- Dr Deepti Shastri (Salem, TN)
- Dr Dhananjay (Bareilly, UP)
- Dr Dhiraj Saxena (Jaipur, Rajasthan)
- Dr DH Gopalan (Chennai, TN)
- Dr Dibyendu Datta (Kolkata, WB)
- Dr Dimpal Patel (Ahmedabad, Gujarat)
- Dr Dinesh Kumar (Delhi)
- Dr Dipali Trivedi (Ahmedabad, Gujarat)
- Dr Dipti Gautam (Mahasamund, CG)
- Dr Dipti Nimje (Nagpur, Maharashtra)
- Dr Divya Mahajan (Chandigarh)
- Dr Durga Paswan (Greater Noida, UP)
- Dr Durgesh Singh (Mirzapur, UP)
- Dr DV Singh (Bareilly, UP)
- Dr Faizal Mohammad (Siddipet, Telangana)
- Dr Fatima M De Souza (Goa)
- Dr Fazal Ur Rehman (Aligarh, UP)
- Dr Feroz Hussain (Guwahati, Assam)
- Dr G Sundar (Vellore, TN)
- Dr GA Jos Hemalatha (Virudhunagar, TN)
- Dr Gajanan L Maske (Yavatmal, Maharashtra)
- Dr Ganesh Khemnar (Kurnool, AP)
- Dr Ganesh Trivedi (Shri Ganganagar, Rajasthan)
- Dr Garima Sharma (Tanda, HP)
- Dr Garima Pardhi (Vidisha, MP)
- Dr Garima Shivhare (Shahbad, Haryana)
- Dr Gaurav Agnihotri (Amritsar, Punjab)

- Dr Gautam A Shroff (Aurangabad, Maharashtra)
- Dr Gayatri Muthiyan (Nagpur, Maharashtra)
- Dr Geetha KN (Mumbai, Maharashtra)
- Dr Ghanshyam Gupta (Jaipur, Rajasthan)
- Dr Ghulam Mohammad Bhat (Srinagar, J&K)
- Dr Gitanjali Arora (Bhubaneswar, Odisha)
- Dr GL Nigam (Banda, UP)
- Dr Gnanavel A (Kanchipuram, TN)
- Dr Gopal Mondal (Barasat, WB)
- Dr Gopal Sharma (Jhalawar, Rajasthan)
- Dr Gouri Shankar Jha (Laheriasarai, Darbhanga, Bihar)
- Dr Gunapriya Raghunath (Chennai, TN)
- Dr Gunwant Chaudhari (Dahod, Gujarat)
- Dr Gursharan S Dhindsa (Faridkot, Punjab)
- Dr Gyan Prakash Mishra (Basti, UP)
- Dr Gyanraj Singh (Jajpur, Odisha)
- Dr Hamid Ansari (Kanpur Dehat, UP)
- Dr Hari Narayan Yadav (Mathura, UP)
- Dr Harish Chaturvedi (Chamba, HP)
- Dr Haritha Nimmagadda (Navi Mumbai, Maharashtra)
- Dr Harpreet Singh Gulati (Jalandhar, Punjab)
- Dr Harsh Chawre (Datia, MP)
- Dr Harsh Mishrikoti P (Belagavi, Karnataka)
- Dr Harsimrajit Kaur (Patiala, Punjab)
- Dr Harsimran Grewal (Patiala, Punjab)
- Dr Hemlata Ambade (Nagpur, Maharashtra)
- Dr Hina Sharma (Udaipur, Rajasthan)
- Dr Hitant Vohra (Ludhiana, Punjab)
- Dr Hrishikesh Jadhav (Sola, Ahmedabad, Gujarat)
- Dr I Gowri (Chevella, Telangana)
- Dr Ila Gujaria (Shivpuri, MP)
- Dr Indra Kumar Patel (Bahraich, UP)
- Dr Indushri (Kannauj, UP)
- Dr Isha Srivastav (Udaipur, Rajasthan)
- Dr Israr Ahmed Khan (Shahdol, MP)
- Dr JP Yadav (Churu, Rajasthan)
- Dr JS Kullar (Amritsar, Punjab)
- Dr J Sreevidya (Chennai, TN)
- Dr Jaba Rajguru (Vadodra, Gujarat)
- Dr Jaedeo Ughade (Parbhani, Maharashtra)
- Dr Jagmohan Sharma (Jaipur, Rajasthan)
- Dr Jagriti Agrawal (Raipur, CG)
- Dr Jaita Chowdhury (Haldia, WB)
- Dr Jami Sagar Prusty (Berhampur, Odisha)
- Dr Jasmeen Shaikh (Hyderabad, Telangana)
- Dr Jasween Kaur (Jalandhar, Punjab)
- Dr Jaswinder Kaur (Ambala, Haryana)
- Dr Javed Ahmad Khan (Srinagar, J&K)
- Dr Javed Akhtar (Patna, Bihar)
- Dr Jaya Prakash (Kamareddy, Telangana)
- Dr Jayasree K (Kozhikode, Kerala)
- Dr Jayasree Reddy (Siddipet, Telangana)
- Dr Jessy Rose George (Kozhikode, Kerala)
- Dr Jeyanthi G (Thirunelveli, TN)
- Dr Jitendra Gupta (Ratlam, MP)
- Dr Jitendra Patel (Ahmedabad, Gujarat)
- Dr Jolly Agarwal (Dehradun, Uttarakhand)
- Dr Joy Ghoshal (Mangalagiri, AP)
- Dr Jwalant Waghmare (Sevagram, Maharashtra)
- Dr Jyoti Gaiwad (Mumbai, Maharashtra)
- Dr Jyoti Ramling Gaikwad (Sanpada, Maharashtra)
- Dr Jyoti Rohilla (Mohali, Punjab)
- Dr Jyotsna Singh (Chandigarh)
- Dr K Manivanan (Kuppam, AP)
- Dr K Shanmuganathan (Puducherry)
- Dr K Udhaya (Tiruchengode, TN)
- Dr Kalpana Ramachandran (Chennai, TN)
- Dr Kalpana Sharma (Udaipur, Rajasthan)
- Dr Kalu Ram Meena (Bikaner, Rajasthan)
- Dr Kalyan Bhattacharya (Kolkata, WB)
- Dr Kamaljeet Kaur (Jalandhar, Punjab)
- Dr Kamil Khan (Lucknow, UP)
- Dr Kanahiya Jee (Barabanki, UP)
- Dr Kanan Shah (Ahmedabad, Gujarat)
- Dr Kanchan Kapoor (Chandigarh)
- Dr Kanika Sachdeva (Amritsar, Punjab)
- Dr Kavita Nanda (Hamirpur, HP)
- Dr Kavita Pahuja (Bikaner, Rajasthan)
- Dr Kiran Kalloor (Palakkad, Kerala)
- Dr Kiran V Padeyappanavar (Belagavi, Karnataka)
- Dr Kirti Nemade (Nagpur, Maharashtra)
- Dr KK Thakur (Doda, J&K)
- Dr KKP Singh (Ranchi, Jharkhand)
- Dr Komala B (Bengaluru)
- Dr Krishnaiah M (Suryapet, Telangana)
- Dr Krishna Gopal (Bareilly, UP)
- Dr Krishna Tiwari (Prayagraj, UP)
- Dr Kulbir Kaur (Amritsar, Punjab)
- Dr Kuldeep (Kannauj, UP)
- Dr Kunal Chawla (Shimla, HP)
- Dr L Hema (Nellore, AP)
- Dr Lakshmikantha (Meppadi, Wayanad, Kerala)
- Dr Lalatendu Swain (Puri, Odisha)
- Dr Lency Davis (Thrissur, Kerala)
- Dr Lenin S (Kanyakumari, TN)
- Dr Lola Das (Thrissur, Kerala)
- Dr M Chatterjee (Raipur, CG)
- Dr M Prasad (Dhanbad, Jharkhand)
- Dr M Siva Kumar (Thiruvannamalai, TN)
- Dr M Sivakumar (Trichi, TN)
- Dr MA Doshi (Karad, Maharashtra)
- Dr Madasi Pranay Kumar (Karimnagar, Telangana)
- Dr Madhusmita Panda (Balasore, Odisha)
- Dr Mahendra Kumar Pant (Dehradun, Uttarakhand)
- Dr Mahesh GM (Chitradurga, Karnataka)
- Dr Mahesh K Sharma (Chandigarh)
- Dr Mahesh Ugale (Latur, Maharashtra)
- Dr Mahita Bojja (Nagarkurnool, Telangana)
- Dr Malamoni Dutta (Kokrajhar, Assam)
- Dr Mallela Padmavati (Hyderabad, Telangana)
- Dr Mamata Sar (Burla, Odisha)
- Dr Mamta Anand (Prayagraj, UP)
- Dr Mamta Kumari (Pawapuri, Bihar)
- Dr Mamta Sharma (Jalandhar, Punjab)
- Dr Maneesha (Mohali, Punjab)
- Dr Mangesh Lone (Mumbai, Maharashtra)
- Dr Mangesh Selukar (Latur, Maharashtra)
- Dr Mani Kathapillai (Chengalpattu, TN)
- Dr Maninder Kaur (Patiala, Punjab)
- Dr Manish Khanna (Firozabad, UP)
- Dr Manish Patil (Ujjain, MP)
- Dr Manisha Nakhate (Navi Mumbai, Maharashtra)
- Dr Manisha R Gaikwad (Bhubaneswar, Odisha)
- Dr Manisha Upadhyay (Azamgarh, UP)
- Dr Manju Bala (Patiala, Punjab)
- Dr Manjunath V Motagi (Indore, MP)
- Dr Manjusha Tabhane (Nagpur, Maharashtra)
- Dr Manjushree Chakroborty (Nagaon, Assam)
- Dr Manoj Sharma (Jhalawar, Rajasthan)
- Dr Maria Kala (Siddipet, Telangana)
- Dr Martin Lucas A (Bengaluru)
- Dr Md Jawed Akhtar (Patna, Bihar)
- Dr Meenakshi Aggarwal (Ludhiana, Punjab)
- Dr Meenakshi Borkar (Mumbai, Maharashtra)
- Dr Meenakshi Khullar (Faridkot, Punjab)
- Dr Meenakshi Parthsarathy (Bengaluru, Karnataka)
- Dr Meetu Agarwal (Faridabad, Haryana)
- Dr Meghana Mishra (Reva, MP)
- Dr Mehandi V Mahajan (Thiruvallur, TN)
- Dr Mehera Bhoir (Mumbai, Maharashtra)
- Dr MG Puranik (Pune, Maharashtra)
- Dr Mini Kariappa (Thrissur)
- Dr Mini Mol (Mumbai, Maharashtra)
- Dr MM Peerzade (Solapur, Maharashtra)
- Dr Mohammad Mujahid Ansari (Shahdol, MP)
- Dr Mohammad Nazeem Khawaja (Baramulla, J&K)
- Dr Mohd Ajmal (Siddharthnagar, UP)
- Dr Monica Jain (Agroha, Haryana)
- Dr Monika Gupta (Bathinda, Punjab)
- Dr Monika Lalit Piplani (Amritsar, Punjab)
- Dr MP Sultana (Nellore, AP)
- Dr Mrinal Barua (Rishikesh, Uttarakhand)
- Dr Mritunjay Pandey (Deoria, UP)
- Dr MS Arathi (Chennai, TN)
- Dr Mubeen Rashid (Kathua, J&K)
- Dr Mudasir Ahmad Khan (Anantnag, J&K)
- Dr Mukesh Mittal (Shivpuri, MP)
- Dr Mukesh Singhla (Rishikesh, Uttarakhand)
- Dr Muktar Hussain (Badaun, UP)
- Dr Mukul Sarma (Tinsukia, Assam)
- Dr Muthukumaravel Narayanaswamy (Ariyur, Puducherry)
- Dr N Bhanu Sudha Parimala (Mangalagiri, AP)
- Dr Navbir Pasricha (Lucknow, UP)
- Dr Nagraj S (Mahabubnagar, Telangana)
- Dr Naina Wakode (Vidisha, MP)
- Dr Namdeo Y Kamdi (Chandrapur, Maharashtra)
- Dr Nandita Dutta (Jalpaiguri, WB)
- Dr Naresh Thaduri (Bhopal, MP)
- Dr Natwar Agrawal (Jabalpur, MP)
- Dr Nava Kalyani (Hyderabad, Telangana)
- Dr Navita Aggarwal (Bhatinda, Punjab)
- Dr Navneet Kumar (Lucknow, UP)
- Dr Neelam Bala (Amritsar, Punjab)
- Dr Neelam Jit Kaur (Patiala, Punjab)
- Dr Neeraj Pandey (Ghazipur, UP)
- Dr Neeru Goyal (Ludhiana, Punjab)
- Dr Neeta Chhabra (Faridabad, Haryana)
- Dr Neetu Arora (Nalhar, Nuh, Haryana)
- Dr Neha Rai (Bhopal, MP)
- Dr Neha Vijay (Alwar, Rajasthan)
- Dr Nidhi Puri (Bilaspur, HP)
- Dr Nilesh Rakate (Bhopal, MP)
- Dr Nilofer Mulla (Mumbai, Maharashtra)
- Dr Nimisha Madhu (Gaya, Bihar)
- Dr Nirmal Kumar K (Vikarabad, Telangana)
- Dr Nirmaladevi M (Coimbatore, TN)
- Dr Nirmalya Saha (Agartala, Tripura)
- Dr Nirupama Gupta (Greater Noida, UP)

- Dr Nisha Yadav (Etawah, UP)
- Dr Nishigandha Sadamate (Vadodara, Gujarat)
- Dr Nita Gathe (Gondia, Maharashtra)
- Dr Nitin R Mudiraj (Sangali, Maharashtra)
- Dr Nityanand Srivastava (Etawah, UP)
- Dr Nivedita Pandey (Israna, Panipat, Haryana)
- Dr Niyati Airen (Srinagar, Uttarakhand)
- Dr Nusrat Jabeen (Jammu, J&K)
- Dr P Ashok (Hyderabad, Telangana)
- Dr P Bapuji (Eluru, AP)
- Dr P David Anand Kumar (Telangana)
- Dr P Sasikala (Tiruchengode, TN)
- Dr Padamjeet Panchal (Patna, Bihar)
- Dr Padmasini S (Chennai, TN)
- Dr Pankaj Maheria (Valsad, Gujarat)
- Dr Pankaj Singh (Jaipur, Rajasthan)
- Dr Pankaj Soni (Mandi, HP)
- Dr Parveen Akhter (Jammu)
- Dr Praveen Sharma (Sri Ganganagar, Rajasthan)
- Dr Patil Shrish (Chitradurga, Karnataka)
- Dr Payal Kasat (Kharagpur, WB)
- Dr Peter Ericson (Hyderabad, Telangana)
- Dr PG Khanwalkar (Bhopal, MP)
- Dr Phalguni Srimani (Kolkata, WB)
- Dr Piyush Kumar (Dehradun, Uttarakhand)
- Dr PK Ramakrishnan (Palakkad, Kerala)
- Dr PN Panshewdikar (Palghar, Maharashtra)
- Dr Pooja (Rohtak, Haryana)
- Dr Poonam Delmotra (Shahbad, Haryana)
- Dr Poonam Verma (Amritsar, Punjab)
- Dr PP Kulkarni (Islampur, Maharashtra)
- Dr Prabhakaran K (Ahmedabad, Gujarat)
- Dr Prabhjot Kaur (Mandi, HP)
- Dr Pradeep Bokariya (Sevagram, Maharashtra)
- Dr Pradeep Kumar (Gaya, Bihar)
- Dr Pradeep Pawar (Mumbai, Maharashtra)
- Dr Prafulla Pralhadrao Nikam (Wardha, Maharashtra)
- Dr Prajakta Kishve (Hyderabad, Telangana)
- Dr Prajna Paramita Samanta (Bhubaneswar, Odisha)
- Dr Prakash Baburao Hosmani (Solapur, Maharashtra)
- Dr Prakash KG (Udaipur, Rajasthan)
- Dr Pramod (Kanpur, UP)
- Dr Pranab Deb Barma (Tripura)
- Dr Prasanna MB (Ernakulam, Kerala)
- Dr Prashant Chaware (Bhopal, MP)
- Dr Prashant E Natekar (Hyderabad)
- Dr Prashant Munjamkar (Bibinagar, Hyderabad)
- Dr Prateek Singha (Nahan, HP)
- Dr Prathistha Potdar (Greater Noida, UP)
- Dr Pratibha Shakya (Lucknow, UP)
- Dr Pratima Jaiswal (Kota, Rajasthan)
- Dr Praveen B Iyer (Mumbai, Maharashtra)
- Dr Praveen Kurrey (Raipur, CG)
- Dr Praveen Ojha (Udaipur, Rajasthan)
- Dr Praveen Singh (Karamsad, Gujarat)
- Dr Preeti Chaudhary (Bhatinda, Punjab)
- Dr Preeti Goswami (Delhi)
- Dr Prerna Gupta (Amausi, Lucknow, UP)
- Dr Pritha S Bhuiyan (Mumbai, Maharashtra)
- Dr Priti Chaudhary (Bhatinda)
- Dr Priti Nemade (Nagpur, Maharashtra)
- Dr Priti Sinha (Meerut, UP)
- Dr Priya P Roy (Karad, Maharashtra)
- Dr Priya Ranganath (Bengaluru, Karnataka)
- Dr PS Chitra (Ariyalur, TN)
- Dr Pulipati Anil Kumar (Vizianagaram, AP)
- Dr Punita (Lucknow, UP)
- Dr Punita Sharma (Amritsar, Punjab)
- Dr Purushotam Rao (Vikarabad, Telangana)
- Dr PV Satya Kumar (Vijayawada, AP)
- Dr R Azhagiri (Chennai, TN)
- Dr R Manoranjitham (Perambalur, TN)
- Dr R Sarah (Madurai, TN)
- Dr Rachna Agarwal (Bharatpur, Rajasthan)
- Dr Rachna Magotra (Jammu)
- Dr Rachna Rastogi (Greater Noida, UP)
- Dr Rajan Singla (Patiala, Punjab)
- Dr Rajashree Biswal (Cuttack, Odisha)
- Dr Rajashree S Raut (Kolhapur, Maharashtra)
- Dr Rajasri Chunder (Budge, Kolkata, WB)
- Dr Rajat Subhra Das (Raebareli, UP)
- Dr Rajeev Panwar (KK Nagar, Chennai, TN)
- Dr Rajiv Ranjan (Ranchi, Jharkhand)
- Dr Rajendra Prasad (Gaya, Bihar)
- Dr Rajendra Singrolay (Ratlam, MP)
- Dr Rajendrakumar D Virupaxi (Belagavi, Karnataka)
- Dr Rajesh Dehankar (Nagpur, Maharashtra)
- Dr Rajesh Maurya (Dehradun, Uttarakhand)
- Dr Rajkumar KR (Gulbarga, Karnataka)
- Dr Rajlaxmi Panda (Berhampur, Odisha)
- Dr Rajveer Singh Chourasia (Bhawanipatna, Odisha)
- Dr Rakesh Gupta (Bareilly, UP)
- Dr Rakesh Kumar Verma (Lucknow, UP)
- Dr Rakesh Mani (Bikaner, Rajasthan)
- Dr Rakesh Mishra (Lucknow, UP)
- Dr Rakesh Shukla (Mirzapur, UP)
- Dr Ram Kumar Singhal (Bharatpur, Rajasthan)
- Dr Ram Prakash Gupta (Greater Noida, UP)
- Dr Randhir S Chauhan (Solan, HP)
- Dr Randhir Sigh Chauhan (Solan, Himachal Pradesh)
- Dr Rani Raphael M (Alappuzha, Kerala)
- Dr Ranjana Barjatya (Ajmer, Rajasthan)
- Dr Ranjeet Kumar (Deoghar, Jharkhand)
- Dr Ranjneet Guha (Patna, Bihar)
- Dr Rashi Mittal (Jaipur, Rajasthan)
- Dr Rashi Nigam (Kanpur, UP)
- Dr Rashmi Deopujari (Vidisha, MP)
- Dr Rashmi Ghai (Hardoi, UP)
- Dr Rashmi Jaiswal (Bhopal, MP)
- Dr Rashmi Malhotra (Rishikesh, Uttarakhand)
- Dr Rashmi Prasad (Patna, Bihar)
- Dr Rashmi S Sinha (Mumbai, Maharashtra)
- Dr Rashmoni Jana (Delhi)
- Dr Ratesh Kumar (Faridabad, Haryana)
- Dr Raveena Singh (Fatehpur, UP)
- Dr Ravi Kant Sharma (Solan, Himachal Pradesh)
- Dr Raviendra Marathe (Akola, Maharashtra)
- Dr Reeha Mahajan (Vijaypur, Jammu, J&K)
- Dr Reena Singla (Mohali, Punjab)
- Dr Rekha More (Mumbai, Maharashtra)
- Dr Rekha Parashar (Dausa, Rajasthan)
- Dr Renu Kumari (Panipat, Haryana)
- Dr Renuka Ahankari (Pune, Maharashtra)
- Dr Renuka Sharma (Greater Noida, UP)
- Dr Richa Gupta (Chandigarh)
- Dr Richa Niranjan (Srinagar, Uttarakhand)
- Dr Rimpi Gupta (Karnal, Haryana)
- Dr Rimple Bansal (Patiala, Punjab)
- Dr Ritesh Shah (Ahmedabad, Gujarat)
- Dr Ritika Gaddewar (Nagpur, Maharashtra)
- Dr Ritika Sharma (Amritsar, Punjab)
- Dr Ritu Gothwal (Churu, Rajasthan)
- Dr Ritu Saloi (Diphu, Assam)
- Dr Ritu Slathia (Rajouri, J&K)
- Dr RK Diwan (Lucknow, UP)
- Dr RK Shrivtastav (Unnao, UP)
- Dr Rohini Karambelkar (Islampur, Maharashtra)
- Dr Rohini Motwani (Bibinagar, Telangana)
- Dr Roli Joshi (Unnao, UP)
- Dr Romi S (Kollam, Kerala)
- Dr Roonmoni Deka (Guwahati, Assam)
- Dr RS Bulagouda (Vijayapura, Karnataka)
- Dr Rubi Saikia (Jorhat, Assam)
- Dr Ruchi Dhuria (Delhi)
- Dr Ruchi Goyal (Patiala, Punjab)
- Dr Ruchi Jain (Jhansi, UP)
- Dr Ruchi Ratnesh (Deoghar, Jharkhand)
- Dr Rup Sekhar Deka (Nalbari, Assam)
- Dr Rupa Chaparrwal (Indore, MP)
- Dr Rupali Kavitake (Alibagh, Maharashtra)
- Dr Ruta Bapat (Navi Mumbai, Maharashtra)
- Dr S Arrchana (Chengalpattu, TN)
- Dr S Babu Rao (Hyderabad, Telangana)
- Dr S Bharathi Rani (Sivagangai, TN)
- Dr S Diwya Lakshmi (Virudhunagar, TN)
- Dr S Karthick Selvaraj (Kanchipuram, TN)
- Dr S Naveen Kumar (Hyderabad, Telangana)
- Dr S Satish Kumar (Dharmapuri, TN)
- Dr S Satishkumar (Kalakuruchi, TN)
- Dr S Sundarapandian (Chengalpattu, TN)
- Dr Sabin Malik (Ernakulam, Kerala)
- Dr Sabita Mishra (Delhi)
- Dr Sachendra Mittal (Jaipur, Rajasthan)
- Dr Sachin Soni (Bilaspur, HP)
- Dr Sadakat Ali (Dehradun, Uttarakhand)
- Dr Sagun Shukla (Shahjanpur, UP)
- Dr Saif Omar (Bihta, Bihar)
- Dr Saikat Roy (Kalyani, Nadia, WB)
- Dr Sajan Skaria (Udaipur, Rajasthan)
- Dr Sajey PS (Alappuzha, Kerala)
- Dr Saju Binu Cherian (Hyderabad, Telangana)
- Dr Saleena N Ali (Alappuzha, Kerala)
- Dr Samala Niveditha (Nagarkurnool, Telangana)
- Dr Samatha Roshini Padala (Siddipet, Telangana)
- Dr Sambhu Prasad (Sasaram, Bihar)
- Dr Sameer Sathe (Datia, MP)
- Dr Sami Ahmed (Jaipur, Rajasthan)
- Dr Samta Gaur (Pali, Rajasthan)
- Dr Sandeep K Sharma (Ambedkar Nagar, UP)
- Dr Sandeep S Mohite (Karad, Maharashtra)
- Dr Sandhya Kurup (Kolanchery, Kerala)
- Dr Sangeeta Bali (Sitapur, UP)
- Dr Sangeeta Chouhan (Jaipur, Rajasthan)
- Dr Sangeeta Gupta (Jammu, J&K)
- Dr Sangeeta M (Bengaluru)
- Dr Sangeeta Naik (Hyderabad, Telangana)
- Dr Sanjana (Bhatinda, Punjab)
- Dr Sanjay Sharma (Sri Ganganagar, Rajasthan)
- Dr Sanjeev Kolagi (Bagalkot, Karnataka)
- Dr Santhini Arulselvi (Karaikal, Puducherry)
- Dr Santosh Kumar (Dholpur, Rajasthan)
- Dr Santoshkumar A Dope (Latur, Maharashtra)

- Dr Sarada Devi (Moinabad, Telangana)
- Dr Saritha S (Hyderabad, Telangana)
- Dr Saroj Sharma (Faridabad, Haryana)
- Dr Saryu Sen (Sikar, Rajasthan)
- Dr Sashi Bhushan (Kuppam, AP)
- Dr Satheesha KS (Mangaluru, Karnataka)
- Dr Satyashree Ray (Koraput, Odisha)
- Dr Saurabh Kulkarni (Aurangabad, Maharashtra)
- Dr Saurjya Ranjan Das (Bhubaneswar, Odisha)
- Dr Savithri Krishnan (Kollam, Kerala)
- Dr Sayantan Das (Kishanganj, Bihar)
- Dr SD Gupta (Bhopal, MP)
- Dr Seema (Amritsar, Punjab)
- Dr Seema Gupta (Jaipur, Rajasthan)
- Dr Seema Gupta (Ludhiana, Punjab)
- Dr Seema Prakash (Udaipur, Rajasthan)
- Dr Seema Sharma (Rajouri, J&K)
- Dr Seema SR (Bengaluru, Karnataka)
- Dr Shaheen Rizvi (Mumbai, Maharashtra)
- Dr Shaifaly Madan Rustagi (Delhi)
- Dr Shailaja Shetty (Bengaluru, Karnataka)
- Dr Shailendra Singh (Banda, UP)
- Dr Shakuntala Pai (Manipal, Karnataka)
- Dr Shalika Sharma (Vijaypur, J&K)
- Dr Shalini Chaudhary (Sonipat, Haryana)
- Dr Shalni Kumar (Delhi)
- Dr Shantanu Nandy (Bankura, WB)
- Dr Shanthini S (Puducherry)
- Dr Sharad Sawant (Mumbai, Maharashtra)
- Dr Sharmisttha Biswas (Kolkata WB)
- Dr Shashi Munjal (Dehradun, Uttarakhand)
- Dr Shavi Garg (Faridabad, Haryana)
- Dr Sheela Sivan (Perinthalmanna, Malappuram, Kerala)
- Dr Shema Nair (Bhopal, MP)
- Dr Sherry Sharma (Jalandhar, Punjab)
- Dr Shibanee Jena (Jajpur, Odisha)
- Dr Shikha (Delhi)
- Dr Shikha Sharma (Agra, UP)
- Dr Shikky Garg (Firozabad, UP)
- Dr Shilpa Bhimalli (Belagavi, Karnataka)
- Dr Shilpa Sonare (Nagpur, Maharashtra)
- Dr Shirin Jahan (Fatehpur, UP)
- Dr Shivaji B Sukre (Parbhani, Maharashtra)
- Dr Shivani Dhingra (Kannauj, UP)
- Dr Shobha Ramnarayan (Kolenchery, Ernakulum, Kerala)
- Dr Shrikant Verma (Raipur, CG)
- Dr Shruthi BN (Bengaluru, Karnataka)
- Dr Shruti Mamidwar (Chandrapur, Maharashtra)
- Dr Shubhangi Bhagwat Ghule (Jalgaon, Maharashtra)
- Dr Shubhpreet Sodhi (Nahan, HP)
- Dr Shweta Asthana (Udaipur, Rajasthan)
- Dr Shweta Swami (Karnal, Haryana)
- Dr Simmi Mehra (Rajkot, Gujarat)
- Dr Simmi Soni (Aziznagar, Telangana)
- Dr Sindhu Chaudhary (Almora, Uttarakhand)
- Dr Sirikonda Parimala (Mahabubnagar, Telangana)
- Dr SK Chavan (Pune, Maharashtra)
- Dr SM Belsare (Talgaon, Pune, Maharashtra)
- Dr Smruti Rekha Mohanty (Bhubaneswar, Odisha)
- Dr Sohinder Kaur (Jhajjar, Haryana)
- Dr Sonali Thomas (Haldwani, Uttarakhand)
- Dr Sonia Singh (Ludhiana, Punjab)
- Dr Sonu (Greater Noida, UP)
- Dr Soumitra Trivedi (Raipur, CG)
- Dr Soumya Chakraborty Bhattachrya (Kohima, Nagaland)
- Dr Sreevidya J (Chennai, TN)
- Dr SS Saiyad (Nadiad, Gujarat)
- Dr Stuti Srivastava (Udaipur, Rajasthan)
- Dr Shubha Shrivastava (Meerut, UP)
- Dr Subhash Gujar (Vadnagar, Gujarat)
- Dr Subhash K Deshpande (Dharwad, Karnataka)
- Dr Subhash Gupta (Shahjahanpur, UP)
- Dr Subhasis Chakraborty (Kolkata, WB)
- Dr Subodh Kumar (Patna, Bihar)
- Dr Suchetra Chaudhary (Ahmadabad, Gujarat)
- Dr Suchit Kumar (Dehradun, Uttarakhand)
- Dr Sudha R (Salem, TN)
- Dr Sudha Rani (Hazaribagh, Jharkhand)
- Dr Sudhakar Kumar Ray (Mathura, UP)
- Dr Sudhir Saxena (Gwalior, MP)
- Dr Sujata K (Kuppam, AP)
- Dr Sujithaa N (Villupurum, TN)
- Dr Sukhinder Baidwain (Nahan, HP)
- Dr Sumalatha Thimmaraju (Hyderabad, Telangana)
- Dr Suman (Rohtak, Haryana)
- Dr Suman Kumari (Gaya, Bihar)
- Dr Suman Yadav (Tanda, HP)
- Dr Sumedha Anjankar (Raipur, CG)
- Dr Sumit Babuta (Jaipur, Rajasthan)
- Dr Sumit Gupta (Kota, Rajasthan)
- Dr Sumit Patil (Bhopal, MP)
- Dr Sumita Agrawal (Dehradun, Uttarakhand)
- Dr Sumita Shukla (Ayodhya, UP)
- Dr Sundar Lal Jethani (Dehradun, Uttarakhand)
- Dr Sunita Bharti (Navi Mumbai, Maharashtra)
- Dr Sunita Gupta (Ahmedabad, Gujarat)
- Dr Sunita Nayak (Patna, Bihar)
- Dr Suniti Pandey (Kanpur, UP)
- Dr Surajit Chatak (Jodhpur, Rajasthan)
- Dr Suranjali Sharma (Faridabad, Haryana)
- Dr Surekha Patil (Jaipur, Rajasthan)
- Dr Surekha W Meshram (Gondia, Maharashtra)
- Dr Suresh Kanta Rathee (Rohtak, Haryana)
- Dr Suresh Kumar (Vellore, TN)
- Dr Suresh Sharma (Sri Ganganagar, Rajasthan)
- Dr Susan Varghese (Kollam, Kerala)
- Dr Sushant Swaroop Das (Bilaspur, HP)
- Dr Susheela Rana (Mandi, HP)
- Dr Sushil Jiwane (Bhopal, MP)
- Rt. Brig (Dr) Sushil Kumar (Faridabad, Haryana)
- Dr Sushma Kushal Kataria (Jodhpur, Rajasthan)
- Dr SVV Nagarajamannar (Rajahmundry, AP)
- Dr Swati Bansal (Karnal, Haryana)
- Dr Swati Saxena (Dehradun, Uttarakhand)
- Dr Swati Yadav (Ghaziabad, UP)
- Dr Sweta Singh (Barabanki, UP)
- Dr T Anitha (Villupurum, TN)
- Dr T Rajan (Puducherry)
- Dr T Sreekanth (Peerancheru, Telangana)
- Dr Tapan Kumar Jana (Murshidabad, WB)
- Dr Taqiuddin Mohammed (Hyderabad, Telangana)
- Dr Tarkeshwar Golghate (Nagpur, Maharashtra)
- Dr TC Singel (Dahod, Gujarat)
- Dr Tejaswi HL (Mandya, Karnataka)
- Dr Tejendra Singh (Mathura, UP)
- Dr Teresa Rani (AP)
- Dr Thanuja Kumari (Telangana)
- Dr Thuslima M (Chennai, TN)
- Dr TK Rajashree (Hyderabad, Telangana)
- Dr Tom J Nallikuzhy (Idukki, Kerala)
- Dr Trupti Balwir (Nagpur, Maharashtra)
- Dr Uday Kumar (Telangana)
- Dr Ujwala Bhanarkar (Kalyani, WB)
- Dr UK Gupta (Jaipur, Rajasthan)
- Dr UK Kulkarni (Belagavi, Karnataka)
- Dr Upendra M (Kothagundum, Telangana)
- Dr Usha KK (Manjeri, Kerala)
- Dr V Anandhi (Trichy, TN)
- Dr V Dharani (Villupuram, TN)
- Dr V Rajapriya (Omandurar, TN)
- Dr V Ravi Kumar (Shimoga, Karnataka)
- Dr V Subhashini (Amalapuram, AP)
- Dr Vaishali Inamdar (Nanded, Maharashtra)
- Dr Vandana Mehta (New Delhi)
- Dr Vandana Sidhu (Amritsar, Punjab)
- Dr Vandana Tiwari (Haldwani, Uttarakhand)
- Dr Vanita Gupta (Hapur, UP)
- Dr Vanita Gupta (Udhampur, J&K)
- Dr Varsha Dahiphale (Ambajogai, Maharashtra)
- Dr Varsha Mokhasi (Bengaluru)
- Dr Vasant Vaniya (Vadodra, Gujarat)
- Dr Vashali Kadam (Mumbai, Maharashtra)
- Dr Vasi Padmaja (Telangana)
- Dr Vedula Sailaja (Hyderabad, Telangana)
- Dr Venkateshwar Reddy (Mehboobnagar, Telangana)
- Dr Vijay Anand S Nagdeve (Raipur, CG)
- Dr Vijay Nayak (Bundi, Rajasthan)
- Dr Vijayamma KN (Kerala)
- Dr Vijisha Phalgunan (Puducherry)
- Dr Vikas Saxena (Ajmer, Rajasthan)
- Dr Vikram Ephram (Yadadri, Telangana)
- Dr Vinay Kumar (Saharanpur, UP)
- Dr Vinay Sharma (Muzaffarnagar, UP)
- Dr Vineet Gohiya (Khandwa, MP)
- Dr Vinod Kumar (Turky, Bihar)
- Dr Vinodini (Secunderabad, Telangana)
- Dr Vinoth S (Chennai, TN)
- Dr Vipin Kumar (Varanasi, UP)
- Dr Virendra Bhdhiraja (Karnal, Haryana)
- Dr Vishal Bhadkaria (Sagar, MP)
- Dr Vishnu Gupta (Muzaffarnagar, UP)
- Dr VK Chimurkar (Wardha, Maharashtra)
- Dr VP Rukhmode (Gondia, Maharashtra)
- Dr X Chandra Philip (Puducherry)
- Dr Yogendra Singh (Gorakhpur, UP)
- Dr Yogesh Diwan (Shimla, HP)
- Dr Yogesh Shridhar Ganorkar (Pune, Maharashtra)
- Dr Yogesh Yadav (Hapur, UP)
- Dr Yuvraj Bhosale (Mumbai, Maharashtra)
- Dr Zafar Sultana (Hyderabad, Telangana)
- Dr Zeba Alam (Patna, Bihar)
- Dr Zeba Khan (Mumbai, Maharashtra)
- Dr Zeenat Akhtar (Jammu, J&K)
- Dr Zia Ul Haq (Hyderabad, Telangana)
- Dr Zuberi Hussain Riyaz (Badnapur, Jalna, Maharashtra)
- Pulkit Jain (Ludhiana, Punjab)

*Editors*

# Reviewers

We extend our gratitude to the following anatomy teachers for their unwavering support and for reviewing various topics in the field.

- Dr Aga Ammar Murthuza (Bengaluru, Karnataka)
- Dr Angela (Kollam, Kerala)
- Dr Anjali Jain (Ludhiana, Punjab)
- Dr Anu Sharma (Ludhiana, Punjab)
- Dr Aparna K Vedapriya (Siddipet, Telangana)
- Dr Archana Rani (Lucknow, UP)
- Dr Arvind Kumar Pankaj (Lucknow, UP)
- Dr Ashok KL (Bengaluru, Karnataka)
- Dr Benjamin W (Palakkad, Kerala)
- Dr Dharmaraj Tamgire (Puducherry)
- Dr Dibyendu Datta (Kolkata, WB)
- Dr Dinesh Kumar V (Puducherry)
- Dr Gaurav Agnihotri (Amritsar, Punjab)
- Dr Gitanjali Arora (Bhubaneswar, Odisha)
- Dr Gunapriya Raghunath (Chennai, Tamil Nadu)
- Dr Hitant Vohra (Ludhiana, Punjab)
- Dr Indira CK (Ernakulam, Kerala)
- Dr Jahira Banu T (Puducherry)
- Dr Jaswinder Kaur (Ambala, Haryana)
- Dr Juned Labbai (Mumbai, Maharashtra)
- Dr K Chandra Kumari (Trivandrum, Kerala)
- Dr Komala B (Bengaluru, Karnataka)
- Dr Kumari TK (Kollam, Kerala)
- Dr Maitreyee Mutalik (Sindhudurg, Maharashtra)
- Dr Mubeena Sheikh (Palakkad, Kerala)
- Dr Nagaraja V Pai (Mumbai, Maharashtra)
- Dr Nusrat Jabeen (Jammu, J&K)
- Dr Payal Kasat (Kharagpur, WB)
- Dr PK Ramakrishnan (Palakkad, Kerala)
- Dr Prajna Paramita Samanta (Bhubaneswar, Odisha)
- Dr Pratibha Shakya (Lucknow, UP)
- Dr Pretty Rathnakar (Mangaluru, Karnataka)
- Dr R Gomathi (Puducherry)
- Dr R Sarah (Madurai, Tamil Nadu)
- Dr Rajashree Biswal (Cuttack, Odisha)
- Dr Rakesh Kumar Diwan (Lucknow, UP)
- Dr Rakesh Kumar Verma (Lucknow, UP)
- Dr Rakhi More (Mumbai, Maharashtra)
- Dr Rashmi Sinha (Mumbai, Maharashtra)
- Dr Ravikiran Gole (Mumbai, Maharashtra)
- Dr Rohini K (Bengaluru, Karnataka)
- Dr S Arivu Selvan (Calicut, Kerala)
- Dr S Naveen Kumar (Hyderabad, Telangana)
- Dr Sabin Malik (Guildford, UK)
- Dr Saleena N Ali (Alappuzha, Kerala)
- Dr Sandhya Kurup (Kolanchery, Kerala)
- Dr Sajay PS (Alappuzha, Kerala)
- Dr Saurjya Ranjan Das (Bhubaneswar, Odisha)
- Dr Shantanu Nandy (Kolkata, WB)
- Dr Sharmila Pal (Jadavpur, Kolkata, WB)
- Dr Sheela Sivan (Perimthalmanna, Kerala)
- Dr Smrutirekha Mohanty (Bhubaneswar, Odisha)
- Dr Sneha John (Mumbai, Maharashtra)
- Dr Sreekumar R (Thiruvananthapuram, Kerala)
- Dr Sreevidya J (Chennai, TN)
- Dr Srividya Sreenivasan (Mumbai, Maharashtra)
- Dr Surendra Babu T (Bengaluru, Karnataka)
- Dr Swapna Chavan Thakur (Mumbai, Maharashtra)
- Dr Swetha B (Bengaluru, Karnataka)
- Dr T Rajini (Bengaluru, Karnataka)
- Dr Taquiuddin Mohammed (Canada)
- Dr Ujwala Bhanarkar (Kalyani, WB)
- Dr V Lokanayaki (Chennai, Tamil Nadu)
- Dr Vandana LR (Thiruvananthapuram, Kerala)
- Dr Vasrha R Bhivate (Mumbai, Maharashtra)
- Dr WMS Johnson (Chennai, Tamil Nadu)
- Dr Yogitha R (Bengaluru, Karnataka)

***Editors***

# Contents

# *eSmartQuiz* – Online MCQ Test

After attending the class, students should go through the "*eSmartQuiz* – Online MCQ test" for the following reasons:

- *Reinforcement of Learning*: The "*eSmartQuiz* – Online MCQ test" provide an opportunity to reinforce learning after attending a class or reading a book. It helps to assess understanding and retention of concepts, to solidify knowledge and identify areas that need further revision or clarification.
- *Assessment of Comprehension*: The "*eSmartQuiz* – Online MCQ test" is an effective tool to assess comprehension of the subject matter and to demonstrate the ability to apply the concepts learned in the class.
- *Enhancement of Attention and Critical Thinking*: The "*eSmartQuiz* – Online MCQ test" will help to make students attentive for the class and to enhance critical thinking skills by selecting the most appropriate answer among the given options.

Each *eSmartQuiz* test consists of 10 MCQs, mostly image-based, and the students can see their scores at the end of each test. These questions will be modified after a certain interval. Use the given links or scan the QR code (given in each chapter) for the test. One student can solve each test only one time.

| *Chapter* | *Link for* **eSmartQuiz** |
|---|---|
| **Head and Neck** | |
| 1. Osteology of Head and Neck | https://forms.gle/L23dCS6nuUdcH4416 |
| 2. Scalp, Temple and Face | https://forms.gle/JCQ9kMV1n5q3hwHd6 |
| 3. Side of the Neck | https://forms.gle/o7xkkfE8nZwp7qUC6 |
| 4. Anterior Region of the Neck | https://forms.gle/VzXQVfSfbTaHJZTn7 |
| 5. Parotid Region | https://forms.gle/uKsU6corLTTnBovz5 |
| 6. Temporal and Infratemporal Regions | https://forms.gle/iP5JkDtKtrRL8r1r8 |
| 7. Submandibular Region | https://forms.gle/3NVu6uePp3ZgbUv57 |
| 8. Structures in the Neck | https://forms.gle/rukg8W5wummqvsnv9 |
| 9. Prevertebral and Paravertebral Regions | https://forms.gle/gVEpDdaTY7kvFWJ99 |
| 10. Back of the Neck | https://forms.gle/nPGqbURZPH2i7hg77 |
| 11. Contents of Vertebral Canal | https://forms.gle/vxZuN9BhChfqYHa36 |
| 12. Cranial Cavity | https://forms.gle/bwgzsWSvQ9HV6KSz9 |
| 13. Contents of the Orbit | https://forms.gle/1KgWiySrEVWFhRCUA |
| 14. Mouth and Pharynx | https://forms.gle/F74Vwpj43aHSBxr86 |
| 15. Nose, Paranasal Sinuses and Pterygopalatine Fossa | https://forms.gle/tMAGush9LAF929FF8 |
| 16. Larynx | https://forms.gle/VyjBKNLUNb4FzEvdA |
| 17. Tongue | https://forms.gle/cT17eXaE9fo1HYKNA |
| 18. Ear | https://forms.gle/618J9JzvQC4Sm9229 |
| 19. Eyeball | https://forms.gle/iVm65VU6LSHKhRsu5 |
| 20. Surface Marking and Radiological Anatomy | https://forms.gle/MEpq8w8CXdjvgRyS8 |

# Index of Competencies

As per the latest NMC Guidelines | Competency Based Medical Education (CBME) Curriculum under Graduate Medical Education Regulation

| Code | Competency | Chapter | Page no. |
|---|---|---|---|
| AN26.1 | Demonstrate anatomical position of skull, identify and locate individual skull bones in skull | 1 | 2 |
| AN26.2 | Describe the features of norma frontalis, verticalis, occipitalis, lateralis and basalis | 1 | 3 |
| AN26.3 | Describe cranial cavity, its subdivisions, foramina and structures passing through them | 1 | 21 |
| AN26.4 | Describe morphological features of mandible | 1 | 31 |
| AN26.5 | Describe features of typical and atypical cervical vertebrae (atlas and axis) | 1 | 47 |
| AN26.7 | Describe the features of the 7th cervical vertebra | 1 | 51 |
| AN27.1 | Describe the layers of scalp, its blood supply, its nerve supply and surgical importance | 2 | 54 |
| AN27.2 | Describe emissary veins with its role in spread of infection from extracranial route to intracranial venous sinuses | 1 | 3 |
| AN28.1 | Describe and demonstrate muscles of facial expression and their nerve supply | 2 | 59 |
| AN28.2 | Describe sensory innervation of face | 2 | 64 |
| AN28.3 | Describe and demonstrate origin/formation, course, branches/tributaries of facial vessels | 2 | 66 |
| AN28.4 | Describe and demonstrate branches of facial nerve with distribution | 2 | 63 |
| AN28.5 | Describe cervical lymph nodes and lymphatic drainage of scalp, face and neck | 2, 8 | 57, 159 |
| AN28.6 | Identify superficial muscles of face, their nerve supply and actions | 2 | 59 |
| AN28.7 | Explain the anatomical basis of facial nerve palsy | 2 | 64 |
| AN28.8 | Explain surgical importance of deep facial vein | 2 | 67 |
| AN28.9 | Describe and demonstrate the parts, borders, surfaces, contents, relations and nerve supply of parotid gland with course of its duct and surgical importance | 5 | 103 |
| AN28.10 | Explain the anatomical basis of Frey's syndrome | 5 | 109 |
| AN29.1 | Describe and demonstrate the boundaries, subdivisions and contents of posterior triangle of neck | 3 | 83 |
| AN29.2 | Describe and demonstrate attachments, nerve supply, relations and actions of sternocleidomastoid | 3 | 81 |
| AN29.4 | Explain anatomical basis of wry neck | 3 | 83 |
| AN29.5 | Describe and demonstrate attachments of: inferior belly of omohyoid, scalenus anterior, scalenus medius, and levator scapulae | 3, 9 | 86, 175 |
| AN30.1 | Describe the cranial fossae and identify related structures | 1, 12 | 21, 205 |
| AN30.2 | Describe and identify major foramina with structures passing through them | 1 | 27 |
| AN30.3 | Describe and identify dural folds and dural venous sinuses | 12 | 193 |
| AN30.4 | Describe clinical importance of dural venous sinuses | 12 | 196 |
| AN30.5 | Explain effect of pituitary tumours on visual pathway | 12 | 203 |
| AN31.1 | Describe and identify extraocular muscles of eyeball, along with a note on its attachment, action and clinical anatomy | 13 | 211 |
| AN31.2 | Describe and demonstrate vessels in the orbit | 13 | 215, 217 |
| AN31.3 | Describe anatomical basis of Horner's syndrome | 8 | 158 |
| AN31.4 | Enumerate components of lacrimal apparatus | 2 | 71 |
| AN32.1 | Describe boundaries and subdivisions of anterior triangle | 4 | 93 |
| AN32.2 | Describe and demonstrate boundaries and contents of digastric and submental triangles | 4 | 93, 96 |
| AN33.1 | Describe and demonstrate extent, boundaries and contents of temporal and infratemporal fossae | 6 | 112 |
| AN33.2 | Describe and demonstrate attachments, direction of fibres, nerve supply and actions of muscles of mastication | 6 | 113 |
| AN33.3 | Describe and demonstrate articulating surface, type and movements of temporomandibular joint | 6 | 120 |
| AN33.4 | Explain the clinical significance of pterygoid venous plexus | 6 | 118 |
| AN33.5 | Describe the features of dislocation of temporomandibular joint | 6 | 123 |
| AN34.1 | Describe and demonstrate the superficial and deep structures, muscles, nerves, vessels, and glands in the submandibular region | 7 | 129 |
| AN34.2 | Describe and demonstrate the morphology, relations and nerve supply of submandibular salivary gland and submandibular ganglion | 7 | 132 |
| AN34.3 | Describe the basis of formation of submandibular stones | 7 | 136 |
| AN35.1 | Describe the parts, extent, attachments, modifications of deep cervical fascia | 3 | 76 |
| AN35.2 | Describe and demonstrate location, parts, borders, surfaces, relations, blood supply and applied anatomy of thyroid gland. Also describe the parathyroid glands in brief | 8 | 138 |

*(Contd.)*

(Contd.)

| Code | Competency | Chapter | Page no. |
|---|---|---|---|
| AN35.3 | Demonstrate and describe the origin, parts, course and branches of subclavian artery | 8 | 147 |
| AN35.4 | Describe and demonstrate origin, course, relations, tributaries and termination of internal jugular and brachiocephalic veins | 8 | 153 |
| AN35.5 | Describe and demonstrate extent, drainage and applied anatomy of cervical lymph nodes | 8 | 159 |
| AN35.6 | Describe and demonstrate the extent, formation, relation and branches of cervical sympathetic chain | 8 | 157 |
| AN35.7 | Describe the course and branches of IX, X, XI and XII nerve in the neck | 8 | 155 |
| AN35.8 | Describe the anatomically relevant clinical features of thyroid swellings | 8 | 142 |
| AN35.9 | Describe the clinical features of compression of subclavian artery and lower trunk of brachial plexus by cervical rib | 8 | 150 |
| AN35.10 | Describe the fascial spaces of neck/pharynx | 3 | 81 |
| AN36.1 | Describe and demonstrate the structures of the vestibule of the mouth and oral cavity proper | 14 | 224 |
| AN36.2 | Describe the: (1) morphology, relations, blood supply and applied anatomy of palatine tonsil, (2) composition of soft palate | 14 | 229, 242 |
| AN36.3 | Describe and demonstrate the muscles, nerve supply, blood supply and lymphatic drainage of the pharynx | 14 | 234 |
| AN36.4 | Describe the components and functions of Waldeyer's lymphatic ring | 14 | 241 |
| AN36.5 | Describe the boundaries and clinical significance of pyriform fossa | 16 | 264 |
| AN36.6 | Describe the anatomical basis of tonsillitis, tonsillectomy, adenoids and peritonsillar abscess | 14 | 243 |
| AN36.7 | Describe the clinical significance of Killian's dehiscence | 14 | 240 |
| AN37.1 | Describe and demonstrate features of nasal septum, lateral wall of nose, their blood supply and nerve supply | 15 | 247 |
| AN37.2 | Describe location and functional anatomy of paranasal sinuses | 15 | 252 |
| AN37.3 | Describe anatomical basis of sinusitis and maxillary sinus tumours | 15 | 254 |
| AN38.1 | Describe the morphology, identify structure of the wall, nerve supply, blood supply and actions of intrinsic and extrinsic muscles of the larynx | 15 | 258 |
| AN38.2 | Describe the anatomical aspects of laryngitis | 16 | 264 |
| AN38.3 | Describe anatomical basis of recurrent laryngeal nerve injury | 16 | 268 |
| AN39.1 | Describe and demonstrate the morphology, nerve supply, embryological basis of nerve supply, blood supply, lymphatic drainage and actions of extrinsic and intrinsic muscles of tongue | 17 | 272 |
| AN39.2 | Explain the anatomical basis of hypoglossal nerve palsy | 17 | 274 |
| AN40.1 | Describe and identify the parts, blood supply and nerve supply of external ear | 18 | 279 |
| AN40.2 | Describe and demonstrate the boundaries, contents, relations and functional anatomy of middle ear and auditory tube | 14, 18 | 242, 284 |
| AN40.3 | Describe the features of internal ear | 18 | 290 |
| AN40.4 | Explain anatomical basis of otitis externa and otitis media | 18 | 286 |
| AN40.5 | Explain anatomical basis of myringotomy | 18 | 282 |
| AN41.1 | Describe and demonstrate parts and layers of eyeball | 19 | 295 |
| AN41.2 | Describe the anatomical aspects of cataract, glaucoma and central retinal artery occlusion | 19 | 300, 301 |
| AN41.3 | Describe the position, nerve supply and actions of intraocular muscles | 19 | 298 |
| AN42.1 | Describe the contents of the vertebral canal | 11 | 187 |
| AN42.2 | Describe and demonstrate the boundaries and contents of suboccipital triangle | 10 | 183 |
| AN42.3 | Describe the position, direction of fibres, relations, nerve supply, actions of semispinalis capitis and splenius capitis | 10 | 179 |
| AN43.1 | Describe and demonstrate the movements with muscles producing the movements of atlanto-occipital joint and atlantoaxial joint. | 9 | 173 |
| AN43.2 | Identify, describe and draw the microanatomy of pituitary gland, thyroid, parathyroid gland, tongue, salivary glands, tonsil, epiglottis, cornea, retina | 8, 12, 14, 17, 19 | 143, 203, 243, 271, 296, 299 |
| AN43.3 | Identify, describe and draw microanatomy of olfactory epithelium, eyelid, lip, sclerocorneal junction, optic nerve, cochlea—organ of Corti, pineal gland | 18, 19 | 292, 298 |
| AN43.4 | Describe the development and developmental basis of congenital anomalies of face, palate, tongue, branchial apparatus, pituitary gland, thyroid gland and eye | 2, 8, 12, 14, 17, 19 | 73, 143, 202, 232, 276, 302 |
| AN43.5 | Demonstrate: (1) Testing of muscles of facial expression, extraocular muscles, muscles of mastication, (2) Palpation of carotid arteries, facial artery, superficial temporal artery, (3) Location of internal and external jugular veins, (4) Location of hyoid bone, thyroid cartilage and cricoid cartilage with their vertebral levels | 20 | 303 |
| AN43.6 | Demonstrate surface projection of: Thyroid gland, parotid gland and duct, pterion, common carotid artery, internal jugular vein, subclavian vein, external jugular vein, facial artery in the face and accessory nerve | 20 | 304 |
| AN43.7 | Identify the anatomical structures in: (1) Plain X-ray skull; (2) AP view and lateral view, (3) Plain X-ray cervical spine—AP and lateral view, (4) Plain X-ray of paranasal sinuses | 20 | 309 |
| AN43.8 | Describe the anatomical route used for carotid angiogram and vertebral angiogram | 20 | 311 |
| AN43.9 | Identify anatomical structures in carotid angiogram and vertebral angiogram | 20 | 311 |

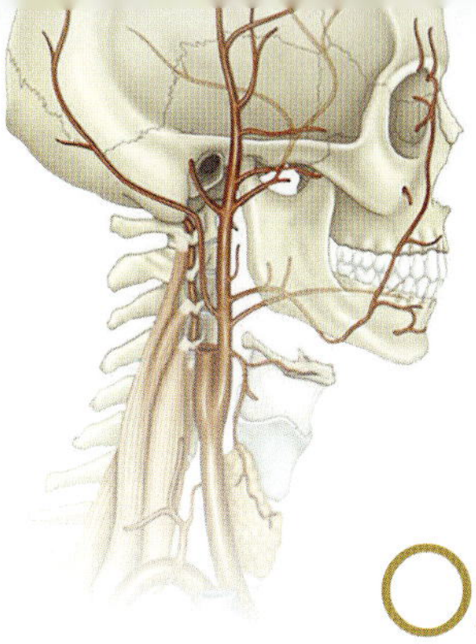

Chapter

1

# Osteology of Head and Neck

The *head* is the globular uppermost part of the body, which is connected with the trunk by the *neck*. The *face* is the anterior aspect of head and the muscles present here express facial movements. The *scalp* overlies the lateral, posterior and superior aspects of skull.

## Functions of Head and Neck

The head and neck region performs the following functions:

1. Protection to brain, endocrine glands and special senses.
2. Gives passage to food and air and connects their upper parts to their respective lower parts.
3. Produces voice for communication.

## Peculiar Features of Human Head and Neck

1. The head comprises skull and lodges the brain covered by meninges, hypophysis cerebri, special senses, teeth and blood vessels. Brain is the highest seat of intelligence.
2. To accommodate the increased volume of nervous tissue, the cranial cavity had to enlarge.
3. Correspondingly, the lower jaw or mandible had to retract.
4. The eyes also had come more anteriorly, on each side of the nose.
5. The external nose also became prominent.
6. The external ear becomes vestigial and chin is pushed forwards to accommodate the broad tongue.
7. Tongue, the organ for speech, is securely placed in the oral cavity for articulation of words, i.e. speech.
8. The vocalisation centre is big to articulate various words and speak distinctly. Speech is a special and chief characteristic of the human.

## Regions of Head and Neck

For study purposes, the head and neck are divided into the following regions:

1. ***Frontal region:*** Lies in front of skull.
2. ***Parietal region:*** Lies on top of skull, formed chiefly by the parietal bones. It is seen from the top.
3. ***Occipital region:*** Forms back of skull.
4. ***Temporal region:*** It is the area above the ears.
5. ***Ocular region:*** It is the region around the large orbital openings, containing the precious eyeball, muscles to move the eyeball, nerves and blood vessels to supply these muscles.
6. ***Auricular region:*** The region of the external ear with external auditory meatus comprises the auricular region.
7. ***Nasal region:*** The region of the external nose, its muscles and the associated cavity comprise the nasal region. Sense of smell is perceived from this region.
8. ***Oral region:*** Comprises upper and lower lips and the angle of the mouth, where the lips join each side. Numerous muscles are present here, to express feelings and emotions. These are parts of the muscles of facial expression. They show feelings, without words.
9. ***Oral cavity:*** It houses the organ of speech and taste. Tongue itself is not swallowed, though everything put on the tongue passes downwards.
10. ***Parotid region:*** Lies on the side of the face. It contains the biggest serous parotid salivary gland, which lies around the external auditory meatus.
11. ***Neck:*** Each half of the neck comprises two triangles between anterior median line and posterior median line.
    a. ***Posterior triangle:*** Lies between sternocleidomastoid, the *neck and chin turning muscle*; trapezius, *the shrugging muscle* and middle one-third of the clavicle. It contains spinal root of accessory nerve, proximal parts of the important brachial plexus, subclavian vessels with its branches and tributaries. Its apex is above and base is below.
    b. ***Anterior triangle:*** Lies between the anterior median line and the anterior border of sternocleidomastoid muscle. Its apex is in lower part of neck, close to sternum and base above. It contains the common carotid artery and branches of external carotid artery, last four cranial nerves, lymph nodes.

**Competency:**
**AN26.1** Demonstrate anatomical position of skull, identify and locate individual skull bones in skull.

### Bones of Head and Neck

The bones of head and neck include:
1. Skull, i.e. cranium with mandible
2. Seven cervical vertebrae
3. Hyoid
4. Six ossicles of the ear.

## SKULL

The skeleton of the head is called the *skull*. It consists of several bones that are joined together to form the ***cranium***. The term skull also includes the mandible or lower jaw, which is a separate bone. However, the two terms, skull and cranium, are often used synonymously (Plate 1.1).

### Parts of Skull

The skull can be divided into two main parts:
1. ***Calvaria*** or *brain box/neurocranium* is the upper part of the cranium, which encloses the brain. It consists of a skull cap/vault (intramembranous ossification) and a base (intracartilaginous ossification).
2. ***Facial skeleton***/viscerocranium constitutes the rest of the skull and includes the mandible.

### Bones of the Skull

The skull consists of 28 bones, including 6 ear ossicles.
1. **Calvaria** or brain box is composed of 14 bones, including three paired ear ossicles.

| *Paired* | *Unpaired* |
|---|---|
| 1. Parietal | 1. Frontal |
| 2. Temporal | 2. Occipital |
| 3. Malleus | 3. Sphenoid |
| 4. Incus | 4. Ethmoid |
| 5. Stapes | |

2. ***Facial skeleton*** is composed of 14 bones.

| *Paired* | *Unpaired* |
|---|---|
| 1. Maxilla | 1. Mandible |
| 2. Zygomatic | 2. Vomer |
| 3. Nasal | |
| 4. Lacrimal | |
| 5. Palatine | |
| 6. Inferior nasal concha | |

### Skull Joints

The joints in the skull are mostly ***sutures***, a few primary cartilaginous joints and three pairs of synovial joints. The sutures can be classified into:
1. Plane suture — edges of bone are flat, e.g. internasal suture.
2. Serrate suture, e.g. coronal suture.
3. Denticulate suture, e.g. lambdoid suture.

**Plate 1.1:** Cranial and facial skeleton

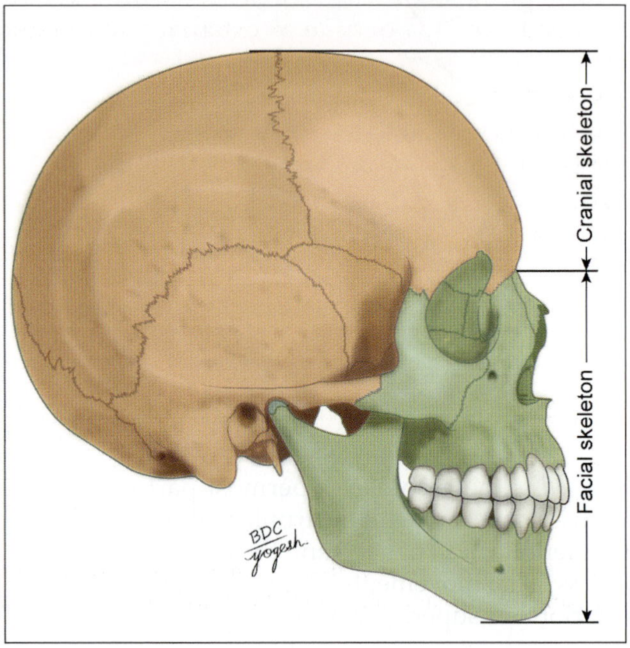


4. Squamous suture, e.g. parietotemporal suture.
5. Schindylesis, e.g. palatomaxillary suture.

***Movable joints of skull:*** Two pairs of synovial joints are present between the ossicles of middle ear. One pair is the largest *temporomandibular joint*.

### Anatomical Position of Skull

Hold the skull in both the hands so that (Fig. 1.1):
1. The orbital cavities are directed forwards
2. The lower margin of the orbit and upper margin of the external acoustic meatus lie in the same horizontal plane (called ***Frankfurt's plane***).

*Note*: ***Reid's base line*** is a horizontal line obtained by joining the infraorbital margin to the centre of external acoustic meatus, i.e. auricular point (Fig. 1.1). It is used in conventional radiography when performing CT imaging.

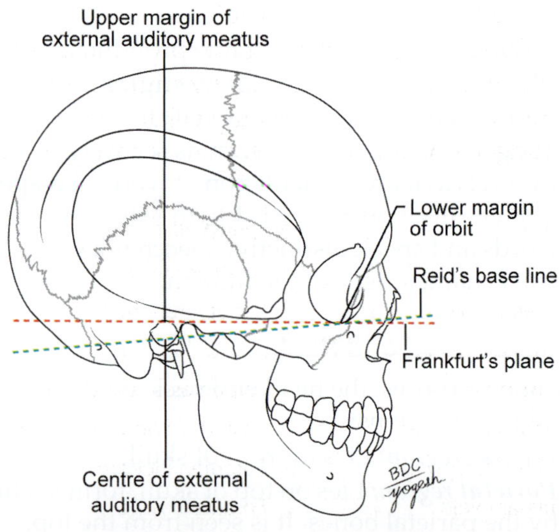


**Fig. 1.1:** Anatomical position of skull

### Methods of Study of the Skull

The skull can be studied as a whole. The whole skull can be studied from the outside or externally in different views:

1. Superior view — norma verticalis
2. Posterior view — norma occipitalis
3. Anterior view — norma frontalis
4. Lateral view — norma lateralis
5. Inferior view — norma basalis.

The whole skull can be studied from the inside or internally after removing the roof of the calvaria or skull cap:

a. Internal surface of the ***cranial vault***.
b. Internal surface of the ***cranial base*** that shows a natural subdivision into anterior, middle and posterior cranial fossae.

***Competency:***
**AN27.2** Describe emissary veins with its role in spread of infection from extracranial route to intracranial venous sinuses

### Peculiarities of Skull Bones

1. Base of skull ossifies in cartilage, while the skull cap ossifies in membrane.
2. At birth, skull comprises one table only. By 4 years or so, two tables are formed. Between the two tables, there are *diploes* (Greek *double*), i.e. spaces containing red bone marrow forming RBCs, granular series of WBCs and platelets. Four diploic veins on each side drain the formed blood cells into neighbouring veins.
3. At birth, the 4 angles of parietal bone have membranous gaps or fontanelles. These allow overlapping of bones during vaginal delivery, if required. These also allow skull bones to increase in size after birth, for housing the delicate brain.
4. Some skull bones have air cells in them and are called pneumatic bones, e.g. frontal and maxilla.
   a. They reduce the weight of skull.
   b. They maintain humidity of inspired air.
   c. They give resonance to voice.
   d. These may get infected resulting in sinusitis.
5. Skull bones are united mostly by sutures.
6. Skull has foramina for 'emissary veins', which connect intracranial venous sinuses with extracranial veins. These try to relieve raised intracranial pressure. Infection may reach through the emissary veins into cranial venous sinuses as these veins are valveless (Table 1.1).
7. Petrous temporal is the densest bone of the body. It lodges internal ear, middle ear, including three ossicles, i.e. malleus, incus and stapes. Ossicles are 'bones within the bone' and are fully formed at birth.
8. Skull lodges brain, meninges, CSF, glands like hypophysis cerebri and pineal, venous sinuses, teeth, special senses like retina of eyeball, taste buds of tongue, olfactory epithelium, cochlear and vestibular nerve endings.

***Competency:***
**AN26.2** Describe the features of norma frontalis, verticalis, occipitalis, lateralis and basalis.

## EXTERIOR OF THE SKULL

### NORMA VERTICALIS

#### Shape

When viewed from above, the skull is usually oval in shape. It is wider posteriorly than anteriorly. The shape may be more nearly circular (Fig. 1.2, Flowchart 1.1).

#### Bones

1. Frontal bone anteriorly.
2. Occipital bone posteriorly.
3. Parietal bone on each side.

#### Sutures

1. ***Coronal suture*** is placed between the frontal and the two parietal bones. The suture crosses the cranial vault from side-to-side (Fig. 1.2).
2. ***Sagittal suture*** is placed in the median plane between the two parietal bones.
3. ***Lambdoid suture*** lies posteriorly between the occipital and the two parietal bones. It is labda-shaped, hence the name.

*Note*: **Metopic** (Latin *forehead)* **suture** is occasionally present in about 3% to 8% of individuals. It lies in the median plane and separates the two halves of the frontal bone. Normally, it fuses at 6 years of age.

**TABLE 1.1: The emissary veins of the skull**

| *Name* | *Foramen of skull* | *Veins outside skull* | *Venous sinus* |
|---|---|---|---|
| 1. Parietal emissary vein | Parietal foramen | Veins of scalp | Superior sagittal sinus |
| 2. Mastoid emissary vein | Mastoid foramen | Veins of scalp | Sigmoid sinus |
| 3. Emissary vein | Hypoglossal canal | Internal jugular vein | Sigmoid sinus |
| 4. Condylar emissary vein | Posterior condylar foramen | Suboccipital venous plexus | Sigmoid sinus |
| 5. 2–3 emissary veins | Foramen lacerum | Pharyngeal venous plexus | Cavernous sinus |
| 6. Emissary vein | Foramen ovale | Pterygoid venous plexus | Cavernous sinus |
| 7. Emissary vein | Foramen caecum | Veins from upper part of nose | Superior sagittal sinus |

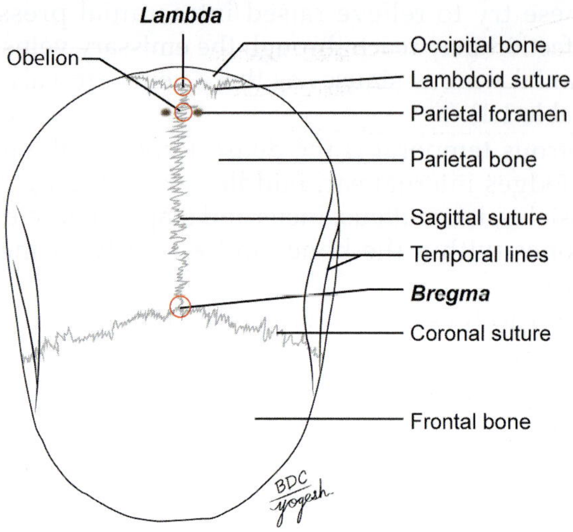


**Fig. 1.2:** Norma verticalis

**Flowchart 1.1:** Features of norma verticalis

**Norma verticalis**
Top view of skull

| *Bones* | *Sutures* | *Features* |
|---|---|---|
| Frontal | Coronal | Vertex |
| Parietal | Sagittal | Bregma |
| Occipital | Lambdoid | Lambda |
| | Metopic (in 3–8%) | Parietal eminence |
| | | Obelion |
| | | Parietal foramen |
| | | – Emissary vein |

### Features (Fig. 1.2)

1. ***Vertex*** is the highest point on sagittal suture.
2. ***Vault*** of skull is the arched roof for the dome of skull.
3. ***Bregma*** is the meeting point between the coronal and sagittal sutures. In the foetal skull, this is the site of a membranous gap, called the *anterior fontanelle*, which closes at 18 to 24 months of age. It allows growth of brain.
4. ***Lambda*** is the meeting point between the sagittal and lambdoid sutures. In the foetal skull, this is the site of the *posterior fontanelle*, which closes at birth—2 to 3 months of age.
5. ***Parietal tuber*** *(eminence)* is the area of maximum convexity of the parietal bone. This is a common site of fracture of the skull.
6. ***Parietal foramen***, one on each side, pierces the parietal bone near its upper border, 2.5 to 4 cm in front of the lambda. The parietal foramen transmits an emissary vein from the veins of scalp to superior sagittal sinus.
7. ***Obelion*** is the point on the sagittal suture between the two parietal foramina.
8. ***Temporal lines*** begin at the zygomatic process of the frontal bone, arch backwards and upwards and cross the frontal bone, the coronal suture and the parietal bone. Over the parietal bone, there are two lines—superior and inferior. Traced anteriorly, they fuse to form a single line. Traced posteriorly, the superior line fades out over the posterior part of the parietal bone, but the inferior temporal line continues downwards and forwards with zygomatic arch.
9. A pair of anterolateral/sphenoidal fontanelle and a pair of posterolateral or mastoid fontanelles are also present. These fontanelles close within 3–4 months after birth.

## NORMA OCCIPITALIS

Norma occipitalis is convex upwards and on each side and is flattened below (Fig. 1.3, Flowchart 1.2).

### Bones

1. Parietal bones above.
2. Squamous part of the occipital bone below.
3. Mastoid part of the temporal bone on each side.

### Sutures

1. ***Lambdoid suture*** lies between the occipital bone and the two parietal bones. Sutural or wormian bones are common along this suture.
2. ***Occipitomastoid suture*** lies between the occipital bone and mastoid part of the temporal bone.
3. ***Parietomastoid suture*** lies between the parietal bone and mastoid part of the temporal bone.

   The posterior part of the ***sagittal suture*** is also seen.

### Features

1. *Lambda, parietal foramina* and *obelion* have been examined in the norma verticalis.
2. ***External occipital protuberance*** is a median prominence in the lower part of this norma. It marks the junction of the head and the neck. The most prominent point on this protuberance is called the *inion*.
3. ***Superior nuchal lines*** are curved bony ridges passing laterally from the protuberance. These also mark the junction of the head and the neck. The area below the superior nuchal lines will be studied with the norma basalis.
4. ***Highest nuchal lines*** are not always present. They are curved bony ridges situated about 1 cm above the superior nuchal lines. They begin from the upper part of the external occipital protuberance and are more arched than the superior nuchal lines.

**Flowchart 1.2:** Features of norma occipitalis

**Norma occipitalis**

| *Bones* | *Sutures* | *Features* |
|---|---|---|
| Parietal | Lambdoid | Lambda |
| Occipital | Occipitomastoid | External occipital protuberance |
| Mastoid part of temporal | Parietomastoid | - Trapezius |
| | | Inion |
| | | Superior nuchal lines |
| | | - Trapezius |
| | | - Sternocleidomastoid |
| | | - Splenius capitis |
| | | Highest nuchal lines |
| | | - Epicranial aponeurosis |
| | | - Occipitalis |

Mastoid foramen: Emissary vein, meningeal branch of occipital artery

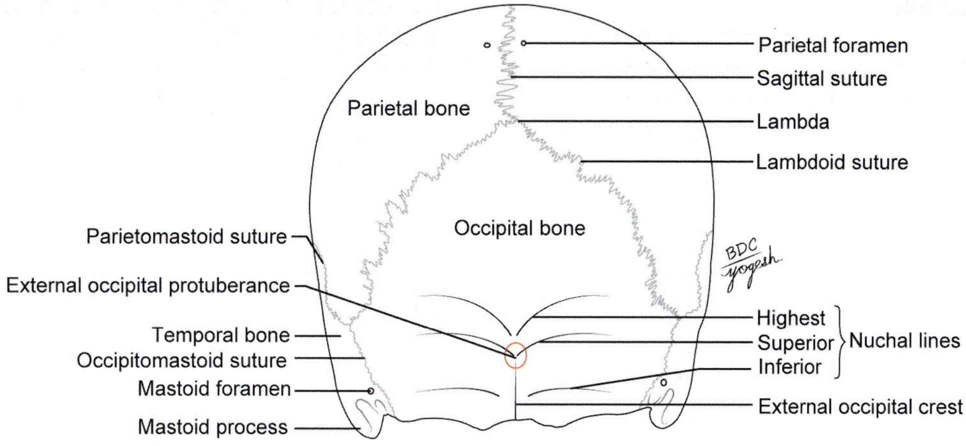


**Fig. 1.3:** Norma occipitalis

5. ***Occipital point*** is a median point, a little above the inion. It is the point farthest from the glabella.
6. ***Mastoid*** (Greek *breast*) ***foramen*** is located on the mastoid part of the temporal bone at or near the occipitomastoid suture. Internally, it opens at the sigmoid sulcus. The mastoid foramen transmits an emissary vein (Table 1.1) and the meningeal branch of the occipital artery.

*Note:* ***Interparietal bone*** (inca bone) is occasionally present. It is a large triangular bone located at the apex of the squamous occipital. This is not a sutural or accessory bone but represents the membranous part of the occipital bone which has failed to fuse with the rest of the bone.

### Attachments

1. The upper part of the external occipital protuberance gives origin to the trapezius, and the lower part gives attachment to the upper end of the ligamentum nuchae.
2. The medial 1/3rd of the superior nuchal line gives origin to the trapezius, and the lateral part provides insertion to the sternocleidomastoid above and to the splenius capitis below.
3. The highest nuchal lines, if present, provide attachment to the epicranial aponeurosis medially, and give origin to the occipitalis or occipital belly of occipitofrontalis muscle laterally. In case of absence of highest nuchal lines, these structures are attached to superior nuchal lines.

## NORMA FRONTALIS

The norma frontalis is roughly oval in outline, being wider above than below (Plate 1.2, Fig. 1.4, Flowchart 1.3).

### Bones

1. *Frontal* bone forms the forehead. Its upper part is smooth and convex, but the lower part is irregular and is interrupted by the orbits and by the anterior bony aperture of nose.
2. Right and left *maxillae* form the upper jaw.
3. Right and left *nasal* bones form the bridge of the nose.
4. *Zygomatic* (Greek *yoke*) bones form the bony prominence of the superolateral part of the cheeks.
5. *Mandible* forms the lower jaw.

### Descriptive Subdivisions

The *norma frontalis* can be studied under the following heads.

1. Frontal region
2. Orbital openings
3. Anterior nasal aperture
4. Lower part of the face.

### Frontal Region

The frontal region presents the following features:

1. ***Superciliary arch*** is a rounded, curved elevation situated just above the medial part of each orbit. It overlies the frontal sinus and is better marked in males than in females.

**Flowchart 1.3:** Features of norma frontalis

***Norma frontalis***

***Frontal region***
- Superciliary arches
- Glabella
- Nasion
- Frontal eminence

***Orbital openings***
- 4 orbital margins
  - Superior: Frontal bone
  - Medial: Frontal bone, Frontal process of maxilla
  - Inferior: Zygomatic bone, maxilla
  - Lateral: Zygomatic and frontal bones
- Supraorbital notch: Supraorbital nerve and vessels

***Nasal aperture***
- Pear-shaped
- Boundaries
  - Nasal bone
  - Nasal notch of maxilla
- Anterior nasal spine
- Rhinion

***Lowest part of face***
- Maxillae
  - Nasal notch
  - Anterior nasal spine
  - Infraorbital foramen: Infraorbital nerve and vessels
  - Processes: Frontal, zygomatic, alveolar
- Zygomatic bone
  - Zygomaticus major and minor
  - Zygomaticofacial foramen

**Plate 1.2:** Norma frontalis

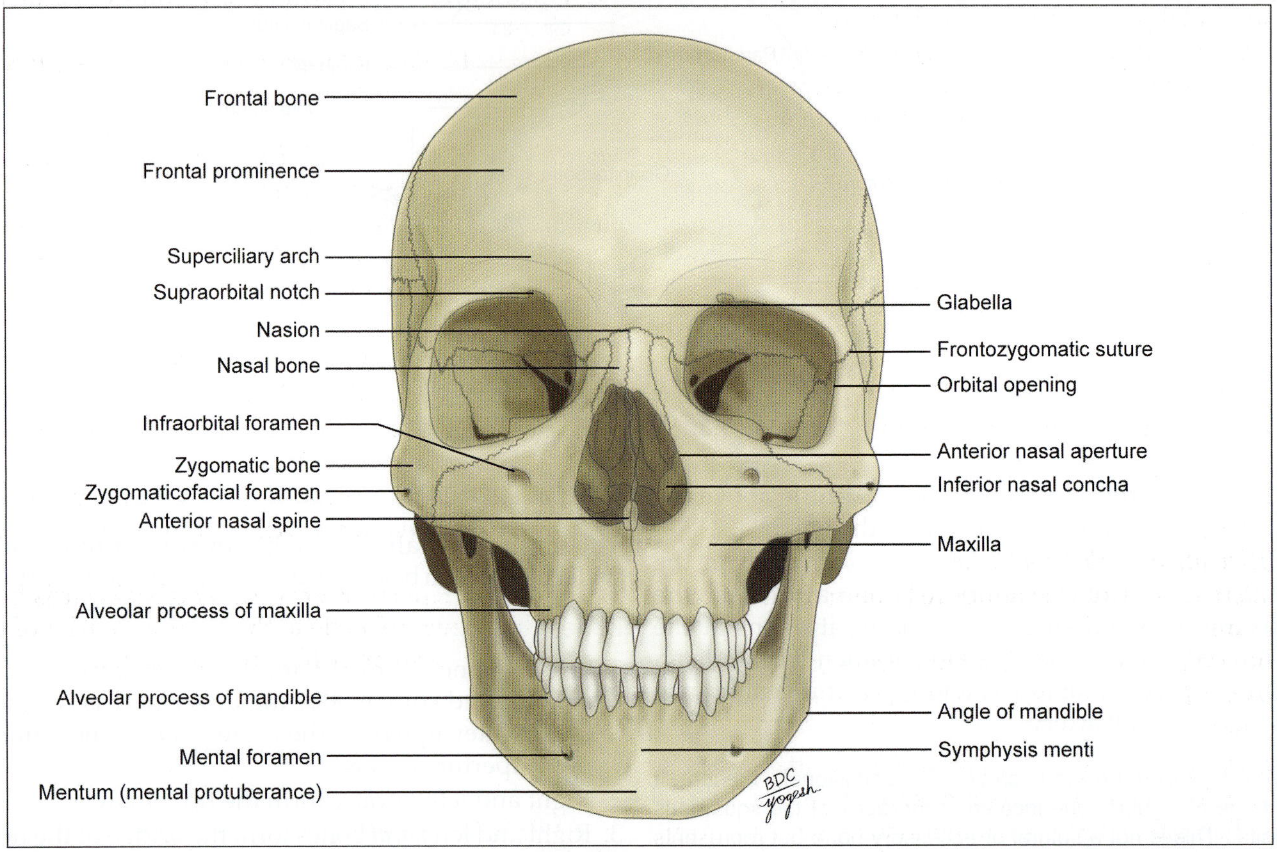


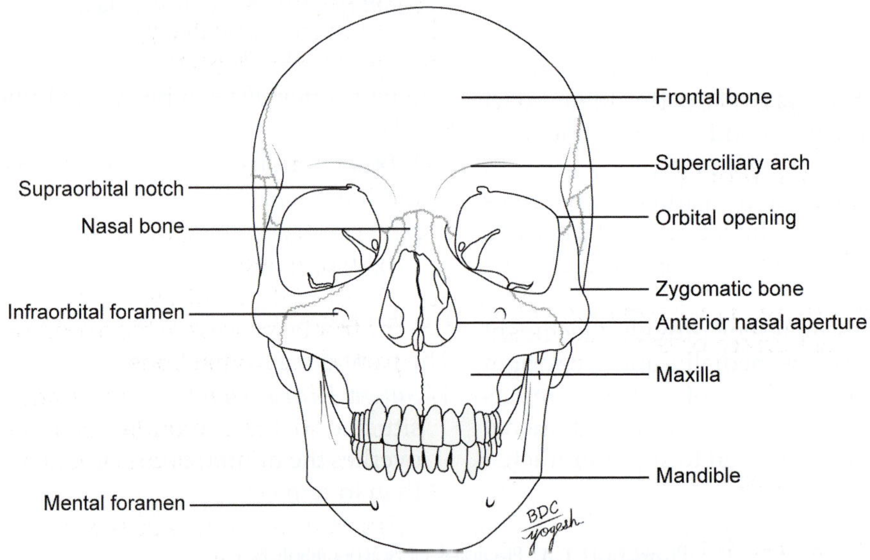


**Fig. 1.4:** Norma frontalis: Walls of orbit, nasal aperture and lower part of face

2. ***Glabella*** is a median elevation connecting the two superciliary arches. Below the glabella, the skull recedes to frontonasal suture at root of the nose.
3. ***Nasion*** is a median point at the root of the nose where the internasal suture meets with the frontonasal suture.
4. ***Frontal tuber*** or *eminence* is a low rounded elevation above the superciliary arch – one on each side. It is more prominent in females and in children.

## Orbital Openings

Each orbital (Latin *circle*) opening is quadrangular in shape and is bounded by the following four margins.

1. ***Supraorbital margin*** is formed by the frontal bone. At the junction of its lateral 2/3rd and its medial 1/3rd, it presents the supraorbital notch or foramen.
2. ***Infraorbital margin*** is formed by the zygomatic bone laterally, and maxilla medially.

3. ***Medial orbital margin*** is ill-defined. It is formed by the frontal bone above, and by the lacrimal crest of the frontal process of the maxilla below.
4. ***Lateral orbital margin*** is formed mostly by the frontal process of zygomatic bone but is completed above by the zygomatic process of frontal bone. *Frontozygomatic suture* lies at their union.

### Anterior Nasal Aperture

The anterior bony aperture of the nose is pear-shaped, being wide below and narrow above.

#### Boundaries

***Above:*** By the lower border of the nasal bones.

***Below:*** By the nasal notch of the body of maxilla on each side.

#### Features

1. *Articulations of the nasal bone:*
   *Anteriorly* — with the opposite bone at the internasal suture.
   *Posteriorly* — with the frontal process of the maxilla.
   *Superiorly* — with the frontal bone at the frontonasal suture.
   *Inferiorly* — the upper nasal cartilage is attached to it.
2. ***Anterior nasal spine*** is a sharp projection in the median plane in the lower boundary of the piriform aperture.
3. ***Rhinion*** is the lowermost point of the internasal suture.

### Lower Part of the Face

The lower part of the face is formed by the following bones:
1. Maxilla forms upper jaw.
2. Zygomatic bone forms malar prominences.
3. Mandible forms lower jaw.

#### Maxilla

Maxilla contributes a large share in the formation of the facial skeleton. The anterior surface of the body of the maxilla presents:
1. *Nasal notch* medially
2. *Anterior nasal spine*
3. ***Infraorbital foramen***, 1 cm below the infraorbital margin
4. ***Incisive fossa*** above the incisor teeth
5. ***Canine fossa*** lateral to the canine eminence.

In addition, three out of four ***processes of the maxilla*** are also seen in this norma.
1. ***Frontal process*** *of the maxilla* is directed upwards. It articulates anteriorly with the nasal bone, posteriorly with the lacrimal bone and superiorly with the frontal bone (Fig. 1.7).
2. ***Zygomatic process*** *of the maxilla* is short but stout and articulates with the zygomatic bone.
3. ***Alveolar process*** *of the maxilla* bears sockets for the upper teeth.

#### Zygomatic Bone (Malar Bone)

1. Zygomatic bone forms the prominence of the cheek.
2. ***Zygomaticofacial foramen*** is seen on its surface.

#### Mandible (Lower Jaw Bone)

Mandible (Latin *to chew*) forms the lower jaw. Its following features are seen in norma frontalis:
1. *Upper border* or *alveolar arch* lodges the lower teeth.
2. *Lower border* or *base* is rounded.
3. Middle point of the base is called the *mental point or **gnathion***.
4. The point on the angle of mandible is called ***gonion***.
5. *Anterior surface* of the body of the mandible presents:
   a. *Symphysis menti*, the *mental protuberance* and the *mental tubercles*, anteriorly.
   b. ***Mental foramen*** below the interval between the two premolar teeth, transmitting the *mental nerve and vessels*.
   c. ***Oblique line*** runs upwards and backwards from the mental tubercle to the anterior border of the *ramus* (Latin branch) of the mandible.

### Sutures of the Norma Frontalis

1. Internasal
2. Frontonasal
3. Nasomaxillary
4. Lacrimomaxillary
5. Frontomaxillary
6. Intermaxillary
7. Zygomaticomaxillary
8. Zygomaticofrontal.

### Attachments

1. The medial part of the superciliary arch gives origin to the corrugator supercilii muscle (Fig. 1.5).
2. Procerus muscle arises from the nasal bone near the median plane.
3. The orbital part of the orbicularis oculi arises from the frontal process of the maxilla and from the nasal part of the frontal bone.
4. Medial palpebral ligament is attached to the frontal process of the maxilla between the frontal and maxillary origins of the orbicularis oculi.
5. Levator labii superioris alaeque nasi arises from the frontal process of the maxilla in front of the orbicularis oculi.
6. Levator labii superioris arises from the maxilla between the infraorbital margin and the infraorbital foramen.
7. Levator anguli oris arises from the canine fossa.
8. Nasalis and the depressor septi arise from the surface of the maxilla bordering the nasal notch.
9. Incisivus labii superioris muscle arises from an area just below the depressor septi. It forms part of orbicularis oris.
10. Zygomaticus major and minor arise from the surface of the zygomatic bone. The zygomaticus minor

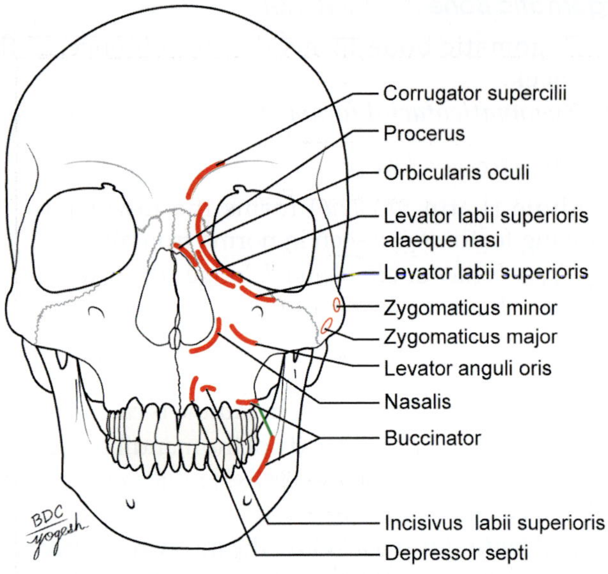


**Fig. 1.5:** Attachments of muscles to the norma frontalis

muscle arises below the zygomaticofacial foramen. The zygomaticus major arises lateral to the minor muscle.

11. Buccinator arises from maxilla and mandible opposite molar teeth and from *pterygomandibular raphe*. It also forms part of orbicularis oris.

### *Structures Passing Through Foramina*

1. *Supraorbital notch or foramen* transmits the *supraorbital nerves and vessels.*
2. *External nasal nerve* emerges between the nasal bone and upper nasal cartilage.
3. *Infraorbital foramen* transmits the *infraorbital nerve* and *vessels.*
4. *Zygomaticofacial foramen* transmits the nerve of the same name, a branch of *maxillary nerve.*
5. *Mental foramen* on the mandible transmits the mental nerve and vessels.

## CLINICAL ANATOMY

The *nasal bone is one of the most commonly fractured bones of the face*. Mandible and parietal eminence are the next bones to be fractured.

## NORMA LATERALIS

**Bones** (Plate 1.3, Figs 1.6a and b, Flowchart 1.4)

1. Frontal
2. Parietal
3. Occipital
4. Temporal
5. Sphenoid
6. Zygomatic
7. Mandible
8. Maxilla
9. Nasal

### Features

### *Temporal Lines*

The *temporal lines* have been studied in the norma verticalis. The inferior temporal line, in its posterior part, turns downwards and forwards and becomes continuous with the ***supramastoid crest*** on the squamous temporal bone near its junction with the mastoid temporal. This crest is continuous anteriorly with the posterior root of the zygomatic arch (Flowchart 1.4, Plate 1.3, Figs 1.6a to c).

### *Zygomatic Arch or Zygoma*

The *zygomatic arch* is a horizontal bar on the side of the head, in front of the ear, a little above the tragus. It is formed by the temporal process of the zygomatic bone in anterior 1/3rd and the zygomatic process of the temporal bone in posterior 2/3rd. The ***zygomaticotemporal suture*** crosses the arch obliquely downwards and backwards.

#### *Features*

1. The arch comprises 2 surfaces (medial and lateral) and 2 borders (upper and lower).
2. Medially, the arch is separated from the side of the skull by a gap, which is deeper in front than behind. The *lateral surface* of the arch is subcutaneous.
3. *Upper border* is continuous with temporal line in front and with supramastoid crest behind. The anterior end of the upper border is called the ***jugal point***.
4. The *posterior end* of the zygomatic arch is attached to the squamous temporal bone by *anterior* and *posterior roots*.
5. The ***tubercle of the root of the zygoma*** lies on its lower border at the junction of the anterior and posterior roots.

**Flowchart 1.4:** Features of norma lateralis

***Norma lateralis***

- ***Temporal lines***
  - Superior
    - Temporal fascia
  - Inferior
    - Temporalis
  - Supramastoid crest
- ***Zygomatic arch***
  - Attachments
    - Masseter[O]
    - Lateral temporomandibular ligament
- ***External acoustic meatus***
  - Formation
    - Tympanic part of temporal bone
    - Squamous part of temporal bone
- ***Mastoid process***
  - Attachments:
    1. Sternocleidomastoid[I]
    2. Splenius capitis
    3. Longissimus capitis
- ***Mastoid notch***
  - Posterior belly of digastric
- ***Styloid process***
  - Styloglossus
  - Stylohyoid
  - Stylopharyngeus
  - Ligaments:
    - Stylohyoid
    - Stylomandibular

Foramina: ***Mastoid foramen:*** Emissary vein, branch of occipital artery
***Zygomaticotemporal foramen:*** Zygomaticotemporal nerve

BDC yogesh

**Plate 1.3:** Norma lateralis

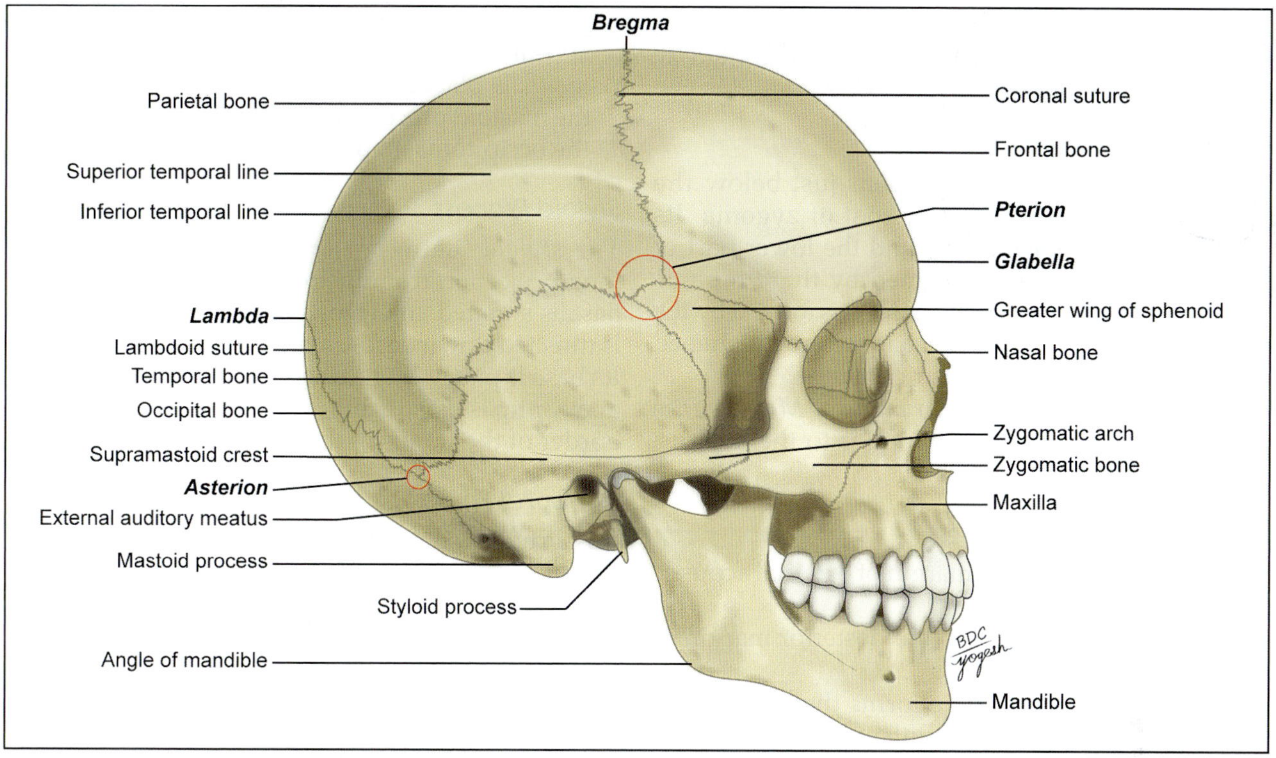


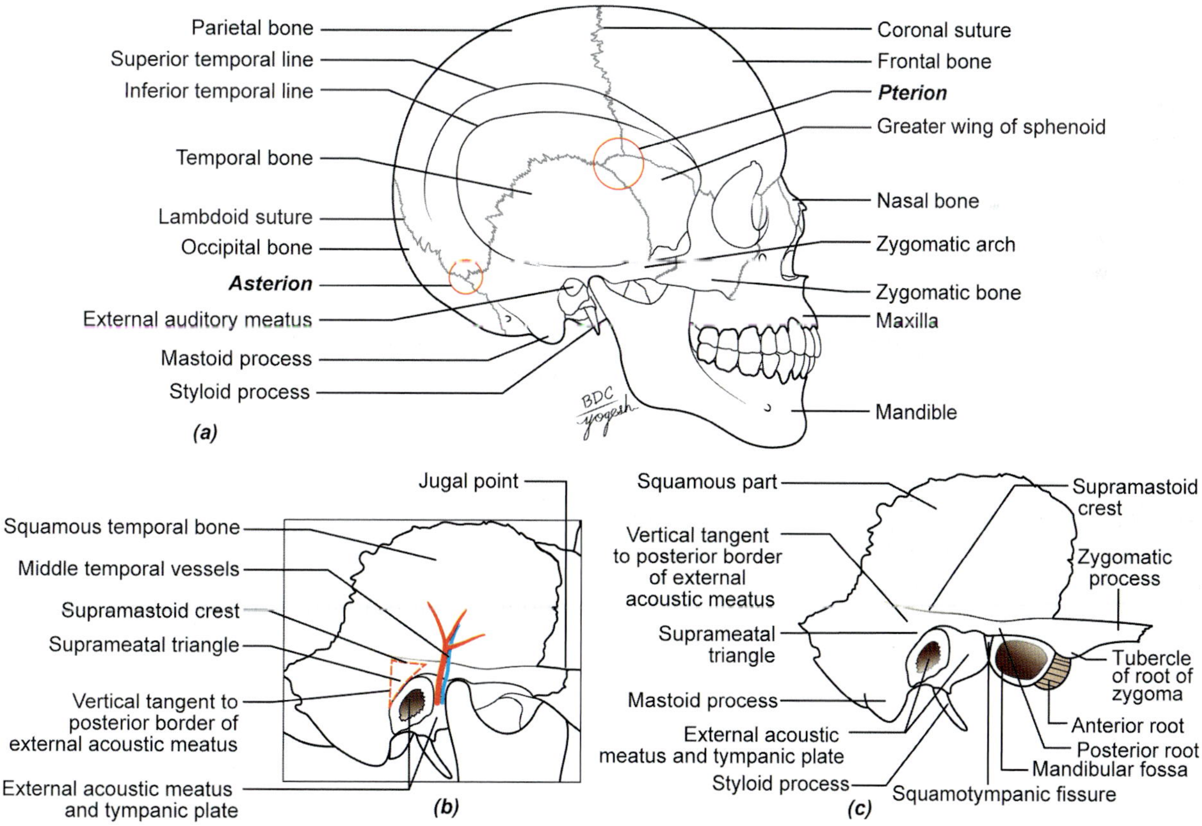


**Figs 1.6a to c:** (a) Norma lateralis, (b) bones forming norma lateralis, and (c) tympanic plate forming margins of external acoustic meatus

6. The ***anterior root*** (articular tubercle) passes medially in front of the *mandibular fossa*. The ***posterior root*** passes backwards along the lateral margin of the mandibular or articular fossa, then above the external acoustic meatus to become continuous with the supramastoid crest.

7. Two projections are visible in relation to these roots.
   a. One is *tubercle of root of zygoma* at its lower border.
   b. Another tubercle is visible just behind the mandibular or articular fossa and is known as ***postglenoid tubercle***.

### External Acoustic Meatus

1. The *external acoustic meatus* opens just below the posterior part of the posterior root of zygoma. Its anterior and inferior margins and the lower part of the posterior margin are formed by the tympanic plate, and the posterosuperior margin is formed by the squamous temporal bone. The margins are roughened for the attachment of auricular cartilage.
2. The ***suprameatal triangle*** *(triangle of Mc-Ewen)* is a small depression posterosuperior to the meatus. (Flowchart 1.5)
   **Boundaries**
   *Superior*: Supramastoid crest
   *Anterior*: Posterosuperior margin of external acoustic meatus
   *Posterior*: Vertical tangent to the posterior margin of the meatus.
   *Clinical aspects*: The triangle forms the lateral wall of the tympanic or mastoid antrum (Fig. 1.9c). The mastoid antrum lies 1.25 cm deep to the suprameatal triangle. This triangle is an important landmark in cortical mastoidectomy.
3. The ***suprameatal spine*** *(of Henle)* may be present on the anteroinferior margin of the triangle. It serves as a surgical landmark while performing middle ear surgeries.

### Mastoid Part of the Temporal Bone

1. The *mastoid part of the temporal bone* lies just behind the external acoustic meatus.
2. The mastoid temporal bone articulates posterosuperiorly with the posteroinferior part of the parietal bone at the horizontal *parietomastoid suture,* and posteriorly with the squamous occipital bone at the *occipitomastoid suture.* These two sutures meet at the lateral end of the lambdoid suture. The ***asterion*** is the point where the parietomastoid, occipitomastoid and lambdoid sutures meet. In infants, the asterion is the site of the ***posterolateral*** **or** ***mastoid fontanelle,*** which closes by 12 months (Fig. 1.3).

**Flowchart 1.5:** Suprameatal triangle

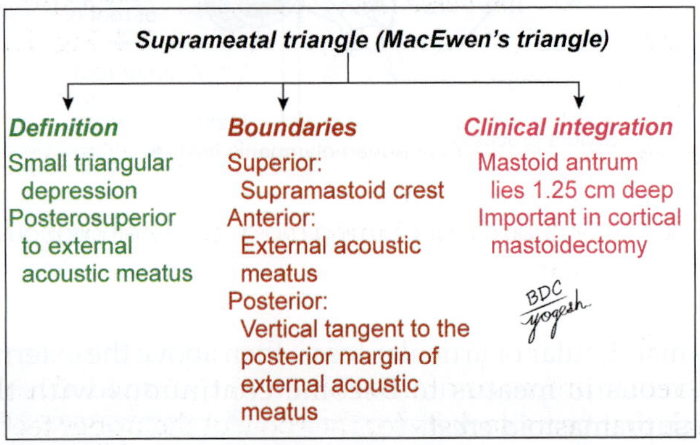


3. The ***mastoid process*** is a breast-like projection from the lower part of the mastoid temporal bone, posteroinferior to the external acoustic meatus. It appears during the 2nd year of life. The *tympanomastoid fissure* is placed on the anterior aspect of the base of the mastoid process. The *mastoid foramen* lies at or near the occipitomastoid suture (Fig. 1.5).

### Styloid Process

The *styloid* (Latin *pen*) *process* is a needle-like thin, long projection from the temporal bone seen in norma basalis situated anteromedial to the mastoid process. It is directed downwards, forwards and slightly medially. Its base is partly ensheathed by the tympanic plate. The apex or tip is usually hidden from view by the posterior border of the ramus of the mandible.

### Temporal Fossa

It is a shallow depression on the side of the skull.

#### Boundaries

1. *Above:* Superior temporal line.
2. *Below:* Upper border of the zygomatic arch laterally, and by the infratemporal crest of the greater wing of the sphenoid bone medially. Through the gap deep to the zygomatic arch, temporal fossa communicates with the infratemporal fossa.
3. *Anterior wall:* Formed by the zygomatic bone and by parts of the frontal and sphenoid bones. This wall separates the fossa from the orbit.
4. *Floor:* The anterior part of the floor is crossed by an H-shaped suture where four bones—frontal, parietal, greater wing of sphenoid and temporal adjoin each other. This area is termed the ***pterion***.

*Note:*

*The* ***pterion*** lies 4 cm above the midpoint of the zygomatic arch and 2.5 cm behind the frontozygomatic suture. Deep to the pterion lie, *middle meningeal vein*, *anterior division of the middle meningeal artery* and *stem of the lateral sulcus of brain (Sylvian point)* (Flowchart 1.6).

On the temporal surface of the zygomatic bone forming the anterior wall of the fossa, there is the *zygomaticotemporal foramen.*

#### Attachments (Fig. 1.7)

1. Temporal fascia is attached to the superior temporal line and to the area between the two temporal lines. Inferiorly, it is attached to the outer and inner lips of the upper border of the zygomatic arch.
2. Temporalis muscle arises from the whole of the temporal fossa.
3. The medial surface and lower border of the zygomatic arch give origin to the masseter.
4. Lateral ligament of the temporomandibular joint is attached to the tubercle of the root of the zygoma.
5. The sternocleidomastoid, splenius capitis and longissimus capitis are inserted from before backwards on the posterior part of the lateral surface of the mastoid process. Posterior belly of digastric arises from mastoid notch. The groove obliquely placed behind mastoid notch is due to occipital artery.

**Flowchart 1.6:** Pterion

**Pterion**

| Definition | Meeting bones | Deep relations | Clinical |
|---|---|---|---|
| H-shaped suture in the floor of temporal fossa | - Frontal<br>- Temporal<br>- Parietal<br>- Greater wing of sphenoid | - MMV<br>- Anterior division of MMA<br>- Stem of lateral sulcus | Fracture of pterion<br>↓<br>Rupture of MMV<br>↓<br>Extradural hematoma<br>↓<br>T/t: Craniotomy |

(MAA: Middle meningeal artery, MMV: Middle meningeal vein)

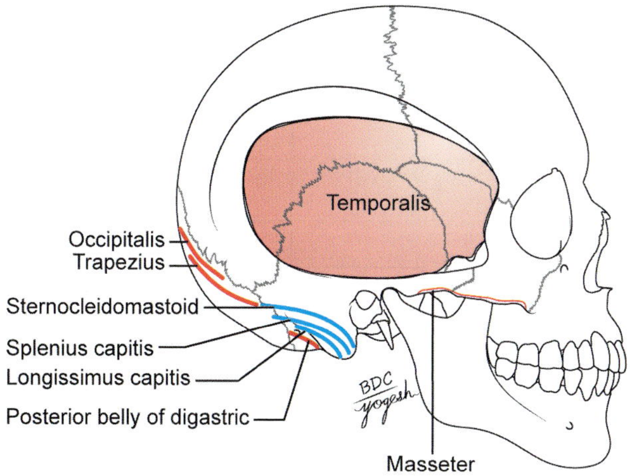


**Fig. 1.7:** Attachments of norma lateralis

6. The *gap* between the zygomatic arch and the side of the skull transmits:
   a. Tendon of the temporalis muscle
   b. Deep temporal vessels
   c. Deep temporal nerves
   d. Zygomaticotemporal vessels and nerve

*Note*: For infratemporal fossa, *see* Chapter 6. For pterygopalatine fossa, *see* Chapter 15.

### Structures Passing Through Foramina

1. *Tympanomastoid fissure* on the anterior aspect of the base of the mastoid process transmits the *auricular branch* of *vagus nerve.*
2. Mastoid foramen transmits:
   a. *Emissary vein* connecting the *sigmoid sinus* with the *posterior auricular vein* (Table 1.1).
   b. Meningeal branch of the occipital artery.
3. *Zygomaticotemporal foramen* transmits the nerve of the same name and a minute artery.

### CLINICAL ANATOMY

***Pterion**, the site of anterolateral fontanelle,* is the thin part of skull. In roadside accidents, the anterior division of middle meningeal artery at pterion (Fig. 1.8) may be ruptured, leading to clot formation between the skull bone and dura mater or extradural haemorrhage (Fig. 1.9). The clot compresses the motor area of brain, leading to

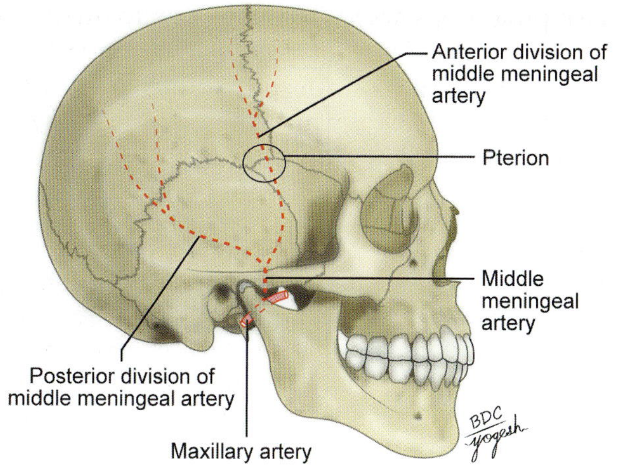


**Fig. 1.8:** Position of anterior division of middle meningeal artery against the pterion

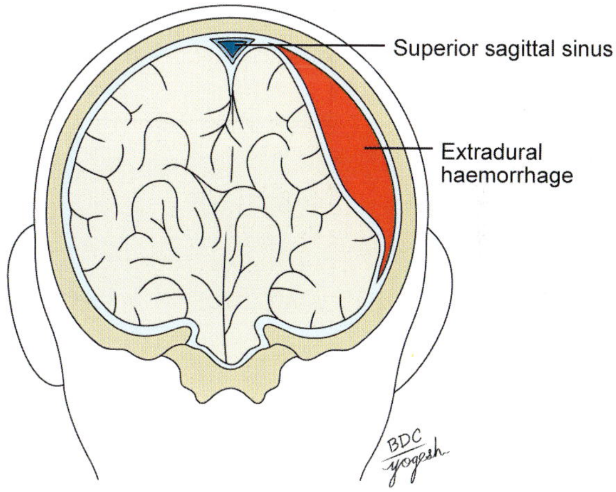


**Fig. 1.9:** Extradural haemorrhage

paralysis of the opposite side. The clot must be sucked out at the earliest by trephining. The head must be protected by a helmet during driving a two-wheeler.

## NORMA BASALIS

The inferior view of the skull is norma basalis. For the descriptive purposes, the norma basalis is divided into anterior, middle and posterior parts by two imaginary transverse lines:

1. ***Anterior transverse line:*** It passes along the posterior margin of the hard palate.
2. ***Posterior transverse line:*** It passes along the anterior margin of the foramen magnum (Plate 1.4, Fig. 1.10).

### Anterior Part of Norma Basalis

The anterior part of norma basalis consists of two parts (Plate 1.5, Flowchart 1.7):

1. Alveolar processes of maxillae or alveolar arch
2. Hard palate

#### Alveolar Arch

Alveolar processes of maxillae form U-shaped alveolar arch that bears sockets for the roots of the upper teeth.

Plate 1.4: Parts of norma basalis

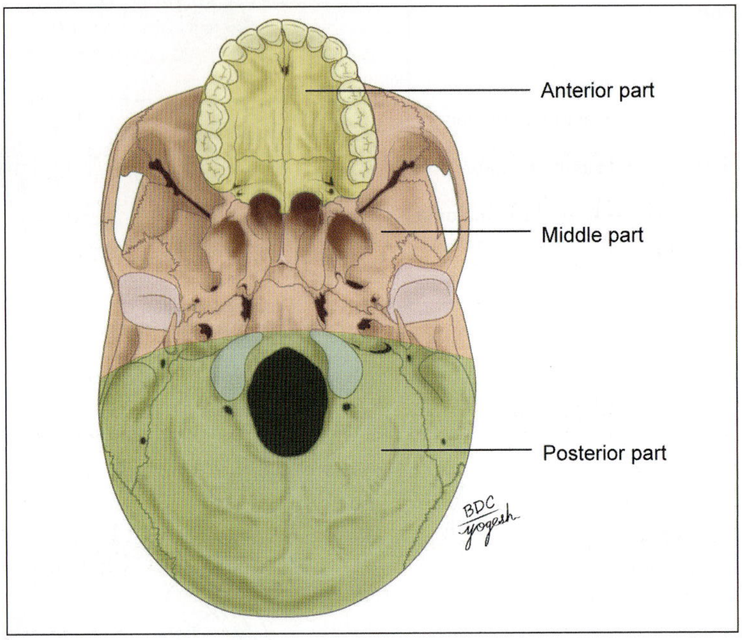


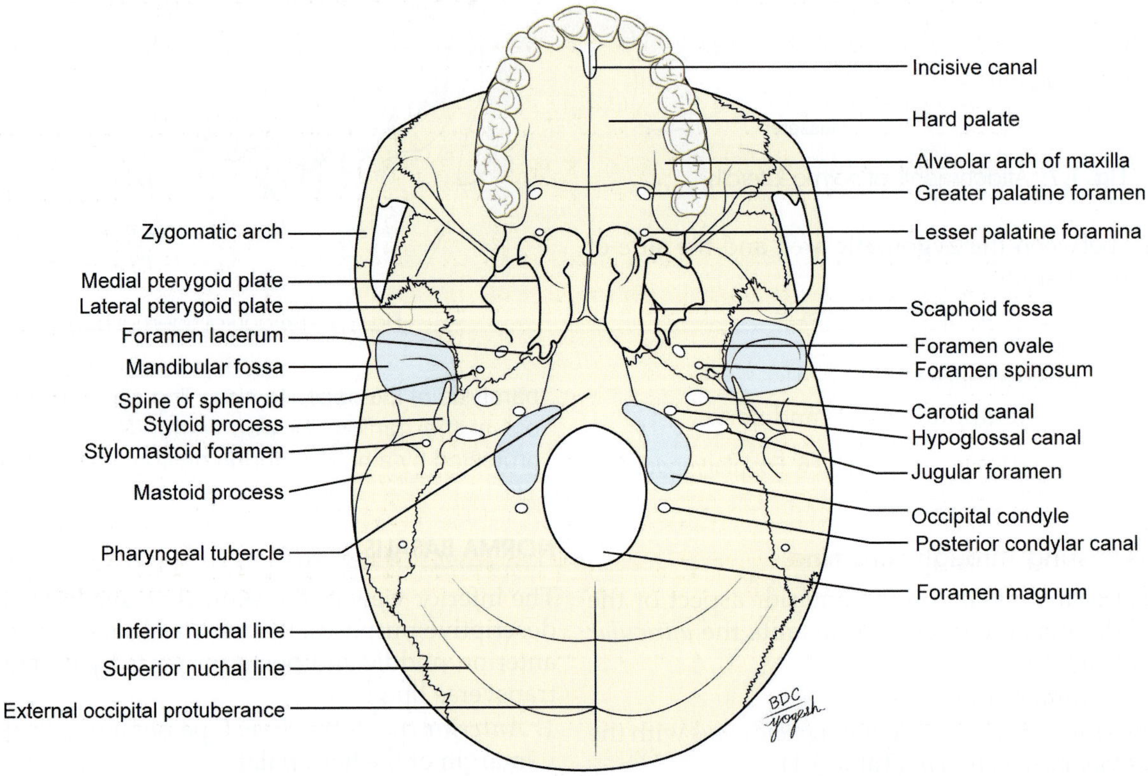


Fig. 1.10: Norma basalis

### Hard Palate

1. *Formation:*
   a. Anterior 2/3rd, by the palatine processes of the maxillae.
   b. Posterior 1/3rd, by the horizontal plates of the palatine bones.
2. *Sutures:* The palate is crossed by a cruciform suture made up of intermaxillary, interpalatine and palatomaxillary sutures.
3. It is arched in all directions. It shows pits for the palatine glands.
4. The *posterior border* of the hard palate is free and presents the ***posterior nasal spine*** in the median plane.
5. The ***palatine crest*** is a curved ridge near the posterior border. It begins behind the greater palatine foramen and runs medially.
6. ***Incisive foramen*** is a deep fossa situated anteriorly in the median plane. Two ***incisive canals,*** right and left,

**Plate 1.5:** Anterior part of norma basalis

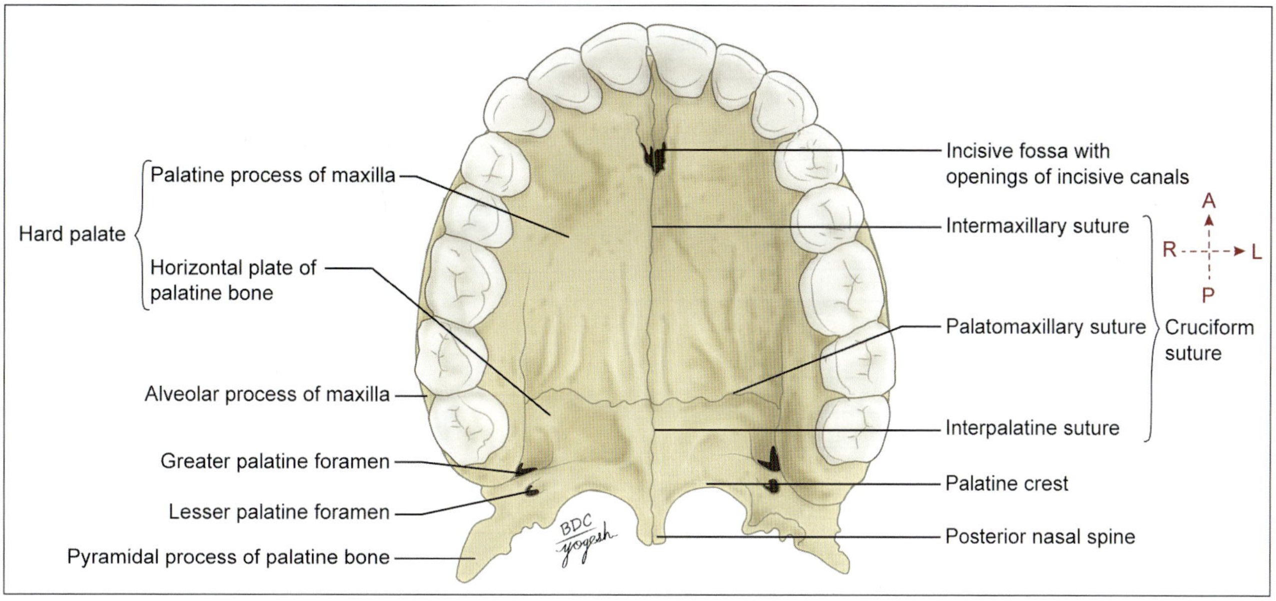


**Flowchart 1.7:** Features of anterior part of norma basalis

***Anterior part of norma basalis***

- ***Alveolar process***
  - Arched border of maxillae
  - 8 sockets for teeth
- ***Hard palate***
  - Formation
    - Maxilla
    - Palatine bone
  - Cruciform suture
  - Posterior border
    - Palatine aponeurosis
  - Posterior nasal spine
    - Musculus uvulae
  - Palatine crest
    - Tensor veli palatini
- ***Foramina***
  - Incisive canal
    - Greater palatine vessels and nerve
    - Nasopalatine nerve
  - Greater palatine foramen
    - Greater palatine vessels and nerve
  - Lesser palatine foramina
    - Lesser palatine nerves and vessels

**Plate 1.6:** Bones of middle part of norma basalis

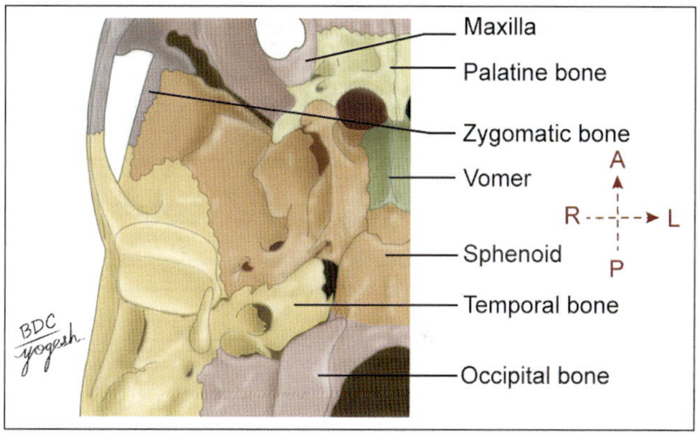


pierce the walls of the incisive foramen, usually one on each side, but occasionally in the median plane, the left being anterior and the right, posterior.

7. ***Greater palatine foramen***, one on each side, is situated just behind the lateral part of the palatomaxillary suture. A groove leads from the foramen towards the incisive fossa.
8. ***Lesser palatine foramina***, two or three in number on each side, lie behind the greater palatine foramen and perforate the pyramidal process of the palatine bone.

## Middle Part of Norma Basalis

The middle part extends from the posterior border of the hard palate to the arbitrary transverse line passing through the anterior margin of the foramen magnum. Middle part of the norma basalis is studied as median and lateral areas (Plates 1.6 and 1.7).

### *Median Area*

1. The median area shows (Flowchart 1.8):
   a. Posterior border of the *vomer*.
   b. A *broad bar of bone* formed by fusion of the posterior part of the body of sphenoid and the basilar part of occipital bone.
2. The ***vomer*** separates the two posterior nasal apertures. Its inferior border articulates with the bony palate. The superior border splits into two ***alae*** and articulates with the ***rostrum*** of the *sphenoid bone* (Fig. 1.11).

**Flowchart 1.8:** Features of median area of middle part of norma basalis

***Middle part of norma basalis: Median part***

- ***Vomer***
  - Separates posterior nasal apertures
  - Alae of vomer
- ***Broad bar of bone***
  - Formation:
    - Body of sphenoid
    - basiocciput
  - Pharyngeal tubercle
    - Superior constrictor
  - Longus capitis
  - Rectus capitis anterior
- ***Canals***
  1. Palatovaginal
     Pharyngeal branches of pterygopalatine ganglion and maxillary artery
  2. Vomerovaginal
     Pharyngeal branch of pterygopalatine ganglion

**Plate 1.7:** Features of middle part of norma basalis

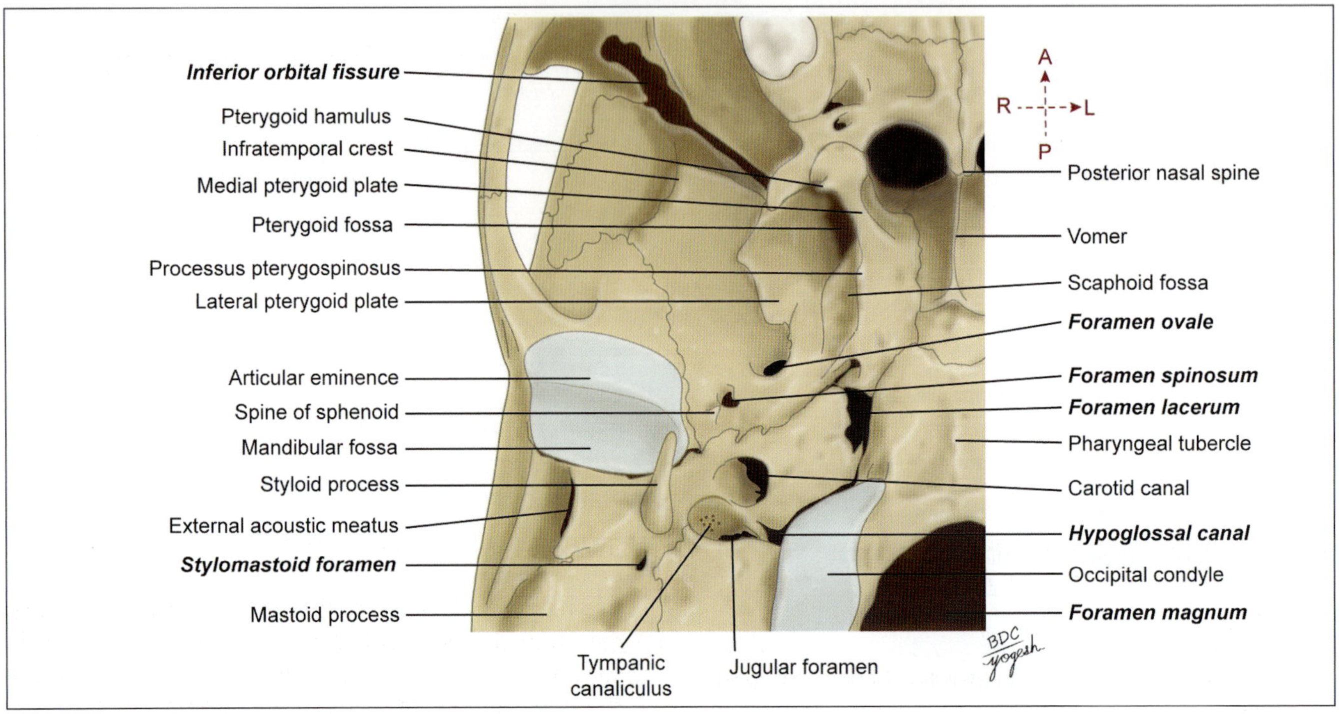


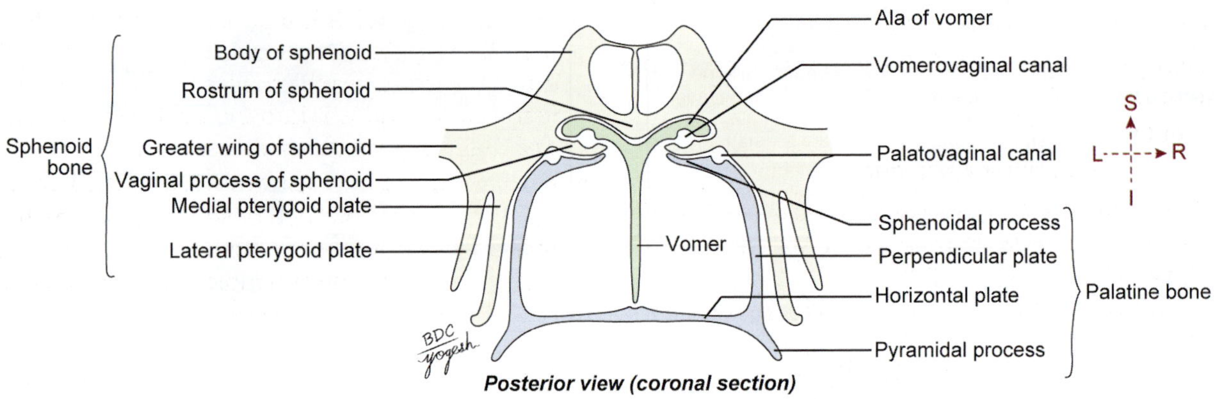


**Fig. 1.11:** Vomerovaginal and palatovaginal canals

3. The broad bar of the bone is marked in the median plane by the ***pharyngeal tubercle,*** a little in front of the foramen magnum (Plate 1.8).

*Note*:

***Palatinovaginal canal:*** The inferior surface of the vaginal process of the medial pterygoid plate is marked by an anteroposterior groove, which is converted into the palatinovaginal canal by the upper surface of the sphenoidal process of the palatine bone. The canal opens anteriorly into the posterior wall of the pterygopalatine fossa (Fig. 1.11).

***Vomerovaginal canal:*** The lateral border of each ala of the vomer comes into relationship with the vaginal process of the medial pterygoid plate, and may overlap it from above to enclose the vomerovaginal canal (Fig. 1.11).

### *Lateral Area*

The lateral area shows (Plate 1.8, Flowchart 1.9)

a. Two parts of the sphenoid bone — pterygoid process and greater wing.
b. Three parts of the temporal bone — petrous temporal, tympanic plate and squamous temporal.

1. **Pterygoid process** projects downwards from the junction of greater wing and the body of sphenoid behind the third molar tooth.

   Inferiorly, it divides into the *medial and lateral pterygoid plates*, which are fused together anteriorly, but are separated posteriorly by the V-shaped *pterygoid fossa.*

   The fused anterior borders of the two plates articulate medially with the perpendicular plate of the palatine bone, and are separated laterally from the posterior surface of the body of the maxilla by the *pterygomaxillary fissure.*

2. **Medial pterygoid plate**

   It is directed backwards. It has medial and lateral surfaces and a free posterior border.

   The upper end of posterior border divides to enclose a triangular depression called the ***scaphoid fossa.***

**Flowchart 1.9:** Features of lateral area of middle part of norma basalis

**Middle part of norma basalis: Lateral area**

| *Medial pterygoid plate* | *Lateral pterygoid plate* | *Greater wing of sphenoid* | *Temporal bone* | *Tegmen tympani* | *Mandibular fossa* |
|---|---|---|---|---|---|
| Longer<br>Posterior border<br>- Pharyngobasilar fascia<br>- Superior constrictor<br>Pterygoid hamulus<br>- Pterygomandibular raphe<br>Scaphoid fossa<br>- Tensor veli palatini | Shorter<br>Lateral surface<br>- Lower head of lateral pterygoid<br>Medial surface<br>- Deep head of medial pterygoid | Infratemporal surface<br>- Upper head of lateral pterygoid<br>Spine of sphenoid<br>- Sphenomandibular ligament<br>- Anterior ligament of malleus<br>- Pterygospinous ligament | Inferior surface of petrous part<br>- Levator veli palatini | Divides squamotympanic fissure into:<br>- Anterior petrosquamous fissure<br>- Posteior petrotympanic fissure | - Forms TMJ<br>- Postglenoid tubercle |

***Foramina:*** ***Foramen spinosum***: Middle meningeal artery, meningeal branch of mandibular nerve, posterior trunk of middle meningeal vein
***Foramen ovale***: Mandibular nerve, accessory meningeal artery, lesser petrosal nerve, emissary vein
***Carotid canal:*** ICA, sympathetic plexus
***Petrotympanic fissure:*** Chorda tympani nerve, anterior ligament of malleus, anterior tympanic artery

The lower end of the posterior border is prolonged downwards and laterally to form the ***pterygoid hamulus***.

3. **Lateral pterygoid plate**

   It is directed backwards and laterally. It has medial and lateral surfaces and a free posterior border.

   The posterior border sometimes has a projection at its middle called the *pterygospinous process*, which projects towards the spine of the sphenoid.

4. **Infratemporal surface of the greater wing of the sphenoid**

   It is pentagonal.

   It shows the following 4 foramina:

   a. ***Foramen ovale*** is large and oval. It is situated posterolateral to the upper end of the posterior border of lateral pterygoid plate.

   b. ***Foramen spinosum*** is small and circular in shape. It is situated posterolateral to the foramen ovale, and is limited posterolaterally by the spine of sphenoid.

   c. Sometimes, there is the ***emissary sphenoidal foramen*** *or foramen of Vesalius*. It is situated between the foramen ovale and the scaphoid fossa. Internally, it opens between the foramen ovale and the foramen rotundum.

   d. At times, there is a ***canaliculus innominatus*** situated between the foramen ovale and the foramen spinosum.

   There is a small, sharp, downward projection between the posterolateral and posteromedial margins called the ***spine of the sphenoid***.

   ***Sulcus tubae*** is the groove between the posteromedial margin of the greater wing of the sphenoid and the petrous temporal bone. It lodges the *cartilaginous part of the auditory tube*. Posteriorly, the groove leads to the bony part of the auditory tube, which lies within the petrous temporal bone.

5. **Inferior surface of the *petrous* part of the temporal bone** is triangular in shape with its apex directed forwards and medially (Greek petrous = *rock*). It lies between the greater wing of the sphenoid and the basiocciput.

   Its *apex* is perforated by the upper end of the carotid canal, and is separated from the sphenoid by the foramen lacerum. The *inferior surface* is perforated by the lower end of the *carotid canal* posteriorly.

   ***Carotid canal*** runs forwards and medially within the petrous temporal bone.

   ***Tegmen tympani:*** It is a part of the petrous temporal bone that is present in the middle cranial fossa. It has a down turned edge, which is seen in the *squamotympanic fissure* and divides it into the posterior *petrotympanic* and anterior *petrosquamous* fissures.

6. ***Foramen lacerum*** is a short, wide canal, 1 cm long.

   Its lower end is bounded posterolaterally by the apex of the petrous temporal, medially by the basiocciput and the body of the sphenoid and anteriorly by the root of the pterygoid process and the greater wing of the sphenoid bone (Fig. 1.13).

7. ***Tympanic part of the temporal bone****, also called the* ***tympanic plate****,* is a triangular curved plate, which lies in the angle between the petrous and squamous parts. Its apex is directed medially and lies close to the spine of the sphenoid.

   The *base or lateral border* is curved, free and roughened.

   Its *anterior surface* forms the posterior wall of the mandibular fossa. The *posterior surface* is concave and forms the anterior wall, floor and lower part of the posterior wall of the bony external acoustic meatus.

   Its *upper border* bounds the petrotympanic fissure.

   The *lower border* is sharp and free.

   Medially, the tympanic plate passes along the anterolateral margin of the lower end of the carotid canal. Laterally, it forms the anterolateral part of the *sheath of the styloid process*. Internally, the tympanic plate is fused to the petrous temporal bone.

8. ***Squamous part of the temporal bone*** forms:

   a. The anterior part of the mandibular/articular fossa, which articulates with the head of the mandible to form the temporomandibular joint.

b. The tubercle of root of zygoma, which is continuous with the anterior root of the zygoma.
c. A small posterolateral part of the roof of the infratemporal fossa.

### Posterior Part of Norma Basalis

The posterior part of norma basalis is studied as median and lateral areas (Plate 1.8, Flowchart 1.10).

#### Median Area

The median area shows the following four features from before backwards:
1. Foramen magnum
2. External occipital crest
3. External occipital protuberance
4. Nuchal lines.

1. ***Foramen magnum*** (Latin *great*) is the largest foramen of the skull. It opens upwards into the posterior cranial fossa, and downwards into the vertebral canal. It is oval in shape, being wider behind than in front where it is overlapped on each side by the occipital condyles.
2. ***External occipital crest*** begins at the posterior margin of the foramen magnum and ends posteriorly and above at the external occipital protuberance.
3. ***External occipital protuberance*** is a projection located at the posterior end of the crest. It is easily felt in the living, in the midline, at the point where the back of the neck becomes continuous with the scalp.
4. ***Nuchal lines*:** These are superior, inferior and the highest. The *superior nuchal lines* begin at the external occipital protuberance and the *inferior nuchal lines* at the middle of the crest. Both of them curve laterally and backwards and then laterally and forwards.

   *Highest nuchal line* is faded and seen above superior nuchal line (occasionally).

#### Lateral Area

The *lateral area* shows:
- Condylar part of the occipital bone
- Squamous part of the occipital bone
- Jugular foramen between the occipital and petrous temporal bones
- Styloid process of the temporal bone
- Mastoid part of the temporal bone.

1. ***Condylar or lateral part of the occipital bone*** presents the following features:
   - ***Occipital condyles*** are oval in shape and are situated on each side of the anterior part of the foramen magnum. Their long axis is directed forwards and medially. They articulate with the superior articular facets of the atlas vertebra to form the *atlanto-occipital joints*.
   - ***Hypoglossal canal*** or *anterior condylar canal* pierces the bone anterosuperior to the occipital condyle, and is directed laterally and slightly forwards.

**Plate 1.8:** Norma basalis – Posterior part labelled

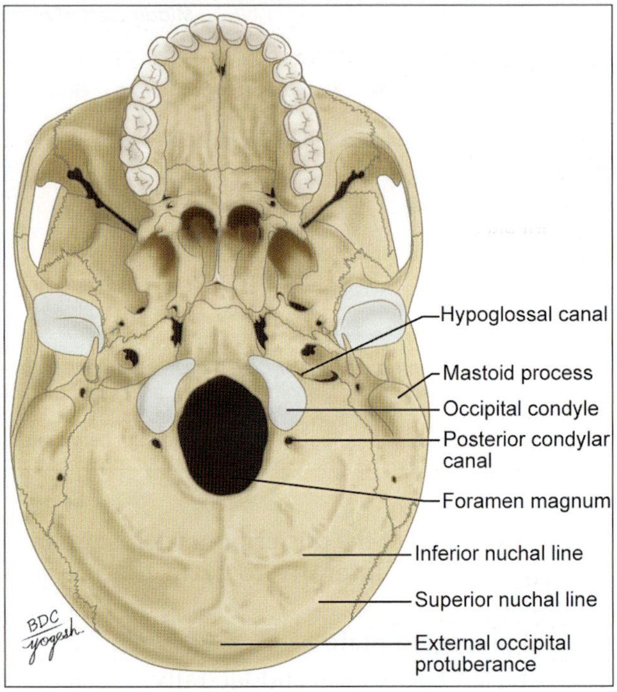


**Flowchart 1.10:** Features of posterior part of norma basalis

***Posterior part of norma basalis***

***Median area***
- External occipital crest
  - Ligamentum nuchae
- External occipital protuberance
- Nuchal lines: Highest, superior, inferior
- Semispinalis capitis
- Obliquus capitis anterior
- Rectus capitis minor
- Rectus capitis major
- Foramen magnum

***Lateral area***
- Occipital condyle
- Hypoglossal canal
  - Hypoglossal nerve
  - Meningeal branches of XIIth nerve and ascending pharyngeal artery
- Posterior condylar canal
  - Emissary vein
- Stylomastoid foramen
  - Facial nerve
  - Stylomastoid branch of posterior auricular artery
- Mastoid process: SCM, splenius capitis, longissimus capitis
- Mastoid notch: Posterior belly of digastric

BDC yogesh

   - ***Condylar canal*** or *posterior condylar canal* is occasionally present in the floor of a condylar fossa present behind the occipital condyle. Superiorly, it opens into the sigmoid sulcus.
   - ***Jugular process of the occipital bone*** lies lateral to the occipital condyle and forms the posterior boundary of jugular foramen.
2. ***Squamous part of occipital bone*** is marked by the superior and inferior nuchal lines mentioned above (Fig. 1.3).
3. ***Jugular foramen*** is large and elongated, with its long axis directed forwards and medially. It is placed at the posterior end of the petro-occipital suture.
4. ***Styloid process*** is described in Chapter 8, page 161.

   ***Stylomastoid foramen*** is situated between the anterior end of mastoid process and root of styloid process.

5. ***Mastoid process***, a component of mastoid part is a large conical projection located posterolateral to the stylomastoid foramen. It is directed downwards and forwards. It forms the lateral wall of the *mastoid notch*.

*Note*:

At the posterior end of the foramen, its anterior wall (petrous temporal) is hollowed out to form ***jugular fossa***, which lodges the superior bulb of the internal jugular vein. The fossa is larger on the right side than on the left.

The lateral wall of the jugular fossa is pierced by a minute canal, the ***mastoid canaliculus*** *(Arnold's canal).* It transmits the auricular branch of vagus nerve or Arnold's nerve.

Near the medial end of the jugular foramen, there is the ***jugular notch***. At the apex of the notch, there is an opening that leads into the ***cochlear canaliculus***.

***Tympanic canaliculus*** opens on or near the thin edge of bone between the jugular fossa and the lower end of the carotid canal.

## Attachments (Fig. 1.12)

1. Palate
2. Posterior border of the hard palate provides attachment to the palatine aponeurosis. The posterior nasal spine gives origin to the musculus uvulae. Palatine crest provides attachment to a part of the tendon of tensor veli palatini muscle.
3. Inferior surface of the basiocciput:
   a. *Pharyngeal tubercle* gives attachment to the raphe, which provides insertion to the upper fibres of the superior constrictor muscle of the pharynx.
   b. The area in front of the tubercle forms the roof of the *nasopharynx* and supports the *pharyngeal tonsil*.
   c. Longus capitis is inserted lateral to the pharyngeal tubercle.
   d. Rectus capitis anterior is inserted a little posterior and medial to the hypoglossal canal.
4. Medial pterygoid plate:
   a. Lower part of the posterior border and the pterygoid hamulus give origin to the superior constrictor of the pharynx.
   b. Upper part of the posterior border is notched by the *auditory* tube.
   c. Pterygomandibular raphe is attached to the tip of the *pterygoid hamulus* at one end and to the mandible behind 3rd molar tooth at the other end.
5. Lateral pterygoid plate:
   a. Its lateral surface gives origin to the larger lower head of lateral pterygoid muscle.
   b. Its medial surface gives origin to the deep head of the medial pterygoid. The small, superficial head of this muscle arises from the *maxillary tuberosity* and the adjoining part of the pyramidal process of the palatine bone.
   c. Pharyngobasilar fascia is attached below to the processus tuberis.

      Processus tuberis/pterygospinous process (Civinini's ligament) is a triangular projection, which is present at the middle of the posterior border of lateral pterygoid plate. It supports the medial end of cartilaginous part of auditory tube.
   d. The pterygospinous process, which is present at the middle of lateral pterygoid plate gives attachment to the ligament of same name.

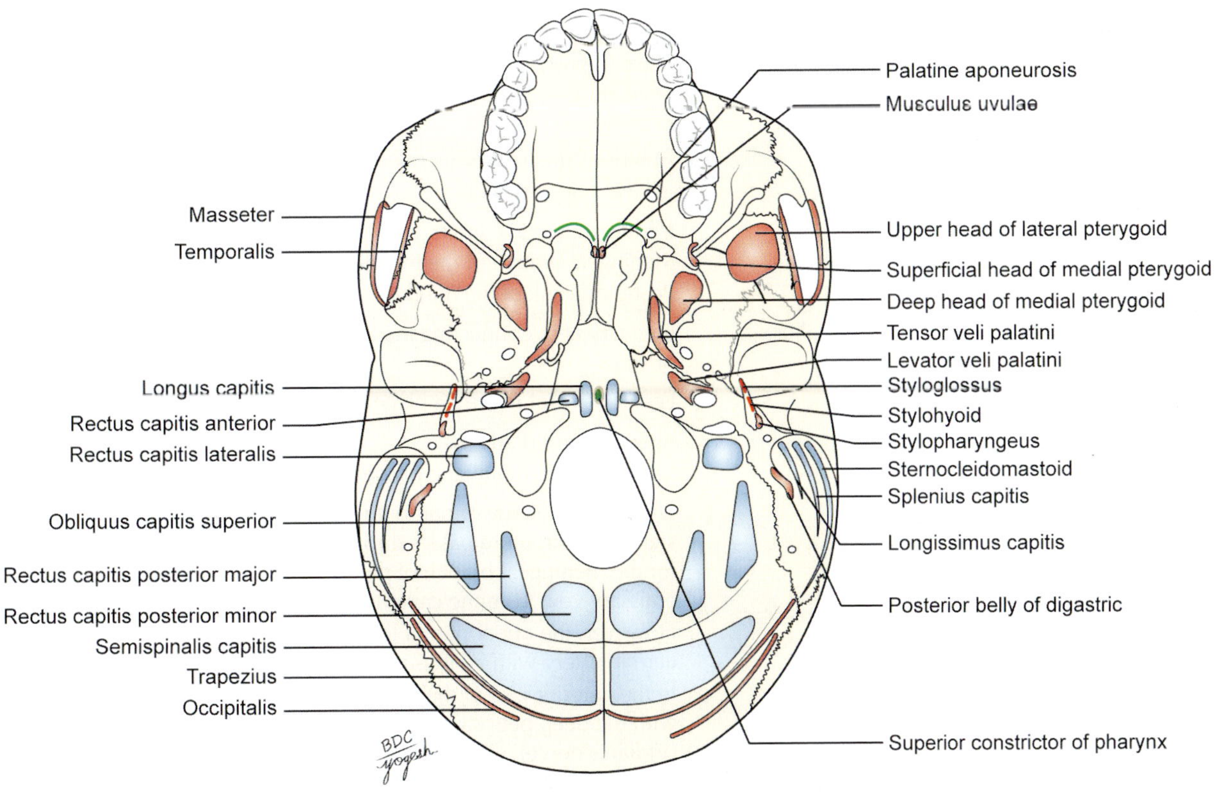


**Fig. 1.12:** Muscles attached to the base of skull

6. Infratemporal surface of the greater wing of the sphenoid: It gives origin to the upper head of the lateral pterygoid muscle, and is crossed by the deep temporal and masseteric nerves.
7. *Spine of the sphenoid:* It is related laterally to the auriculotemporal nerve, and medially to the chorda tympani nerve and auditory tube.

   Its *tip* provides attachment to sphenomandibular ligament, anterior ligament of malleus and pterygo-spinous ligament.

   Its *anterior aspect* gives origin to the most posterior fibres of the tensor veli palatini and tensor tympani muscles.
8. Inferior surface of petrous temporal bone: It gives origin to the levator veli palatini.
9. Margins of the foramen magnum: It provides attachment to:
   a. Anterior atlanto-occipital membrane, anteriorly.
   b. Posterior atlanto-occipital membrane, posteriorly.
   c. Alar ligaments on the roughened medial surface of each occipital condyle.
10. Ligamentum nuchae is attached to the external occipital protuberance and crest.
11. Rectus capitis lateralis is inserted into the inferior surface of the jugular process of the occipital bone
12. Squamous part of the occipital bone: The area between the superior and inferior nuchal lines provides insertion medially to the semispinalis capitis, and laterally to the obliquus capitis superior muscle.

    The area below the inferior nuchal line provides insertion medially to the rectus capitis posterior minor, and laterally to the rectus capitis posterior major.
13. Mastoid notch gives origin to the posterior belly of digastric muscle.

The structures passing through various foramina of skull are listed in Table 1.2.

**TABLE 1.2: Structures passing through foramina of skull**

| *Foramen* | *Structures* |
|---|---|
| Incisive foramen | Terminal parts of the greater palatine vessels from the palate to the nose<br>Terminal part of the nasopalatine nerve from the nose to the palate |
| Greater palatine foramen | Greater palatine vessels (Fig. 1.12)<br>Anterior palatine nerve ( both of which run forwards in the groove that passes forwards from the foramen) |
| Lesser palatine foramina | Middle and posterior palatine nerves |
| Palatinovaginal canal | Pharyngeal branch from the pterygopalatine ganglion<br>A small pharyngeal branch of the maxillary artery |
| Vomerovaginal canal (if patent) | Pharyngeal branch from pterygopalatine ganglion and vessels |
| Foramen ovale | **M**andibular nerve (Fig. 1.11)<br>**A**ccessory meningeal artery<br>**L**esser petrosal nerve<br>**E**missary vein connecting the cavernous sinus with the pterygoid plexus of veins<br>Anterior trunk of middle meningeal vein (occasionally)<br>[*Mnemonic*—**MALE**] |
| Foramen spinosum | Middle meningeal artery<br>Meningeal branch of the mandibular nerve or nervus spinosus<br>Posterior trunk of the middle meningeal vein |
| Emissary sphenoidal foramen (foramen of Vesalius) | Emissary vein connecting the cavernous sinus with the pterygoid plexus of veins |
| Canaliculus innominatus (if present) | Lesser petrosal nerve (in place of foramen ovale) |
| Carotid canal | Internal carotid artery<br>Venous and sympathetic plexuses around the artery |
| Foramen lacerum (Fig. 1.13) | During life, the lower part of the foramen is filled with cartilage, and no significant structure passes through the whole length of the canal, except for the meningeal branch of the ascending pharyngeal artery and an emissary vein from the cavernous sinus.<br>However, the upper part of the foramen is traversed by the internal carotid artery with venous and sympathetic plexuses around it.<br>In the anterior part of the foramen, the greater petrosal nerve unites with the deep petrosal nerve to form the nerve of the pterygoid canal (Vidian's nerve), which leaves the foramen by entering the pterygoid canal in the anterior wall of the foramen lacerum (Figs 1.15a and b). |

*(Contd.)*

**TABLE 1.2: Structures passing through foramina of skull** *(Contd.)*

| *Foramen* | *Structures* |
|---|---|
| Medial end of the petrotympanic fissure | Chorda tympani nerve<br>Anterior ligament of malleus<br>Anterior tympanic artery |
| Foramen magnum<br>(Fig. 1.14, Flowchart 1.11) | Through the narrow anterior part:<br>a. Apical ligament of dens<br>b. Vertical band of cruciate ligament<br>c. Membrana tectoria<br>Through wider posterior part:<br>a. Lowest part of medulla oblongata<br>b. Three meninges<br>Through the subarachnoid space pass:<br>a. Spinal accessory nerves<br>b. Vertebral arteries with its sympathetic plexus<br>c. Posterior spinal arteries<br>d. Anterior spinal artery |
| Hypoglossal or anterior condylar canal | Hypoglossal nerve<br>Meningeal branch of the hypoglossal nerve (These are the sensory fibres of first cervical spinal nerve supplying the dura mater of posterior cranial fossa)<br>Meningeal branch of the ascending pharyngeal artery<br>Emissary vein connecting the sigmoid sinus with the internal jugular vein |
| Posterior condylar canal | Emissary vein connecting the sigmoid sinus with suboccipital venous plexus |
| Jugular foramen<br>*Note*: The glossopharyngeal notch near the medial end of the jugular foramen lodges the inferior ganglion of the glossopharyngeal nerve<br>(Fig. 1.15, Flowchart 1.12) | Through the anterior part:<br>a. Inferior petrosal sinus<br>b. Meningeal branch of the ascending pharyngeal artery<br>Through the middle part: IX, X and XI cranial nerves<br>Through the posterior part:<br>a. Internal jugular vein<br>b. Meningeal branch of the occipital artery. |
| Mastoid canaliculus (Arnold's canal) (lies in the lateral wall of the jugular fossa) | Auricular branch of the vagus (Arnold's nerve) |
| Tympanic canaliculus (on the thin edge of partition between the jugular fossa and carotid canal) | Tympanic branch of glossopharyngeal nerve (Jacobson's nerve) to the middle ear cavity |
| Stylomastoid foramen | Facial nerve<br>Stylomastoid branch of the posterior auricular artery |
| External nasal foramen | External nasal nerve |
| Inferior orbital fissure | Zygomatic nerve; orbital branches of pterygopalatine ganglion; infraorbital nerve and vessels |
| Infraorbital foramen | Infraorbital nerve and vessels |
| Petrotympanic fissure | Chorda tympanic nerve, anterior ligament of malleus and anterior tympanic artery |
| Pterygoid canal | Nerve to pterygoid canal and vessels |
| Pterygomaxillary fissure | Maxillary nerve |
| Pterygopalatine fossa | Pterygopalatine ganglion |
| Supraorbital foramen | Supraorbital nerve and vessels |
| Zygomatic foramen | Zygomatic nerve |
| Zygomaticofacial foramen | Zygomaticofacial nerve |
| Zygomaticotemporal foramen | Zygomaticotemporal nerve |

*Note*: Auricular branch of the vagus (Arnold's nerve) passes laterally through the bone, crosses the facial canal and emerges at the tympanomastoid fissure. The nerve is extracranial at birth, but becomes surrounded by bone as the tympanic plate and mastoid process develop (also called Alderman's nerve).

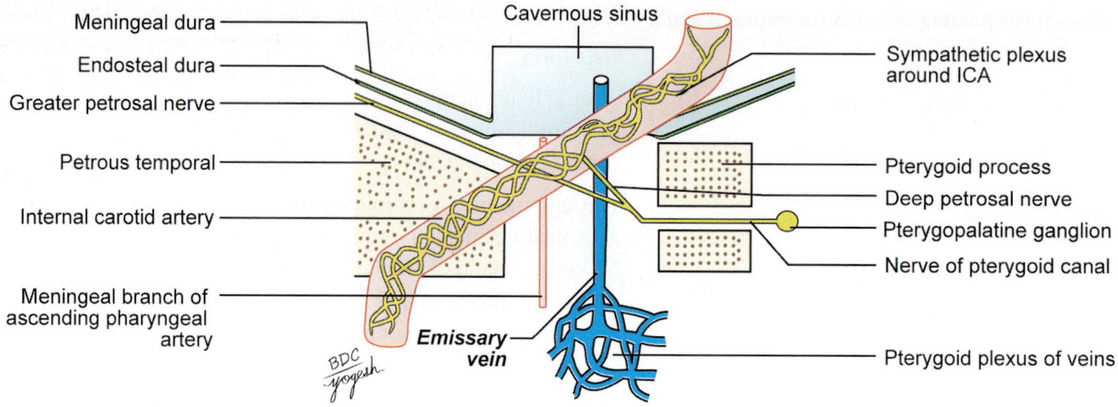


**Fig. 1.13:** Structures related to the foramen lacerum

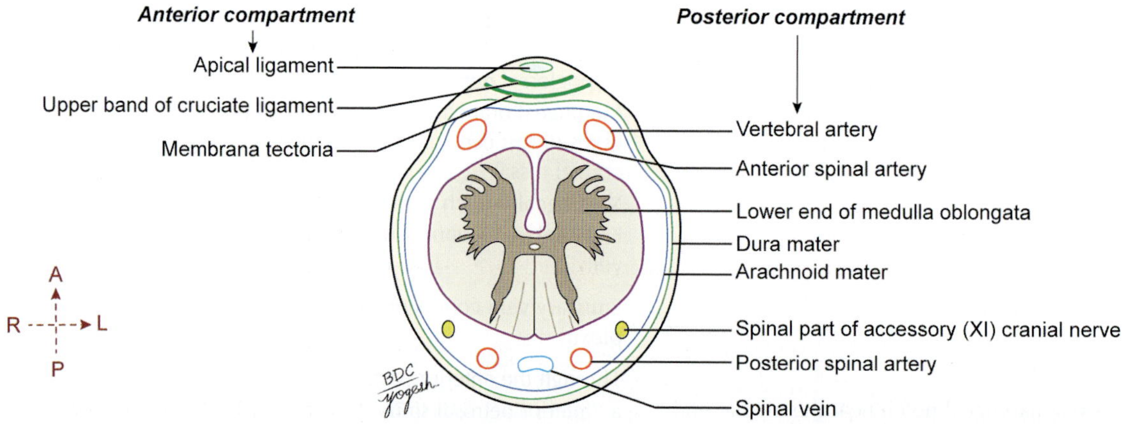


**Fig. 1.14:** Structures passing through foramen magnum

**Flowchart 1.11:** Foramen magnum

***Compartments of foramen magnum***

Divided by alar ligament

***Anterior***
- Apical ligament
- Upper band of cruciate ligament
- Membrana tectoria

***Posterior***
- Lower end of medulla oblongata
- Meninges
- Structures passing through subarachnoid space
  - Spinal part of XI cranial nerve
  - Two vertebral arteries
  - Sympathetic plexus
  - Anterior and posterior spinal arteries

**Flowchart 1.12:** Jugular foramen

***Compartments of jugular foramen***

***Anterior***
- Inferior petrosal sinus
- Meningeal branch of ascending pharyngeal artery

***Intermediate***
- IX nerve
- X nerve
- XI nerve

***Posterior***
- Internal jugular vein
- Meningeal branch of occipital artery

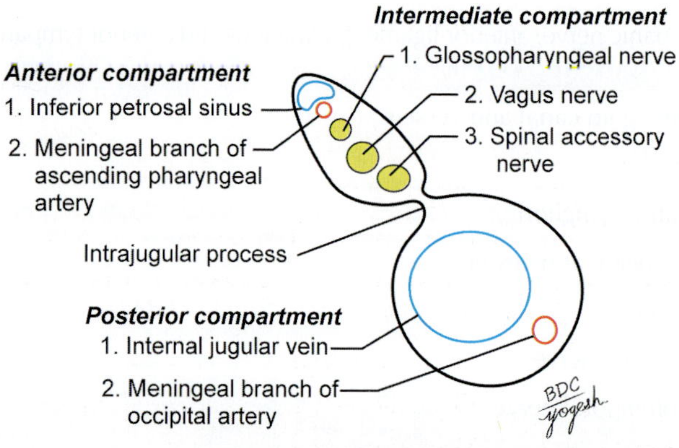


**Fig. 1.15:** Jugular foramen

## INTERIOR OF THE SKULL

- The cranium is lined internally by ***endocranium***, which is continuous with the pericranium through the foramina and sutures (Plate 1.10, Fig. 1.16, Flowchart 1.13).
- The *thickness* of the cranial vault is variable. The bones covered with muscles, i.e. temporal and posterior cranial fossae, are thinner than those covered with scalp. Further, the bones are thinner in females than in males, and in children than in adults.
- Most of the cranial bones consist of:
  a. An *outer table* of compact bone, which is thick, resilient and tough.
  b. An *inner table* of compact bone, which is thin and brittle.
  c. The *diploe* that consists of spongy bone filled with red marrow, in between the two tables.

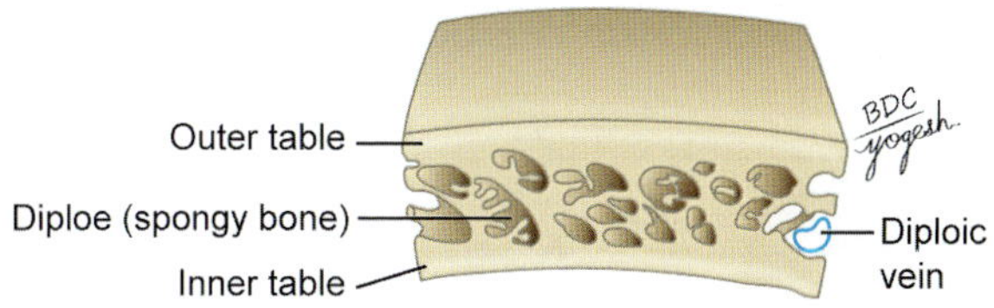


**Fig. 1.16:** Structure of cranial bones

*Note*: The skull bones derive their blood supply mostly from the meningeal arteries from inside and very little from the arteries of the scalp. Blood supply from the outside is rich in those areas where muscles are attached, e.g. the temporal fossa and the suboccipital region. The blood from the diploes is drained by four diploic veins on each side draining into venous sinuses (Table 1.3 and Fig. 1.17).

Many bones, like vomer (Latin *ploughshare*), pterygoid plates, do not have any diploe.

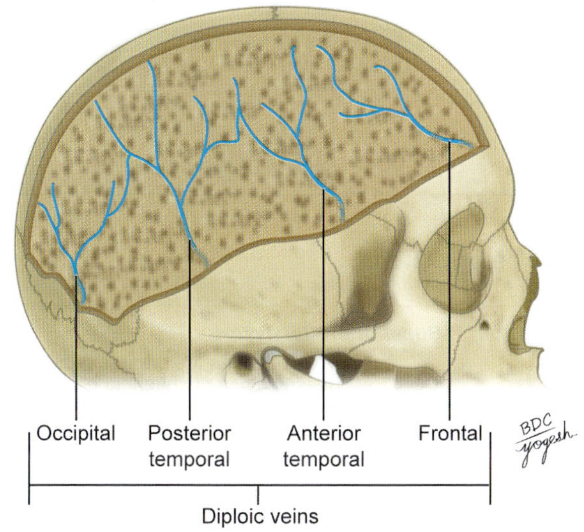


**Fig. 1.17:** Diploic veins

## INTERNAL SURFACE OF CRANIAL VAULT

The shape, the bones present and the sutures uniting them have been described with the norma verticalis. It shows the following features (Plate 1.9):

1. The *inner table* is thin and brittle. It presents *markings* produced by meningeal vessels, venous sinuses, arachnoid granulations and to some extent by cerebral gyri. It also presents raised ridges formed by the attachments of the dural folds.
2. The ***frontal crest*** lies anteriorly in the median plane. It projects backwards.
3. The ***sagittal sulcus*** runs from before backwards in the median plane. It becomes progressively wider posteriorly. It lodges the superior sagittal sinus.
4. The ***granular foveolae*** are deep, irregular, large, pits situated on each side of the sagittal sulcus. They are formed by arachnoid granulations. They are larger and more numerous in aged persons.
5. ***Vascular markings:*** The groove for the anterior branch of the middle meningeal artery, and the accompanying vein runs upwards 1 cm behind the coronal suture. Smaller grooves for the branches from the anterior and posterior branches of the middle meningeal vessels run upwards and backwards over the parietal bone.
6. The ***parietal foramina*** open near the sagittal sulcus 2.5 to 3.75 cm in front of the lambdoid suture.
7. The *impressions for cerebral gyri* are less distinct. These become very prominent in cases of raised intracranial tension.

***Competencies:***

**AN26.3** Describe cranial cavity, its subdivisions, foramina and structures passing through them.

**AN30.1** Describe the cranial fossae and identify related structures.

## INTERNAL SURFACE OF THE BASE OF SKULL

The interior of the base of skull presents natural subdivisions into the anterior, middle and posterior cranial fossae. The dura mater is firmly adherent to the floor of fossae and is continuous with pericranium through the foramina and fissures (Plate 1.10, Fig. 1.18, Flowchart 1.13).

### Anterior Cranial Fossa

It is separated from the middle cranial fossa by the free *posterior border* of the *lesser wing of the sphenoid*, the *anterior clinoid process* and the *anterior margin of the sulcus chiasmaticus* (Plate 1.11).

#### Floor

It is formed by:

1. *Cribriform plate of the ethmoid bone*
2. *Body of the sphenoid or jugum sphenoidale*
3. *Orbital plate of the frontal bone*
4. *Lesser wing of the sphenoid.*

**TABLE 1.3: Diploic veins**

| *Vein* | *Foramen* | *Drainage* |
|---|---|---|
| Frontal diploic vein | Supraorbital foramen | Drain into supraorbital vein |
| Anterior temporal or parietal diploic vein | In the greater wing of sphenoid | Sphenoparietal sinus or in anterior deep temporal vein |
| Posterior temporal or parietal diploic vein | Mastoid foramen | Transverse sinus |
| Occipital diploic vein (largest) | Foramen in occipital bone | Occipital vein or confluence of sinuses |
| Small unnamed diploic veins | Pierce inner table of skull close to the margins of superior sagittal sinus | Venous lacunae |

**Plate 1.9:** Internal surface of the vault of the skull (calvaria or skull cap)

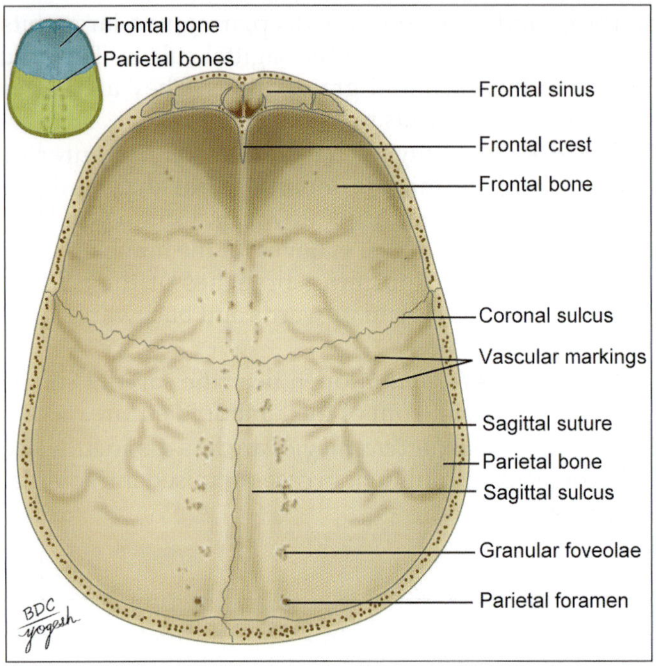


**Plate 1.10:** Cranial fossae and bones forming the interior of the skull

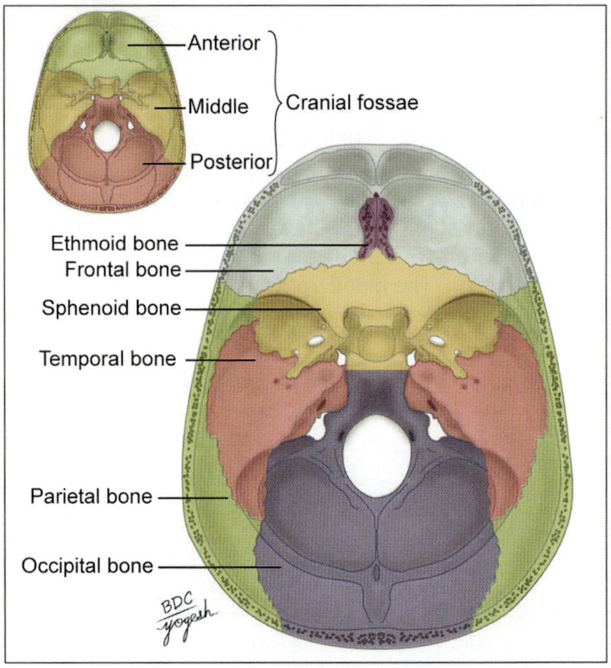


**Flowchart 1.13:** Features of interior of the base of skull

***Anterior cranial fossa***

***Features***
- Frontal crest
  - Falx cerebri
- Crista galli
  - Falx cerebri
- Jugum sphenoidale
- Cribriform plate of ethmoid
- Orbital plate of frontal bone
- Lesser wing of sphenoid
  - Free posterior border
  - Anterior clinoid process
  Free margin of tentorium cerebelli

***Foramina***
- Foramen caecum
  - Emissary vein
- Anterior ethmoidal canal
  - Anterior ethmoidal nerve and vessels
- Posterior ethmoidal canal
  - Posterior ethmoidal vessels
- Optic canal
  - Optic nerve
  - Ophthalmic artery

***Superior orbital fissure***

Lies between the greater and lesser wings of sphenoid bone
Divided into 3 parts by tendinous ring

***Lateral part***
- Lacrimal nerve
- Frontal nerve
- Trochlear nerve
- Superior ophthalmic vein

***Middle part***
- Upper and lower divisions of oculomotor nerve
- Nasociliary nerve
- Abducent nerve

***Medial part***
- Inferior ophthalmic vein
- Sympathetic nerves

***Median area of middle cranial fossa***

Body of sphenoid

***Features***
- Sulcus chiasmaticus
- Sella turcica
  - Occupies pituitary gland
  - Tuberculum sellae
  - Middle clinoid process
  - Dorsum sellae
  - Posterior clinoid process
- Carotid groove

***Attachments***
- Posterior clinoid process
- Tuberculum sellae and dorsum sellae
  - Diaphragma sellae

***Foramen***
- Optic canal
  - Optic nerve
  - Ophthalmic artery
- Carotid groove
  - Internal carotid artery

***Lateral area of middle cranial fossa***

***Features***
- Greater wing of sphenoid
- Groove for middle meningeal vessels
- Trigeminal impression
- Hiatus for greater and lesser petrosal nerves
- Arcuate eminence
- Tegmen tympani

***Foramina***
- Foramen spinosum: Middle meningeal artery, nervous spinosus
- Foramen ovale: Mandibular nerve, accessory meningeal artery, lesser petrosal nerve, emissary vein
- Foramen rotundum: Maxillary nerve
- Foramen lacerum: Emissary vein
- Superior orbital fissure

***Median area of posterior cranial fossa***

***Features***
- Clivus
- Foramen magnum
- Internal occipital protuberance
- Internal occipital crest
- Vermian fossa
- Groove for transverse sinus
- Cerebellar fossa

***Relations and foramina***
- Clivus: Related to pons, medulla, basilar venous plexus
- Attachments
  1. Apical ligament of dens
  2. Vertical band of cruciate ligament
  3. Membrana tectoria
- Internal occipital crest
  1. Falx cerebelli
- Foramen magnum

***Lateral area of posterior cranial fossa***

***Features***
- Condylar part of occipital bone
  - Jugular tubercle
- Posterior surface of petrous part of temporal bone
- Mastoid part of temporal bone
  - Sigmoid sulcus

***Foramina***
- Hypoglossal canal
  - 12th nerve
  - Meningeal branch of ascending pharyngeal artery
  - Emissary vein
- Condylar canal: Emissary vein
- Internal acoustic meatus
  - VII and VIII nerves
  - Labyrinthine vessels
- Jugular foramen
- Mastoid foramen: Emissary vein

Plate 1.11: Features of anterior cranial fossa

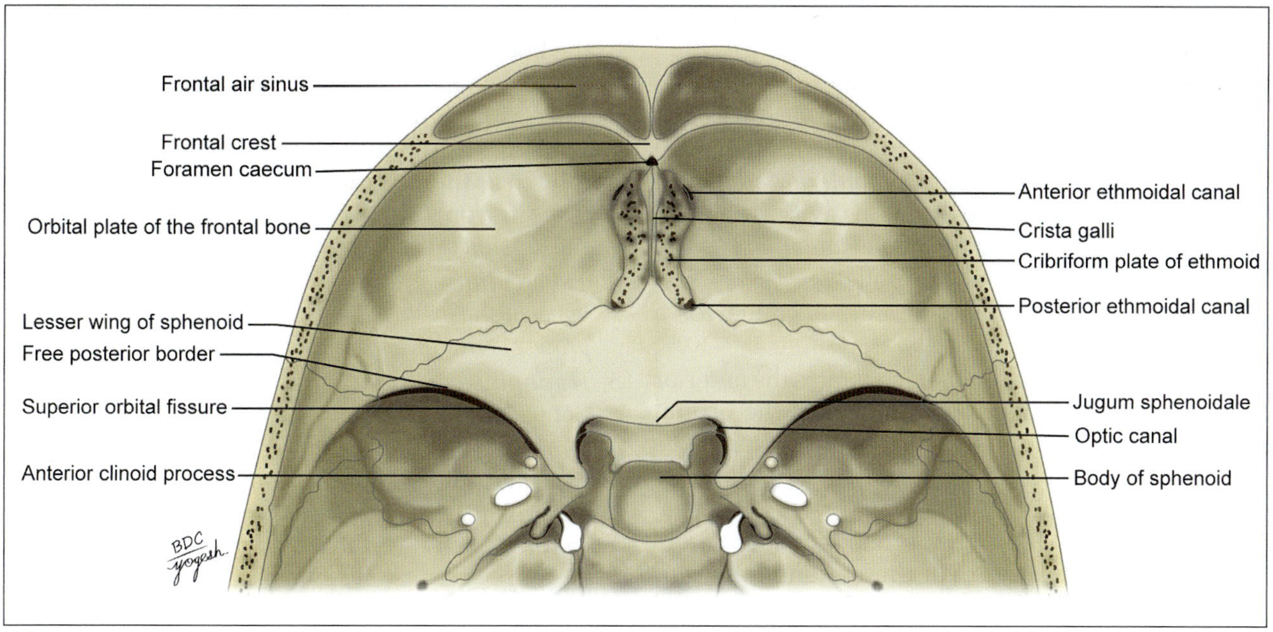


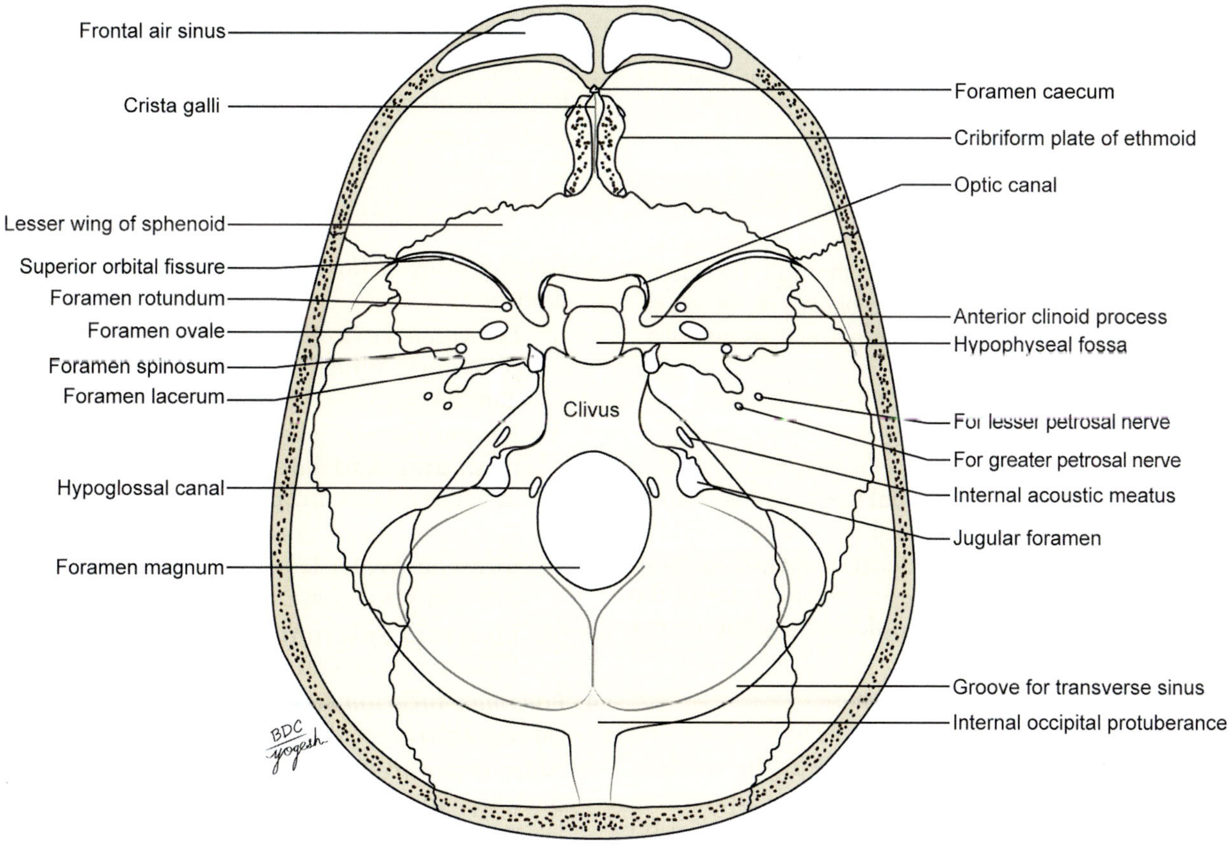


Fig. 1.18: Features of cranial fossae

### Features

1. ***Cribriform plate of the ethmoid bone*** separates the anterior cranial fossa from the nasal cavity. It is quadrilateral in shape.
   a. *Anterior* margin articulates with the frontal bone at the *frontoethmoidal suture,* which is marked in the median plane by the ***foramen caecum***. This foramen is usually blind, but is occasionally patent.
   b. *Posterior margin* articulates with the jugum sphenoidale. At the posterolateral corners of cribriform plane, one sees the ***posterior ethmoidal canals***.

c. Its *lateral margins* articulate with the orbital plate of the frontal bone: The suture between them presents the ***anterior ethmoidal canal*** placed behind the crista galli.

Anteriorly, the cribriform plate has a midline projection called the ***crista galli*** (Latin *cock's comb*). On each side of the crista galli, there are foramina through which the *anterior ethmoidal nerve and vessels* pass to the nasal cavity. The plate is also perforated by *numerous foramina* for the passage of olfactory nerve rootlets.

2. ***Jugum sphenoidale*** separates the anterior cranial fossa from the sphenoidal sinuses.
3. ***Orbital plate of the frontal bone*** separates the anterior cranial fossa from the orbit. It supports the orbital surface of the frontal lobe of the brain, and presents reciprocal impressions. The *frontal air sinus* may extend into its anteromedial part.
4. ***Lesser wing of the sphenoid*** is broad medially where it is continuous with the jugum sphenoidale and tapers laterally. The free *posterior border* fits into the *stem of the lateral sulcus of the brain*. It ends medially as a prominent projection, the ***anterior clinoid process***. Inferiorly, the posterior border forms the upper boundary of the *superior orbital fissure*. Medially, the lesser wing is connected to the body of the sphenoid by ***anterior and posterior roots***, which enclose the ***optic canal***.

### CLINICAL ANATOMY

Fracture of the anterior cranial fossa may cause bleeding and discharge of cerebrospinal fluid through the nose. It may also cause a condition called *black eye*, which is produced by seepage of blood into the eyelid, as frontalis muscle has no bony origin.

## Middle Cranial Fossa

It is deeper than the anterior cranial fossa, and is shaped like a butterfly, being narrow and shallow in the middle; and wide and deep on each side. It is separated from the posterior cranial fossa by the superior border of the petrous temporal bone, and the dorsum sellae of the sphenoid (Plate 1.12).

### Floor

Floor is formed by body of sphenoid in the median region and by greater wing of sphenoid, squamous temporal and anterior surface of petrous temporal on each side.

### Features

***Median area:*** The body of the sphenoid presents the following features:

1. ***Sulcus chiasmaticus*** or *optic groove* leads, on each side, to the optic canal. The optic chiasma does not occupy the sulcus, it lies at a higher level well behind the sulcus.
2. ***Optic canal*** leads to the orbit. It is bounded laterally by the lesser wing of the sphenoid, in front and behind by the two roots of the lesser wing, and medially by the body of sphenoid.
3. ***Sella turcica*** (pituitary fossa or hypophyseal fossa): The upper surface of the body of the sphenoid is hollowed out in the form of a Turkish saddle, and is known as the *sella turcica*. It consists of the *tuberculum sellae* in front, the *hypophyseal fossa* in the middle and the *dorsum sellae* behind.
4. ***Tuberculum sellae*** separates the optic groove from the *hypophyseal fossa*. Its lateral ends form the *middle clinoid process*, which may join the anterior clinoid process.
5. ***Hypophyseal fossa*** lodges the hypophysis cerebri. Beneath the floor of fossa lie the sphenoidal air sinuses.
6. ***Dorsum sellae*** is a transverse plate of bone projecting upwards; it forms the back of the saddle. The superolateral angles of the dorsum sellae are expanded to form the *posterior clinoid processes*.

#### Lateral area

1. The lateral area is deep and lodges the temporal lobe of the brain.
2. ***Superior orbital fissure*** opens anteriorly into the orbit. It is *bounded* above by the lesser wing, below by the greater wing, and medially by the body of the sphenoid. Its medial end is wider than the lateral. The long axis of the fissure is directed laterally, upwards and forwards. The lower border is marked by a small projection, which provides attachment to the *common tendinous ring of Zinn*. The ring divides the fissure into three parts.
3. ***Greater wing of the sphenoid*** presents the following features:
   a. ***Foramen rotundum*** leads anteriorly to the pterygopalatine fossa containing pterygopalatine ganglia.
   b. ***Foramen ovale*** lies posterolateral to the foramen rotundum and lateral to the lingula. It leads inferiorly to the infratemporal fossa.
   c. ***Foramen spinosum*** lies posterolateral to the foramen ovale. It also leads, inferiorly, to the infratemporal fossa.
   d. ***Emissary sphenoidal foramen*** or foramen of Vesalius carries an emissary vein.
4. ***Foramen lacerum*** lies at the posterior end of the carotid groove, posteromedial to the foramen ovale.
5. ***Anterior surface of the petrous temporal bone*** presents the following features:
   a. *Trigeminal impression* lies near the apex, behind the foramen lacerum. It lodges the trigeminal ganglion within its dural cave.
   b. *Hiatus and groove for the greater petrosal nerve* are present lateral to the trigeminal impression. They lead to the foramen lacerum.
   c. *Hiatus* and *groove for the lesser petrosal nerve* lie lateral to the hiatus for the greater petrosal nerve. They lead to the foramen ovale or to canaliculus innominatus to relay in otic ganglion.

Plate 1.12: Features of middle cranial fossa

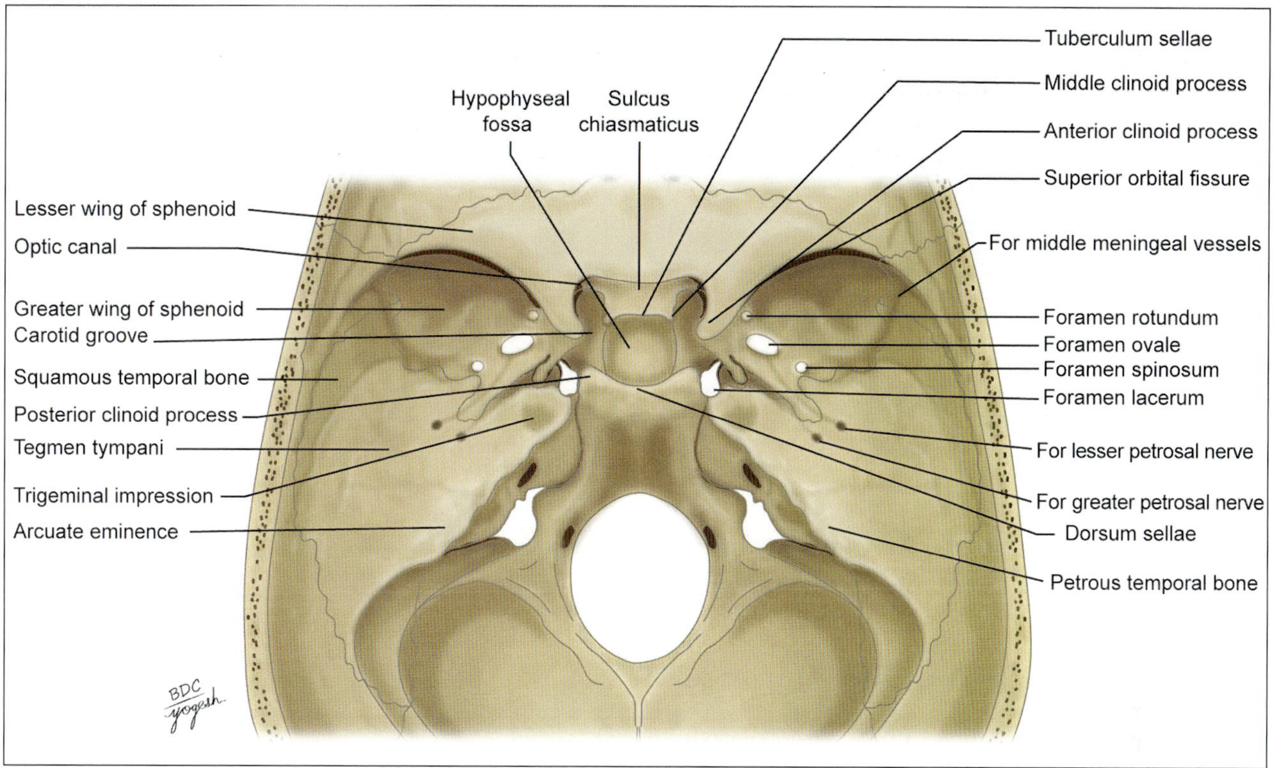


d. Still more laterally there is the *arcuate eminence* produced by the superior semicircular canal.

e. ***Tegmen tympani*** is a thin plate of bone anterolateral to the arcuate eminence. It forms a continuous sloping roof for the tympanic antrum, for the tympanic cavity and for the canal for the tensor tympani. The lateral margin of the tegmen tympani is turned downwards; it forms the lateral wall of the bony auditory tube. Its lower edge is seen in the squamotympanic fissure and divides it into the petrosquamous and petrotympanic fissures.

6. ***Cerebral surface of the squamous temporal bone*** is concave. It shows impressions for the temporal lobe and grooves for branches of the middle meningeal vessels.

## CLINICAL ANATOMY

Fracture of the middle cranial fossa produces:

a. Bleeding and discharge of CSF through the ear.

b. Bleeding through the nose or mouth may occur due to involvement of the sphenoid bone.

c. The seventh and eighth cranial nerves may be damaged, if the fracture also passes through the internal acoustic meatus. If a semicircular canal is damaged, vertigo may occur.

## Posterior Cranial Fossa

This is the largest and deepest of the three cranial fossae. The posterior cranial fossa contains the *hindbrain*, which consists of the *cerebellum behind and the pons and medulla in front* (Plate 1.13).

### Floor

It is formed by clivus, foramen magnum and part of temporal and occipital bones.

### Features

#### Median area

1. ***Clivus*** is the sloping surface in front of the foramen magnum. It is formed by fusion of the posterior part of the body of the sphenoid, including the dorsum sellae with the basilar part of the occipital bone or basiocciput. It is related to the *basilar plexus of veins*, and supports the pons and medulla.
2. On each side, the clivus is separated from the petrous temporal bone by the *petro-occipital fissure*, which is grooved by the inferior petrosal sinus, and is continuous behind with the jugular foramen.
3. ***Foramen magnum*** lies in the floor of the fossa. The anterior part of the foramen is narrow because it is *overlapped* by the medial surfaces of the occipital condyles.
4. ***Squamous part of the occipital bone*** shows the following features:
   a. ***Internal occipital protuberance*** lies opposite the external occipital protuberance. It is related to the confluence of sinuses, and is grooved on each side by the beginning of transverse sinuses.
   b. ***Internal occipital crest*** runs in the median plane from the internal occipital protuberance to the

Plate 1.13: Features of the posterior cranial fossa

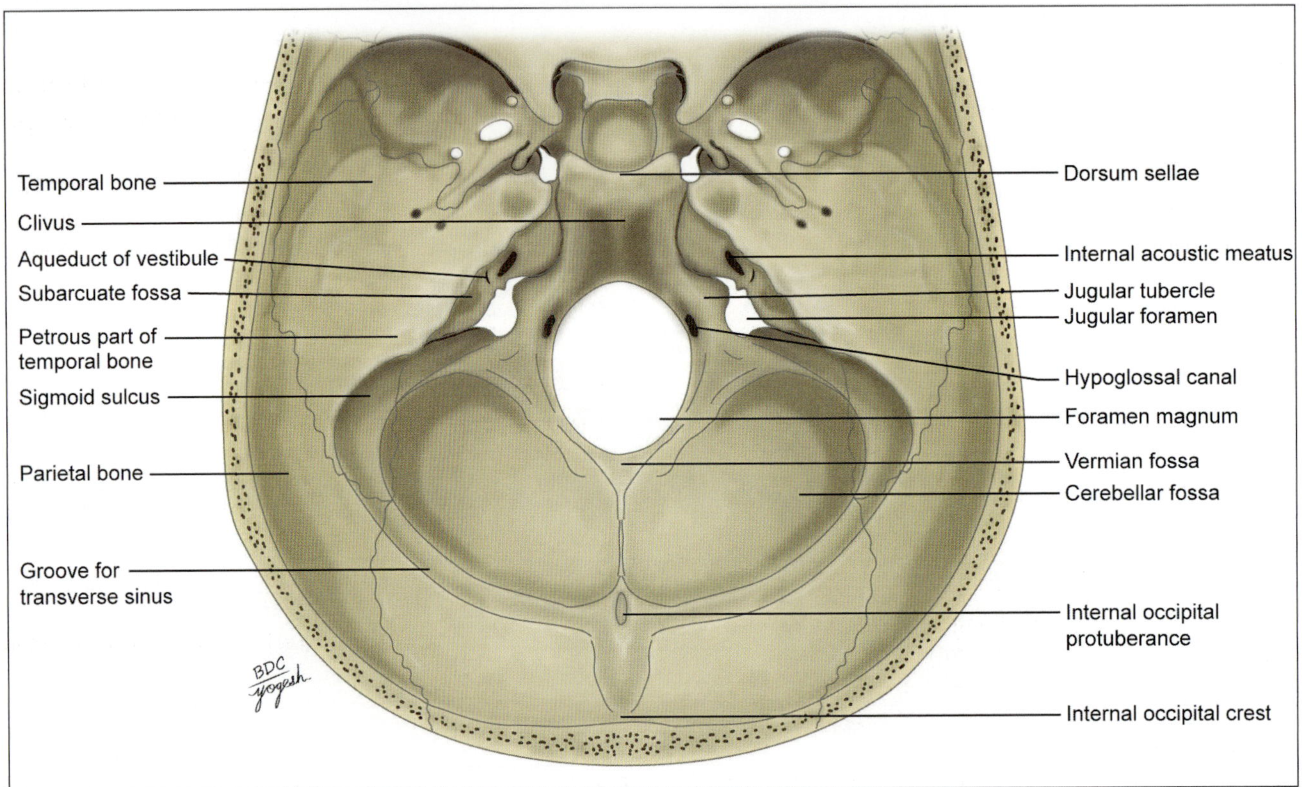


foramen magnum where it forms a shallow depression, the *vermian fossa*.

c. ***Transverse sulcus*** is quite wide and runs laterally from the internal occipital protuberance to the mastoid angle of the parietal bone where it becomes continuous with the sigmoid sulcus. The transverse sulcus lodges the *transverse sinus*. The right transverse sulcus is usually wider than the left and is continuous medially with the superior sagittal sulcus.

d. On each side of the internal occipital crest, there are *deep fossae*, which lodge the cerebellar hemispheres.

### *Lateral area*

1. ***Condylar part of the occipital bone*** is marked by the following features:
   a. ***Jugular tubercle*** lies over the occipital condyle.
   b. ***Hypoglossal canal*** (anterior condylar canal) pierces the bone posteroanterior to the jugular tubercle and runs obliquely forwards and laterally along the line of fusion between the basilar and the condylar parts of the occipital bone.
   c. *Condylar canal* (posterior condylar canal) opens in the lower part of the sigmoid sulcus, which indents the jugular process of occipital bone.
2. ***Posterior surface of the petrous part of the temporal bone*** forms the anterolateral wall of the posterior cranial fossa. The following features may be noted:
   a. ***Internal acoustic meatus*** opens above the anterior part of the jugular foramen. It is about 1 cm long and runs transversely in a lateral direction. It is closed laterally by a perforated plate of bone known as *lamina cribrosa*, which separates it from the internal ear.
   b. The orifice of the *aqueduct of the vestibule* is a narrow slit lying behind the internal acoustic meatus.
   c. The *subarcuate fossa* lies below the arcuate eminence, lateral to the internal acoustic meatus. It lodges the flocculus of the cerebellum.
3. ***Jugular foramen*** lies at the posterior end of the petro-occipital fissure. The upper margin is sharp and irregular, and presents the *glossopharyngeal notch*. The lower margin is smooth and regular.
4. *Mastoid part of the temporal bone* forms the lateral wall of the posterior cranial fossa just behind the petrous part of the bone. Anteriorly, it is marked by the *sigmoid sulcus*, which begins as a downward continuation of the transverse sulcus at the mastoid angle of the parietal bone, and ends at the jugular foramen. The sigmoid sulcus lodges the *sigmoid sinus*, which become the internal jugular vein at the jugular foramen. The sulcus is related anteriorly to the *tympanic antrum*. The *mastoid foramen* opens into the upper part of the sulcus.

## CLINICAL ANATOMY

Fracture of the posterior cranial fossa causes bruising over the mastoid region extending down over the sternocleidomastoid muscle.

## ATTACHMENTS AND RELATIONS: INTERIOR OF THE SKULL

### Attachment on Vault

1. The frontal crest gives attachment to the falx cerebri.
2. The lips of the sagittal sulcus give attachment to the falx cerebri.

### Anterior Cranial Fossa

1. The crista galli gives attachment to the falx cerebri.
2. The orbital surface of the frontal bone supports the frontal lobe of the brain.
3. The anterior clinoid processes give attachment to the free margin of the tentorium cerebelli.

### Middle Cranial Fossa

1. The middle cranial fossa lodges the *temporal lobe of the cerebral hemisphere.*
2. The tuberculum sellae provides attachment to the *diaphragma sellae*
3. The hypophyseal fossa lodges the *hypophysis cerebri.*
4. Upper margin of the dorsum sellae provides attachment to the diaphragma sellae, and the posterior clinoid process to anterior end of the attached margin of tentorium cerebelli
5. One *cavernous sinus* lies on each side of the body of the sphenoid. The internal carotid artery passes through the cavernous sinus.
6. The superior border of the petrous temporal bone is grooved by the *superior petrosal sinus* and provides attachment to the *attached margin of the tentorium cerebelli*. It is grooved in its medial part by the *trigeminal nerve* (trigeminal impression).

### Posterior Cranial Fossa

1. The posterior cranial fossa contains the hindbrain, which consists of the cerebellum behind, and the pons and medulla in front (Plate 1.13).
2. The lower part of the clivus provides attachment from above downwards to: Membrana tectoria, upper vertical band of cruciate ligament and apical ligament (MCA).
3. The internal occipital crest gives attachment to the falx cerebelli.
4. The jugular tubercle is grooved by the *ninth, tenth and eleventh cranial nerves* as they pass to the jugular foramen.
5. The subarcuate fossa on the posterior surface of petrous temporal bone lodges the *flocculus of the cerebellum*.

***Competency:***
**AN30.2** Describe and identify major foramina with structures passing through them.

### Structures Passing Through Foramina

The following foramina seen in the cranial fossae have been dealt with under the norma basalis: Foramen ovale, foramen spinosum, emissary sphenoidal foramen, foramen lacerum, foramen magnum, jugular foramen, hypoglossal canal and posterior condylar canal. Additional foramina seen in the cranial fossae are listed in Table 1.4.

**TABLE 1.4: Additional foramina seen in the cranial fossae and structures passing through them**

| ***Foramen*** | ***Structures*** |
|---|---|
| Foramen caecum | Usually blind, but occasionally it transmits emissary vein to superior sagittal sinus from upper part of nose |
| Posterior ethmoidal canal | Vessels of the same name. Note that the posterior ethmoidal nerve does not pass through the canal |
| Anterior ethmoidal canal | Corresponding nerve and vessels |
| Foramina of cribriform plate | Olfactory nerve rootlets |
| Optic canal (Fig. 1.19) | Optic nerve, Ophthalmic artery ] with meninges |
| Superior orbital fissure (Fig. 1.19) | Lateral part<br>1. Lacrimal nerve<br>2. Frontal nerve<br>3. Trochlear nerve<br>4. Superior ophthalmic vein<br>Middle part<br>1. Upper and lower divisions of the oculomotor nerve<br>2. Nasociliary nerve in between the two divisions of the oculomotor<br>3. The abducent nerve, inferolateral to the foregoing nerves<br>Medial part<br>1. Inferior ophthalmic vein<br>2. Sympathetic nerves from the plexus around the internal carotid artery |
| Foramen rotundum | Maxillary nerve |
| Internal acoustic meatus | Seventh and eighth cranial nerves<br>Labyrinthine vessels |
| External opening of vestibular aqueduct | Endolymphatic duct |

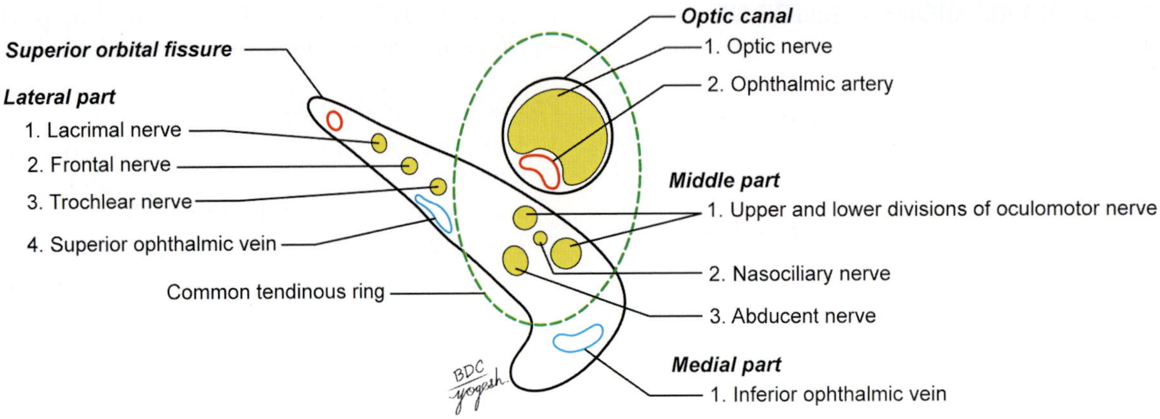


**Fig. 1.19:** Superior orbital fissure and optic canal

## FOETAL SKULL/NEONATAL SKULL

### Features of Foetal of Newborn Skull (Fig. 1.20)

1. The foetal or newborn skull is large in proportion to the other parts of skeleton.
2. *Facial skeleton* is small as compared to calvaria. In foetal skull, the facial skeleton is 1/7th of calvaria; in adults, it is half of calvaria.

   *Anatomical justification:* The facial skeleton is small due to rudimentary mandible and maxillae, non-eruption of teeth and small size of maxillary sinus and nasal cavity. The large size of calvaria is due to precocious growth of brain.
3. *Base of the skull* is short and narrow, though internal ear is almost of adult size, the petrous temporal has not reached the adult length.
4. *Structure of bones*: The bones of cranial vault are smooth and unilamellar; there is no diploe. The tables and diploes appear by 4th year of age.
5. *Bony prominences*
   - Frontal and parietal tubera are prominent.
   - Glabella, superciliary arches and mastoid processes are not developed.
6. *Paranasal air sinuses:* These are rudimentary or absent.
7. *Temporal bone*
   - The internal ear, tympanic cavity, tympanic antrum and ear ossicles are of adult size.
   - The tympanic part is represented by an incomplete tympanic ring.
   - Mastoid process is absent, it appears during the later part of second year.
   - External acoustic meatus is short and straight. Its bony part is unossified and represented by a fibrocartilaginous plate.
   - Tympanic membrane faces more downwards than laterally due to the absence of mastoid process.
   - Stylomastoid foramen is exposed on the lateral surface of the skull because mastoid portion is flat.
   - Styloid process lies immediately behind the tympanic ring and has not fused with the remainder of the temporal bone.
   - Mandibular fossa is flat and placed more laterally, and the anterior root/articular tubercle has not developed.
   - The subarcuate fossa is very deep and prominent.
   - Facial canal is short.
8. *Orbits:* These are large. The germs of developing teeth lies close to the orbital floor. Orbit comprises base or an outer opening with upper, lower, medial and lateral walls. Its apex lies at the optic foramen/canal. It also has superior and inferior orbital fissures.

### OSSIFICATION

- Two halves of frontal bone are separated by metopic suture.
- The mandible is also present in two halves. It is a derivative of 1st branchial arch.
- Occipital bone is in four parts (squamous one, condylar two and basilar one).
- The four bony elements of temporal bone are separate, except for the commencing union of the tympanic part with the squamous and petrous parts. The second centre for styloid process has not appeared.
- Unossified membranous gaps, a total of 6 fontanelles at the angles of the parietal bones are present.
- Squamous suture between parietal and squamous temporal bones is present.

## POSTNATAL GROWTH OF SKULL

The growth of calvaria and facial skeleton proceeds at different rates and over different periods. Growth of calvaria is related to growth of brain, whereas that of the facial skeleton is related to the development of dentition, muscles of mastication and of the tongue. The rates of growth of the base and vault are also different.

### Growth of the Vault

1. *Rate:* Rapid during 1st year, and then it slows up to the 7th year when it is almost of adult size.
2. *Growth in breadth:* This growth occurs at the sagittal suture, sutures bordering greater wings, occipitomastoid suture, and the petro-occipital suture at the base.

3. *Growth in height*: This growth occurs at the fronto-zygomatic suture, pterion, squamosal suture and asterion.
4. *Growth in anteroposterior diameter:* This growth occurs at the coronal and lambdoid sutures.

### Growth of the Base

The base grows in anteroposterior diameter at three cartilaginous plates situated between the occipital and sphenoid bones, between the pre- and post-sphenoids, and between the sphenoid and ethmoid.

### Growth of the Face

1. Growth of orbits and ethmoid is completed by 7th year.
2. In the face, the growth occurs mostly during first year, although it continues till puberty and even later.

### Thickening of Bones

1. Two tables and diploe appear by 4th year. Differentiation reaches maximum by about 35 years, when the diploic veins produce characteristic marking in the radiographs.
2. Mastoid process appears during 2nd year, and the mastoid air cells during 6th year.

### Obliteration of Sutures of the Vault

1. Obliteration begins on the inner surface between 30 and 40 years, and on the outer surface between 40 and 50 years.
2. The timings are variable, but it usually takes place first in the lower part of the coronal suture, next in the posterior part of the sagittal suture and then in the lambdoid suture.
3. Obliteration of suture and age
   - Sagittal suture: 35 years
   - Coronal suture: 38–41 years
   - Vomero-ethmoid suture: 45 years
   - Lambdoid suture: Before 50 years
   - Sphenoparietal and sphenofrontal suture: 65 years
   - Temporosphenoid suture: 70 years

### In Old Age

The skull generally becomes thinner and lighter but in small proportion of cases, it increases in thickness and weight. The most striking feature is reduction in the size of mandible and maxillae due to loss of teeth and absorption of alveolar processes. This causes decrease in the vertical height of the face and a change in the angles of the mandible, which become more obtuse.

### Closure of Fontanelles

Anterior fontanelle (bregma) closes by 18 months, mastoid fontanelle by 12 months, posterior fontanelle (lambda) by 2–3 months and sphenoidal fontanelle also by 2–3 months.

*Note*: ***Wormian or sutural bones:*** These are small irregular bones found in the region of the fontanelles, and are formed by additional ossification centres. They are most common at the lambda and at the asterion; common at the pterion (epipteric bone); and rare at the bregma (Os Kerckring). Wormian bones are common in hydrocephalic skulls.

## CLINICAL ANATOMY

***Fontanelles***

- Fontanelles are soft membranous gaps present in the skull vault of newborn.
- There are 6 fontanelles at birth as follows (Figs 1.20a and b):
- *Anterior fontanelle* between frontal and parietal bones. Anterior fontanelle is the largest fontanelle. It lies at the bregma.
- *Posterior fontanelle* between occipital and parietal bones. It lies at the lambda.
- *Anterolateral (sphenoid) fontanelle* between greater wing of sphenoid, squamous temporal, frontal and parietal bones. It lies at the pterion.
- *Posterolateral (mastoid) fontanelle* between parietal, occipital, squamous temporal and occipital bones. It lies at the asterion.
- *Closure of fontanelle* (*Ref. 42nd edn, Gray's Anatomy*)
  - Anterolateral and posterior fontanelles close within 2–3 months after birth.
  - Posterolateral fontanelles close by the end of first year.
  - Anterior fontanelle closes by 18–24 months of age.

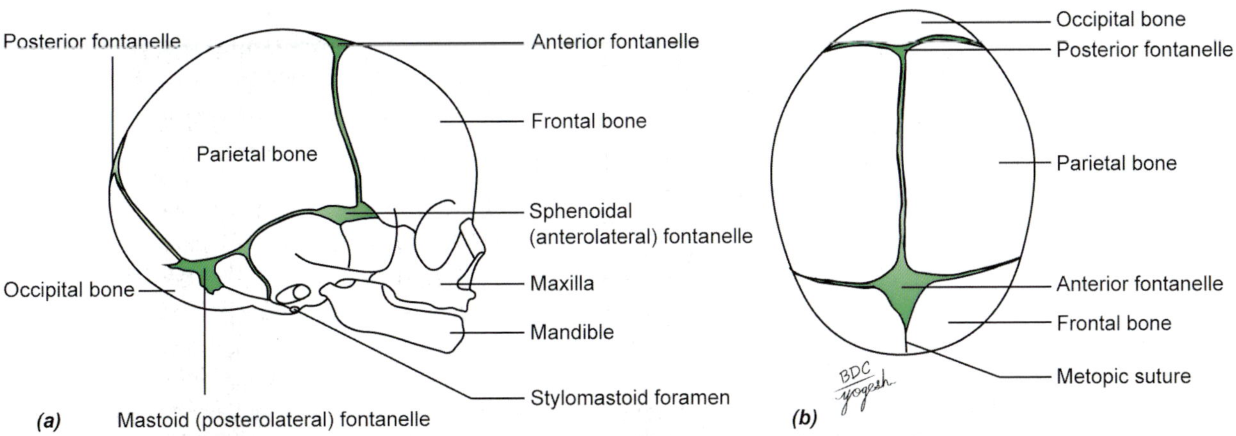


**Figs 1.20a and b:** Fontanelles of skull: (a) Lateral aspect and (b) superior aspect

- *Function of fontanelles*
  - Allow moulding of skull during the birth passage of body.
  - Permit growth of skull bones to increase the cranial capacity.
  - Accommodate developing brain.
- *Clinical aspects*
  1. Closure of fontanelles gives an idea about the age of the newborn.
  2. The anterior fontanelle is largest and of great clinical significance. Appearance of anterior fontanelle gives an idea of intracranial pressure.
     - Bulging fontanelles indicate increased intracranial pressure.
     - Depressed fontanelles indicate dehydration cases.
  3. If fontanelles fuse early, brain growth is stunted; such children are less intelligent.
  4. Bones override at the fontanelle helping to decrease size of head during vaginal delivery.
  5. ***Caput succedaneum*** is soft tissue swelling on any part of skull due to rupture of capillaries during delivery. Skull becomes normal within a few days in postnatal life (Fig. 1.21).

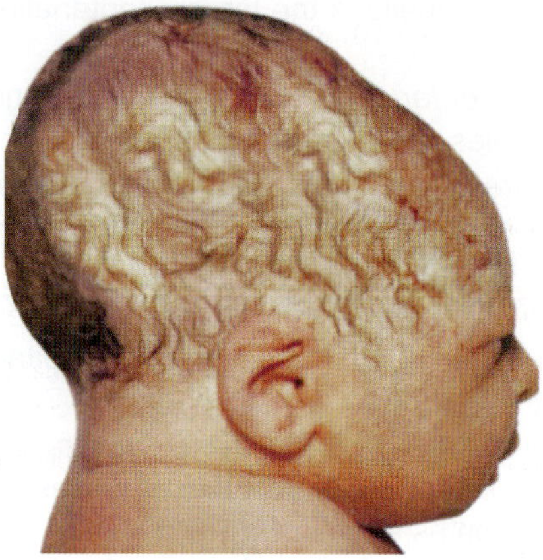

**Fig. 1.21:** Caput succedaneum

## SEX DIFFERENCES IN THE SKULL

There are no sex differences until puberty. The postpubertal differences are listed in Table 1.5.

**TABLE 1.5: Sex differences in the skull**

| *Features* | *Males* | *Females* |
|---|---|---|
| 1. Weight | Heavier | Lighter |
| 2. Size | Larger | Smaller |
| 3. Capacity | Greater in males | 10% less than males |
| 4. Walls | Thicker | Thinner |
| 5. Muscular ridges, glabella, superciliary arches, temporal lines, mastoid processes, superior nuchal lines and external occipital protuberance | More marked | Less marked |
| 6. Tympanic plate | Larger and margins are more roughened | Smaller and margins are less roughened |
| 7. Supraorbital margin | More rounded | Sharp |
| 8. Forehead | Sloping (receding) | Vertical |
| 9. Frontal and parietal tubera | Less prominent | More prominent |
| 10. Vault | Rounded | Somewhat flattened |

## CRANIOMETRY

*Craniometry* is the process of recording various measurements of the skull.

### Cephalic Index

It expresses the shape of the head, and is the proportion of breadth to length of the skull. Thus:

$$\text{Cephalic index} = \frac{\text{Maximum cranial breath}}{\text{Maximum cranial length}} \times 100$$

The length or the longest diameter is measured from the glabella to the occipital point, the breadth or the widest diameter is measured usually a little below the parietal tubera.

*Note: Human races may be:*
1. *Dolichocephalic* or long-headed when the index is 75 or less.
2. *Mesaticephalic* when the index is between 76 and 80.
3. *Brachycephalic* or short-headed or round-headed when the index is above 80.
4. Dolichocephaly is a feature of primitive races, like Eskimos, Negroes, etc.
5. Brachycephaly through mesaticephaly has been a continuous change in the advanced races, like the Europeans.

### Facial Angle

This is the angle between two lines drawn from the nasion to the basion or anterior margin of foramen magnum and a line drawn from basion to the prosthion or central point on upper incisor alveolus (Fig. 1.9).

Facial angle is a rough index of the degree of development of the brain because it is the angle between facial skeleton, i.e. viscerocranium, and the calvaria, i.e. neurocranium, which are inversely proportional to each other. The angle is the smallest in the most evolved races of man, it is larger in lower races, and still larger in anthropoids.

*Note:*

**Abnormal crania**

1. ***Oxycephaly or acrocephaly, tower-skull, or steeple skull*** is an abnormally tall skull. It is due to premature closure of the suture between presphenoid and postsphenoid in the base, and the coronal suture in skull cap, so that the skull is very short anteroposteriorly. Compensation is done by the upward growth of skull for the enlarging brain.

2. ***Scaphocephaly or boat-shaped skull*** is due to premature synostosis in the sagittal suture; as a result, the skull is very narrow from side-to-side but greatly elongated.

**Competency:**
**AN26.4** Describe morphological features of mandible.

## MANDIBLE

The *mandible*, or the lower jaw, is the largest and the strongest bone of the face. It develops from the *1st pharyngeal arch*.

It is a horseshoe-shaped bone. It consists of three parts (Plate 1.14, Figs 1.22 and 1.23, Flowchart 1.14):

- *Body* – horizontally placed
- *Two rami* – vertically placed.

### BODY OF MANDIBLE

Each half of the body has:
*Two surfaces*: External and internal
*Two borders*: Superior border or alveolar process and inferior border or base of the mandible.

***Outer surface*** presents the following features:

1. ***Symphysis menti*** is the line at which the right and left halves of the bone meet each other. It is marked by a faint ridge.
2. ***Mental protuberance*** (*mentum* = chin) is a median triangular projecting area in the lower part of the midline. The inferolateral angles of the protuberance form the *mental tubercles*.
3. ***Mental foramen*** lies below the interval between the premolar teeth.
4. The *oblique line* is the continuation of the sharp anterior border of the ramus of the mandible. It runs downwards and forwards towards the mental tubercle.
5. The *incisive fossa* is a depression that lies just below the incisor teeth.

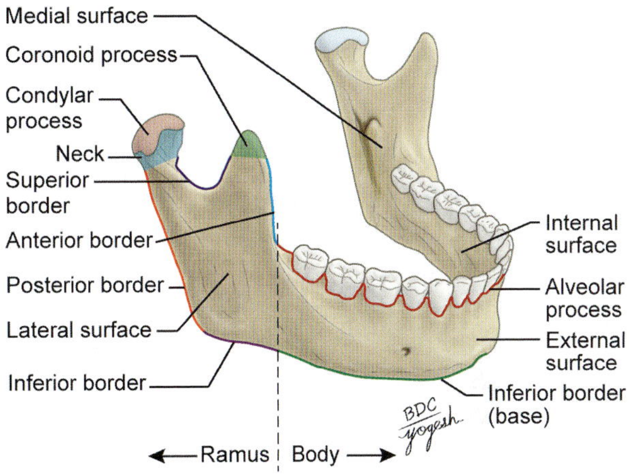


**Fig. 1.22:** Parts of mandible

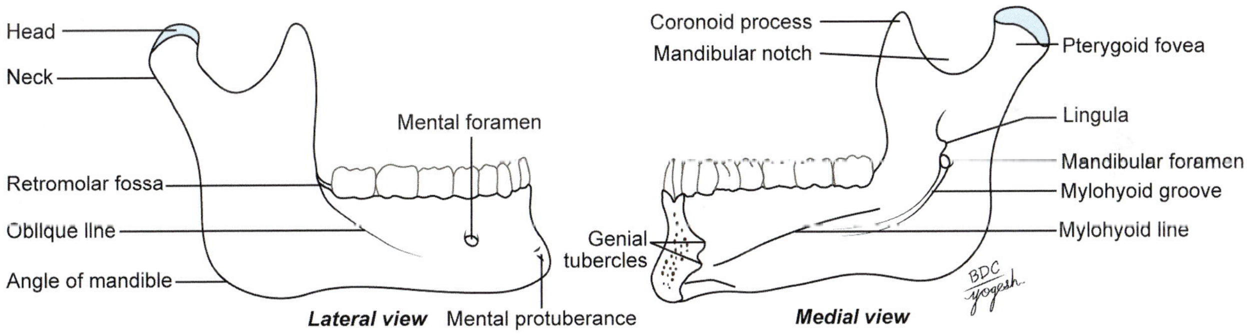


**Fig. 1.23:** Mandible (lateral and medial views)

**Flowchart 1.14:** Mandible

***Body of mandible***

- ***External surface***
  - Symphysis menti
  - Mental protuberance
  - Mental tubercle
  - Mental foramen
  - Oblique line
  - Incisive fossa
  - ***Attachments***
  - Oblique line:
    - Buccinator
    - Depressor anguli oris
    - Depressor labii inferioris
  - Incisive fossa
    - Mentalis
    - Orbicularis oris
- ***Inner surface***
  - Mylohyoid line
    - Mylohyoid
    - Superior constrictor
    - Pterygomandibular raphe
  - Mylohyoid groove
  - Submandibular fossa
  - Sublingual fossa
  - Genial tubercles
    - Genioglossus
    - Geniohyoid
  - Digastric fossa
    - Anterior belly of digastric
- ***Borders***
  - Alveolar border
    - Sockets for 8 teeth
  - Lower border
    - Platysma

***Ramus of mandible***

- ***2 Surfaces***
  - ***Lateral surface***
    - Rough
    - Masseter
  - ***Medial surface***
    - Mandibular foramen
      Inferior alveolar nerve and vessels
  - Lingula
    - Sphenomandibular ligament
  - Mylohyoid groove
  - Medial pterygoid
- ***4 Borders***
  - ***Anterior border***
    - Sharp
    - Temporalis
  - ***Posterior border***
    - Round
  - ***Superior border***
    - Mandibular notch
    - Masseteric nerves and vessels
  - ***Inferior border***
    - Stylomandibular ligament
- ***2 Processes***
  - ***Coronoid process***
    - Flat, triangular
    - Temporalis
  - ***Condylar process***
    - Head of mandible
      Forms TMJ
  - Neck
    - Lateral temporo-mandibular ligament
  - Pterygoid fovea
    - Lateral pterygoid

***Mental foramen:*** Mental nerves and vessels

BDC yogesh

Plate 1.14: Mandible

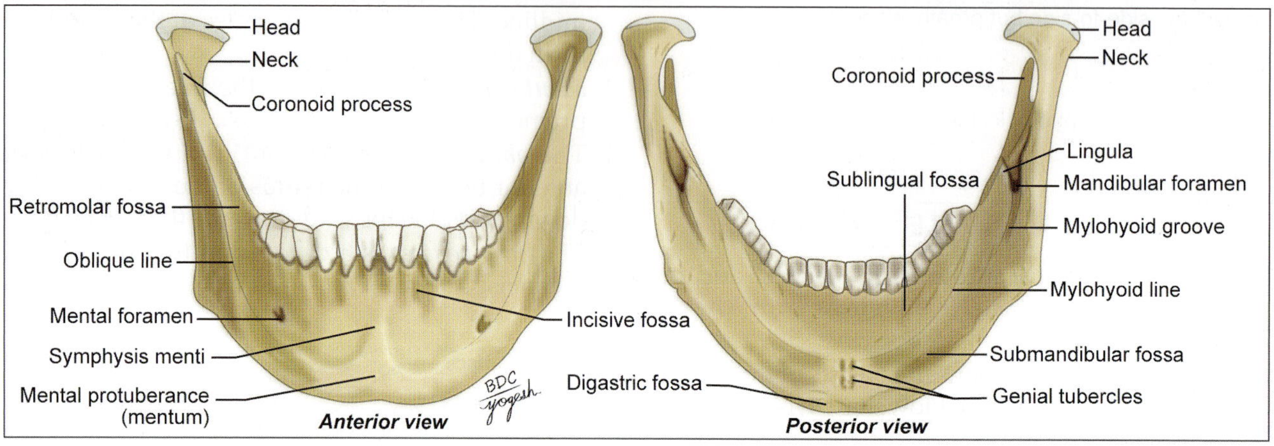


***Inner surface*** presents the following features:

1. ***Mylohyoid line*** is a prominent ridge that runs obliquely downwards and forwards from below the third molar tooth to the median area below the genial tubercles (*see* below). The mylohyoid groove (present on the ramus) extends onto the body below the posterior end of the mylohyoid line.
2. Below the mylohyoid line, the surface is slightly hollowed out to form the ***submandibular fossa,*** which lodges the submandibular gland.
3. Above the mylohyoid line, there is the *sublingual fossa* in which the sublingual gland lies.
4. The posterior surface of the symphysis menti is marked by four small elevations called the *superior and inferior* ***genial tubercles***.

***Upper or alveolar border*** bears sockets for the teeth.

***Lower border*** of the mandible is also called the *base.* Near the midline, the base shows an oval depression called the *digastric fossa*.

## RAMUS

The ramus is quadrilateral in shape and has:

- *Two surfaces* — lateral and medial
- *Four borders* — upper, lower, anterior and posterior
- *Two processes* — coronoid and condyloid.

- ***Lateral surface*** is flat and bears a number of oblique ridges.
- ***Medial surface*** presents the following features:
  1. ***Mandibular foramen*** lies a little above the centre of ramus at the level of occlusal surfaces of the teeth. It leads into the *mandibular canal,* which descends into the body of the mandible and opens at the *mental foramen* (Fig. 1.23).
  2. The anterior margin of the mandibular foramen is marked by a sharp tongue-shaped projection called the ***lingula***. The lingula is directed towards the head or condyloid process of the mandible.
  3. The *mylohyoid groove* begins just below the mandibular foramen, and runs downwards and forwards to be gradually lost over the submandibular fossa.
- ***Upper border*** of the ramus is thin and is curved downwards forming the *mandibular notch.*
- ***Lower border*** is the backward continuation of the base of the mandible. Posteriorly, it ends by becoming continuous with the posterior border at the *angle* of the mandible (Fig. 1.23).
- ***Anterior border*** is thin, while the *posterior border* is thick.
- ***Coronoid process*** (Greek *crow's beak*) is a flattened triangular upward projection from the anterosuperior part of the ramus. Its anterior border is continuous with the anterior border of the ramus. The posterior border bounds the mandibular notch.
- ***Condyloid process*** (Latin *knuckle-like*) is a strong upward projection from the posterosuperior part of the ramus. Its upper end is expanded from side-to-side to form the ***head***. The head is covered with fibrocartilage and articulates with the temporal bone to form the temporomandibular joint. The constriction below the head is the ***neck***. Its anterior surface presents a depression called the ***pterygoid fovea***.

## ATTACHMENTS AND RELATIONS OF THE MANDIBLE

### Muscles

1. The oblique line on the lateral side of the body gives origin to the buccinator as far forwards as the anterior border of the first molar tooth. In front of this origin, the depressor labii inferioris and the depressor anguli oris arise from the oblique line below the mental foramen (Figs 1.24a and b).
2. The incisive fossa gives origin to the mentalis and mental slips of the orbicularis oris.
3. The parts of both the inner and outer surfaces just below the alveolar margin are covered by the mucous membrane of the mouth.
4. Mylohyoid line gives origin to the mylohyoid muscle.
5. Superior constrictor muscle of the pharynx arises from an area above the posterior end of the mylohyoid line.
6. *Upper genial tubercle* gives origin to the genioglossus, and the *lower tubercle* to geniohyoid.

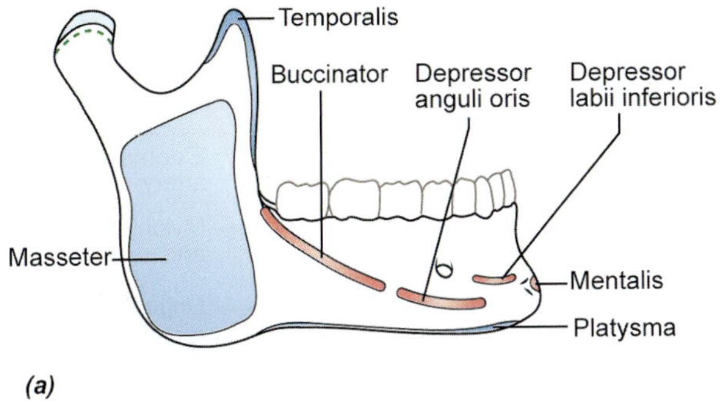


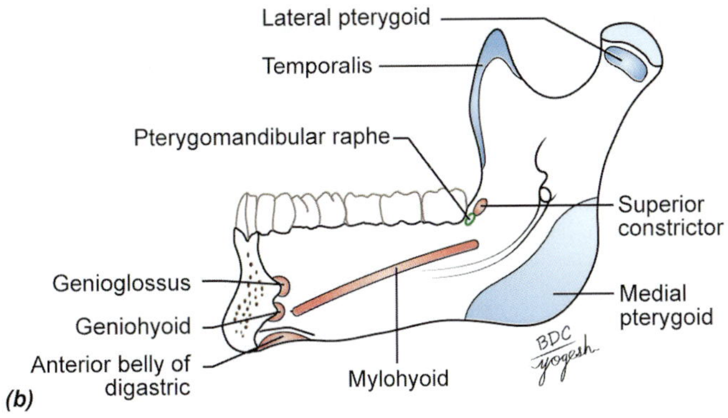


**Figs 1.24a and b:** Attachments of the mandible: (a) Lateral surface of the right half of the mandible and (b) inner surface of right half of the mandible

7. Anterior belly of the digastric muscle arises from the digastric fossa.
8. Platysma is inserted into the lower border.
9. Whole of the lateral surface of ramus except the posterosuperior part provides insertion to the masseter muscle.
10. Medial pterygoid muscle is inserted on the medial surface of the ramus, on the roughened area below and behind the mylohyoid groove.
11. Temporalis is inserted into the apex and medial surface of the coronoid process. The insertion extends downwards on the anterior border of the ramus.
12. Lateral pterygoid muscle is inserted into the pterygoid fovea on the anterior aspect of the neck.

### Ligaments

1. Pterygomandibular raphe is attached immediately behind the third molar tooth in continuation with the origin of superior constrictor.
2. Deep cervical fascia (investing layer) is attached to the whole length of lower border.
3. Sphenomandibular ligament is attached to the lingula.
4. The lateral surface of neck provides attachment to the lateral ligament of the temporomandibular joint.
5. Stylomandibular ligament is attached to the angle of the mandible.

## NERVES AND VESSELS RELATED TO THE MANDIBLE (Figs 1.25a and b)

1. The mental foramen transmits the *mental nerve and vessels*.
2. The *inferior alveolar nerve and vessels* enter the *mandibular canal through the mandibular foramen*, and run forwards within the canal.
3. The *mylohyoid nerve and vessels* lie in the *mylohyoid groove*.
4. The *lingual nerve* is related to the medial surface of the ramus in front of the mylohyoid groove.
5. The area above and behind the mandibular foramen is related to the *inferior alveolar nerve and vessels* and to the *maxillary artery*.
6. The *masseteric nerve and vessels* pass through the mandibular notch.
7. The *auriculotemporal nerve* and *superficial temporal artery* are related to the medial side of the neck of mandible.
8. Facial artery is palpable on the lower border of mandible at anteroinferior angle of masseter.

*Note*: Facial and maxillary arteries are not accompanied by respective nerves. The lingual nerve does not get company of its artery.

***Structures related to mandible***

1. Salivary glands: Parotid, submandibular and sublingual.
2. Lymph nodes: Parotid, submandibular and submental.
3. Arteries (7): Maxillary, superficial temporal, masseteric, inferior alveolar, mylohyoid, mental and facial.
4. Nerves (6): Lingual, auriculotemporal, masseteric, inferior alveolar, mylohyoid and mental.
5. Muscles of mastication: Insertions of temporalis, masseter, medial pterygoid and lateral pterygoid.
6. Ligaments: Lateral ligament of temporomandibular joint, stylomandibular ligament, sphenomandibular and pterygomandibular raphe.

[*Mnemonics*

***Nerves related to mandible $M^3$LIA:*** **$M^3$**– masseteric nerve, mental nerve and nerve to mylohyoid; **L**– lingual nerve; **I**– inferior alveolar nerve, **A**– auriculotemporal nerve.

***Arteries related to mandible: $M^4$IFS:*** **$M^4$**– masseteric, maxillary, mental arteries and artery to mylohyoid; **I**– inferior alveolar artery, **F**– facial artery, **S**– superficial temporal artery].

## OSSIFICATION

The mandible is the *second bone, next to the clavicle, to ossify* in the body. Its greater part ossifies *in membrane*. The parts ossifying in *cartilage* include the *incisive part* below the incisor teeth, the *coronoid and condyloid processes* and the *upper half of the ramus* above the level of the mandibular foramen.

Each half of the mandible ossifies from only one *centre*, which appears at about the *6th week* of intrauterine life in the mesenchymal *sheath of Meckel's cartilage* near the future mental foramen. Meckel's cartilage is the skeletal element of 1*st pharyngeal arch*.

At birth, the mandible consists of two halves connected at the *symphysis menti* by fibrous tissue. Bony union takes place during the first year of life.

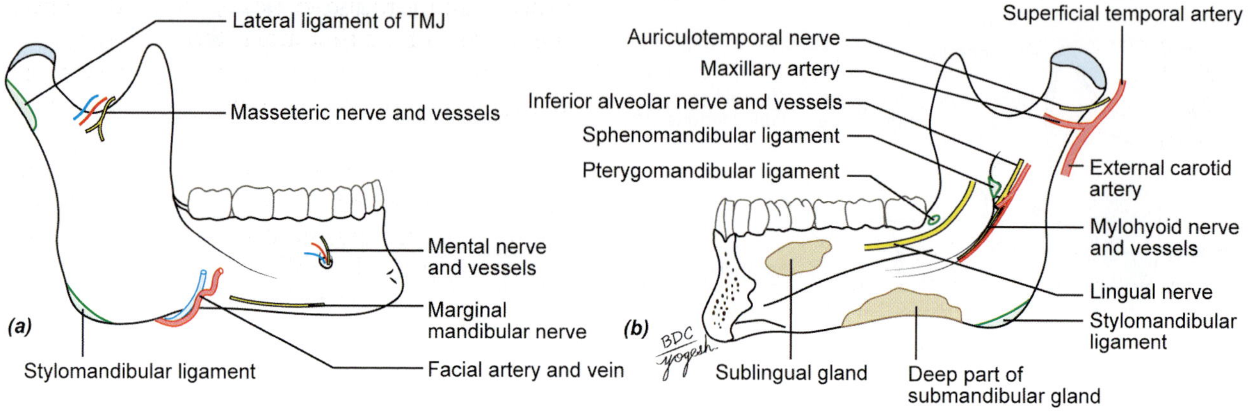


**Figs 1.25a and b:** Relations of the mandible: (a) Lateral surface of the right half of the mandible and (b) inner surface of right half of the mandible

## AGE CHANGES IN THE MANDIBLE

The mandible shows considerable changes with age. The changes are observed in the following points (Fig. 1.26, Table 1.6):

1. Position of mental foramen
2. Angle of mandible
3. Relationship between condylar and coronoid processes
4. Location of mandibular canal
5. Alveolar process and teeth.

## CLINICAL ANATOMY

- The mandible is commonly fractured at the canine socket where it is weak.
- Involvement of the inferior alveolar nerve in the callus may cause neuralgic pain, which may be referred to the areas of distribution of the buccal and auriculotemporal nerves. If the nerve is damaged, the areas supplied by these nerves become insensitive.
- The next common fracture of the mandible occurs at the angle and neck of mandible. Toothache of lower jaw referred to external auditory meatus, as both are supplied by branches of mandibular division of trigeminal nerve.

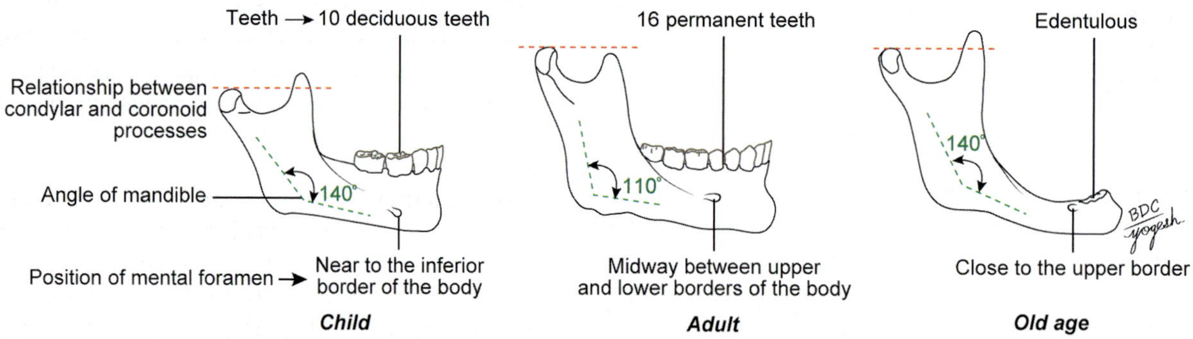


**Fig 1.26:** Age changes in the mandible

**TABLE 1.6: Age changes in mandible**

| Feature | In children | In adult | In old age |
|---|---|---|---|
| Angle of mandible | 140° | 110° | 140° |
| Direction of mental foramen | Upward and backward | Horizontally backward | Forward |
| Position of mental foramen | Near the inferior border of the body | Midway between upper and lower borders of the body | Close to the upper border |
| Alveolar process | Rudimentary | Well-developed | Absorbed to form alveolar ridge, edentulous |
| Teeth | Ten deciduous teeth | 16 permanent teeth | Edentulous |
| Relationship between condylar and coronoid processes | Coronoid process lies at a higher level than condylar process | Condylar process lies at a higher level than the coronoid process | Coronoid process lies at higher level than the condylar process |
| Height of body | Gradually increases | Maximum | Gradually decreases |
| Position of mandibular canal | Runs near the lower border | Runs parallel to the mylohyoid line | Runs close to the upper border |

## MAXILLA

Maxilla (cheek) is the second largest bone of the face, the first being the mandible. The two maxillae form the whole of the upper jaw (Plate 1.15).

### SIDE DETERMINATION

1. Anterior surface ends medially into a deeply concave border, called the *nasal notch*. Posterior surface is convex.
2. Alveolar border with sockets for upper teeth faces downwards with its convexity directed outwards. Frontal process is the longest process, which is directed upwards.
3. Medial surface is marked by a large irregular penning, the *maxillary hiatus*/antrum of Highmore for maxillary air sinus.

### FEATURES

Each maxilla consists of (Plate 1.15):
1. Body
2. Four processes: Frontal, zygomatic, palatine and alveolar.

#### Body of Maxilla

It is pyramidal in shape, with its base directed medially at the nasal surface, and the apex directed laterally at the zygomatic process. It has four surfaces and encloses a large cavity, the *maxillary sinus* described in Chapter 15, page 252.

It has four surfaces:
1. Anterior or facial,
2. Posterior or infratemporal,
3. Superior or orbital and
4. Medial or nasal.

#### *Anterior or Facial Surface*

1. Anterior surface forms a part of norma frontalis.
2. Above the incisor teeth, there is a slight depression, the *incisive fossa*, which gives origin to depressor septi. Incisivus labii superioris (part of orbicularis oris) arises from the alveolar margin below the fossa, and the *nasalis* superolateral to the fossa along the nasal notch.
3. Lateral to canine eminence, there is a larger and deeper depression, the *canine fossa*, which gives origin to levator anguli oris.
4. Above the canine fossa, there is *infraorbital foramen*, which transmits *infraorbital nerve and vessels*.
5. Levator labii superioris arises between the infraorbital margin and infraorbital foramen.
6. Medially, the anterior surface ends in a deeply concave border, the nasal notch, which terminates below into a process that, along with the corresponding process of the opposite maxilla, forms the anterior nasal spine. Anterior surface bordering the nasal notch gives origin to nasalis and depressor septi.

#### *Posterior or Infratemporal Surface*

1. It forms the anterior wall of *infratemporal fossa*, and is separated from anterior surface by the zygomatic process and a rounded ridge, which descends from the process of the first molar tooth.
2. Near the centre of the surface open two or three *alveolar canals* for *posterior superior alveolar nerve and vessels*.
3. Posteroinferiorly, there is a rounded eminence, the ***maxillary tuberosity***, which articulates superomedially with pyramidal process of palatine bone, and gives origin laterally to the superficial head of medial pterygoid muscle.
4. Above the maxillary tuberosity, the smooth surface forms anterior wall of *pterygopalatine fossa*, and is grooved by *maxillary nerve*.

#### *Superior or Orbital Surface*

1. Superior surface is smooth, triangular and slightly concave, and forms the greater part of the *floor of orbit*.
2. The surface presents *infraorbital groove* leading forwards to *infraorbital canal*, which opens on the anterior surface as *infraorbital foramen*. The groove, canal and foramen transmit the *infraorbital nerve and vessels*. Near the midpoint, the canal gives off laterally a branch, the *canalis sinuous*, for the passage of *anterior superior alveolar nerve and vessels*.
3. Inferior oblique muscle of eyeball arises from a depression just lateral to lacrimal notch at the anteromedial angle of the surface.

#### *Medial or Nasal Surface*

1. Medial surface forms a part of the *lateral wall of nose*.
2. *Posterosuperiorly*, it displays a large irregular opening of the maxillary sinus, the *maxillary hiatus*.
3. Below the hiatus, the smooth concave surface forms a part of *inferior meatus of nose*.
4. Behind the hiatus, the surface articulates with perpendicular plate of palatine bone, enclosing the *greater palatine canal*, which runs downwards and forwards, and transmits *greater palatine vessels and the anterior, middle and posterior palatine nerves*.
5. In front of the hiatus, there is *nasolacrimal groove*, which is converted into the nasolacrimal canal by articulation with the *descending process of lacrimal bone* and the *lacrimal process of inferior nasal concha*. The canal transmits *nasolacrimal duct to the inferior meatus of nose*.
6. More anteriorly, an oblique ridge forms the *conchal crest* for articulation with the inferior nasal concha.
7. Above the conchal crest, the shallow depression forms a part of the *atrium of middle meatus* of nose.

#### Processes of Maxilla

It has four processes: Frontal, zygomatic, palatine and alveolar (Plate 1.15).

#### *Zygomatic Process*

The zygomatic process is a pyramidal lateral projection that articulates with the zygomatic bone.

Plate 1.15: Right maxilla

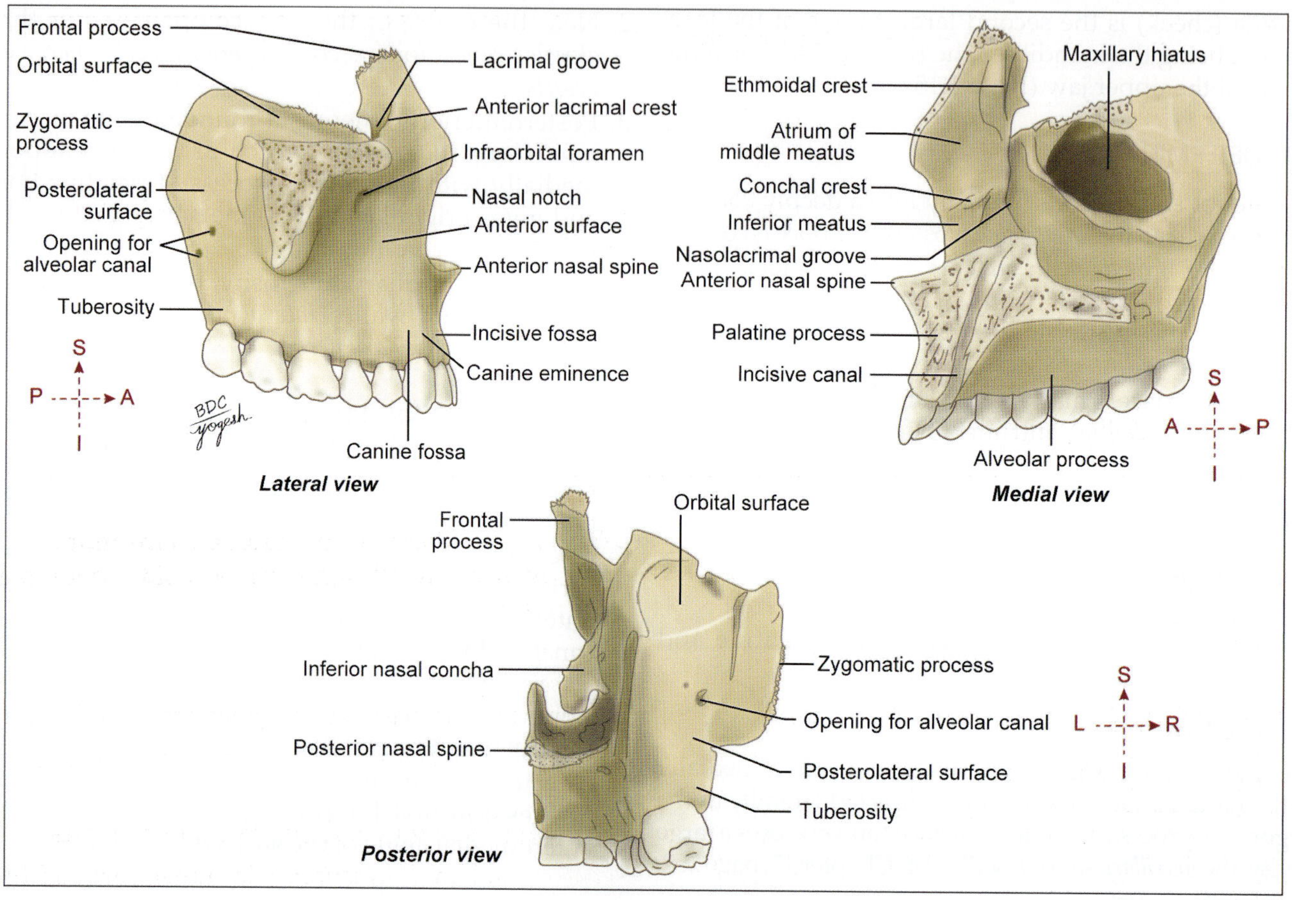


### Frontal Process

1. The frontal process projects upwards to *articulate* above with the frontal bone, in front with nasal bone and behind with lacrimal bone.
2. *Lateral surface* is divided by a vertical ridge, the ***anterior lacrimal crest***, into a smooth anterior part and a grooved posterior part.
3. The anterior lacrimal crest gives attachment to lacrimal fascia and the medial palpebral ligament. The anterior smooth area gives origin to the orbital part of orbicularis oculi and levator labii superioris alaeque nasi. The posterior grooved area forms the anterior half of the floor of *lacrimal groove*.
4. *Medial surface* of the frontal process has horizontal *ethmoidal crest* that articulates with middle nasal concha. The area below the ethmoidal crest is hollowed out to form the atrium of the middle meatus of nose.

### Alveolar Process

1. The alveolar process forms half of the alveolar arch, and bears sockets for the roots of upper 8 teeth.
2. Buccinator arises from the posterior part of its outer surface up to the 1st molar tooth.

### Palatine Process

1. Palatine process is a thick horizontal plate projecting medially to form a part of the hard.
2. Its medial border is raised superiorly to form the *nasal crest*. The groove between the nasal crests of two maxillae receives lower border of vomer; anterior part of the ridge is high and is known as *incisor crest*, which terminates anteriorly into the anterior nasal spine.
3. Incisive canal traverses near the anterior part of the medial border.

*Note*: The maxilla and premaxilla ossify from primary ossification centres that appear in 7th week of intrauterine life and three secondary ossification centres that appear in 8th week after birth. The premaxilla fuse with alveolar process almost immediately after the ossification. There is no evidence of a separate centre of ossification for the incisor-bearing portion of the maxilla (premaxilla). A small maxillary sinus is present at birth which enlarges until the eruption of permanent dentition.

## PARIETAL BONE

Two parietal bones form a large part of the roof and sides of vault of skull. Each bone is roughly quadrilateral in shape with its convexity directed outwards (Plate 1.16).

### SIDE DETERMINATION

Outer surface is convex and smooth, inner surface is concave and depicts vascular markings.

Anteroinferior angle is pointed and shows a groove for anterior division of middle meningeal artery.

### FEATURES

Parietal bone has two surfaces, four borders and four angles (Plate 1.16).

**Plate 1.16:** Parietal bone (medial and lateral views)

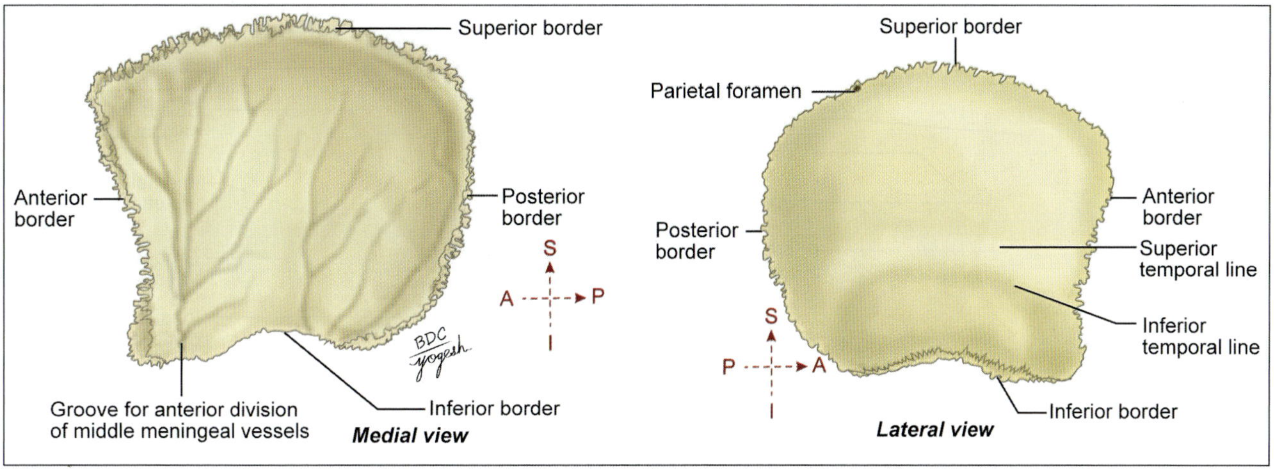


### Surfaces

1. Outer convex
2. Inner concave

### Borders

1. Superior or sagittal
2. Inferior or squamosal
3. Anterior or frontal
4. Posterior or occipital

### Angles

1. Anterosuperior or frontal
2. Anteroinferior or sphenoidal
3. Posterosuperior or occipital
4. Posteroinferior or mastoid

   At each of the four angles, are four fontanelles. These are:

   a. One anterior fontanelle
   b. One posterior fontanelle
   c. Two anterolateral or sphenoidal fontanelles
   d. Two posterolateral or mastoid fontanelles.

Details can be studied from *norma verticalis* and *norma lateralis* and *inner aspect of skull cap*.

## OCCIPITAL BONE

Single occipital bone occupies posterior and inferior parts of the skull (Plate 1.17).

### ANATOMICAL POSITION

It is concave forwards and encloses the largest foramen of skull, foramen magnum, through which cranial cavity communicates with the vertebral canal. On each side of foramen magnum is the occipital condyle, which articulates with atlas vertebra.

### FEATURES

Occipital bone is divided into three parts (Plate 1.17):

1. Squamous part – expanded plate of the bone that lies behind the foramen magnum.
2. Basilar part – lies in front of foramen magnum.
3. Condylar or lateral part – on each side of foramen magnum.

### Squamous Part

Comprises two surfaces, three angles and four borders.

*Surfaces:* External convex surface and internal concave surface.

*Angles:* One superior angle and two lateral angles.

*Borders:* Two lambdoid borders in upper part and two mastoid borders in lower part.

### Basilar Part

The basilar part of occipital bone is called basiocciput. It articulates with basisphenoid to form the base of skull. It is quadrilateral in shape and comprises two surfaces and four borders.

*Surfaces* are superior and inferior.

*Borders* are anterior, posterior and two lateral, on each side.

### Condylar Part

It comprises:

- Superior surface
- Inferior surface which shows occipital condyles and hypoglossal canal.

The details can be read from descriptions of *norma occipitalis* and *posterior cranial fossa*.

## FRONTAL BONE

Frontal bone forms the forehead, most of the roof of orbit, and most of the floor of anterior cranial fossa. Its parts are squamous, orbital and nasal parts (Plate 1.18).

### ANATOMICAL POSITION

Squamous part is vertical and is convex forwards. Two orbital plates are horizontal thin plates projecting backwards. Nasal part is directed forwards and downwards.

**Plate 1.17:** Occipital bone (#: posterior condylar canal)

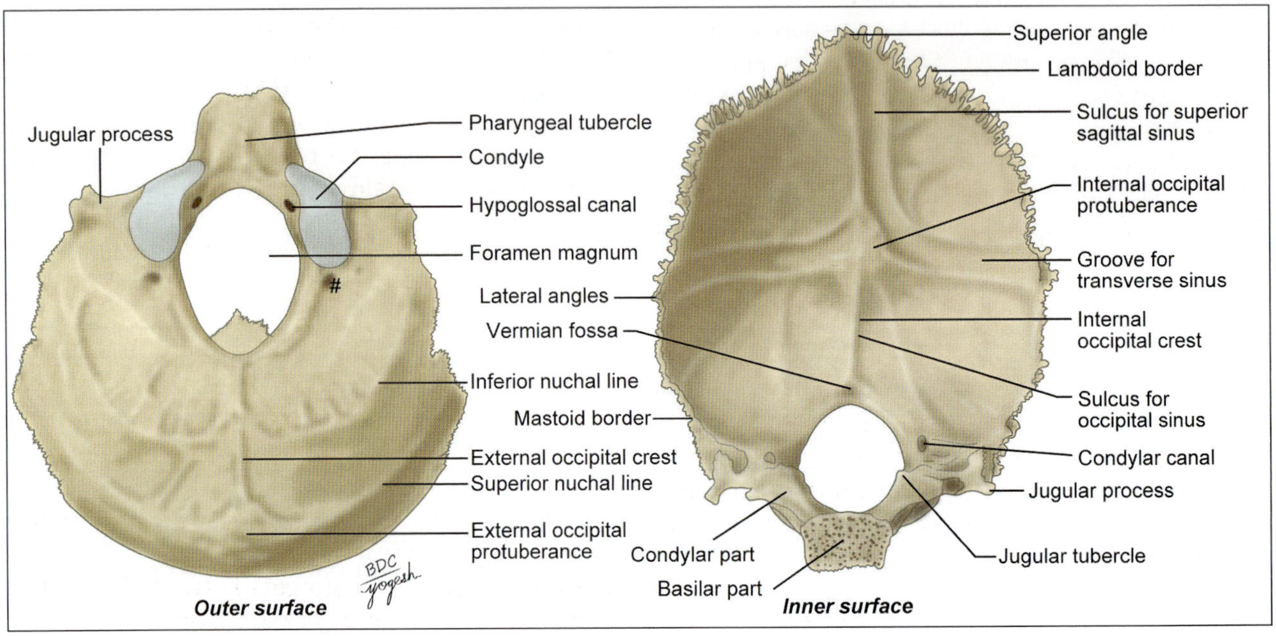


**Plate 1.18:** Frontal bone

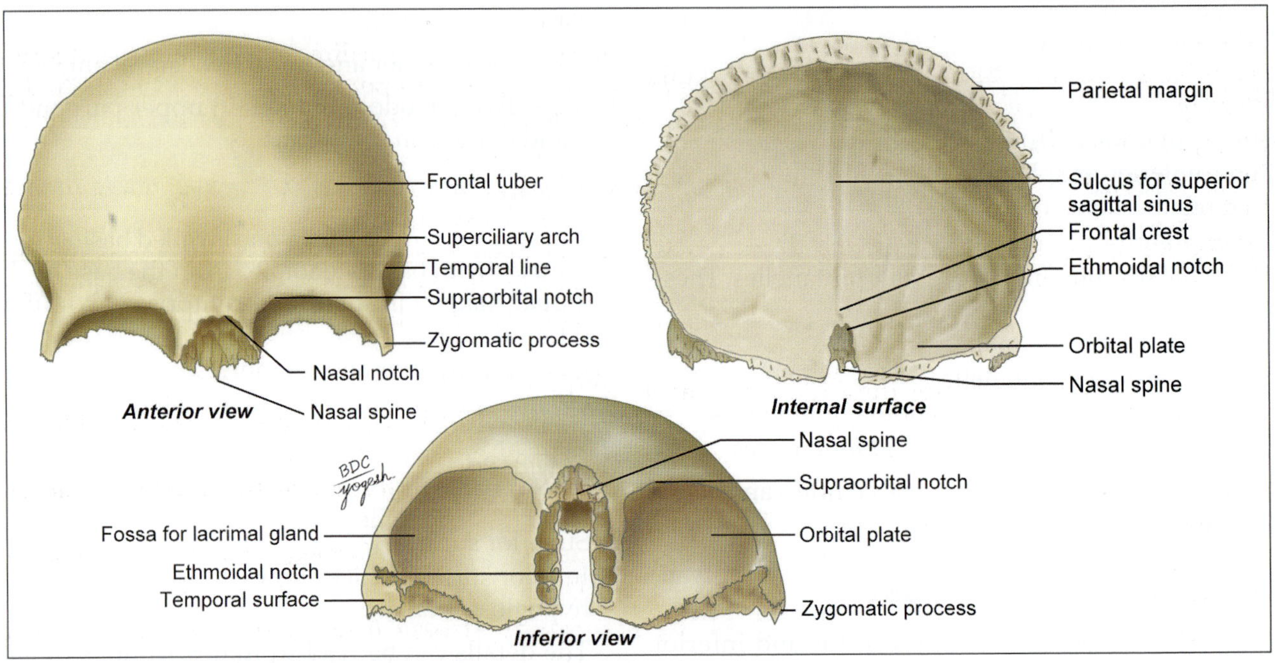


## Squamous Part

The squamous part presents two surfaces, two borders and encloses a pair of frontal air sinuses.

### Outer Surface

It is smooth and shows:

1. Frontal tuberosity
2. Superciliary arches
3. Glabella
4. Frontal air sinus is a cavity within outer and inner tables of frontal bone, divided by a bony septum into two parts
5. Metopic suture
6. Upper or parietal border: Articulates with parietal bone
7. Lower or orbital border: Free, presents supra-orbital notch foramen
8. Zygomatic process
9. Temporal line and temporal surfaces.

### Inner Surface

It is concave and presents:

1. Sagittal sulcus
2. Frontal crest

### Orbital Parts (Plates)

Orbital plates are separated from each other by a wide gap – the ethmoidal notch.

Orbital or inferior surface of the plate is smooth and presents lacrimal fossa anterolaterally and trochlear spine anteromedially.

Ethmoidal notch is occupied by cribriform plate of ethmoid bone. On each side of notch are small air spaces, which articulate with the labyrinth of ethmoid to complete ethmoidal air sinuses. At the margins are anterior and posterior ethmoidal canals.

### Nasal Part

Lies between two supraorbital margins. The margins of the nasal notch on each side articulate with nasal, frontal process of maxilla and lacrimal bones.

Details can be studied from descriptions of *norma frontalis, norma lateralis, inner aspect of skull cap and anterior cranial fossa*.

## TEMPORAL BONE

Temporal bones are situated at the sides and base of skull (Plate 1.19).

### SIDE DETERMINATION

- Plate-like squamous part is directed upwards and laterally.
- Strong zygomatic process is directed forwards.
- Petromastoid part, triangular in shape, is directed medially.
- External acoustic meatus, enclosed between squamous and tympanic parts, is directed laterally.

### FEATURES

The temporal bone consists of the following parts (Plate 1.19):

1. Squamous
2. Mastoid
3. Petrous
4. Tympanic
5. Styloid process.

### Squamous Part

It is expanded, thin, translucent portion of the bone. It shows the following features:

1. *Temporal or external surface:* It forms the greater part of the temporal fossa. It gives origin to the temporalis muscle.
2. *Groove for middle temporal vessels* is a vertical groove that ascends upward from the external acoustic meatus.
3. *Supramastoid crest* is a curved ridge that ascends upward and backward from the anterior part of the external acoustic meatus. It gives attachment to the *temporal fascia* and marks the posterior boundary of the temporal fossa.
4. *Auricularis posterior* muscle arises from the space between the supramastoid crest and the line of the squamomastoid suture.
5. *Suprameatal spine* is a bony projection on the medial side of the suprameatal triangle.
6. *Internal surface* is concave. It is marked by irregular impressions for the temporal gyri and presents grooves for the middle meningeal vessels.

### Zygomatic Process of the Temporal Bone

It forms an elongated bony process. It articulates with the temporal process of the zygomatic bone to form the *zygomatic arch*. It consists of

*Two roots: anterior and posterior*

Elongated thin anterior part.

1. *Roots of the zygomatic process* are anterior and posterior, and they converge to meet at a point to form a tubercle known as the *tubercle of the root of the zygoma*. It gives attachment to the *lateral temporomandibular ligament*.
2. At the tubercle, the process is twisted and the thin anterior part projects forward from it.
3. The *anterior root of the zygoma* projects horizontally lateralward and its inferior surface is convex and smooth. It forms a thickened bar of the bone in front of the articular fossa and is known as the *articular tubercle (eminence)*.
4. The *posterior root* is directed downward and forward. It is continuous behind with the supramastoid crest and in front with the superior border of the thin anterior part of the zygoma.
5. The thin anterior part of the zygomatic process is subcutaneous.
6. The medial surface and inferior border of zygomatic process give origin to *masseter* muscle. Its superior border gives attachment to the *temporal fascia*.

### Mandibular Fossa

It is formed partly by the squamous part and partly by the tympanic part. It consists of:

a. an *articular part* formed by the squamous part of the temporal bone, and
b. a *nonarticular part* formed by the tympanic part of the bone.

1. *Squamotympanic fissure* separates the articular part from the tympanic part medially.
2. The downturned anterolateral portion of the *tegmen tympani* projects into this fissure and subdivides it into *petrotympanic and petrosquamosal fissures*.
3. *Petrotympanic fissure* communicates with the tympanic cavity. It transmits *anterior ligament of the malleus* and *anterior tympanic branch* of the maxillary artery. It has *anterior canaliculus* for the chorda tympani nerve at its medial end. This canal transmits the *chorda tympani nerve*.

### Mastoid Part

It is thick. It presents the following features:

1. *External surface* is convex.

**Plate 1.19:** Right temporal bone

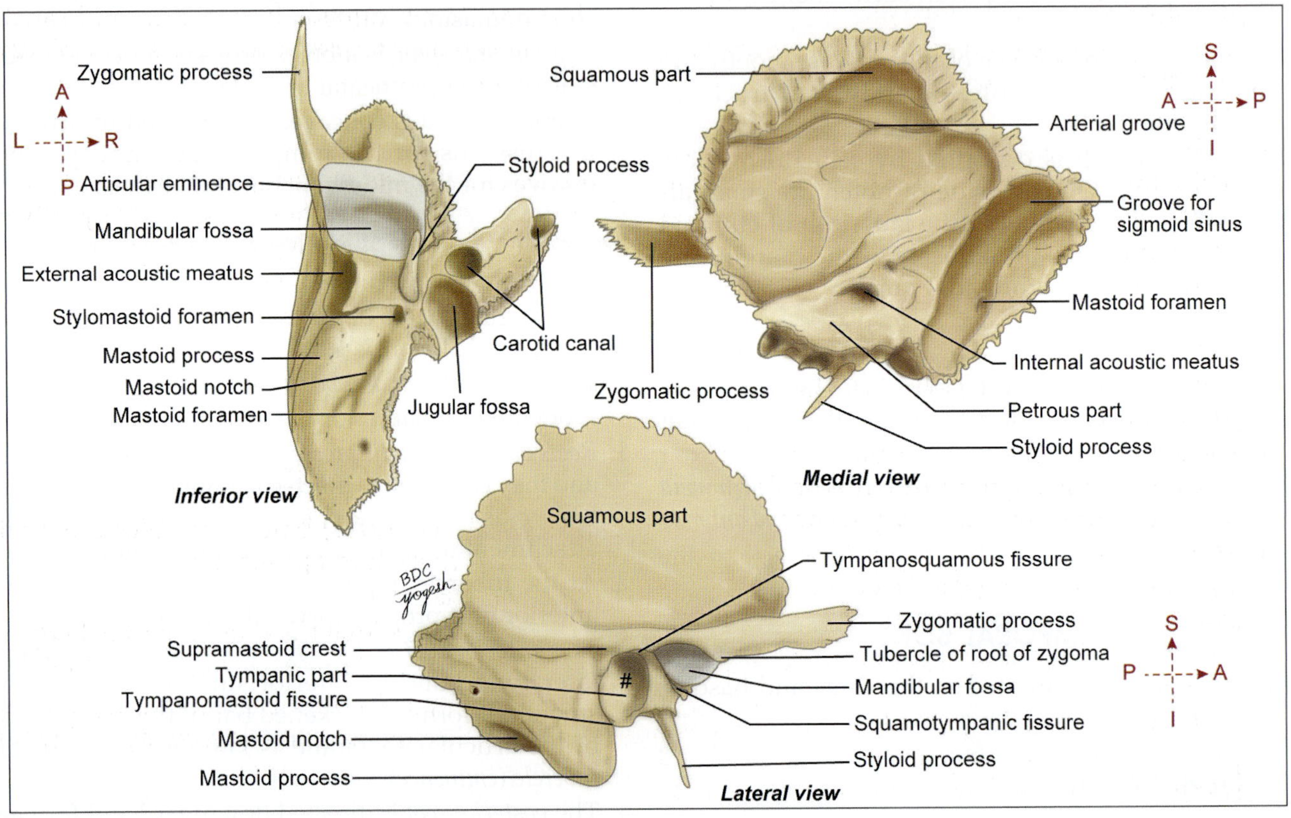


2. It forms a conical projection known as the ***mastoid process***. It gives
   i. Origin to *occipital belly of the occipitofrontalis*
   ii. Insertion to the sternocleidomastoid, splenius capitis and longissimus capitis (from above downward).
3. ***Mastoid notch*** on the medial aspect of the mastoid process gives origin to the *posterior belly of the digastric* muscle.
4. *Groove* located below the digastric lodges the *occipital artery*.
5. *Mastoid foramen* lies below the groove for the occipital artery and close to the posterior border of the mastoid process.
6. The internal surface of the mastoid part is marked by a deep curved groove for sigmoid sinus. The mastoid foramen opens into its floor.
7. **Section of the mastoid part**
   1. It contains a number of irregular *mastoid air cells*.
   2. *Mastoid or tympanic antrum*: It is a large irregular space situated at the upper and anterior portions of the mastoid part.

## Petrous Part

It forms a cylindrical process of bone. It lies between the greater wing of the sphenoid and the occipital bone at the base of the skull.

1. *Base* of the petrous part is fused with the squamous and the mastoid parts, and the apex articulates with the petrosal process of the sphenoid. It is directed upward, forward and medially.
2. *Anterior surface* of the petrous part lies in the middle cranial fossa and is marked by impressions for the temporal lobe of the brain. Immediately behind the apex, this surface presents a depression known as the *trigeminal impression*. It lodges the *trigeminal ganglion*. Behind the trigeminal impression, there is an eminence known as the *arcuate eminence*. It is formed by the *superior semicircular canal* of the internal ear.
3. *Tegmen tympani*
   - On the lateral side of the anterior surface, there is a thin plate of bone called the *tegmen tympani*. It forms the roof of the tympanic antrum, tympanic cavity and the canals for the tensor tympani and the auditory tube.
   - Laterally, the tegmen tympani is bend itself and descends downward on the medial side of the squamous part and forms the lateral wall of the auditory tube.
   - Its anterolateral portion projects into the squamotympanic fissure.
   - On the anterior part of the tegmen tympani, there is a faint groove that leads posteriorly into an *opening for the greater superficial petrosal nerve*.
   - Lateral to this opening, there is another *opening for the lesser petrosal nerve*.
   - *Posterior surface* forms the anterior part of the posterior cranial fossa.
4. *Internal acoustic meatus* is a circular aperture. It extends laterally for about 1 cm.

5. Bottom of the internal auditory meatus is closed by *perforated plate* of bone for the transmission of nerve rootlets of vestibulocochlear nerve.
6. *Inferior surface* of the petrous part is faced downward. Close to the apex, it gives origin to the levator veli palatini muscle.
   - It shows a circular opening of the *carotid canal*, which transmits the *internal carotid artery* with its plexus of sympathetic nerves.
   - Behind the carotid opening there is *jugular fossa*, which lodges the *superior bulb of the internal jugular vein*.
   - At the jugular fossa, there is *tympanic canaliculus* that transmits the *tympanic branch of the glossopharyngeal nerve*.
   - *Jugular surface*: It is a small quadrilateral articular area behind the jugular fossa. It articulates with the jugular process of the occipital bone.
   - *Mastoid canaliculus*: It a small foramen on the lateral wall of the jugular fossa. It transmits the *auricular branch of the vagus nerve*.
   - *Styloid process*: It is a slender process that projects downward.
   - *Stylomastoid foramen*: It lies behind the styloid process. It gives passage to the *facial nerve* and *stylomastoid branch of the posterior auricular artery*.
7. *Superior border* of the petrous part presents a narrow *groove for the superior petrosal sinus* and the margins of the groove give attachment to the *tentorium cerebelli*.
8. *Posterior border* and basilar part of the occipital bone forms a *groove for the inferior petrosal sinus*.
9. *Anterior border* is divided into two parts, a lateral and a medial part; the lateral part joins with the squamous part at the petrosquamosal suture and its medial part articulates with the greater wing of the sphenoid.

### Tympanic Part

It is a plate of bone that lies between the squamous and the mastoid parts. In front, it articulates with the squamous part at the *squamotympanic fissure*, and behind, with the mastoid process at the *tympanomastoid fissure*. The tympanomastoid fissure transmits the *auricular branch of the vagus nerve*. Internally, it is fused with the petrous part of the temporal bone.

It presents the following features:

1. *Anterior surface* forms the posterior nonarticular part of the mandibular fossa and lodges a portion of the parotid gland.
2. *Posterior surface* is concave. It forms the anterior and part of the posterior wall and the floor of the external acoustic meatus. The medial part of this surface has a circular *tympanic sulcus*, which gives attachment to the *tympanic membrane*.
3. *Lateral margin* forms the margin of the bony external ear. It gives attachment to the cartilaginous part of the external ear.
4. *Superior border* articulates with the squamous part medially at the *squamotympanic fissure*.
5. *Lower border* extends from the carotid canal to the styloid process. It forms a *sheath of styloid process*.

### Styloid Process

Styloid (Greek *pillar form*) process is long pointed process directed downwards, forwards and medially between parotid gland and internal jugular vein (Plate 1.19).

- Its base is related to facial nerve
- Its apex is crossed by external carotid artery
- It gives attachment to three muscles and two ligaments.

## SPHENOID BONE

Sphenoid (Greek *wedge*) bone resembles a bat with outstretched wings. It comprises (Plate 1.20):

- A body in the centre.
- Two lesser wings from the anterior part of body.
- Two greater wings from the lateral part of body.
- Two pterygoid (wing-like) processes, directed downwards from the junction of body and greater wings.

### BODY OF SPHENOID

It comprises six surfaces and encloses a pair of sphenoidal air sinuses.

#### Superior or Cerebral Surface

It articulates with ethmoid bone anteriorly and basilar part of occipital bone posteriorly. It shows:

1. Jugum sphenoidale
2. Sulcus chiasmaticus
3. Tuberculum sellae
4. Sella turcica
5. Dorsum sellae
6. Clivus

#### Inferior Surface

1. Rostrum of sphenoid
2. Sphenoid conchae
3. Vaginal processes of medial pterygoid plate.

#### Anterior Surface

Sphenoidal crest articulates with perpendicular plate of ethmoid to form a small part of septum of nose.

Opening of sphenoidal air sinus is seen. Sphenoidal conchae close the sphenoid air sinuses leaving the openings. Each half of anterior surface has two parts—superolateral and inferomedial.

The superolateral depression articulates with labyrinth of ethmoid to complete the posterior ethmoidal air sinuses. The inferomedial smooth triangular area forms the posterior part of the root of the nose.

#### Posterior Surface

It articulates with basilar part of occipital bone.

#### Lateral Surfaces

Carotid sulcus, a broad groove curved like letter 'f' for lodging cavernous sinus and internal carotid artery. Below the sulcus, it articulates with greater wing of sphenoid laterally and with pterygoid process, which is directed downwards.

#### Sphenoidal Air Sinuses

These are asymmetrical air sinuses in the body of sphenoid, and are closed by sphenoidal conchae. The sinus opens into the lateral wall of nose in the sphenoethmoidal recess above the superior concha.

### GREATER WINGS

These are two strong processes that curve laterally and upwards from the sides of the body. It has three surfaces.

#### Superior or Cerebral Surface

It forms the floor of middle cranial fossa and presents from before backwards:

1. Foramen rotundum
2. Foramen ovale
3. Emissary sphenoidale foramen
4. Foramen spinosum.

#### Lateral Surface

A horizontal ridge, the infratemporal crest divides this surface into upper or temporal surface and a lower or infratemporal surface. It is pierced by foramen ovale and foramen spinosum. Its posterior part presents spine of sphenoid.

#### Orbital Surface

Forms the posterior wall of the lateral wall of orbit. Its medial border bears a small tubercle for attachment of a common tendinous ring for the origin of recti muscles of the eyeball. Below the medial end of superior orbital fissure, the grooved area forms the posterior wall of the pterygopalatine fossa and is pierced by foramen rotundum. Borders are surrounding the greater wing of sphenoid.

### LESSER WINGS

Lesser wings are two triangular plates projecting laterally from the anterosuperior part of the body. It comprises:

- A base forming medial end of the wing. It is connected to the body by two roots which enclose the optic canal.
- Tip forms the lateral end of the wing.
- Superior surface forming floor of anterior cranial fossa.
- Inferior surface forming upper boundary of superior orbital fissure.
- Anterior border articulates with the posterior border of orbital plate of frontal bone.
- Posterior border is free and projects into the stem of lateral sulcus of brain. Medially, it terminates into the anterior clinoid process.

#### Superior Orbital Fissure

It is a triangular gap through which middle cranial fossa communicates with the orbit. The structures passing through it are put in list of foramina and structures passing through them.

### PTERYGOID PROCESSES

One pterygoid (Greek *wing*) process on each side projects downwards from the junction of the body with the greater wing of sphenoid (Plate 1.20).

Each pterygoid process divides inferiorly into the medial and lateral pterygoid plates. The plates are fused together in their upper parts, but are separated in their lower parts by the pterygoid fissure. Posteriorly, the pterygoid plates enclose a 'V-shaped interval', the pterygoid fossa. The medial pterygoid plate in its upper part presents a scaphoid fossa. *Refer* to *norma basalis* for medial and lateral pterygoid plates

## ETHMOID BONE

Ethmoid (Greek *sieve*) is a very light cuboidal bone situated in the anterior base of cranial cavity between the two orbits (Plate 1.21).

It forms:

1. Part of nasal septum
2. Part of medial wall of orbit
3. Lateral walls of the nasal cavity

Ethmoid bone comprises:

1. Cribriform plate
2. Perpendicular plate
3. A pair of labyrinth

### CRIBRIFORM PLATE

It is a horizontal perforated bony lamina, occupying ethmoidal notch of frontal bone. It contains foramina for olfactory nerve rootlets.

#### Crista Galli

Crista galli is a median, tooth-like upward projection in the floor of anterior cranial fossa. Foramen transmitting anterior ethmoidal nerve to nasal cavity is situated by the side of crista galli.

### PERPENDICULAR PLATE

It is a thin lamina projecting downwards from the undersurface of the cribriform plate, forming upper part of nasal septum.

**Plate 1.20:** Sphenoid bone

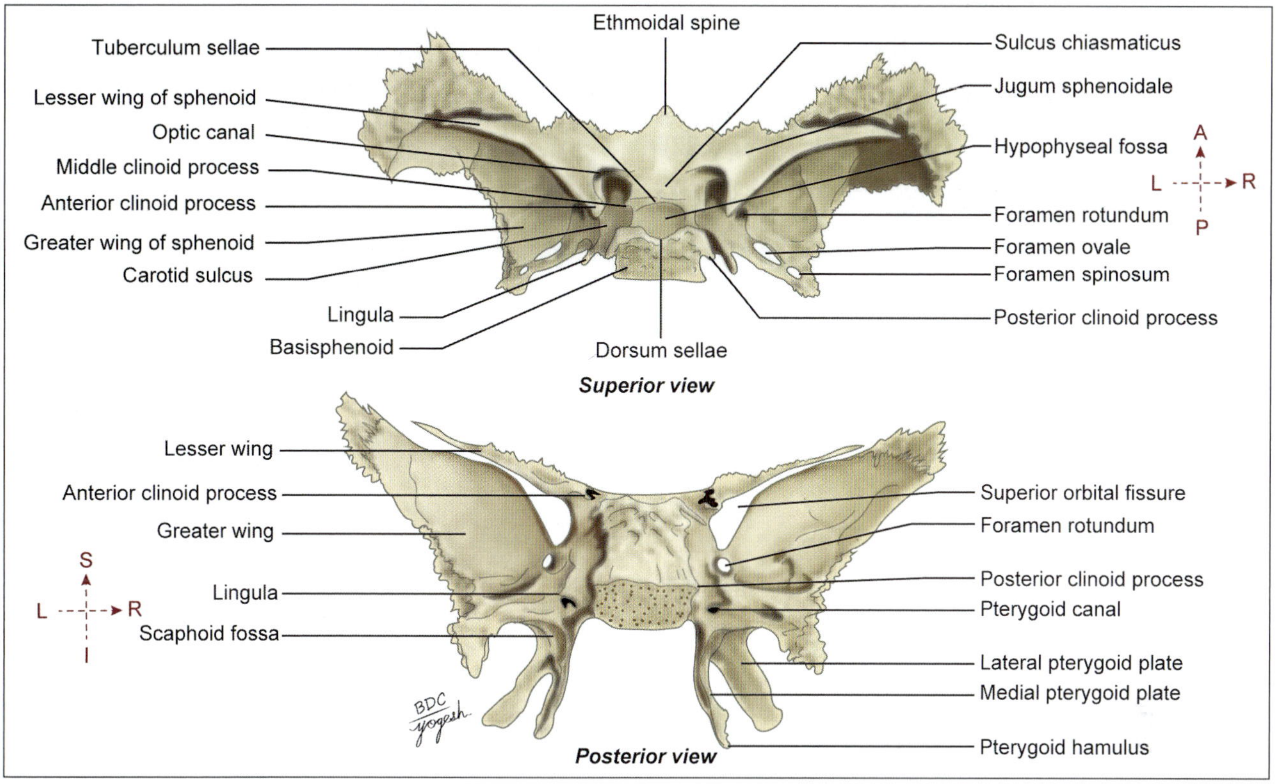


**Plate 1.21:** Right ethmoid bone

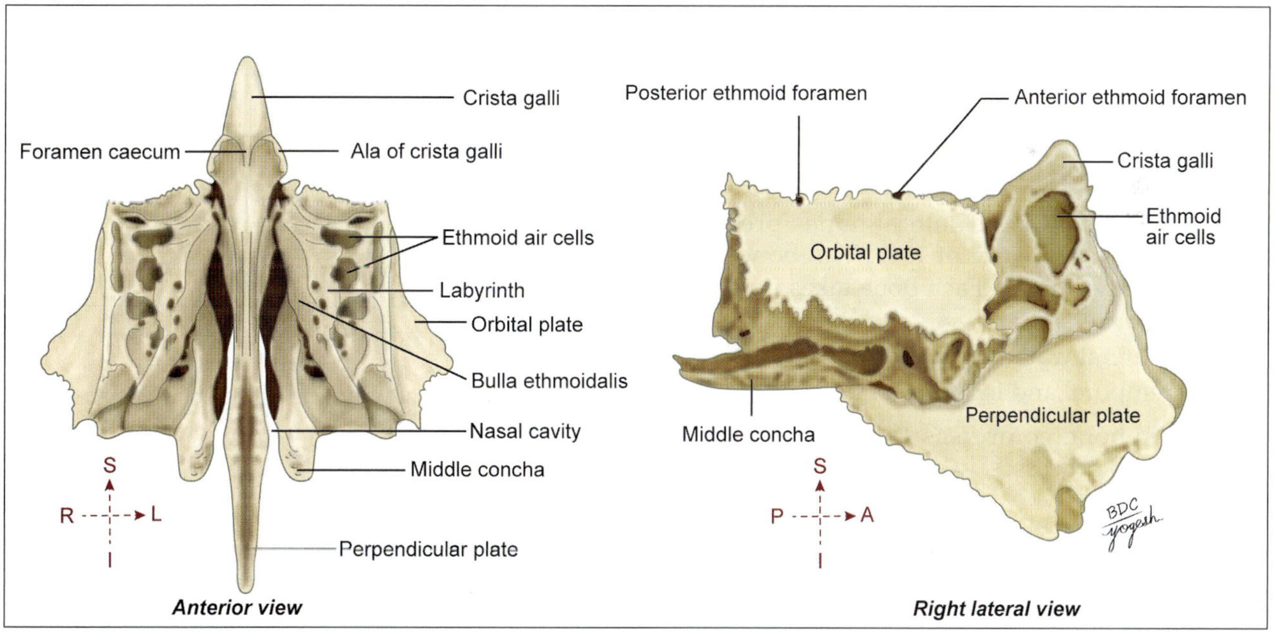


## LABYRINTHS

These are two light cubical masses situated on each side of the perpendicular plate, suspended from the undersurface of the cribriform plate (Plate 1.21). Each labyrinth also encloses large number of 'air cells' arranged in three groups—the anterior, middle and posterior ethmoidal air sinuses. Its surfaces are:

- Anterior surface articulates with frontal process of maxilla to complete anterior ethmoidal air cells.
- Posterior surface articulates with sphenoidal concha to complete posterior ethmoidal air cells.
- Superior surface articulates with orbital plate of frontal bone.
- Inferior surface articulates with nasal surface of maxilla.
- Lateral surface forms medial wall of orbit.
- Medial surface presents small superior nasal concha, middle nasal concha, superior meatus below superior concha and middle meatus below middle concha.

## VOMER

Vomer (Latin *plough share*) is a single thin, flat bone forming posteroinferior part of the nasal septum. It comprises:

- Right and left surfaces marked by nasopalatine nerves which course downwards and forwards (Plate 1.22).
- Superior border splits into two alae with a groove occupied by rostrum of sphenoid.
- Inferior border articulates with nasal crests of maxillae and palatine bones.
- Anterior, longest border, articulates with perpendicular plate of ethmoid above and with septal cartilage below.
- Posterior border is free and separates the two posterior nasal openings.

**Plate 1.22:** Right vomer

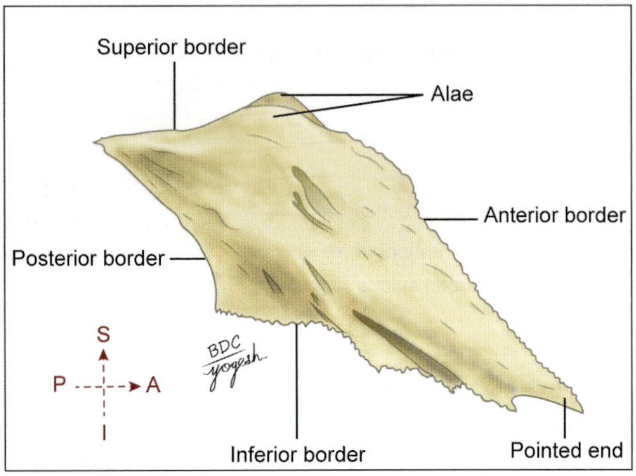


## INFERIOR NASAL CONCHAE

The inferior nasal conchae are two curved bony laminae, these are horizontally placed in the lower part of lateral walls of the nose. Between this concha and floor of the nose lies the inferior meatus of the nose. It comprises two surfaces, two borders and two ends.

- Medial convex surface is marked by vascular grooves.
- Lateral concave surface forms the medial wall of inferior meatus of the nose.
- Superior border is irregular and articulates with lacrimal, maxilla, ethmoid and palatine bones (Plate 1.23).
- Inferior border is free, thick and spongy.
- Posterior end is more pointed than the anterior end.

**Plate 1.23:** Right inferior nasal concha

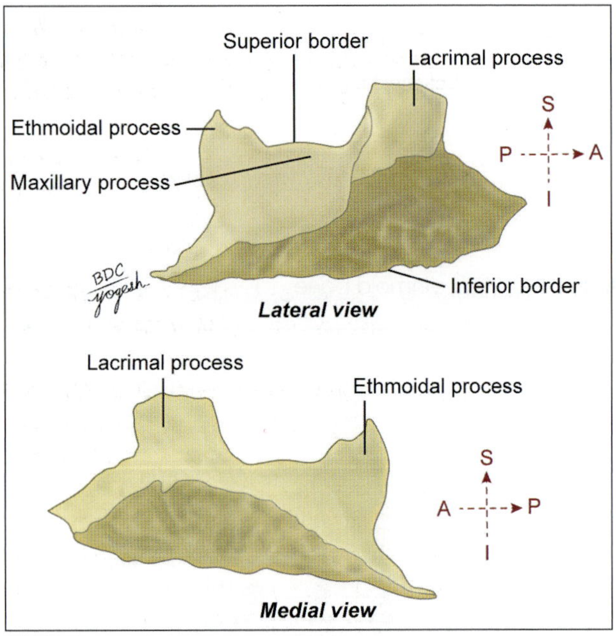


## ZYGOMATIC BONES

These are two small quadrilateral bones present in the upper and lateral part of face. The bone forms prominence of the cheeks. Each bone takes part in the formation of (Plate 1.24):

- Floor and lateral wall of the orbit
- Walls of temporal and infraorbital fossae.

Zygomatic bone comprises three surfaces, four borders and two processes.

### Surfaces

1. Lateral surface presenting zygomaticofacial foramen.
2. Temporal surface is smooth and concave and presents zygomaticotemporal foramen.
3. Orbital surface is also smooth and concave with one or two zygomatico-orbital foramen on this surface and this leads to zygomaticofacial and zygomaticotemporal foramina.

### Borders

1. Anterosuperior or orbital
2. Anteroinferior or maxillary
3. Posterosuperior or temporal border
4. Posteroinferior border

### Processes

1. Frontal process, which is directed upwards.
2. Temporal process, which is directed backwards.

## NASAL BONES

Nasal bones are two small oblong bones, which form the bridge of the nerve.

Each nasal bone has two surfaces and four borders (Plate 1.25).

### Surfaces

1. The outer surface is convex from side-to-side.
2. The inner surface is concave from side-to-side and is traversed by a vertical groove for anterior ethmoidal nerve.

### Borders

1. Superior border is thick and serrated and articulates with nasal part of frontal bone.

**Plate 1.24:** Right zygomatic bone

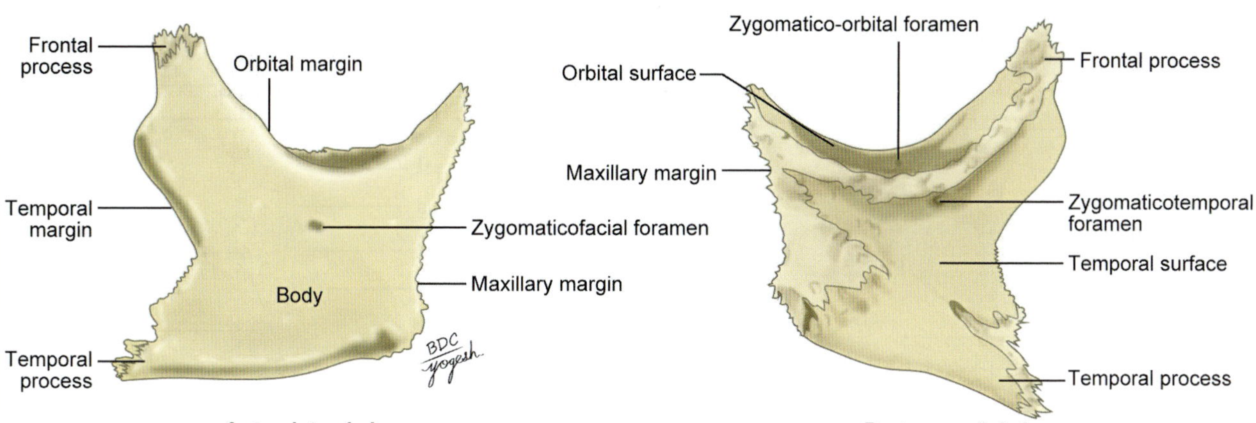


***Anterolateral view*** ***Posteromedial view***

**Plate 1.25:** Nasal bones

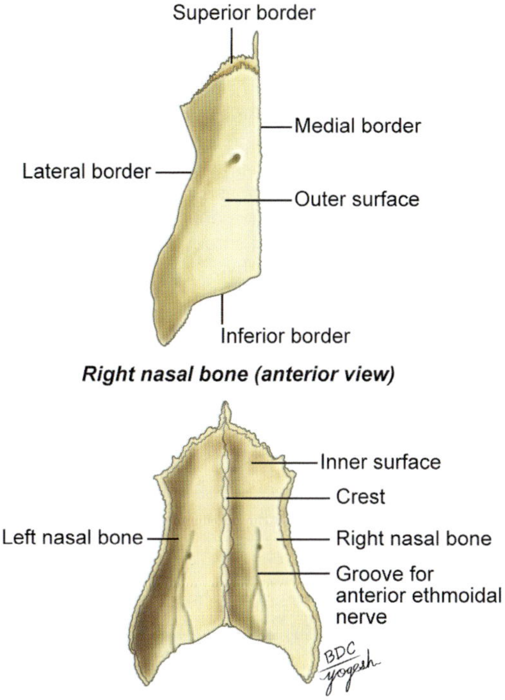


***Right nasal bone (anterior view)***

***Nasal bones (posterior view)***

2. Inferior border is thin and notched and articulates with superior nasal cartilage.
3. Medial border articulates with opposite nasal bone.
4. Lateral border articulates with frontal process of maxilla.

## LACRIMAL BONES

Lacrimal bones are extremely delicate and smallest of the skull bones. These form the anterior part of the medial part of the orbit. Each lacrimal bone comprises two surfaces and four borders (Plate 1.26)

### Surfaces

1. Lateral or orbital surface is divided by posterior lacrimal crest into anterior and posterior parts. The anterior grooved part forms posterior half of the floor of lacrimal groove for lacrimal sac. The posterior smooth part forms part of medial wall of orbit.

**Plate 1.26:** Right lacrimal bone (lateral view)

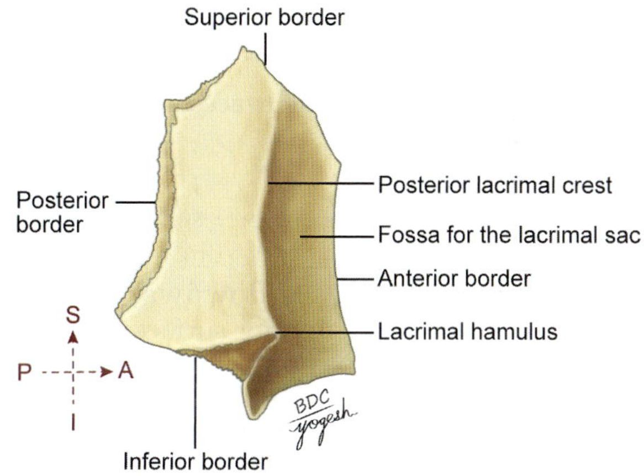


2. Medial or nasal surface forms a part of middle meatus of the nose.

### Borders

1. Anterior border articulates with frontal process of maxilla.
2. Posterior border with orbital plate of ethmoid.
3. Superior border with frontal bone.
4. Inferior border with orbital surface of maxilla.

## PALATINE BONES

Palatine bones are two L-shaped bones present in the posterior part of nasal cavity. Each bone forms:

- Lateral wall and floor of nasal cavity (Plate 1.27).
- Roof of mouth cavity
- Floor of the orbit
- Parts of pterygopalatine fossa.

Each palatine bone has two plates and three processes.

**Plate 1.27:** Right palatine bone

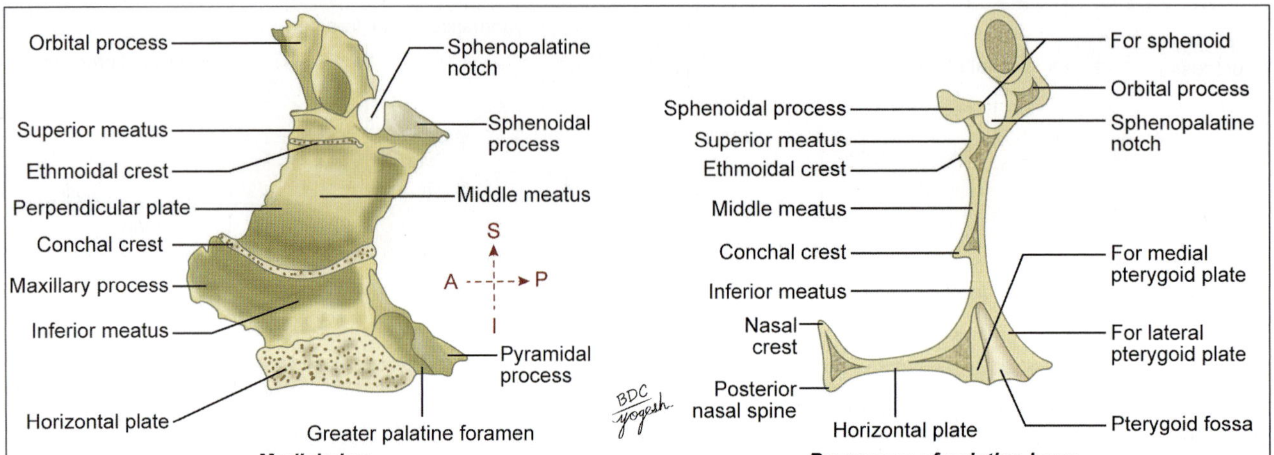


***Medial view*** | ***Processes of palatine bone***

## Plates

1. Horizontal plate forms posterior one-fourth part of bony palate. It has two surfaces and four borders.
2. Perpendicular plate of palatine bone is oblong in shape and comprises two surfaces and four borders *(refer to norma basalis)*.

## Processes

### Pyramidal

Pyramidal process projects downwards from the junction of two plates. Its inferior surface is pierced by lesser palatine foramina.

### Orbital

Orbital process projects upwards and laterally from the perpendicular plate. Its orbital surface is triangular and forms the posterior part of the floor of the orbit.

### Sphenoidal

Sphenoidal process projects upwards and medially from the perpendicular plate. Its lateral surface articulates with medial pterygoid plate.

**Flowchart 1.15:** Hyoid bone

***Hyoid bone***
U-shaped bone

| ***Body*** | ***2 Greater cornua*** | ***2 Lesser cornua*** |
|---|---|---|
| Quadrilateral<br>Anterior surface<br>- Geniohyoid<br>- Mylohyoid<br>- Hyoglossus<br>Posterior surface<br>- Concave<br>Upper border<br>- Genioglossus<br>- Thyrohyoid membrane<br>Lower border<br>- Pretracheal fascia<br>- Sternohyoid<br>- SBOH | Flattened bars<br>Medial end<br>- Hyoglossus<br>- Middle constrictor<br>Medial border<br>- Thyrohyoid membrane<br>- Stylohyoid<br>Lateral border<br>- Thyrohyoid | Small conical piece of bone<br>Tip:<br>- Stylohyoid ligament<br>Middle constrictor |

(SBOH: Superior belly of omohyoid)

## HYOID BONE

The hyoid (Greek *U-shaped*) bone is U-shaped. It is situated in the anterior midline of the neck between the chin and the thyroid cartilage (Plate 1.28, Flowchart 1.15).

At rest, it lies at the level of the 3rd cervical vertebra behind and the base of the mandible in front.

It is kept suspended in position by muscles and ligaments.

The hyoid bone provides attachment to the muscles of the floor of the mouth and to the tongue above, to the larynx below and to the epiglottis and pharynx behind (Fig. 1.27).

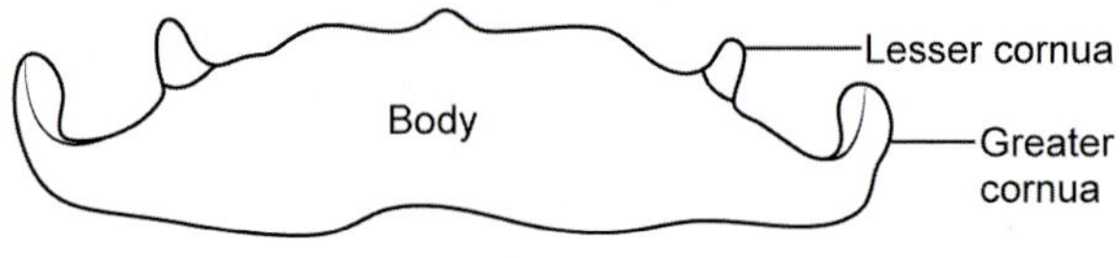


***Anterior view***

**Fig. 1.27:** Features of hyoid bone

### Parts of Hyoid Bone

The hyoid bone consists of the following parts (Plate 1.28, Fig. 1.27):

1. Body
2. Pair of greater cornua
3. Pair of lesser cornua

### Body

It has two surfaces—anterior and posterior, and two borders—upper and lower.

The *anterior surface* is convex and is directed forwards and upwards. It is often divided by a median ridge into two lateral halves.

The *posterior surface* is concave and is directed backwards and downwards.

Each lateral end of the body is continuous posteriorly with the greater horn or cornua. However, till middle life, the connection between the body and greater cornua is fibrous.

**Plate 1.28:** Hyoid bone

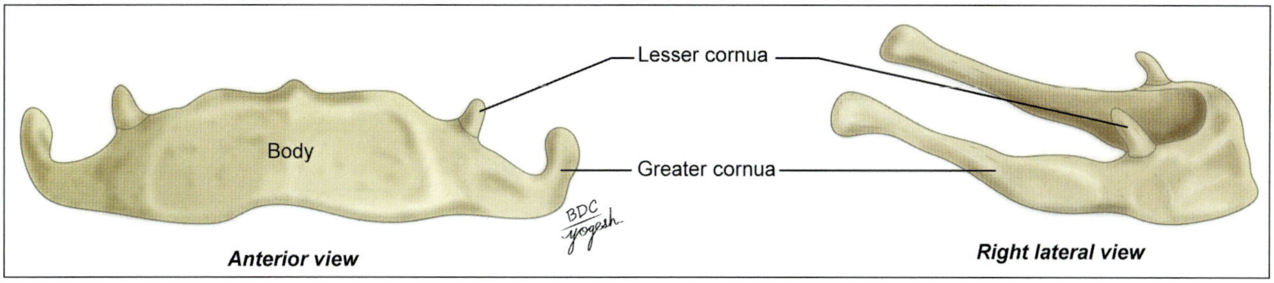


### Greater Cornua

These are flattened from above downwards. Each cornua tapers posteriorly but ends in a tubercle. It has two surfaces—upper and lower, two borders—medial and lateral and a tubercle.

### Lesser Cornua

These are small conical pieces of bone that project upwards from the junction of the body and greater cornua. The lesser cornua are connected to the body by fibrous tissue. Occasionally, they are connected to the greater cornua by synovial joints, which usually persist throughout life but may get ankylosed.

## ATTACHMENTS ON THE HYOID BONE

1. Anterior surface of the body provides insertion to the geniohyoid and mylohyoid muscles and gives origin to a part of the hyoglossus, which extends to the greater cornua (Fig. 1.28).
2. *Upper border* of the body provides insertion to the lower fibres of the genioglossi and attachment to the thyrohyoid membrane.
3. *Lower border* of the body provides attachment to the pretracheal fascia. In front of the fascia, the *sternohyoid* is inserted medially and the superior belly of omohyoid laterally.
4. Below the omohyoid, there is the linear attachment of the thyrohyoid, extending back to the lower border of the greater cornua.
5. *Medial border* of the greater cornua provides attachment to the thyrohyoid membrane, two slips each of stylohyoid muscle and digastric pulley.
6. *Lateral border* of the greater cornua provides insertion to the thyrohyoid muscle anteriorly. The investing fascia is attached throughout its length.
7. The lesser cornua provides attachment to the stylohyoid ligament at its tip. The middle constrictor muscle arises from its posterolateral aspect extending onto the greater cornua.

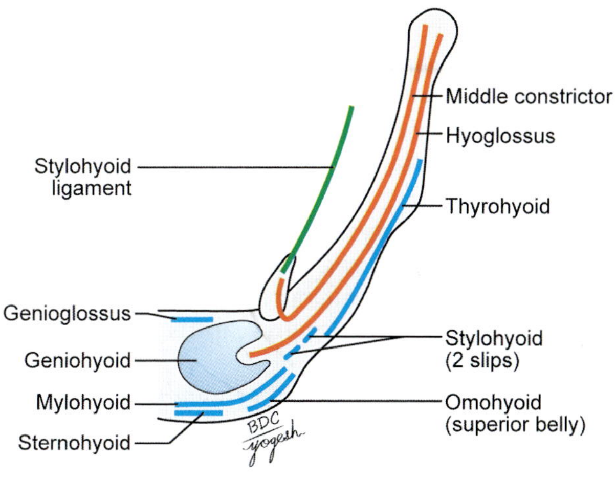


**Fig. 1.28:** Attachments of the hyoid bone

## DEVELOPMENT

Upper part of body and lesser cornua develop from 2nd branchial arch, while lower part of body and greater cornua develop from the 3rd arch.

### CLINICAL ANATOMY

- Hyoid fractures are common in throttling and strangulation.
- Palpation of greater cornua of hyoid bone: It can be palpated in the relaxed neck, at the anterior border of sternocleidomastoid muscle, midway between the mastoid process and the laryngeal prominence.

*Competency:*

**AN26.5** Describe features of typical and atypical cervical vertebrae (atlas and axis).

# CERVICAL VERTEBRAE

## IDENTIFICATION

The cervical vertebrae are identified by the presence of foramina transversaria.

There are seven cervical vertebrae, out of which the 3rd to 6th are ***typical***, while the 1st, 2nd and 7th are ***atypical*** (Plate 1.29).

## TYPICAL CERVICAL VERTEBRAE

### Body

1. The body is *small* and *broader* from side-to-side than from before backwards.

**Plate 1.29:** Articulated cervical vertebrae (right lateral view)

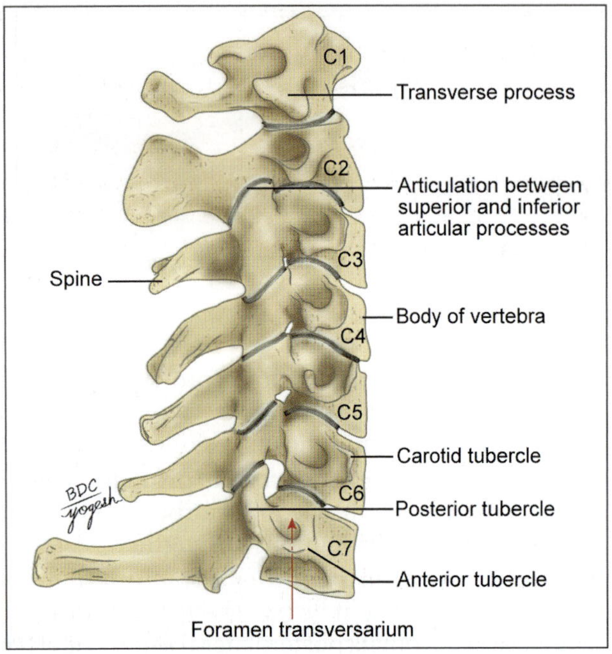


2. Its *superior surface* is concave transversely with upward projecting lips on each side. The anterior border of this surface may be bevelled.
3. The *inferior surface* is saddle-shaped, being convex from side-to-side and concave from before backwards. The lateral borders are bevelled and form synovial joints with the projecting lips of the next lower vertebra. The anterior border projects downwards and may hide the intervertebral disc.
4. The *anterior and posterior surfaces* resemble those of other vertebrae (Plate 1.30, Fig. 1.29, Flowchart 1.16).

## Vertebral Foramen

Vertebral foramen is larger than the body. It is triangular in shape because the pedicles are directed backwards and laterally.

## Vertebral Arch

1. ***Pedicles*** are directed backwards and laterally. The superior and inferior vertebral notches are of equal size.
2. ***Laminae*** are relatively long and narrow, being thinner above than below.
3. The *superior and inferior articular processes* form articular pillars, which project laterally at the junction of pedicle and the lamina. The superior articular facets are flat. They are directed backwards and upwards. The inferior articular facets are also flat but are directed forwards and downwards.
4. The ***transverse processes*** are pierced by foramina transversaria. Each process has *anterior* and *posterior roots*, which end in tubercles joined by the *costotransverse bar*.

   *Note*: The ***costal element*** is represented by the *anterior root, anterior tubercle, the costotransverse bar and the posterior tubercle*. Posterior root represents the transverse process.

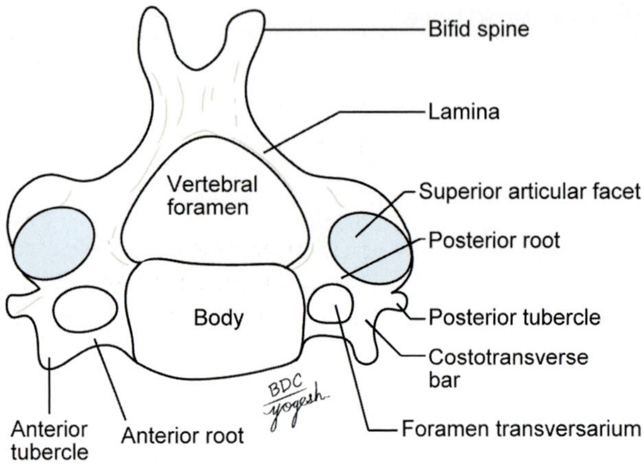


**Fig. 1.29:** Typical cervical vertebra seen from above

**Flowchart 1.16:** Typical cervical vertebra

***Typical cervical vertebra***
3rd to 6th vertebre

***Body***
Broader from side-to-side
Superior surface
- Concave with upward projecting lateral lips
Inferior surface
- Beveled lateral margins
Anterior and posterior surfaces
- Flat

***Vertebral foramen***
- Large, triangular
***Pedicles***
- Superior and inferior vertebral notches
***Laminae***
- Longer, thinner
***Spinous process***
- Bifid

***Articular facets***
Superior: Directed upward and backward
Inferior: Directed downward and forward
***Transverse process***
- Anterior and posterior tubercles
- Costotransverse bar

***Foramen transversarium:*** Vertebral artery and vein, branches of inferior cervical sympathetic ganglion

The anterior tubercle of the 6th cervical vertebra is large and is called the ***carotid tubercle*** because the common carotid artery can be compressed against it.

5. ***Spine*** is short and bifid. The notch is filled up by the ligamentum nuchae.

## Attachments and Relations

1. The anterior and posterior longitudinal ligaments are attached to the upper and lower borders of the body in front and behind, respectively. On each side of the anterior longitudinal ligament, the vertical part of the longus colli is attached to the anterior surface. The posterior surface has two or more foramina for passage of *basivertebral veins*.
2. The upper borders and lower parts of the anterior surfaces of the laminae provide attachment to the ligamenta flava.
3. The *foramen transversarium* transmits the *vertebral artery*, the *vertebral veins* and a *branch from the inferior cervical ganglion*. The *anterior tubercles* give origin to the scalenus anterior, the longus capitis and the oblique part of the longus colli.
4. The *costotransverse bars* are grooved by the *anterior primary rami* of the corresponding cervical nerves.
5. The *posterior tubercles* give origin to the scalenus medius, scalenus posterior, levator scapulae. The

Plate 1.30: Typical cervical vertebra (4th cervical vertebra)

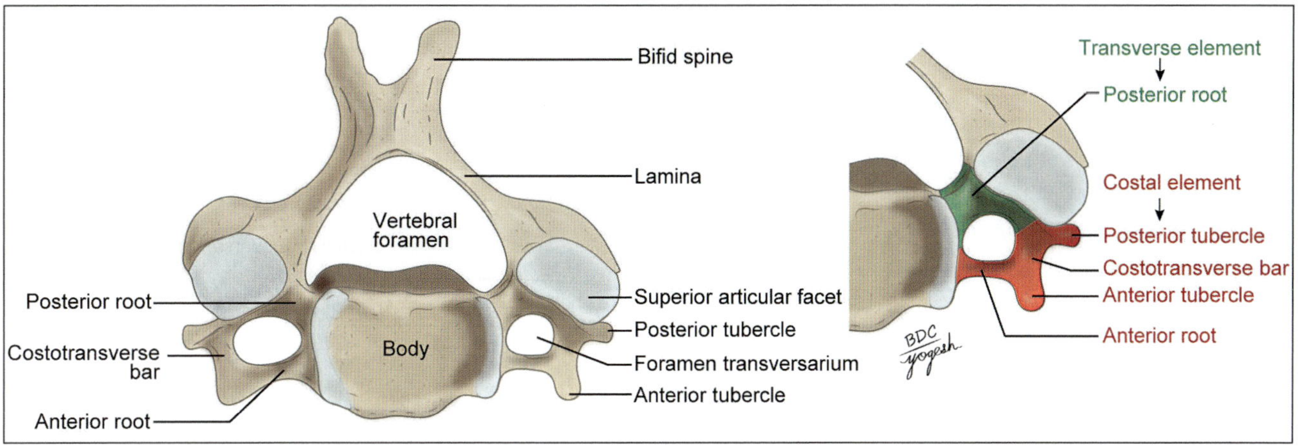


splenius cervicis, the longissimus cervicis and the iliocostalis cervicis are inserted into posterior tubercles.

6. The spine gives attachments to the deep muscles of the back of the neck—spinalis cervicis, semispinalis cervicis and thoracis and multifidus.

## OSSIFICATION

A typical cervical vertebra ossifies from three primary and six secondary centres.

There is one *primary centre* for each half of the neural arch during 9 to 10 weeks of foetal life and one for the *centrum* in 3 to 4 months of foetal life. The two halves of the neural arch fuse posteriorly with each other during the 1st year. Synostosis at the neurocentral synchondrosis occurs during the 3rd year.

The *secondary centres, two* for the annular epiphyseal discs for the peripheral parts of the upper and lower surfaces of the body, *two* for the tips of the transverse processes and *two* for the bifid spine, appear during puberty and fuse with the rest of the vertebrae by 25 years.

## FIRST CERVICAL VERTEBRA

It is called the ***atlas*** (Tiltan, who supported the heaven).

It can be identified by the following features:

1. It is ring-shaped. It has neither a body nor a spine (Plate 1.31, Figs 1.30 and 1.31, Flowchart 1.17).
2. The atlas has a short anterior arch, a long posterior arch, right and left lateral masses and transverse processes.
3. ***Anterior arch*** is marked by a median *anterior tubercle* on its anterior aspect. Its posterior surface bears an *oval facet* that articulates with the *dens.*
4. ***Posterior arch*** forms about 2/5th of the ring and is much longer than the anterior arch. Its posterior surface is marked by a median posterior tubercle. The upper surface of the arch is marked behind the lateral mass by a *groove*. Each *lateral mass* shows the following important features.

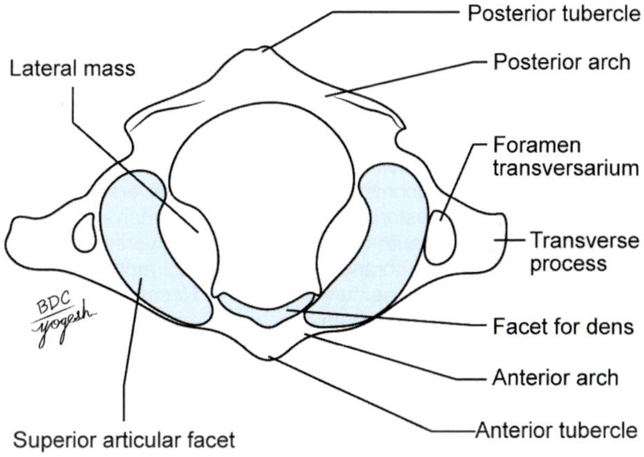


Fig. 1.30: Atlas vertebra

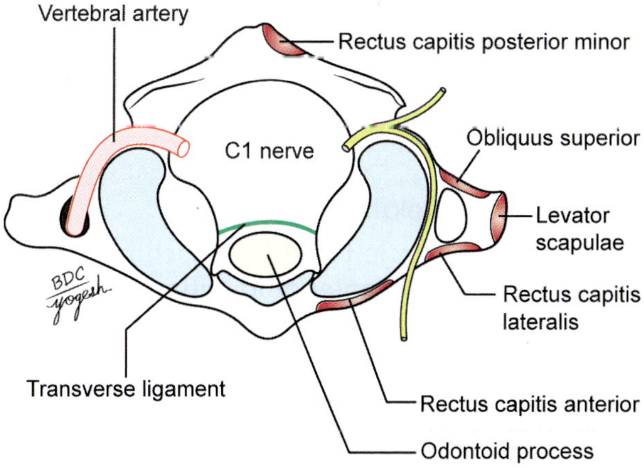


Fig. 1.31: Relations of atlas vertebra

a. Its upper surface bears the *superior articular facet.* This facet is elongated (forwards and medially), concave and is directed upwards and medially. It articulates with the corresponding condyle of the occipital bone to form an atlanto-occipital joint.

b. The lower surface is marked by the *inferior articular facet*. This facet is nearly circular, more or less flat and is directed downwards, medially and backwards. It articulates with

**Plate 1.31:** Atlas vertebra

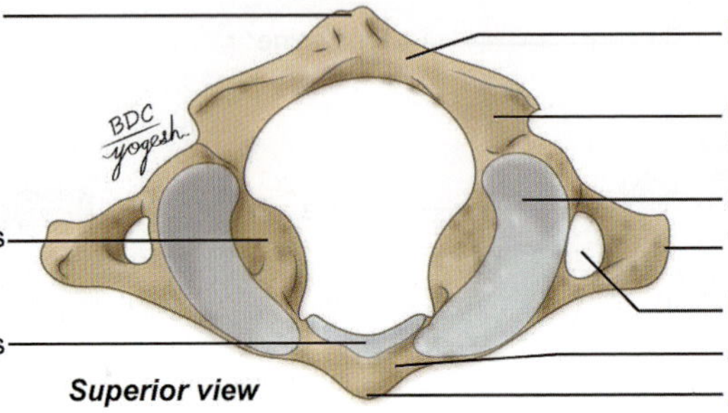


**Flowchart 1.17:** 1st cervical vertebra

***1st cervical vertebra***

Atlas, ring-like, no body, no spine

***Anterior arch***
Convex anteriorly
Anterior tubercle
Facet for odontoid process
Attachments
- Anterior atlanto-occipital membrane
- Anterior longitudinal ligament

***Posterior arch***
Rod-like
Groove on upper surface lodges vertebral artery and C1 spinal nerve
Attachments
- Posterior atlanto-occipital membrane
- Ligamentum flava
- Ligamentum nuchae
- Rectus capitis posterior minor

***Lateral mass***
- Superior articular facets for occipital condyles
- Inferior articular facets for axis
- Transverse process
- Foramen transversarium
Attachments
- Rectus capitis lateralis
- Obliquus capitis superior
- Levator scapulae

the corresponding facet on the axis vertebra to form an atlantoaxial joint.

c. The medial surface of the lateral mass is marked by a small roughened tubercle.

d. The *transverse process* projects laterally from the lateral mass. The transverse process is pierced by the foramen transversarium.

### Attachments and Relations (Fig. 1.31)

1. The anterior tubercle provides attachment (in the median plane) to the anterior longitudinal ligament, and provides insertion on each side to the upper oblique part of longus colli.
2. The upper border of the anterior arch gives attachment to the anterior atlanto-occipital membrane.
3. The lower border of the anterior arch gives attachment to the lateral fibres of the anterior longitudinal ligament.
4. The posterior tubercle provides attachment to the ligamentum nuchae in the median plane and gives origin to the rectus capitis posterior minor on each side.
5. The groove on the upper surface of the posterior arch is occupied by the *vertebral artery* and by the *first cervical nerve*. Behind the groove, the upper border of the posterior arch gives attachment to the posterior atlanto-occipital membrane.
6. The lower border of the posterior arch gives attachment to the highest pair of ligamenta flava.
7. The tubercle on the medial side of the lateral mass gives attachment to the transverse ligament of the atlas.
8. The anterior surface of the lateral mass gives origin to the rectus capitis anterior.
9. The transverse process gives origin to the rectus capitis lateralis from its upper surface anteriorly, obliquus capitis superior from its upper surface posteriorly, levator scapulae from its lateral margin and lower border and insertion to obliquus capitis inferior from its lower surface of the tip. Its posterior tubercle gives insertion to splenius cervicis.

**OSSIFICATION**

Atlas ossifies from three centres, one for each lateral mass with half of the posterior arch, one for the anterior arch. The centres for the lateral masses appear during 7th week of intrauterine life and unite posteriorly at about 3 years. The centre for anterior arch appears at about 1st year and unites with the lateral mass at about 7 years.

## SECOND CERVICAL VERTEBRA

This is called the *axis* (Latin *axile*). It is identified by the presence of the dens or *odontoid* (Greek *tooth*) process, which is a strong, tooth-like process projecting upwards from the body. The dens is usually believed to represent the centrum or body of the atlas, which has fused with the centrum of the axis (Plate 1.32, Fig. 1.32).

### Body and Dens

1. The *superior surface* of the body is fused with the ***dens*** and is encroached upon on each side by the superior articular facets. The dens articulates anteriorly with oval fact on posterior surface of the anterior arch of the atlas, and posteriorly with the transverse ligament of the atlas.
2. The *inferior surface* has a prominent anterior margin, which projects downwards.
3. The *anterior surface* presents a median ridge on each side of which there are hollowed-out impressions.

### Vertebral Arch

1. The ***pedicles*** are concealed superiorly by the superior articular processes. The inferior surface presents a deep

Plate 1.32: Axis vertebra

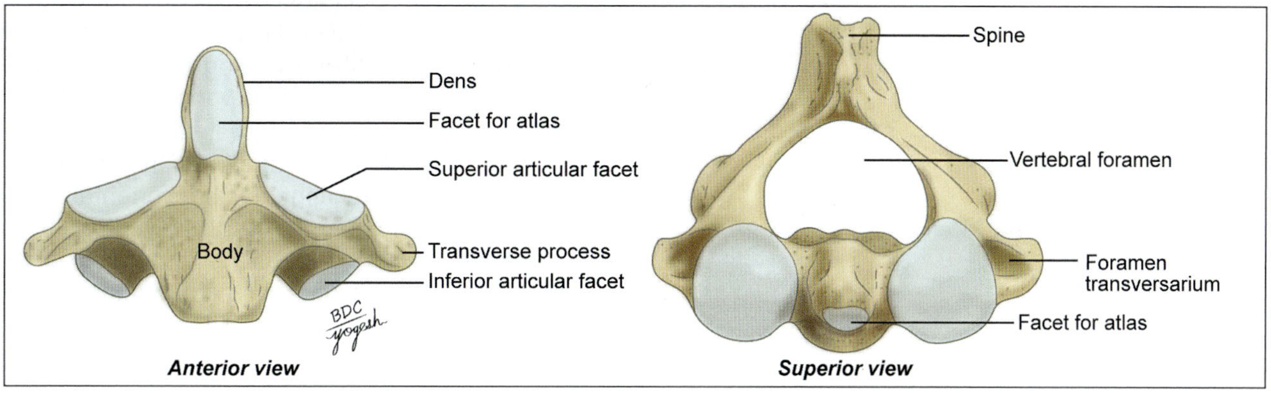


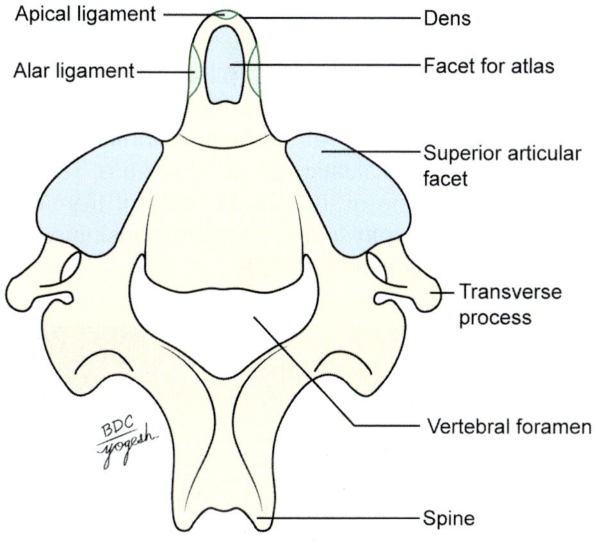


Fig. 1.32: Axis vertebra

and wide *inferior vertebral notch*, placed in front of the inferior articular process. The superior vertebral notch is very shallow and is placed on the upper border of the lamina, behind the superior articular process.

2. The ***laminae*** are thick and strong.
3. ***Articular facets***: Each *superior articular facet* occupies the upper surfaces of the body and of the massive pedicle. Laterally, it overhangs the foramen transversarium. It is a large, flat, circular facet that is directed upwards and laterally. It articulates with the inferior facet of the atlas vertebra to form the atlantoaxial joint. Each *inferior articular facet* lies posterior to the transverse process and is directed downwards and forwards to articulate with the third cervical vertebra.
4. The ***transverse processes*** are very small and represent the true posterior tubercles only. The foramen transversarium is directed upwards and laterally.
5. The ***spine*** is large, thick and very strong. It is deeply grooved inferiorly. Its tip is bifid, terminating in two rough tubercles.

### Attachments

1. The dens provides attachment at its apex to the apical ligament, and on each side, below the apex to the alar ligaments.
2. The anterior surface of the body receives the insertion of the longus colli. The anterior longitudinal ligament is also attached to the anterior surface.
3. The posterior surface of the body provides attachment, from below upwards, to the (A) posterior longitudinal ligament, (B) the membrana tectoria and (C) the vertical limb of the cruciate ligament.
4. The laminae provide attachment to the ligamenta flava.
5. The transverse process gives origin by its tip to the levator scapulae, the scalenus medius anteriorly and the splenius cervicis posteriorly. The *intertransverse muscles* are attached to the upper and lower surfaces of the process.
6. The spine gives attachment to the ligamentum nuchae, the semispinalis cervicis, the spinalis cervicis, the interspinalis and the multifidus and origin to rectus capitis posterior major and the obliquus capitis inferior.

*Competency:*
AN26.7 Describe the features of the 7th cervical vertebra.

## SEVENTH CERVICAL VERTEBRA

It is also known as the ***vertebra prominens*** because of its long spinous process, the tip of which can be felt through the skin at the lower end of the nuchal furrow. Its spine is thick, long and nearly horizontal. It is not bifid but ends in a tubercle (Plate 1.33).

The transverse processes are comparatively large in size, the posterior root is larger than the anterior. The anterior tubercle is absent. The foramen transversarium is relatively small, sometimes double, or may be entirely absent. It does not transmit the vertebral artery.

### Attachments

1. The tip of the *spine* provides attachment to the ligamentum nuchae, trapezius, rhomboid minor, serratus posterior superior, splenius capitis, spinalis cervicis, semispinalis thoracis, interspinales and the multifidus.
2. *Transverse process:* The *foramen transversarium* usually transmits only an accessory vertebral vein. The *posterior tubercle* provides attachment to the

**Plate 1.33:** C7 vertebra

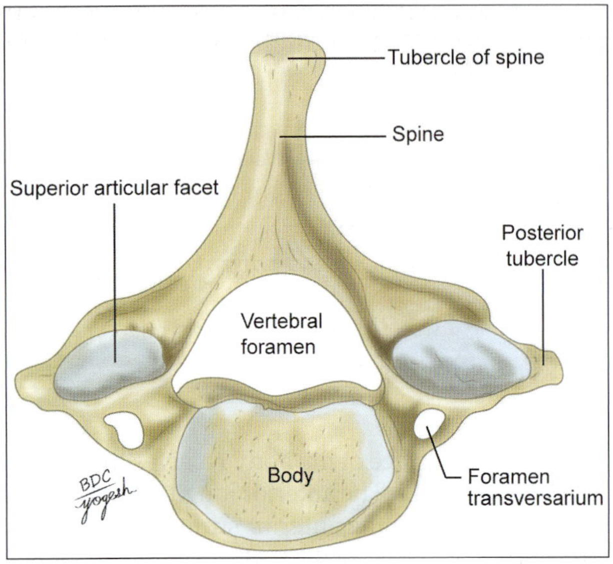


suprapleural membrane. The lower *border* provides attachment to the first pair of levatores costarum.

3. The anterior root of the transverse process may sometimes be separate. It then forms a *cervical rib* of variable size.

## OSSIFICATION

Its ossification is similar to that of a typical cervical vertebra. In addition, separate centre for each costal process appears during 6th month of intrauterine life and fuses with the body and transverse process during 5th to 6th years of life.

## CLINICAL ANATOMY

- The costal element of 7th cervical vertebra may get enlarged to form a ***cervical rib*** (Fig. 1.33). A cervical rib is an additional rib arising from the C7 vertebra and usually gets attached to the 1st rib near the insertion of scalenus anterior. If the rib is more than 5 cm long, it usually displaces the brachial plexus and the subclavian artery upwards. The symptoms are tingling pain along the inner border of the forearm and hand including weakness and even paralysis of the muscles of the palm.
- The intervertebral foramina of the cervical vertebrae lie anterior to the joints between the articular processes. Arthritic changes in these joints, if occur, cause tiny projections or osteophytes. These osteophytes may press on the anteriorly placed cervical spinal nerves in the foramina causing pain along the course and distribution of these nerves.
- The joints in the lateral parts of adjacent bodies of cervical vertebrae are called Luschka's joints. The intervertebral foramen lies between Luschka's joints and facet joints. The cervical nerve roots may get pressed by osteophytes in these joints causing pain (Fig. 1.34).
- The vertebral artery coursing through the foramen transversarium lies lateral to Luschka's joints. The osteophytes of Luschka's joints may cause distortion of the vertebral artery leading to vertebrobasilar insufficiency. This may cause vertigo, dizziness, etc.
- Prolapse of the intervertebral disc occurs at the junction of different curvatures. So, the common site is lower cervical and upper lumbar vertebral regions. In the cervical region, the disc involved is above or below 6th cervical vertebra. The nerve roots affected are C6 and C7. There is pain and numbness along the lateral side of forearm and hand. There may be wasting of muscles of thenar eminence.
- During judicial hanging, the odontoid process usually breaks to hit upon the vital centres in the medulla oblongata (Fig. 1.35).
- Atlas may fuse with the occipital bone. This is called *occipitalisation of atlas* and this may at times compress the spinal cord, which requires surgical decompression.
- The pharyngeal and retropharyngeal inflammations may cause decalcification of atlas vertebra. This may lead to loosening of the attachments of transverse ligament, which may eventually yield, causing *sudden death* from *dislocation of dens*.

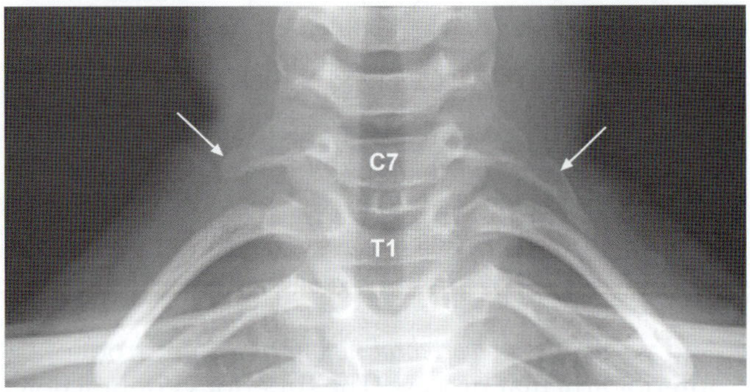


**Fig. 1.33:** Bilateral cervical ribs

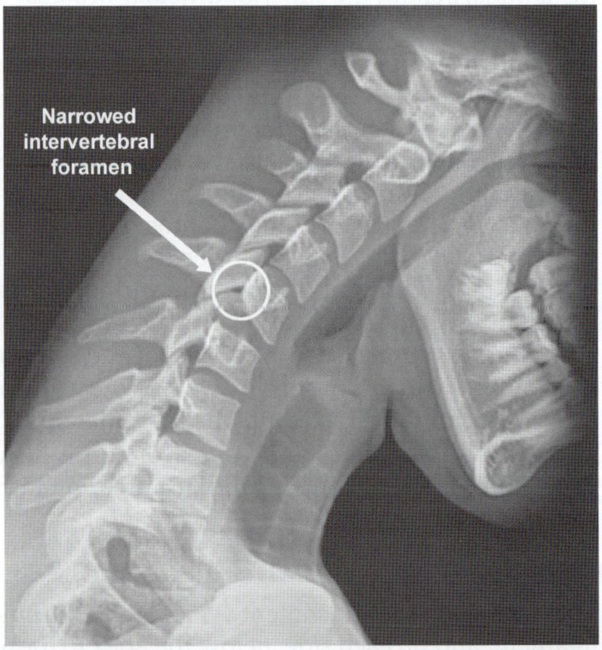


**Fig. 1.34:** Pressure on the cervical nerve due to bony changes

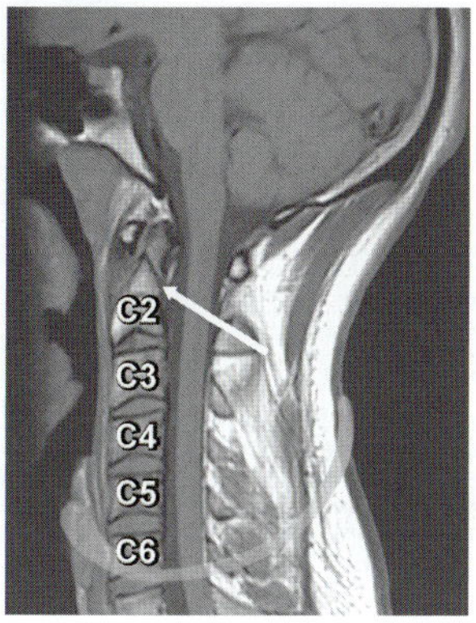


Fig. 1.35: Fracture of the odontoid process during hanging (fracture marked by arrow)

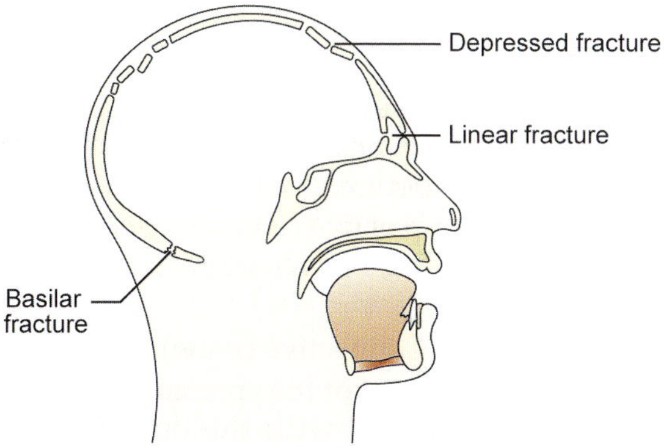


Fig. 1.36: Types of fracture of the skull

- Fractures of skull may be depressed, linear and basilar (Fig. 1.36).
- Hangman's fracture occurs due to fracture of the pedicles of axis vertebra. As the vertebral canal gets enlarged, the spinal cord does not get pressed.

VIDEO

Video 3.1 **Bones of Skull:** Introduction, Bones of skull, Anterior cranial fossa, Middle cranial fossa, Posterior cranial fossa, Orbit, Mandible, Foramina, Norma frontalis, Hyoid bone, Cervical vertebrae.

### *Facts to Remember*

- Eight bones in the calvaria and 14 facial bones make up the skull.
- Most of the joints are 'suture' type of joints. The joint between teeth and gums is gomphosis. There is a pair of temporomandibular joints, which is of synovial variety.
- The bony ossicles are malleus, incus and stapes and are 'bone within bone', as these are present in the petrous temporal bone. Between these three ossicles are two synovial joints.
- Diploe veins contain manufactured RBCs, granulocytes and platelets. These drain into the neighbouring veins.
- Paranasal sinuses give resonance to the voice, besides humidifying and warming up the inspired air.

### BDC's Anatomy *e*-book

1. Principles governing fractures of the skull
2. Age changes in maxilla
3. Ossification of cranial bones
4. Development of neurocranium
5. Further reading
6. Viva voce

Chapter

2

# Scalp, Temple and Face

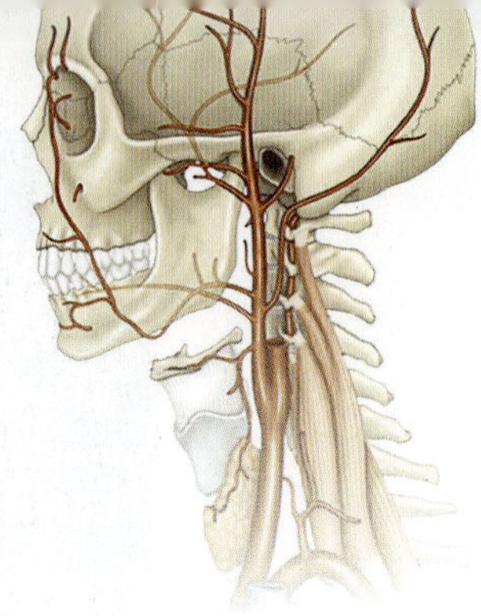

Face is the most prominent part of the body. Facial muscles, being the muscles of facial expression, express a variety of emotions like happiness, joy, sadness, anger, frowning, grinning. The face, therefore, is an *index of mind*.

***Competency:***
**AN27.1** Describe the layers of scalp, its blood supply, its nerve supply and surgical importance.

## SCALP AND SUPERFICIAL TEMPORAL REGION

### SCALP

The soft tissues covering the cranial vault form the scalp (Flowchart 2.1).

#### Extent of Scalp

The scalp extends as follows (Fig. 2.1):
*Anteriorly* — up to supraorbital margins.
*Posteriorly* — up to external occipital protuberance and superior nuchal lines.
*On each side* — up to the zygomatic arch and external acoustic meatus.

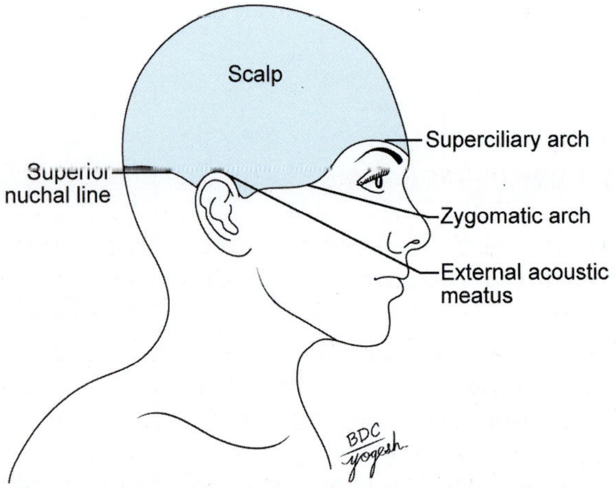


**Fig. 2.1:** Extent of the scalp (*Note*: Some authors consider that the scalp extends up to the superior temporal line)

#### Structure

Conventionally, the superficial temporal region is studied with the scalp, and the following description, therefore, will cover both regions.

The scalp is made up of five layers (*mnemonic*: **SCALP**) (Plate 2.1, Figs 2.2 to 2.4, Flowchart 2.2).

1. **S**kin
2. Superficial fascia (**C**onnective tissue)
3. Deep fascia in the form of the epicranial **a**poneurosis or galea aponeurotica with the occipitofrontalis muscle
4. **L**oose areolar tissue
5. **P**ericranium

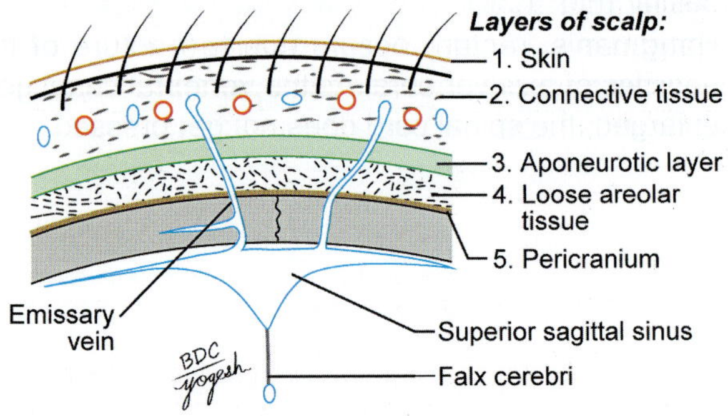


**Fig. 2.2:** Layers of the scalp

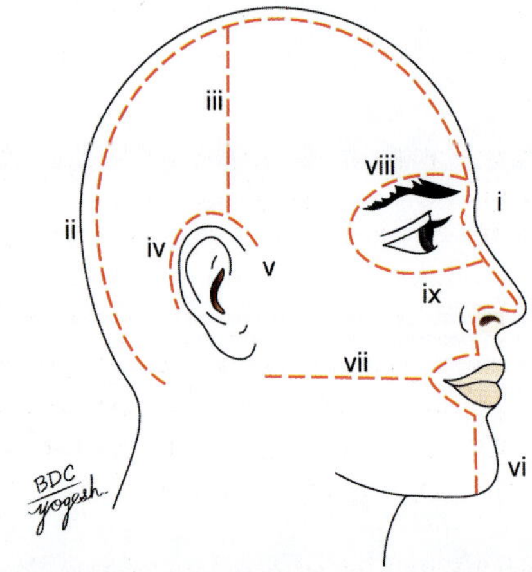


**Fig. 2.3:** Lines of dissection for scalp, face and eyelids

Plate 2.1: Layers of the scalp

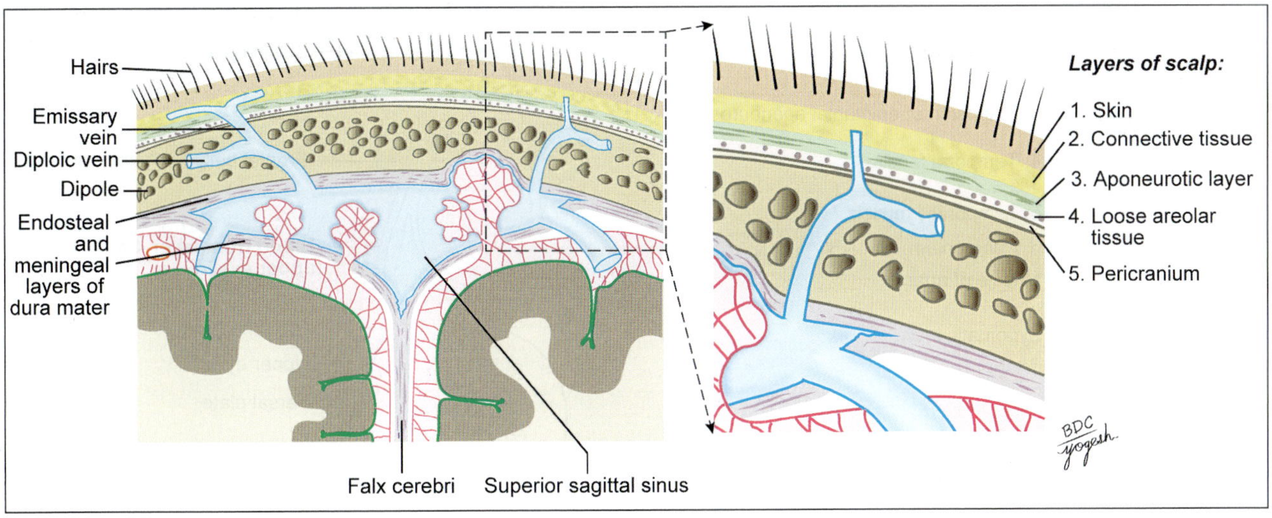


Flowchart 2.1: Scalp

**Scalp**
Tissue covering the skull

- ***Extent***
  - Anterior: Supraorbital margin
  - Posterior: External occipital protuberance, superior nuchal line
  - On each side: Zygomatic arch
- ***Layers***
  - Skin
  - Subcutaneous connective tissue
  - Epicranial aponeurosis
  - Loose areolar tissue
  - Pericranium
- ***Arterial supply***
  - Supratrochlear
  - Supraorbital
  - Superficial temporal
  - Posterior auricular
  - Occipital artery
- ***Nerve supply***
  - ***In front of auricle***
    - Sensory: Supratrochlear, Supraorbital, Zygomaticotemporal, Auriculotemporal
    - Motor: Temporal branch of facial nerve
  - ***Behind the auricle***
    - Sensory: Great auricular (C2, C3), Lesser occipital (C2), Greater occipital (C2), Third occipital (C3)
    - Motor: Posterior auricular branch of facial nerve

***Clinical integration:*** Sebaceous cyst, surgical layers of scalp, black eye, dangerous area of scalp, safety-valve haematoma, cephalohaematoma, caput succedaneum, scalp wound bleeding, gaping wound of scalp.

Flowchart 2.2: Layers of scalp

**Layers of scalp**

- ***Skin***
  - Hairy
  - Adherent to epicranial aponeurosis
  - Numerous hair follicles and sebaceous glands
- ***Subcutaneous connective tissue***
  - Superficial fascia
  - Dense connective tissue
  - Passage for blood vessels and nerves
- ***Epicranial aponeurosis***
  - Called galea aponeurotica
  - Gives insertion to frontalis and occipitalis
- ***Loose areolar tissue***
  - Anteriorly extends into the upper eyelid
  - Posteriorly extends up to superior nuchal line
  - Gives passage to emissary vein
- ***Pericranium***
  - Periosteum of cranial bones
  - Loosely attached to bones

1. ***Skin*** of scalp is hairy. It is adherent to the epicranial aponeurosis through the dense superficial fascia. It has more number of sweat glands and sebaceous glands.
2. The **connective tissue** (*superficial fascia*) is more fibrous and dense in the centre than at the periphery of the head. It contains many blood vessels. It binds the skin to the subjacent aponeurosis and provides the proper medium for the passage of vessels and nerves to the skin.
3. The ***occipitofrontalis muscle*** has two bellies, occipital or occipitalis and frontal or frontalis, both of which are inserted into the epicranial aponeurosis (Fig. 2.5). The *occipital bellies* are small and separate. Each arises from the lateral 2/3rd of the superior nuchal line and is supplied by the *posterior auricular* branch of the *facial nerve*.

   The *frontal bellies* are longer, wider and partly united in the median plane. Each arises from the skin of the upper eyelid and forehead, mingling with the orbicularis oculi and the corrugator supercilia (Fig. 2.6). It is supplied by the *temporal branch* of the facial nerve.

   The muscle raises the eyebrows and causes horizontal wrinkles in the skin of the forehead.

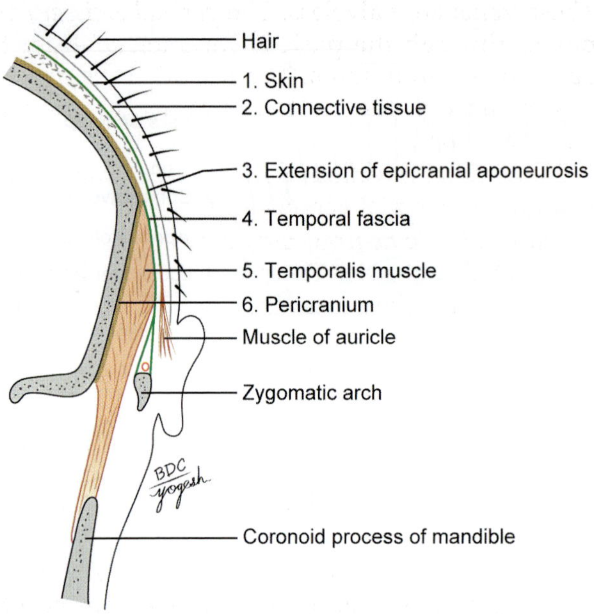


**Fig. 2.4:** Layers of superficial temporal region

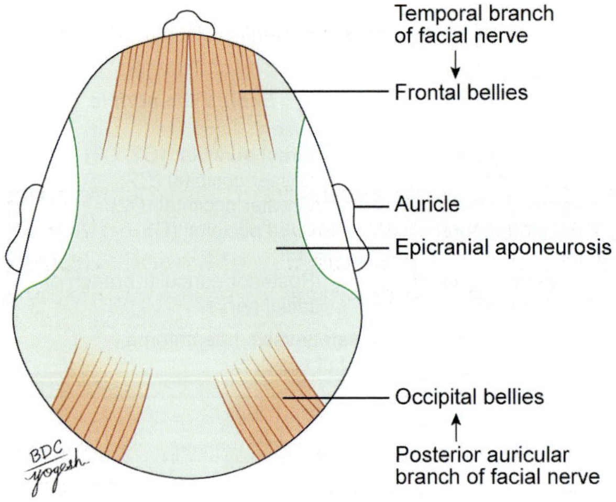


**Fig. 2.5:** Bellies of the occipitofrontalis muscle

4. The ***epicranial aponeurosis***, or ***galea aponeurotica*** is freely movable on the pericranium along with the overlying and adherent skin and fascia. Anteriorly, it receives the insertion of the frontalis; posteriorly, it receives the insertion of the occipitalis and is attached to the external occipital protuberance and the highest/superior nuchal lines in between the occipital bellies. On each side, the aponeurosis is attached to the superior temporal line but sends down a thin expansion that passes over the temporal fascia and is attached to the zygomatic arch.

   *Note*: The first three layers of scalp are called ***surgical layers of the scalp***. These are called 'scalp proper' also.

5. The layer of ***loose areolar tissue*** extends anteriorly into the eyelids because the frontalis muscle has no bony attachment; posteriorly to the highest and superior nuchal lines; and on each side to the superior temporal lines. It gives passage to the emissary veins which connect extracranial veins to intracranial venous sinuses.

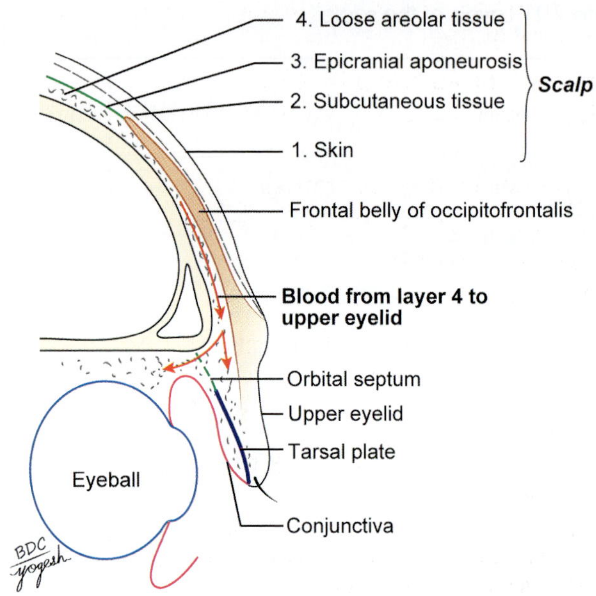


**Fig. 2.6:** Schematic section through the scalp and upper eyelid to show how fluids can pass from the subaponeurotic space or layer of loose areolar tissue of the scalp into the eyelid, and into the subconjunctival area. Note that this is possible because the frontalis muscle has no bony attachment

6. The ***pericranium*** is a periosteum of the skull bones. It is loosely attached to the surface of the bones but is firmly adherent to their sutures where the sutural ligaments bind the pericranium to the endocranium.

## DISSECTION

Place 2–3 wooden blocks under the head to raise it about 10–12 cm from the table. Fig. 2.3 shows a median incision in the skin of scalp extending from root of the nose (i), to the prominent external occipital protuberance (ii). Give a coronal incision across the previous incision from root of one auricle to the other (iii). Extend the incision from the auricle to the mastoid process posteriorly (iv) and to root of zygomatic arch anteriorly (v). Reflect the skin in four flaps. Usually, the skin is so adherent to the subjacent connective tissue and aponeurotic layers that these all come off together. Dissect the layers, including the nerves, vessels, lymphatics and identify these structures in the cadaver.

## SUPERFICIAL TEMPORAL REGION

It is the area between the superior temporal line and the zygomatic arch. This area contains the following six layers (Fig. 2.4):

1. Skin
2. Superficial fascia
3. Thin extension of epicranial aponeurosis which gives origin to extrinsic muscles of the auricle
4. Temporal fascia
5. Temporalis muscle
6. Pericranium.

Tempus means time. Greying of hair first starts here.

## Arterial Supply of Scalp and Superficial Temporal Region

In front of the auricle (Fig. 2.7):

1. Supratrochlear
2. Supraorbital
3. Superficial temporal arteries

Behind the auricle:

1. Posterior auricular
2. Occipital (tortuous) arteries.

*Note*: The supratrochlear and supraorbital arteries are branches of the ophthalmic artery which in turn is a branch of the internal carotid artery. The superficial temporal is a smaller terminal branch of the external carotid artery.

The posterior auricular and occipital arteries are branches of the external carotid artery.

Thus, the scalp has a *rich blood supply* derived from both the internal and the external carotid arteries, the two systems anastomosing over the temple.

## Venous Drainage

The veins of the scalp accompany the arteries and have similar names.

1. The ***supratrochlear*** and ***supraorbital veins*** unite at the medial angle of the eye forming the ***angular*** vein which continues down as the ***facial vein***.
2. The ***superficial temporal vein*** descends in front of the tragus, enters the parotid gland and joins the maxillary vein to form the ***retromandibular* vein**. This vein divides into two divisions.
   a. The ***anterior division*** of the retromandibular vein unites with the facial vein to form the *common facial vein* which drains into the internal jugular vein.
   b. The ***posterior division*** of the retromandibular vein unites with the *posterior auricular vein* to form the *external jugular vein* which ultimately drains into the *subclavian vein*. The occipital veins terminate in the suboccipital venous plexus.
3. ***Emissary veins*** connect the extracranial veins with the intracranial venous sinuses to equalise the pressure. These veins are valveless. The *parietal emissary vein* passes through the parietal foramen to enter the superior sagittal sinus. The *mastoid emissary vein* passes through the mastoid foramen to reach the sigmoid sinus.

   Extracranial infections may spread through these veins to intracranial venous sinuses.
4. ***Diploic veins*** start from the cancellous bone within the two tables of skull. These carry the newly formed blood cells into the general circulation. There are four veins on each side.
   a. The *frontal diploic vein* emerges at the supraorbital notch and open into the supraorbital vein.
   b. *Anterior temporal diploic vein* ends in anterior deep temporal vein or sphenoparietal sinus.
   c. *Posterior temporal diploic vein* ends in the transverse sinus.
   d. The *occipital diploic vein* opens either into the occipital vein or into the transverse sinus near the median plane.

***Competency:***

**AN28.5** Describe cervical lymph nodes and lymphatic drainage of scalp, face and neck.

## Lymphatic Drainage

The anterior part of the scalp drains into the preauricular or ***parotid lymph nodes***, situated on the surface of the parotid gland. The posterior part of the scalp drains into the posterior auricular or mastoid and occipital lymph nodes.

## Nerve Supply

The scalp and temple are supplied by 10 nerves on each side. Out of these, five nerves (four sensory and one motor) enter the scalp in front of the auricle. The remaining five nerves (again four sensory and one motor) enter the scalp behind the auricle (Fig. 2.7 and Table 2.1).

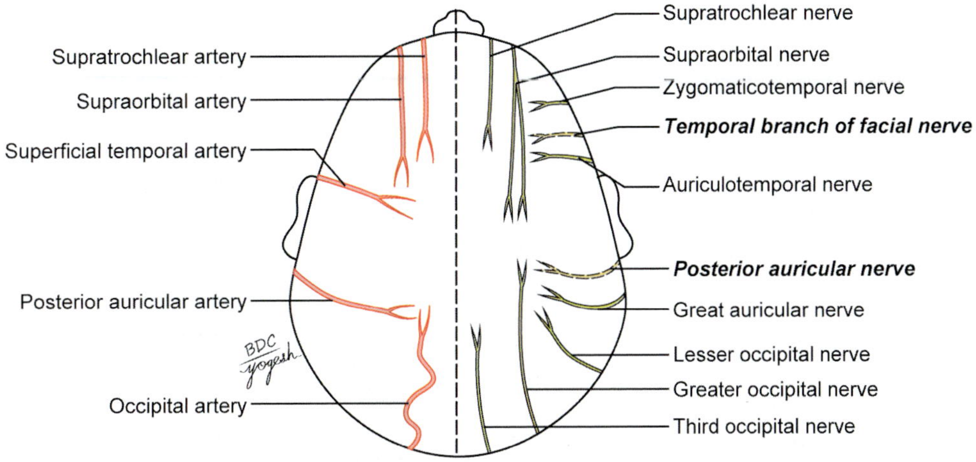


**Fig. 2.7:** Arterial and nerve supply of scalp and superficial temporal region

TABLE 2.1: Nerves of the scalp and superficial temporal region

| *In front of auricle* | *Behind the auricle* |
|---|---|
| ***Sensory nerves*** Supratrochlear, branch of the frontal nerve (ophthalmic division of trigeminal nerve) | ***Sensory nerves*** Posterior division of great auricular nerve (C2, C3) from cervical plexus |
| Supraorbital, branch of frontal nerve (ophthalmic division of trigeminal nerve) | Lesser occipital nerve (C2), from cervical plexus |
| Zygomaticotemporal, branch of zygomatic nerve (maxillary division of trigeminal nerve) | Greater occipital nerve (C2, dorsal ramus) |
| Auriculotemporal branch of mandibular division of trigeminal nerve | Third occipital nerve (C3, dorsal ramus) |
| ***Motor nerve*** Temporal branch of facial nerve | ***Motor nerve*** Posterior auricular branch of facial nerve |

## CLINICAL ANATOMY

- Because of the abundance of sebaceous glands, the scalp is a common site for ***sebaceous cysts*** (Fig. 2.8).
- Collection of blood in the layer of loose connective tissue causes generalised swelling of the scalp. The blood may extend anteriorly into the root of the nose and into the eyelids (as frontalis muscle has no bony origin) resulting in ***black eye***. The posterior limit of such haemorrhage is not seen (Fig. 2.9). If bleeding is due to local injury, the posterior limit of haemorrhage is seen.
- ***Wounds*** of the scalp gape when the epicranial aponeurosis is divided transversely. Such wound needs stitching of layer of aponeurosis carefully (Fig. 2.10).
- Wounds of the scalp ***bleed profusely*** because the vessels are prevented from retracting by the fibrous fascia in second layer of scalp. Bleeding can be arrested by applying pressure at the site of injury by a tight cotton bandage against the bone.
- Because of the density of fascia, subcutaneous haemorrhages are never extensive and the inflammations in this layer cause little swelling but much pain.
- Because the pericranium is adherent to sutures, collections of fluid deep to the pericranium known as ***cephalhaematoma*** take the shape of the bone concerned when there is fracture of particular bone.
- ***Safety-valve haematoma***: Fractures of cranial vault cause escape of intracranial haematoma into sub-aponeurotic space of the scalp through fracture lines. Thus, it prevents compression of cerebrum. This process of collection of blood in sub-aponeurotic space (fourth layer) is called safety-valve hematoma.
- ***Dangerous area of scalp***: The layer of loose areolar tissue is a dangerous area of the scalp because emissary veins connect the veins of this layer with the dural venous sinuses. Hence, any infection of loose areolar tissue layer easily spreads to dural venous sinuses. It may lead to thrombosis of the dural venous sinuses which may be fatal.
- Because of the spread of blood, compression of brain is not seen and so this layer is also called ***safety layer***.
- Since the blood supply of scalp and superficial temporal region is very rich; avulsed portions need not be cut away. They can be replaced in position and stitched: They usually take up and heal well.
- ***Healing of avulsed scalp***: As the scalp and superficial temporal region is richly supplied by anastomosing vessels, the avulsed portion need not to be cut. It can be placed on position and stitched. It usually heals.
- ***Caput succedaneum***: It is a subcutaneous oedema of the scalp produced during delivery. It occurs due to interference in venous return during the passage of the head through the birth canal. It usually subsides in few days on its own.

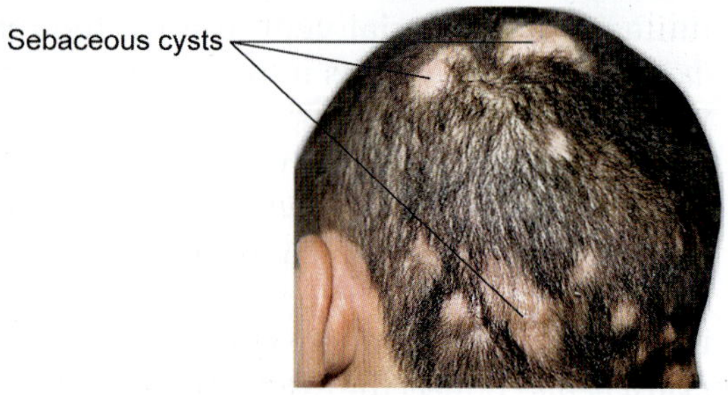


Fig. 2.8: Bilateral sebaceous cysts

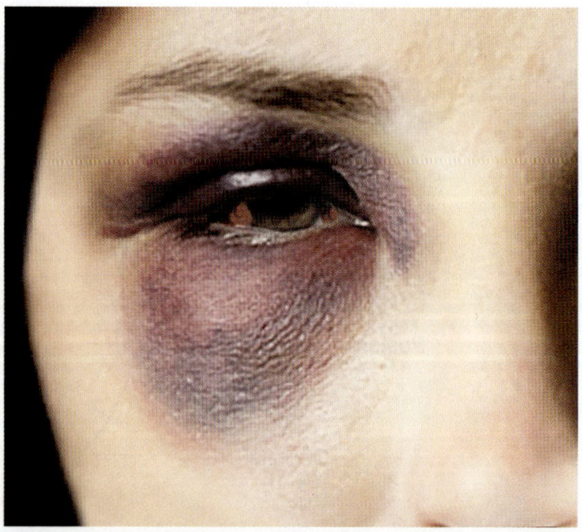

Fig. 2.9: Right eye—black eye due to injury to the scalp

Head and Neck ■ 2

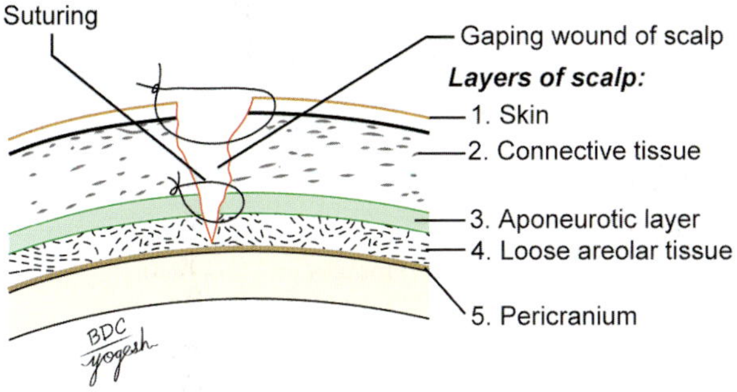


**Fig. 2.10:** Suturing of gaping wound of scalp

## FACE

The face, or countenance, extends superiorly from the adolescent position of hairline, inferiorly to the chin and the base of the mandible and on each side to the auricle. The forehead is, therefore, common to both the face and the scalp.

### SKIN OF THE FACE

1. The facial skin is *very vascular*. Rich vascularity makes the face blush and blanch. Wounds of the face bleed profusely but heal rapidly. The results of plastic surgery on the face are excellent for the same reason.
2. The facial skin is *rich in sebaceous and sweat glands*. Sebaceous glands keep the face oily but also cause *acne* in young adults. Sweat glands help in regulation of the body temperature.
3. *Laxity* of the greater part of the skin facilitates rapid spread of oedema. Renal oedema appears first in the eyelids and face before spreading to other parts of the body.
4. Boils in the nose and ear are acutely painful due to the *fixity* of the skin to the underlying cartilage.
5. Facial skin is very *elastic and thick* because the facial muscles are inserted into it. The wounds of the face, therefore, tend to gape.

### SUPERFICIAL FASCIA

It contains:
1. Facial muscles, all of which are inserted into the skin
2. Vessels and nerves, to the muscles and to the skin
3. Variable amount of fat. Fat is absent from the eyelids but is well developed in the checks, forming the buccal pads that are very prominent in infants in whom they help in sucking.

*Note*: The *deep fascia is absent* from the face, except over the parotid gland where it forms the parotid fascia, and over the buccinator where it forms the *buccopharyngeal fascia*.

### CLEAVAGE LINES OF SKIN IN THE FACE

The cleavage lines or ***Langer lines*** of skin tension are topological lines that are produced due to the parallel orientation of collagen fibres in the dermis and the underlying muscle [Karl Langer, Austrian anatomist, 1819–1887]. The orientation of the cleavage line in the skin of face is region-specific (Fig. 2.11).

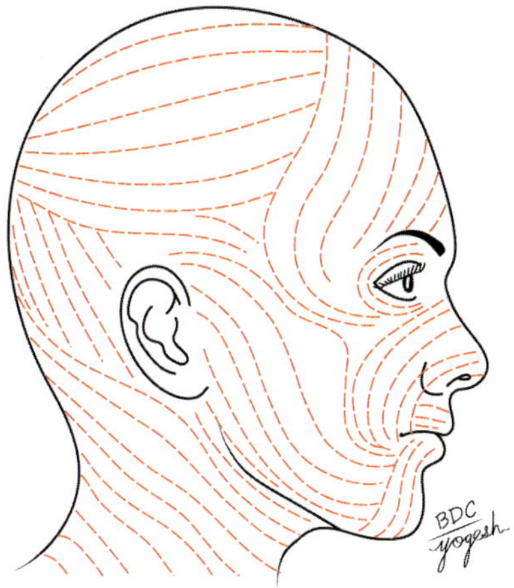

**Fig. 2.11:** The distribution of relaxed skin tension lines in the head and neck region

***Natural wrinkle lines:*** They result from repeated folding of skin perpendicular to the long axis of the underlying contracting muscle of facial expressions. Wrinkle lines become prominent in elderly due to loss of skin elasticity.

*Note*: To excise the lesions of the skin (scars, pigmented patches, or skin cancers), the incisions given along the natural wrinkle lines or cleavage lines produce less scarring.

**DISSECTION**

Give a median incision from the root of nose, across the dorsum of nose, centre of philtrum of upper lip, to centre of lower lip to the chin (vi). Give a horizontal incision from the angle of the mouth to posterior border of ramus of the mandible (vii). Reflect the lower flap towards and up to the lower border of mandible. Direct and reflect the upper flap till the auricle. Subjacent to the skin, the facial muscles are directly encountered as these are inserted in the skin. Identify the various functional groups of facial muscles. Trace the various motor branches of facial nerve emerging from the anterior border of parotid gland to supply these muscles. Amongst these motor branches on the face are the sensory branches of the three divisions of the trigeminal nerve. Try to identify all these with the help of their course given in the text.

***Competencies:***

**AN28.1** Describe and demonstrate muscles of facial expression and their nerve supply.

**AN28.6** Identify superficial muscles of face, their nerve supply and actions.

### FACIAL MUSCLES

The facial muscles are subcutaneous muscles (Plates 2.2, and 2.3, Figs 2.12 to 2.14).

#### Peculiarities

1. Since these muscles are inserted into skin, they bring out various facial expressions. So, these are secondarily known as muscles of facial expression. These have small motor units.

**Plate 2.2:** Muscles of the facial expression (anterior view)

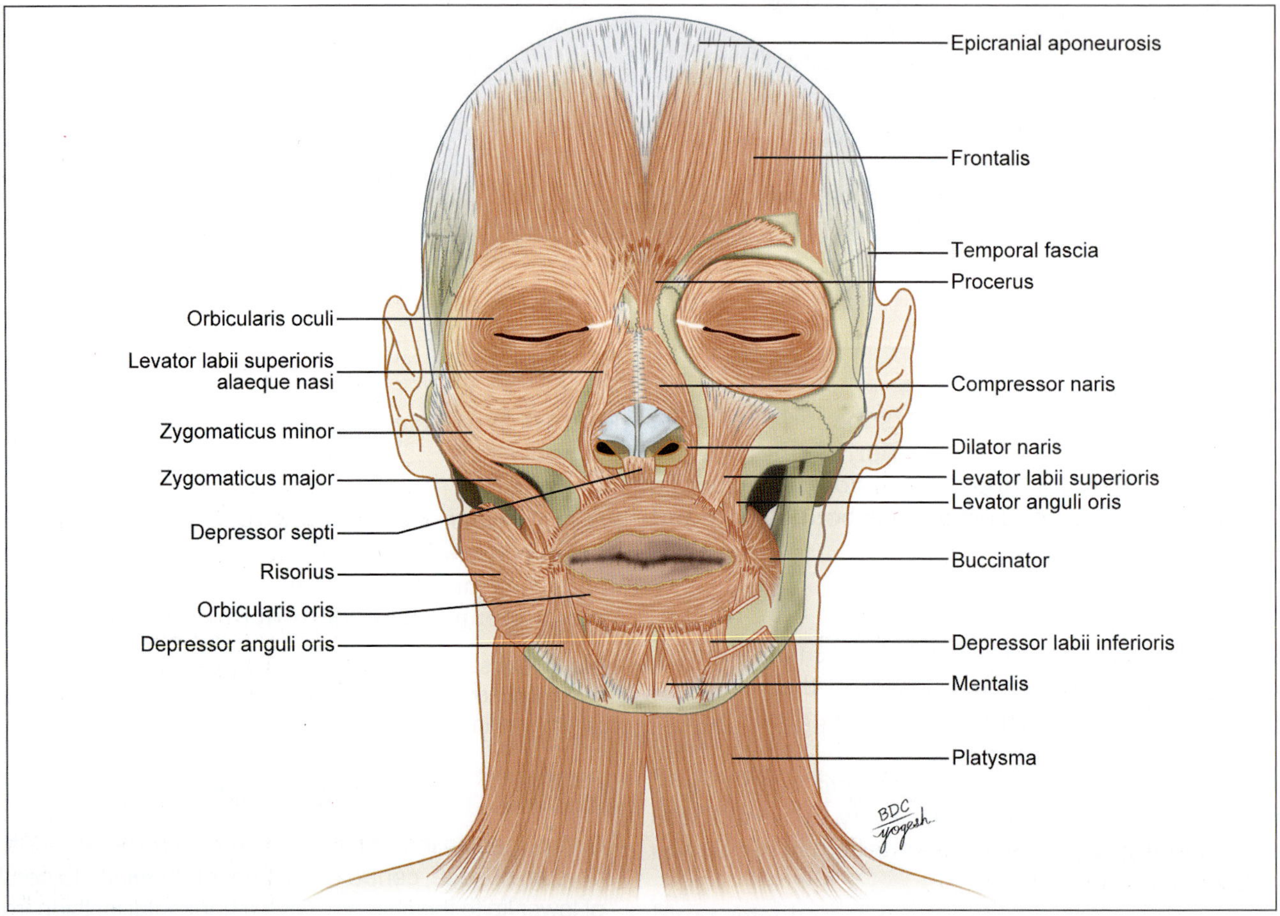


**Plate 2.3:** Muscles of the facial expression (lateral view, note: levator anguli oris is not soon in this view as it lies in deeper plane)

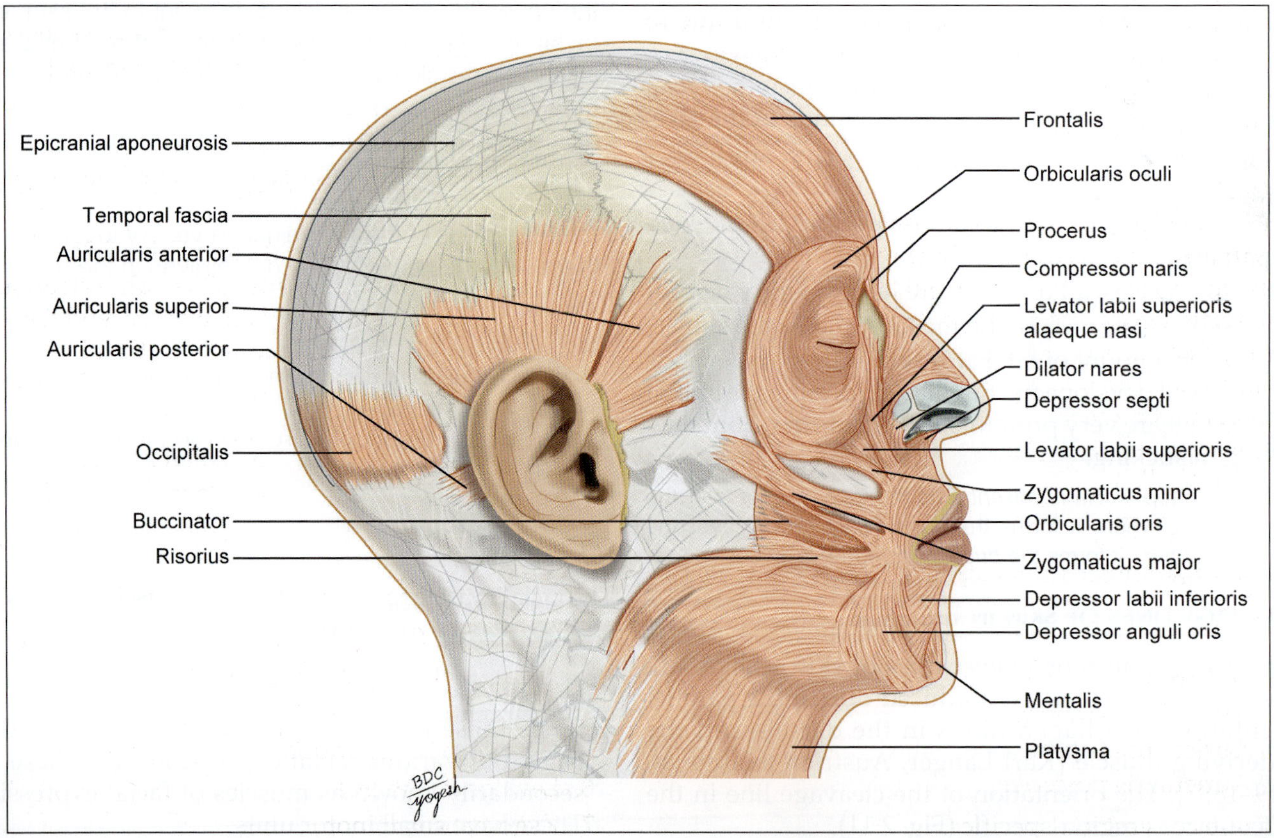

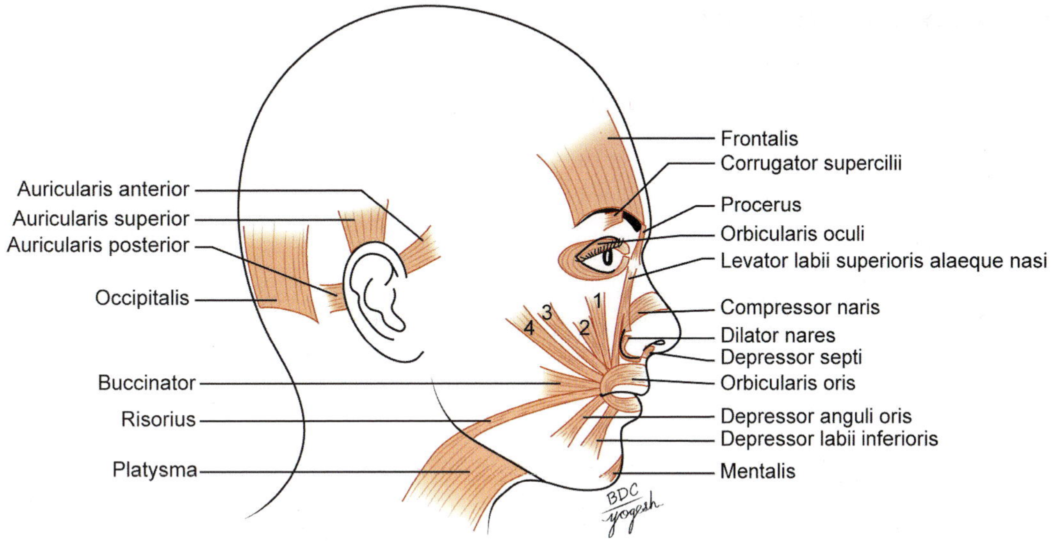


**Fig. 2.12:** Muscles of facial expression (lateral view, 1: levator labii superioris, 2: levator anguli oris, 3: Zygomaticus minor, 4: Zygomaticus major)

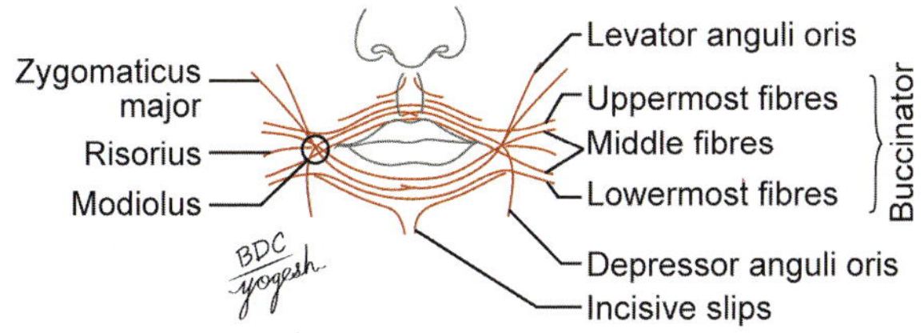


**Fig. 2.13:** Orbicularis oris and buccinator muscles: Arrangement of fibres and formation of modiolus

2. *Embryologically*, they develop from the mesoderm of the 2nd branchial arch, and are, therefore, supplied by the facial nerve.
3. *Morphologically*, they represent the best remnants of the *panniculus carnosus*, a continuous subcutaneous muscle sheet seen in some animals. All of them are inserted into the skin.
4. *Topographically*, the muscles are grouped under the following six heads.
5. *Functionally*, most of these muscles may be regarded primarily as regulators of the three openings situated on the face, namely the palpebral fissures, the nostrils and the oral fissure. Each opening has a single sphincter and a variable number of dilators. Sphincters are naturally circular and the dilators radial in their arrangement. These muscles are better developed around the eyes and mouth than around the nose (Table 2.2).

### Muscle of the Scalp

Occipitofrontalis—described in scalp.

### Muscles of the Auricle

Situated around the ear:

1. Auricularis anterior
2. Auricularis superior
3. Auricularis posterior

These are vestigial muscles.

**TABLE 2.2: Functional groups of facial muscles**

| *Opening* | *Sphincter* | *Dilators* |
|---|---|---|
| A. Palpebral fissure | Orbicularis oculi | 1. Levator palpebrae superioris<br>2. Frontalis part of occipitofrontalis |
| B. Oral fissure | Orbicularis oris | All the muscles around the mouth, except the orbicularis oris, the sphincter and the mentalis, which does not mingle with orbicularis oris |
| C. Nostrils | Compressor naris | 1. Dilator naris<br>2. Depressor septi<br>3. Medial slip of levator labii superioris alaeque nasi |

### Muscles of the Eyelids/Orbital Openings

1. Corrugator (Latin *to wrinkle*) supercilii (Fig. 2.12 and Table 2.3)
2. Orbicularis oculi (Fig. 2.12 and Table 2.3)
3. Levator palpebrae superioris (an extraocular muscle, supplied by sympathetic fibres and the third cranial nerve) is described in Chapter 13.

### Muscles Around Nasal Opening

1. Procerus
2. Compressor naris
3. Dilator naris
4. Depressor septi

### Muscles Around the Mouth

1. Orbicularis oris
2. Buccinator (Latin *cheek*)
3. Levator labii superioris alaeque nasi
4. Zygomaticus major
5. Levator labii superioris
6. Levator anguli oris
7. Zygomaticus minor

**TABLE 2.3: The facial muscles** (Figs 2.12 to 2.15)

| *Name* | *Origin* | *Insertion* | *Actions* |
|---|---|---|---|
| **Muscles of eyelid/orbital opening** | | | |
| Corrugator supercilii | Medial end of superciliary arch | Skin of mid-eyebrow | Vertical lines on forehead, as in frowning |
| Orbicularis oculi | | | |
| a. Orbital part, on and around the orbital margin | Medial part of medial palpebral ligament, frontal process of maxilla and nasal part of frontal bone | Concentric rings return to the point of origin | Protects eye from bright light, wind and rain. Causes forceful closure of eyelids |
| b. Palpebral part, in the lids | Lateral part of medial palpebral ligament | Lateral palpebral raphe | Closes lids gently as in blinking and sleeping |
| c. Lacrimal part, lateral and deep to the lacrimal sac | Lacrimal fascia and posterior lacrimal crest, forms sheath for lacrimal sac | Pass laterally in front of tarsal plates of both eyelids | Dilates lacrimal sac for sucking of lacrimal fluid into the sac, directs lacrimal puncta into lacus lacrimalis; supports the lower lid |
| **Muscles around nasal opening** | | | |
| Procerus | Nasal bone and upper part of superior nasal cartilage | Skin of forehead between eyebrows and on bridge of the nose | Causes transverse wrinkles |
| Compressor naris | Maxilla just lateral to nose | Aponeurosis across dorsum of nose | Nasal aperture compressed |
| Dilator naris | Maxilla over the lateral incisor | Alar cartilage of nose | Nasal aperture dilated |
| Depressor septi | Maxilla over the medial incisor | Lower mobile part of nasal septum | Nose pulled inferiorly |
| **Muscles around the mouth** | | | |
| Orbicularis oris (comprises four quadrants: Upper, lower, right and left. Each quadrant consists of big pars peripheralis and small pars marginalis) | Pars peripheralis comprises of extrinsic fibres converging modiolus where these form triangular sheets going to each lip. Pars marginalis: These fibres arise from modiolus | The triangular sheets go to each lip, where these fibres interdigitate with opposite side fibres<br>These fibres extend to vermilion zone where these interdigitate with fibres of opposite side | Closes lips and protrudes lips, numerous extrinsic muscles make it most versatile for various types of grimaces<br>This part is associated with speech and helps in producing musical tones |
| Buccinator, the muscle of the cheek<br>Pierced by:<br>a. Parotid duct, and<br>b. Buccal branch of mandibular nerve | 1. Upper fibres, from maxilla opposite molar teeth<br>2. Lower fibres, from mandible, opposite molar teeth<br>3. Middle posterior fibres, from pterygomandibular raphe attached to pterygoid hamulus and inner aspect of mandible behind 3rd molar tooth | 1. Upper fibres, straight to the upper lip<br>2. Lower fibres, straight to the lower lip<br>3. Middle fibres decussate upper fibres go to lower lip, while lower fibres reach the upper lip | Flattens cheek against gums and teeth; prevents accumulation of food in the vestibule. This is the *whistling muscle* |
| Levator labii superioris alaeque nasi | Frontal process of maxilla | Upper lip and ala of nose | Lifts upper lip and dilates cartilage of nose the nostril |
| Zygomaticus major | Posterior aspect of lateral surface of zygomatic bone | Skin at the angle of the mouth | Pulls the angle upwards and laterally as in smiling and laughing |
| Levator labii superioris | Infraorbital margin of maxilla | Skin of upper lateral half of the upper lip | Elevates the upper lip, forms nasolabial groove |
| Levator anguli oris | Maxilla just below infraorbital foramen | Skin of angle of the mouth | Elevates angle of mouth, forms nasolabial groove |
| Zygomaticus minor | Anterior aspect of lateral surface of zygomatic bone | Upper lip medial to its angle | Elevates the upper lip |
| Depressor anguli oris | Oblique line of mandible below first molar, premolar and canine teeth | Skin at the angle of mouth and fuses with orbicularis oris | Draws angle of mouth downwards and laterally |
| Depressor labii inferioris | Anterior part of oblique line of mandible | Lower lip at midline, fuses with muscles from opposite side | Draws lower lip downward |
| Mentalis | Mandible inferior to incisor teeth | Skin of chin | Elevates and protrudes lower lip as it wrinkles skin on chin |
| Risorius | Fascia on the masseter muscle | Skin at the angle of the mouth | Retracts angle of mouth |
| **Muscle of the neck** | | | |
| Platysma | Upper parts of pectoral and deltoid fasciae<br>Fibres run upwards and medially | Anterior fibres, to the base of the mandible; posterior fibres, to the skin of the lower face and lip and may be continuous with the risorius | Releases pressure of skin on the subjacent veins; depresses mandible; pulls the angle of the mouth downwards as in horror or fright |

*Modiolus:* It is a compact, mobile fibromuscular structure present at about 1.25 cm lateral to the angle of the mouth opposite the upper second premolar tooth. The five muscles interlacing to form the modiolus are zygomaticus major, buccinator, levator anguli oris, risorius and depressor anguli oris.

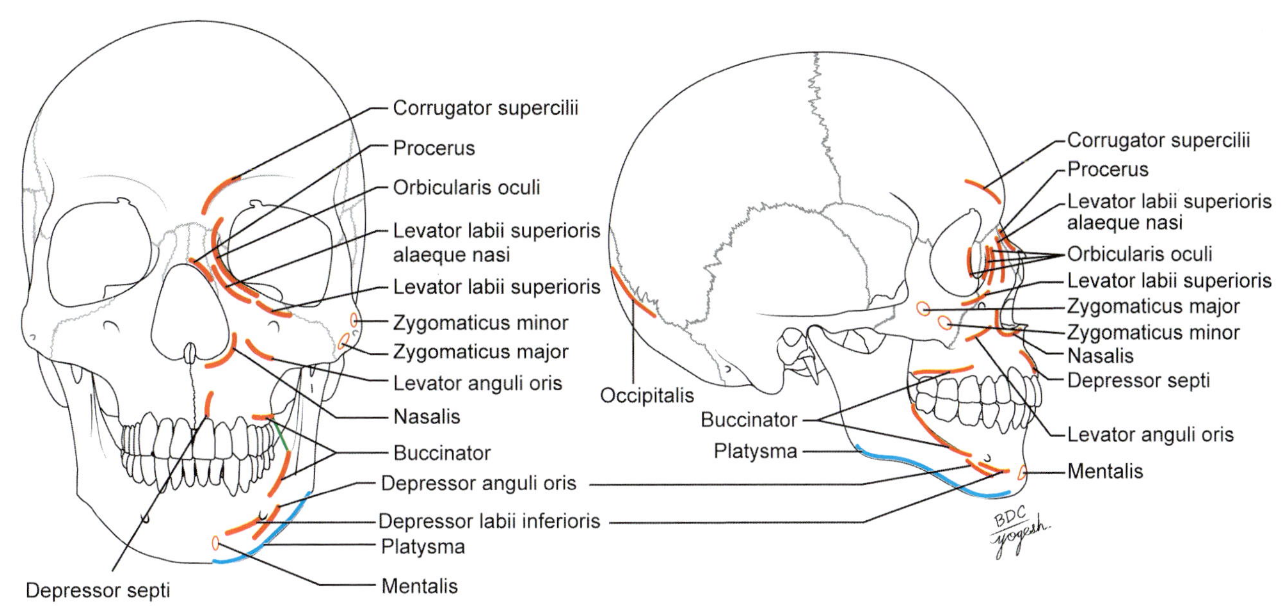


**Fig. 2.14:** Attachments of muscles of facial expression

8. Depressor anguli oris
9. Depressor labii inferioris
10. Mentalis (Latin *chin*)
11. Risorius (Latin *laughter*)

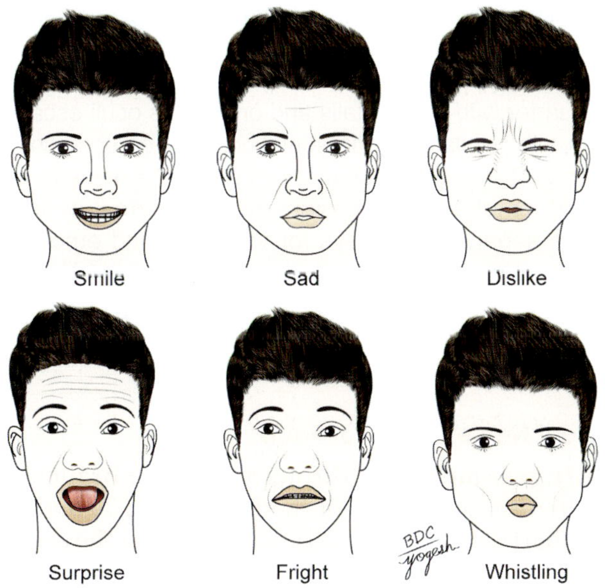


**Fig. 2.15:** Some common facial expressions

*Note*: A few of the *common facial expressions* and the muscles producing them are given below (Fig. 2.15):

1. *Surprise:* Frontalis
2. *Dislike:* Corrugator supercilii and procerus
3. *Anger:* Dilator naris and depressor septi
4. *Smiling and laughing:* Zygomaticus major
5. *Grinning:* Risorius
6. *Sadness:* Levator labii superioris and levator anguli oris
7. *Grief:* Depressor anguli oris
8. *Closing the mouth:* Orbicularis oris
9. *Whistling/kissing:* Buccinator and orbicularis oris
10. *Doubt:* Mentalis
11. *Horror, terror and fright:* Platysma

### Muscle of the Neck

Platysma (Greek *broad*).

Origin, insertion and actions of these muscles are given in Table 2.3.

*Competency:*
**AN28.4** Describe and demonstrate branches of facial nerve with distribution.

## NERVE SUPPLY OF FACE

### Motor Nerve Supply

The *facial nerve* is the motor nerve of the face. Its five terminal branches, temporal, zygomatic, buccal, marginal mandibular and cervical emerge from the parotid gland and diverge to supply the various facial muscles as follows:

1. Temporal — crosses zygomatic arch gives branches for frontalis, auricular muscles, orbicularis oculi.
2. Zygomatic — crosses zygomatic bone and gives branches for orbicularis oculi (lower eyelid part).
3. Buccal — supplies muscles of the cheek and upper lip.
4. Marginal mandibular — supplies muscles of lower lip.
5. Cervical — innervates platysma.

[*Mnemonic*: ***Five branches of the facial nerve (VII)*** (**T**en **Z**ebras **B**it **M**y **C**at): **T**emporal; **Z**ygomatic; **B**uccal; **M**arginal mandibular; **C**ervical]

*Note*: Branches of the facial nerve can be simulated by putting your right wrist on the right ear and spreading five digits: The thumb over the temporal region, the index finger on the zygomatic bone, middle finger on the upper lip, the ring finger on the lower lip and the little finger over the neck (Figs 2.16a and b).

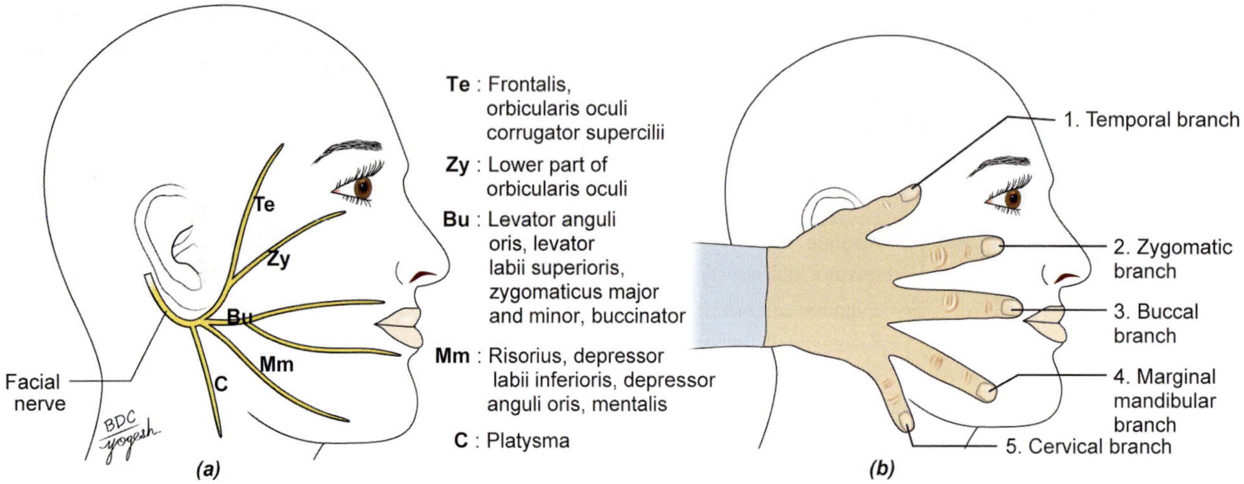


**Figs 2.16a and b:** Terminal branches of the facial nerve and their distribution

*Competency:*
**AN28.7** Explain the anatomical basis of facial nerve palsy.

## CLINICAL ANATOMY

- ***Clinical testing of muscle of facial expressions:*** The facial nerve is examined by testing the following facial muscles (Figs 2.17a to d).
  a. *Frontalis:* Ask the patient to look upwards without moving his head, and look for the normal horizontal wrinkles on the forehead.
  b. *Dilators of mouth:* Showing the teeth.
  c. *Orbicularis oculi:* Tight closure of the eyes.
  d. *Buccinator:* Puffing the mouth and then blowing forcibly as in whistling.
- ***Bell's palsy***: Infranuclear lesion (Fig. 2.18) of the facial nerve, at the stylomastoid foramen is known as *Bell's palsy*, upper and lower quarters of the muscles of face on the same side get paralysed with atrophy of the facial muscles. It also causes loss of taste in most of anterior 2/3rd of the tongue.
  – The face becomes asymmetrical and is drawn up to the normal side.
  – The affected side is motionless. Wrinkles disappear from the forehead.
  – The eye cannot be closed leading to keratitis.
  – Any attempt to smile draws the mouth to the normal side.
  – During mastication, food accumulates between the teeth and the cheek.
  – Articulation of labials is impaired. Tears flow out from the eye.

  Saliva flows down from the angle of mouth.
- ***Supranuclear facial nerve palsy***: In supranuclear lesions of the facial nerve; usually a part of hemiplegia, with injury of corticonuclear fibres, only the lower quarter of the opposite side of face is paralysed. The upper quarter with the frontalis and orbicularis oculi escapes due to its bilateral representation in the cerebral cortex (Fig. 2.19). Only voluntary movements are affected and emotional expressions remain normal as there are separate pathways for voluntary and emotional movements. There is no atrophy of facial muscles.

*Competency:*
**AN28.2** Describe sensory innervation of face.

### Sensory Nerve Supply of Face

The ***trigeminal nerve*** through its three branches is the chief sensory nerve of the face (Figs 2.20 and 2.21, Flowchart 2.3 and Table 2.4). The skin over the angle of the jaw and over the parotid gland is supplied by the great auricular nerve (C2, C3).

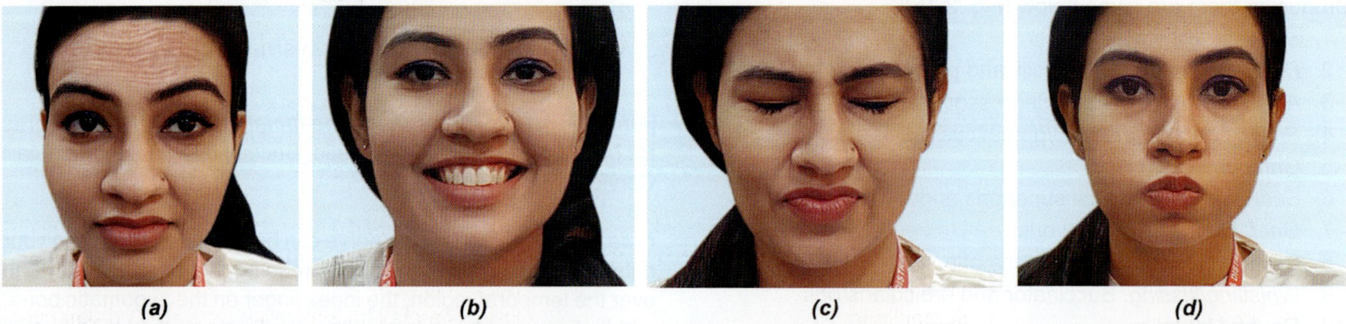


**Figs 2.17a to d:** (a) Test for frontalis, (b) test for dilators of mouth, (c) test for orbicularis oculi, and (d) test for buccinator

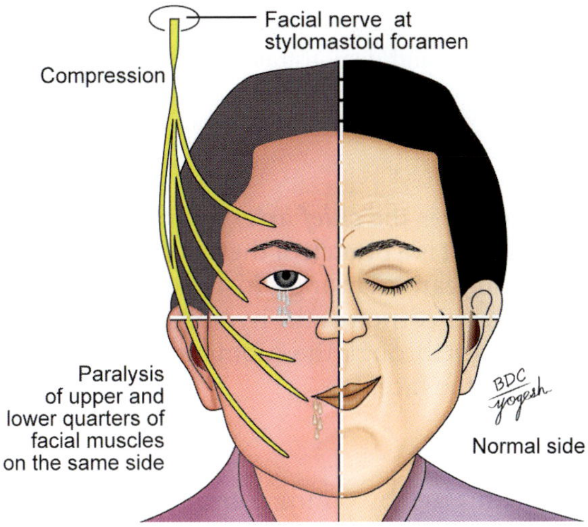


**Fig. 2.18:** Infranuclear lesion of right facial nerve or Bell's palsy

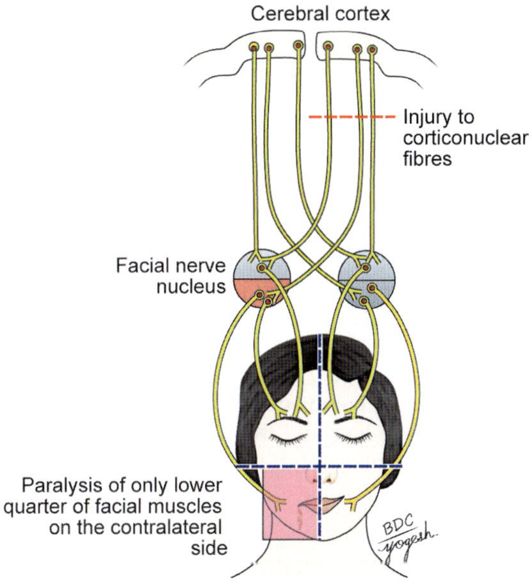


**Fig. 2.19:** Supranuclear lesion of left facial nerve

**Flowchart 2.3:** Sensory nerve supply of face

***Sensory nerve supply of face***

| ***Ophthalmic nerve*** | ***Maxillary nerve*** | ***Mandibular nerve*** | ***Cervical nerves*** |
|---|---|---|---|
| Supratrochlear | Infraorbital | Auriculo-temporal | Great auricular |
| Supraorbital | Zygomatico-facial | Buccal | Transverse cutaneous nerve of neck |
| Lacrimal | Zygomatico-temporal | Mental | Lesser occipital |
| Infratrochlear | | | Supraclavicular |
| External nasal | | | |

***Clinical integration:*** Trigeminal neuralgia (tic douloureuse)

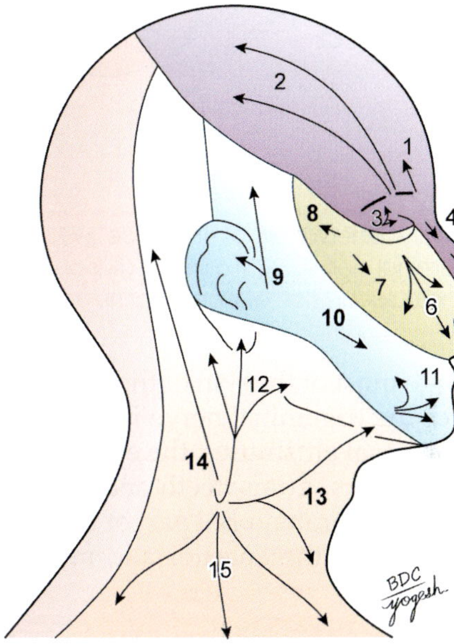

**Fig. 2.20:** The sensory nerves of the face and neck: (1) Supratrochlear, (2) supraorbital, (3) palpebral branch of lacrimal, (4) infratrochlear, (5) external nasal, (6) infraorbital, (7) zygomaticofacial, (8) zygomaticotemporal, (9) auriculotemporal, (10) buccal, (11) mental, (12) great auricular, (13) transverse cutaneous nerve of neck, (14) lesser occipital and (15) supraclavicular

**TABLE 2.4: Cutaneous nerves of the face**

| *Source* | *Cutaneous nerve* | *Area of distribution* |
|---|---|---|
| a. Ophthalmic division of trigeminal nerve | 1. Supratrochlear nerve | Upper eyelid and forehead |
| | 2. Supraorbital nerve | Upper eyelid, frontal air sinus, scalp |
| | 3. Lacrimal nerve | Lateral part of upper eyelid |
| | 4. Infratrochlear nerve | Medial parts of both eyelids |
| | 5. External nasal nerve | Lower part of dorsum and tip of nose |
| b. Maxillary division of trigeminal nerve | 6. Infraorbital nerve | Lower eyelid, side of nose and upper lip |
| | 7. Zygomaticofacial nerve | Upper part of cheek |
| | 8. Zygomaticotemporal nerve | Anterior part of temporal region |
| c. Mandibular division of trigeminal nerve | 9. Auriculotemporal nerve | Upper two-thirds of lateral side of auricle, temporal region |
| | 10. Buccal nerve | Skin of lower part of cheek |
| | 11. Mental nerve | Skin over chin |
| d. Cervical plexus | 12. Anterior division of great auricular nerve (C2, C3) | Skin over angle of the jaw and over the parotid gland |
| | 13. Upper and lower divisions of transverse (anterior) cutaneous nerve of neck (C2, C3) | Lower margin of the lower jaw and upper part of neck |
| | 14. Lesser occipital | Back of auricle |
| | 15. Supraclavicular | Front of thorax till 2nd costal cartilage and skin over upper ½ of deltoid muscle |

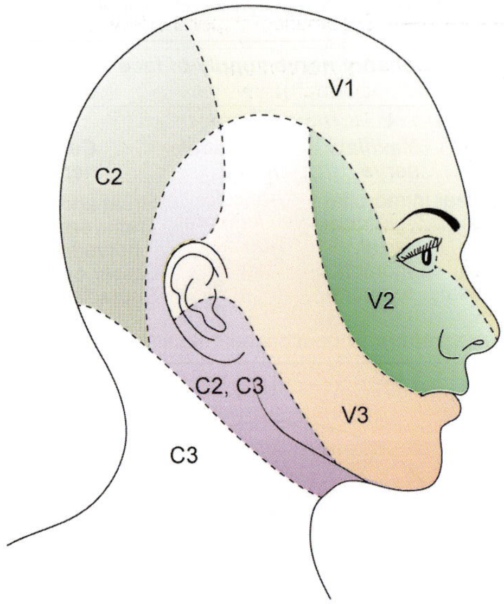


Fig. 2.21: Sensory innervation of the face (V1: Ophthalmic division of trigeminal nerve, V2: Maxillary division of trigeminal nerve, V3: Mandibular division of trigeminal nerve)

In addition to most of the skin of the face, the sensory distribution of the trigeminal nerve is also to the nasal cavity, the paranasal air sinuses, the eyeball, the mouth cavity, palate, cheeks, gums, teeth and anterior 2/3rd of tongue and the supratentorial part of the dura mater, including that lining the anterior and middle cranial fossae (Fig. 2.16).

## CLINICAL ANATOMY

- The sensory distribution of the trigeminal nerve explains why ***headache*** is a uniformly common symptom in involvements of the nose (common cold, boils), the paranasal air sinuses (sinusitis), infections and inflammations of teeth and gums, refractive errors of the eyes and infection of the meninges as in meningitis.
- ***Trigeminal neuralgia*** (***tic douloureux***) may involve one or more of the three divisions of the trigeminal nerve. It causes attacks of very severe burning and scalding pain along the distribution of the affected nerve. Pain is relieved either: (a) By injecting 90% alcohol into the affected division of the trigeminal ganglion, or (b) by sectioning the affected nerve, the main sensory root, or the spinal tract of the trigeminal nerve which is situated superficially in the medulla. The procedure is called medullary tractotomy.

## ARTERIES OF THE FACE

### Features

The face is richly vascular. It is supplied by:
1. The facial artery,
2. The transverse facial artery and
3. Arteries that accompany the cutaneous nerves, which are small branches of ophthalmic, maxillary and superficial temporal arteries (Fig. 2.22, Flowchart 2.4).

*Competency:*
**AN28.3** Describe and demonstrate origin/formation, course, branches/tributaries of facial vessels.

### Facial Artery (Facial Part)

The facial artery is the ***chief artery of the face*** (Fig. 2.22, Flowchart 2.4). It is a branch of the external carotid artery given off in the carotid triangle just above the level of the tip of the greater cornua of the hyoid bone. In its cervical course, it passes through the submandibular region and finally enters the face.

### Course

1. It enters the face by winding around the base of the mandible, and by piercing the deep cervical fascia, at the anteroinferior angle of the masseter muscle. It can be palpated here and is called '**anaesthetist's artery**'.
2. First, it runs upwards and forwards to a point 1.25 cm lateral to the angle of the mouth. Then, it ascends as angular artery by the side of the nose up to the medial angle of the eye, where ***angular artery*** terminates by supplying the lacrimal sac; and by anastomosing with the dorsal nasal branch of the ophthalmic artery.

   The course of the artery in the neck is described in submandibular region.

*Note*: The facial artery is very ***tortuous***. The tortuosity of the artery prevents its walls from being unduly stretched during movements of the mandible, the lips and the cheeks. It lies between the superficial and deep muscles of the face.

### Branches

The anterior branches on the face are large and named. They are:
1. ***Inferior labial***, to the lower lip.
2. ***Superior labial***, to the upper lip and the anteroinferior part of the nasal septum.
3. ***Lateral nasal***, to the ala and dorsum of the nose.

The posterior branches are *small* and unnamed.

**Flowchart 2.4:** Facial artery

***Facial artery***

| ***Beginning*** | ***Termination*** | ***Course*** | ***Branches*** |
|---|---|---|---|
| Branch of external carotid artery<br>Arises at the level of greater cornua of hyoid bone | Continues as angular artery near the angle of eye | Winds around the base of mandible<br>Runs obliquely in the face towards the medial angle of eye<br>Tortuous course | Inferior labial<br>Superior labial<br>Lateral nasal<br>Angular |

***Clinical integration:*** Pulsation of facial artery: at the base of mandible along the anteroinferior angle of masseter or 1.25 cm lateral to the angle of mouth

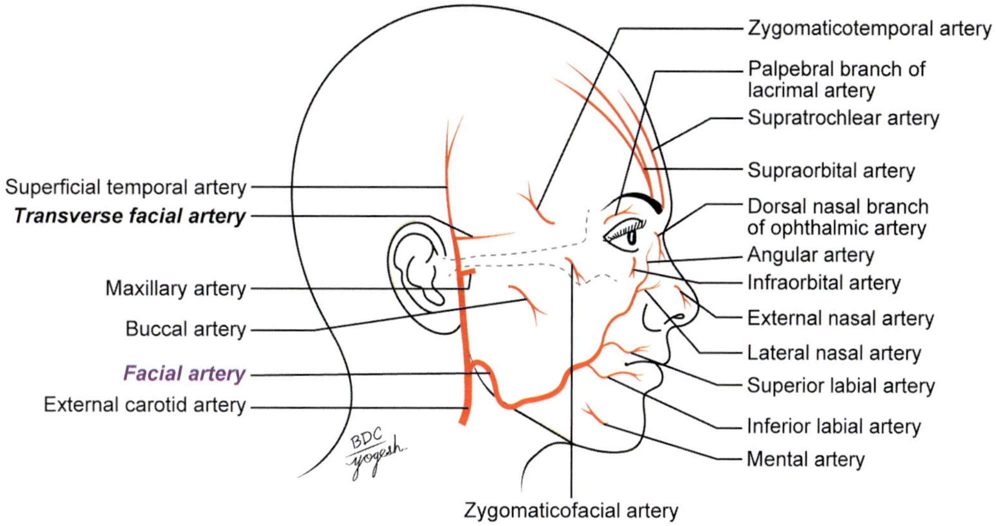


**Fig. 2.22:** Arteries of the face

### Anastomoses

1. The large anterior branches anastomose with similar branches of the opposite side and with the mental artery. In the lips, anastomoses are large, so that cut arteries spurt from both ends.
2. Small posterior branches anastomose with the transverse facial and infraorbital arteries.
3. At the medial angle of the eye, terminal branches of the facial artery anastomose with branches of the ophthalmic artery. This is, therefore, a site for anastomoses between the branches of the external and internal carotid arteries.

## CLINICAL ANATOMY

- Pulsation of facial artery: It can be felt at two sites:
  1. At the base of mandible along the anteroinferior angle of masseter.
  2. At about 1.25 cm lateral to the angle of mouth.
- Rich vascularity of the face helps in rapid healing of wounds.

### Transverse Facial Artery

This small artery is a branch of the *superficial temporal artery* (Fig. 2.22). After emerging from the parotid gland, it runs forwards over the masseter between the parotid duct and the zygomatic arch, accompanied by the upper buccal branch of the facial nerve. It supplies the parotid gland and its duct, masseter and the overlying skin and ends by anastomosing with neighbouring arteries.

## DISSECTION

Tortuous facial artery enters the face at the lower border of mandible. Dissect its course from the anteroinferior angle of masseter muscle running to the angle of mouth till the medial angle of eye, reflecting off some of the facial muscles, if necessary.

Straight facial vein runs on a posterior plane than the artery.

Identify buccopharyngeal fascia on the external surface of buccinator muscle. Clean the deeply placed buccinator muscle situated lateral to the angle of mouth.

Identify parotid duct, running across the cheek 2 cm below the zygomatic arch. The duct pierces buccal pad of fat, buccopharyngeal fascia, buccinator muscle, mucous membrane of the mouth to open into its vestibule opposite second upper molar tooth.

*Competency:*
**AN28.8** Explain surgical importance of deep facial vein.

## VEINS OF THE FACE

1. The veins of the face accompany the arteries and drain into:
   a. Common facial vein
   b. Retromandibular vein.

   These veins communicate with the cavernous sinus.
2. The veins on each side form a ***'W-shaped' arrangement***. Each corner of the 'W' is prolonged upwards into the scalp and downwards into the neck (Fig. 2.23).
3. The ***facial vein*** is the largest vein of the face with no valves. It begins as the angular vein at the medial angle of the eye. It is formed by the union of the supratrochlear and supraorbital veins. The angular vein continues as the facial vein, running downwards and backwards behind the facial artery, but with a straighter course. It crosses the anteroinferior angle of the masseter, pierces the deep fascia, crosses the submandibular gland and joins the anterior division of the retromandibular vein below the angle of the mandible to form the common facial vein. The latter drains into the internal jugular vein. It is represented by a line drawn just behind the facial artery. The other veins drain into neighbouring veins.

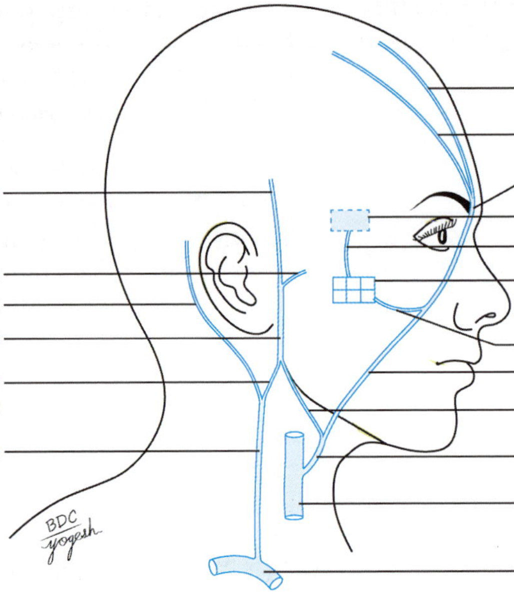


**Fig. 2.23:** The veins of the scalp, face and their deep connections with the cavernous sinus and the pterygoid plexus of veins

4. *Deep connections* of the facial vein include:
   a. A communication between the supraorbital and superior ophthalmic veins.
   b. Another connection with the pterygoid plexus through the ***deep facial* vein** which passes backwards over the buccinator. The connection between facial vein and cavernous sinus is shown in Fig. 2.23.

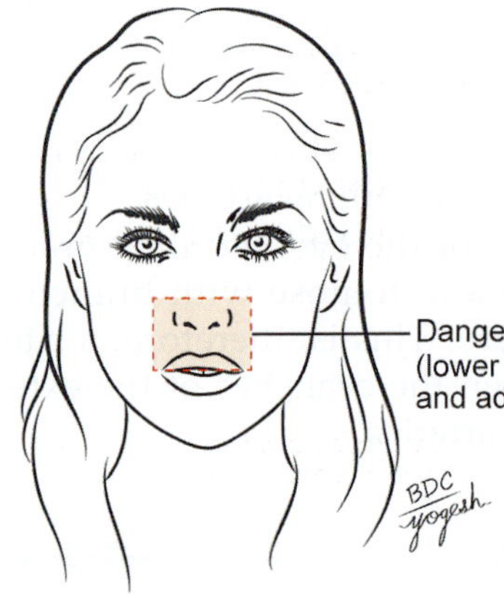


**Fig. 2.24:** Dangerous area of the face (stippled). Spread of infection from this area can cause thrombosis of the cavernous sinus

## CLINICAL ANATOMY

***Dangerous area of face:***

- The dangerous area of face is the lower part of nose, upper lip and adjoining parts of cheek (Fig. 2.24)
- ***Anatomical basis:***
  The venous blood from this area is drained by facial vein. This facial vein has two peculiarities that make this area as dangerous area of face:
  1. Facial vein is devoid of valves.
  2. Facial vein communicates with the cavernous sinus through
     i. Angular vein and supraorbital vein that communicate with superior ophthalmic vein (which is tributary of cavernous sinus).
     ii. Deep facial vein that communicates with pterygoid veinous plexus (which has communication with cavernous sinus via emissary veins).
  3. Facial vein rests on the facial muscles which facilitates the spread of infection and emboli from facial vein to the cavernous sinus.

  Thus, the infection from the dangerous area of the face may spread intracranially to the cavernous sinus.

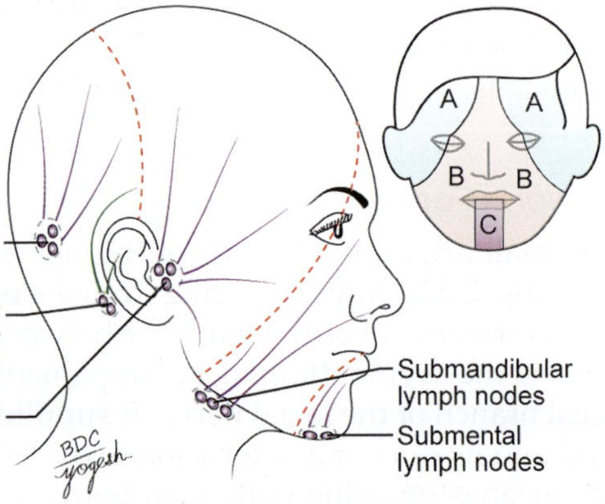


**Fig. 2.25:** The lymph nodes and lymphatic territories of the face. Area A drains into the preauricular nodes, area B drains into the submandibular nodes and area C drains into the submental nodes

## LYMPHATIC DRAINAGE OF THE FACE

The face has three lymphatic territories (Fig. 2.25):

1. ***Upper territory***, including the greater part of the forehead, lateral halves of eyelids, conjunctiva, lateral part of the cheek and parotid area, drains into the *preauricular parotid nodes*.
2. ***Middle territory***, including a strip over the median part of the forehead, external nose, upper lip, lateral

part of the lower lip, medial halves of the eyelids, medial part of the cheek and the greater part of lower jaw, drains into the *submandibular nodes*.

3. ***Lower territory***, including the central part of the lower lip and the chin, drains into the *submental nodes*.

### Labial, Buccal and Molar Mucous Glands

The labial and buccal mucous glands are numerous. They lie in the submucosa of the lips and cheeks. The molar mucous glands, four or five, lie on the buccopharyngeal fascia around the parotid duct. All these glands open into the vestibule of the mouth.

## EYELIDS OR PALPEBRAE

1. The space between the two eyelids is the ***palpebral fissure*** (Fig. 2.26). The two lids are fused to form the medial and lateral angles or ***canthi*** of the eye.
2. At the inner canthus, there is a small triangular space, the ***lacus lacrimalis***. Within it, there is an elevated ***lacrimal caruncle***, made up of modified skin and skin glands.
3. Lateral to the caruncle, the bulbar conjunctiva is pinched up to form a vertical fold called the ***plica semilunaris***.
4. Each eyelid is attached to the margins of the orbital opening. Its free edge is broad and has a rounded outer lip and a sharp inner lip. The outer lip presents two or more rows of eyelashes or cilia, except in the boundary of the lacus lacrimalis.
5. At the point where eyelashes cease, there is a ***lacrimal papilla*** on the summit of which there is the ***lacrimal punctum***. Near the inner lip of the free edge, there is a row of openings of the tarsal glands.
6. The free margin of both eyelids is subdivided into: Lateral 5/6th, the ciliary part with eyelashes and medial 1/6th, the lacrimal part, which lacks cilia.

### Structure

Each lid is made up of the following layers from without inwards (Fig. 2.27):

1. Skin
2. Superficial fascia
3. Orbicularis oculi (palpebral part)
4. Tarsal plate and palpebral fascia
5. Palpebral conjunctiva.

*Note*:

1. ***Skin*** is thin, loose and easily distensible by oedema fluid or blood.
2. ***Superficial fascia*** is without any fat. It contains the palpebral part of the orbicularis oculi. Deep to the muscle is loose areolar tissue which is continuous with loose areolar tissue of the scalp.
3. ***Palpebral fascia*** of the two lids forms the ***orbital septum***. Its thickenings form ***tarsal plates*** or *tarsi* in the lids and the ***palpebral ligaments*** at the angles (Plate 2.4, Fig. 2.28).

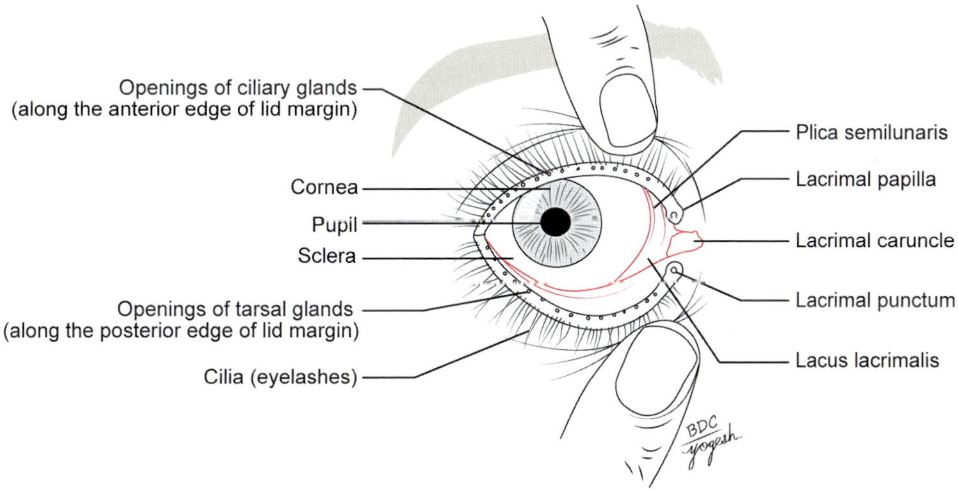


**Fig. 2.26:** Features of the palpebral fissure

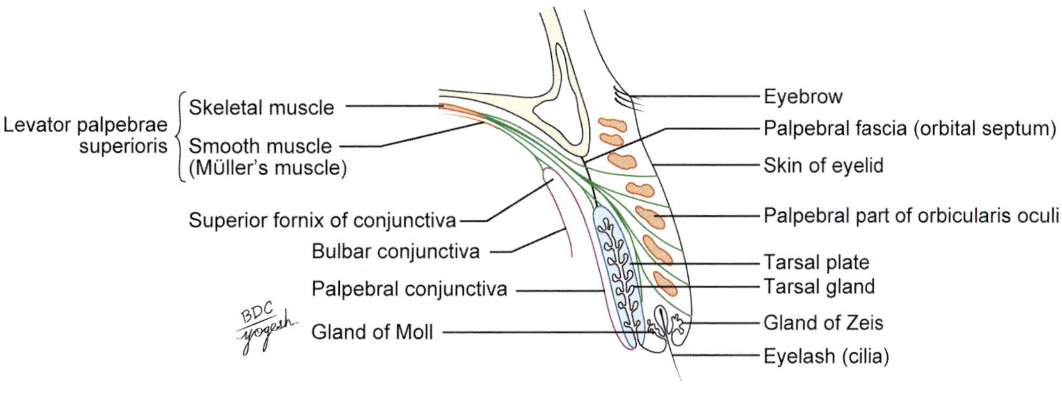


**Fig. 2.27:** Structure of the eyelid (sagittal section of upper eyelid)

**Plate 2.4:** Tarsal plates and palpebral fascia

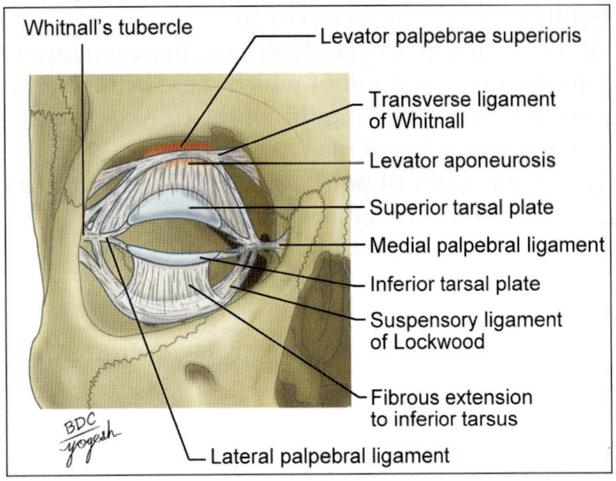


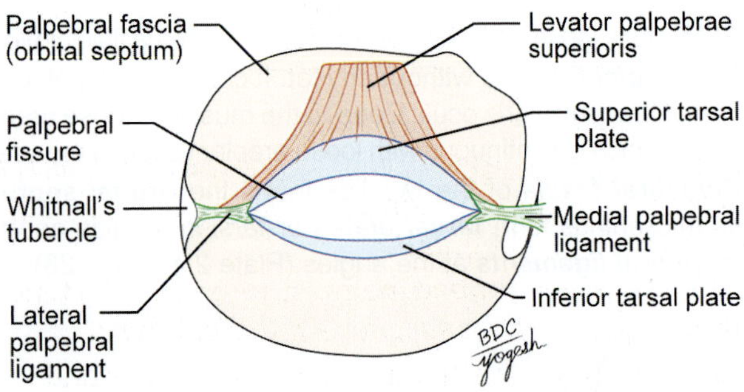


**Fig. 2.28:** Tarsal plates and palpebral fascia

Tarsi are thin plates of condensed fibrous tissue located near the lid margins. They give stiffness to the lids.

The palpebral fascia (orbital septum) is pierced by:

a. Palpebral part of lacrimal gland
b. Fibres of levator palpebrae superioris
c. Vessels and nerves entering the face from the orbit.

4. The upper tarsus receives two tendinous slips from the ***levator palpebrae superioris***, one from voluntary part and another from involuntary part or ***Müller's muscle***.
5. ***Tarsal glands*** or ***meibomian glands*** are embedded in the posterior surface of the tarsi; their ducts open in a row behind the cilia.
6. The ***conjunctiva*** lines the posterior surface of the tarsus.
7. Apart from the usual glands of the skin and mucous glands in the conjunctiva, the larger glands found in the lids are:
   a. Large sebaceous glands also called ***Zeis glands*** at the lid margin associated with cilia.
   b. Modified sweat glands or ***Moll's glands*** at the lid margin closely associated with Zeis glands and cilia.
   c. Sebaceous or *tarsal glands* are also known as *meibomian glands*.

## Blood Supply

The eyelids are supplied by:

1. The superior and inferior palpebral branches of the ophthalmic artery.
2. The lateral palpebral branch of the lacrimal artery.

They form an arcade in each lid.

The veins drain into the ophthalmic and facial veins.

## Nerve Supply

The upper eyelid is supplied by the lacrimal, supraorbital, supratrochlear and infratrochlear nerves from lateral to medial side.

The lower eyelid is supplied by the infraorbital and infratrochlear nerves.

## Lymphatic Drainage

The medial halves of the lids drain into the submandibular nodes, and the lateral halves into the preauricular nodes.

## CLINICAL ANATOMY (Plate 2.5)

- The ***Müller's muscle*** or involuntary part of levator palpebrae superioris is supplied by sympathetic fibres from the superior cervical ganglion. Paralysis of this muscle leads to partial ***ptosis***. This is part of the ***Horner's syndrome***.
- ***Conjunctivitis*** is one of the commonest diseases of the eye. It may be caused by infection or by allergy. The palpebral conjunctiva is examined for anaemia and for conjunctivitis; the bulbar conjunctiva for jaundice.
- Foreign bodies are often lodged in a groove situated 2 mm from the edge of each eyelid.
- ***Chalazion*** is inflammation of a tarsal gland, causing a localised swelling pointing inwards.
- ***Ectropion*** is due to eversion of the lower lacrimal punctum. It usually occurs in old age due to laxity of skin.
- ***Trachoma*** is a contagious granular conjunctivitis caused by the trachoma virus. It is regarded as the commonest cause of blindness.
- ***Stye*** or ***hordeolum*** is a suppurative inflammation of one of the glands of Zeis. The gland is swollen, hard and painful and the whole of the lid is oedematous. The pus points near the base of one of the cilia.
- ***Blepharitis*** is inflammation of the eyelids, especially of the lid margin.

## DISSECTION

Give a circular incision around the roots of eyelids (Fig. 2.3 – viii and ix). This will separate the orbital part of orbicularis oculi from the palpebral parts. Carefully reflect the palpebral part towards the palpebral fissure. Identify the structures present beneath the muscle as given in the text.

The upper and lower eyelids are movable curtains that protect the eyes from foreign bodies and bright light. They keep the cornea clean and moist. The upper eyelid is larger and more movable than the lower eyelid.

Plate 2.5: Some diseases of eyelids

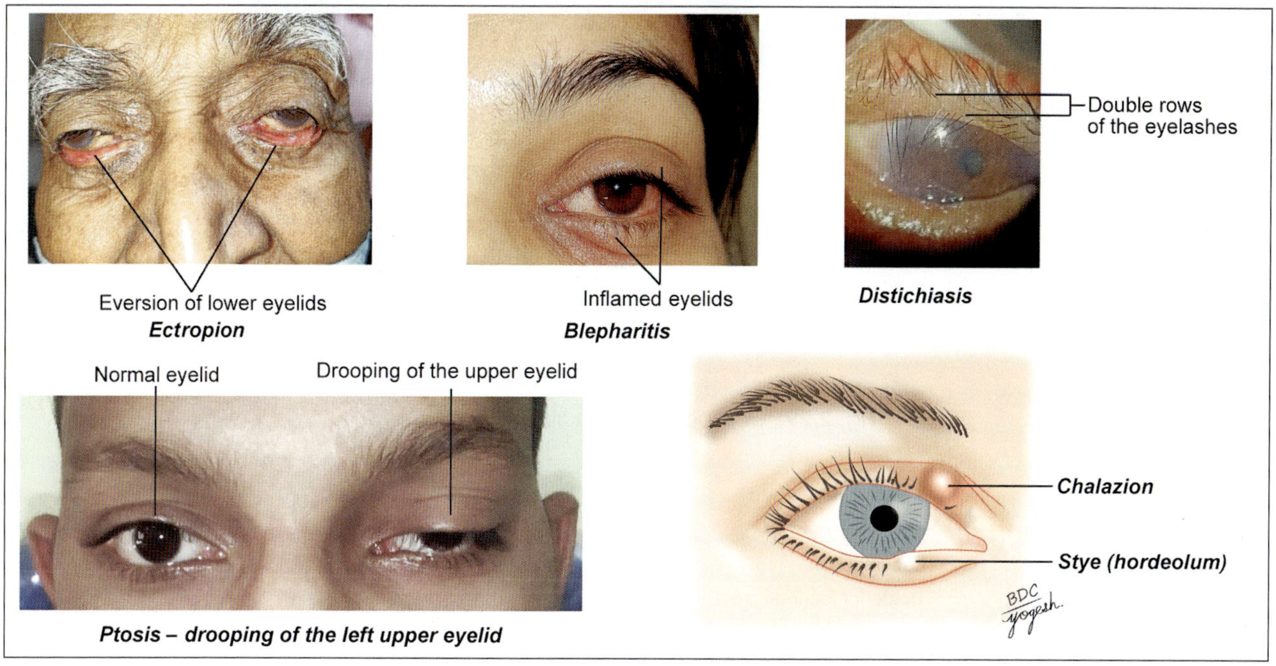


(*Image courtesy*: Dr Rohit Rao)

**Competency:**
**AN31.4** Enumerate components of lacrimal apparatus.

## LACRIMAL APPARATUS

### COMPONENTS

The structures concerned with secretion and drainage of the lacrimal or tear fluid constitute the lacrimal apparatus. It is made up of the following parts (Figs 2.29 and 2.30, Flowchart 2.5):

1. Lacrimal gland and its ducts
2. Conjunctival sac
3. Lacrimal puncta
4. Lacrimal canaliculi
5. Lacrimal sac
6. Nasolacrimal duct.

### Lacrimal Gland

It is a ***serous gland*** situated chiefly in the lacrimal fossa on the anterolateral part of the roof of the bony orbit and partly on the upper eyelid. Small *accessory lacrimal glands* are found in the conjunctival fornices. These are also called ***Krause's gland***.

The gland is 'J' shaped, being indented by the tendon of the *levator palpebrae superioris* muscle. It has:

a. An *orbital part* that is larger and deeper and
b. A *palpebral part* smaller and superficial, lying within the eyelid (Fig. 2.29).

***Ducts of lacrimal gland:*** About 12 *ducts* pierce the conjunctiva of the upper lid and open into the conjunctival sac near the superior fornix. Most of the ducts of the orbital part pass through the palpebral part.

*Note*: Removal of the palpebral part of the lacrimal gland is functionally equivalent to removal of the entire gland. After removal, the conjunctiva and cornea are moistened by accessory lacrimal glands, if present.

***Nerve supply:*** The gland is supplied by the lacrimal branch of the ophthalmic artery and by the *lacrimal nerve*. The nerve has both sensory and secretomotor fibres. Flowchart 2.6 shows the secretomotor fibres for lacrimal gland (Fig. 2.31, Flowchart 2.6).

Flowchart 2.5: Parts of lacrimal apparatus

***Parts of lacrimal apparatus***
Production, secretion, and drainage of tears

***Lacrimal gland***
J-shaped
Has two parts
- Orbital
- Palpebral
12 ducts
↓
Open into superior fornix
Secretes lacrimal fluid

***Conjunctival sac***
Lies between palpebral and bulbar conjunctiva
2 fornices
- Superior
- Inferior

***Lacrimal puncta and canaliculi***
Puncta:
Small openings at lacrimal papillae
Canaliculi:
- One in each eyelid
- 10 mm long
- 2 parts: Vertical and horizontal
Dilatation as ampulla
Open into lacrimal sac

***Lacrimal sac***
Fibroelastic sac
12 mm x 5 mm
Lies in lacrimal fossa
Continues downward as nasolacrimal duct

***Nasolacrimal duct***
18 mm long
Direction: Downward, backward, laterally
Opens into inferior meatus of nose
Guarded by valve of Hasner

BDC yogesh

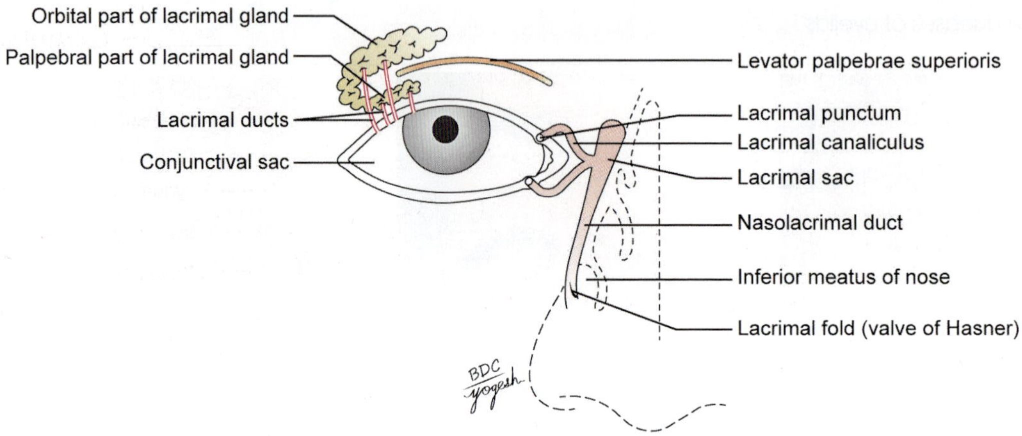


**Fig. 2.29:** Components of lacrimal apparatus

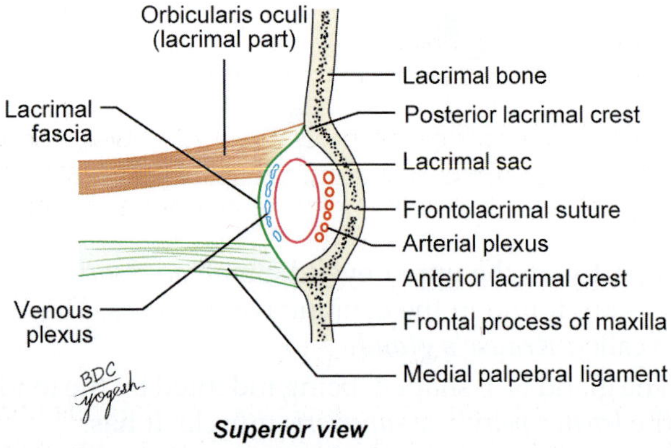


**Fig. 2.30:** Relations of the lacrimal sac (horizontal section passing through the medial part of the orbit)

***Functions:*** Lacrimal glands secrete about 1–15 ml of lacrimal fluid per day. Most of it evaporates, and rest is drained into the lacrimal sac.

*Function of lacrimal fluid*

1. Keep the cornea moist which is essential for its transparency.
2. Nourishes the cornea.
3. Flushes the conjunctival sac.
4. Prevents infection by the action of its lysozymes.
5. Medium for expression with shedding of tears during grief, sorrow and extreme emotional happiness.

## Conjunctival Sac

The conjunctiva lining the deep surfaces of the eyelids is called ***palpebral conjunctiva*** and that lining the front of the eyeball is called ***bulbar conjunctiva*** (Figs 2.29 and 2.30). The potential space between the palpebral and bulbar parts is the ***conjunctival sac.***

The lines along which the palpebral conjunctiva of the upper and lower eyelids is reflected onto the eyeball are called the superior and inferior ***conjunctival fornices.***

*Note:* The *palpebral conjunctiva* is thick, opaque, highly vascular and adherent to the tarsal plate. The *bulbar conjunctiva* covers the sclera. It is thin, transparent and loosely attached to the eyeball. Over the cornea, it is represented by the anterior epithelium of the cornea.

**Flowchart 2.6:** Nerve supply of the lacrimal gland

***Parasympathetic fibres***

Lacrimatory nucleus
↓
Facial nerve
↓
Nervous intermedius
↓
Geniculate ganglion
↓
Greater petrosal nerve
↓
***Pterygopalatine ganglion***
↓ Relay
Postganglionic fibres

***Sympathetic fibres***

T1 segment of spinal cord
↓
Superior cervical sympathetic ganglion
↓ Relay
Postganglionic fibres
↓
Plexus around internal carotid artery
↓
Pterygopalatine ganglion

Both pathways:

↓
Zygomatic nerve
↓
Zygomaticotemporal nerve
↓
***Lacrimal gland***

## Lacrimal Puncta

These are small openings on the lid margin at the top of the laminal papillae. ***Lacrimal papilla*** is a small conical projection at the medial end of free margin of the eyelids.

## Lacrimal Canaliculi

These are one in each eyelid, and it is about 10 mm long. Each canaliculus begins at the lacrimal punctum. It has two parts:

1. Vertical part: 2 mm long
2. Horizontal part: 8 mm long

There is an ampulla (dilated part) in each canaliculus.

## Lacrimal Sac

It is a membranous sac, 12 mm long and 5 mm wide, situated in the lacrimal groove behind the medial palpebral ligament. Its upper end is blind. The lower end is continuous with the nasolacrimal duct.

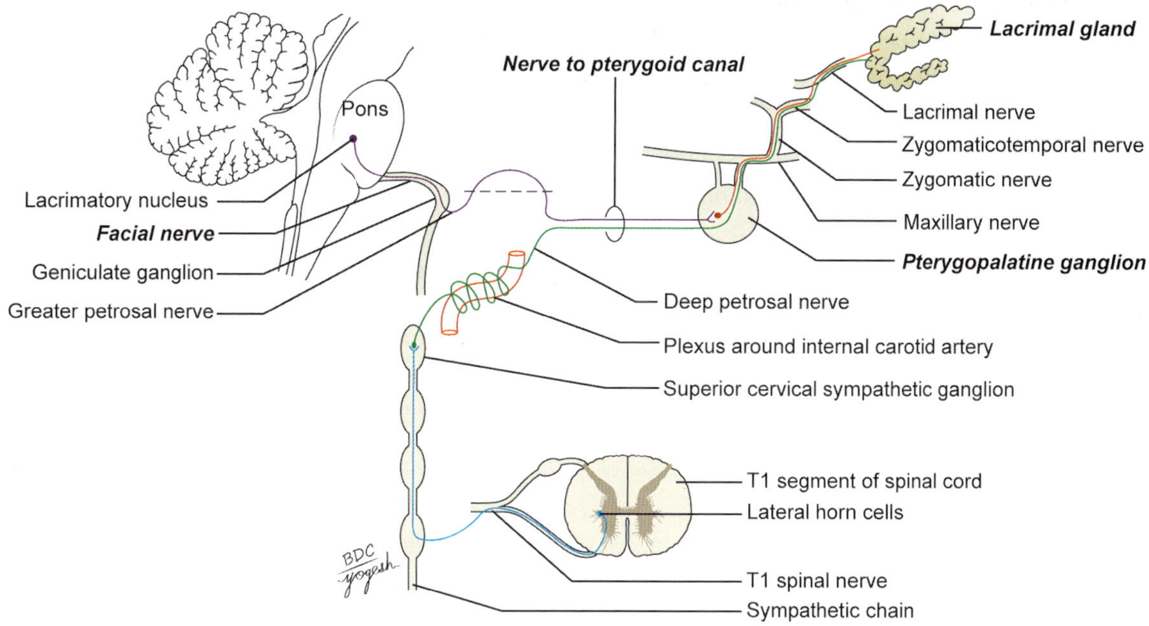


**Fig. 2.31:** Innervation of lacrimal gland (schematic representation, Purple line: Preganglionic parasympathetic fibres, Red line: Postganglionic parasympathetic fibres, Blue line: Preganglionic sympathetic fibres, Green line: Postganglionic sympathetic fibres, *Note*: Greater petrosal nerve enter the middle cranial fossa and enters the foramen lacerum where it forms nerve to pterygoid canal. Middle cranial fossa shown by black dotted line)

The sac is related anteriorly to the medial palpebral ligament and to the orbicularis oculi. Medially, the lacrimal groove separates it from the nose. Laterally, it is related to the lacrimal fascia and the lacrimal part of the orbicularis oculi which helps in dilatation of lacrimal sac for efficient drainage of lacrimal fluid (Fig. 2.30).

### Nasolacrimal Duct

It is a membranous passage, 18 mm long. It begins at the lower end of the lacrimal sac, runs downwards, backwards and laterally and *opens into the inferior meatus of the nose*. A fold of mucous membrane called the ***valve of Hasner***, forms an imperfect valve at the lower end of the duct.

*Note:* ***Factors helping drainage of tears*:**
1. Capillary action of lacrimal canaliculi
2. Blinking of eyelids that spreads the tears in conjunctival sac
3. Drying of tears
4. Inward direction of puncta during blinking
5. Conjunction of lacrimal part of orbicularis oculi pulls the lacrimal fascia that dilates the lacrimal sac.

## CLINICAL ANATOMY

- Inflammation of the lacrimal sac is called ***dacryocystitis***.
- The ducts of lacrimal gland open through its palpebral part into the conjunctival sac. Because of this arrangement, the removal of palpebral part necessitates the removal of the orbital part as well.
- Excessive secretion of the lacrimal fluid overflowing on the cheeks is called ***epiphora***. Epiphora may result due to obstruction in the lacrimal fluid pathway, either at the level of punctum or canaliculi or nasolacrimal duct.

## DISSECTION

On the lateral side of the upper lid, cut the palpebral fascia. This will show the presence of the lacrimal gland deep in this area. Its palpebral part is to be traced in the upper eyelid. On the medial ends of both the eyelids, look for lacrimal papilla. Palpate and dissect the medial palpebral ligament binding the medial ends of the eyelids. Try to locate the small lacrimal sac behind this ligament.

***Competency:***
**AN43.4** Describe the development and developmental basis of congenital anomalies of face, palate, tongue, branchial apparatus, pituitary gland, thyroid gland and eye. (Development of face is given here. For the development of other structures, please refer to respective chapters.)

## DEVELOPMENT OF FACE

The face develops from five mesodermal processes that appear in 4th week surrounding the stomodeum.

These processes are (Fig. 2.32):
1. Frontonasal process (unpaired)
2. Maxillary process (paired)
3. Mandibular process (paired).

Facial development takes place between 4th and 8th weeks.

The various parts of the face are derived as follows:
1. *Lower lip*: Bilateral mandibular process fuses in the midline to form a lower lip and jawbone.
2. *Upper lip*:
   - Central part (philtrum) of upper lip is derived from medial nasal process.

- Lateral parts of upper lip are derived from bilateral maxillary processes.

*Note*: The ectoderm (skin) of maxillary process overgrows and covers central part (philtrum) of the upper lip; hence, skin of the upper lip is supplied by maxillary nerve (Fig. 2.33).

3. Muscles of the face are derived from *second pharyngeal arch*, hence supplied by the facial nerve.

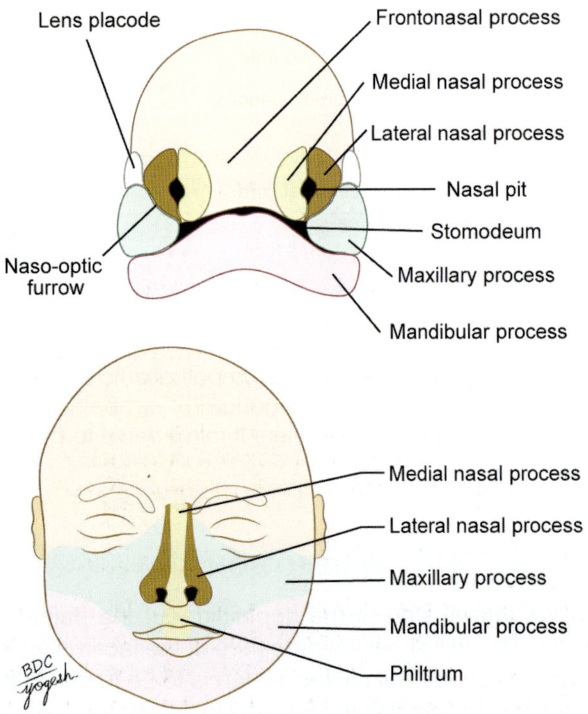


**Fig. 2.32:** Development of the face

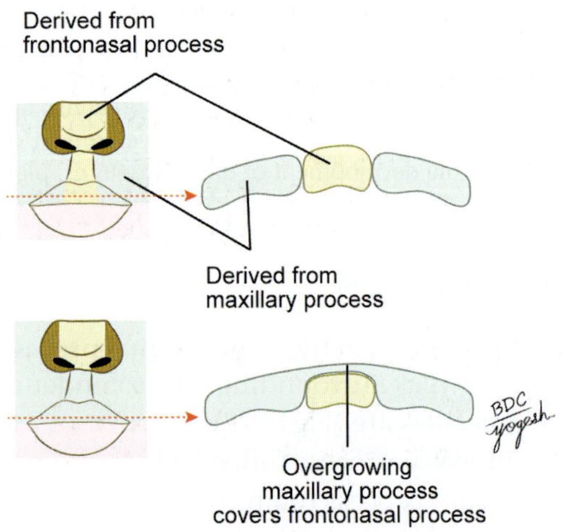


**Fig. 2.33:** Formation of the upper lip. The ectoderm of the maxillary process overgrows the frontonasal process. Hence, skin of the upper lip is supplied by the maxillary nerve

4. *Cheeks*: The maxillary and mandibular processes undergo fusion from the lateral side and form smaller stomodeum or normal oral fissure, where fused part forms cheeks.
5. External nose is derived as follows:
   - Bridge of nose from frontonasal process.
   - Dorsum and tip of the nose from fused medial nasal processes.
   - Ala of nose from lateral nasal processes.
   - Anterior nares (nostrils) from nasal pit.
   - Nasal cavity from nasal sacs.
   - Posterior nares (choanae) from rupture of bucconasal membrane.

VIDEO

**Video 3.2 Scalp and Face:** Scalp, Face

### *Facts to Remember*

- Caput succedaneum is the most common form of birth trauma of the scalp.
- Impulses from skin of the face reach the three branches of trigeminal nerve, whereas the muscles of facial expression are supplied by the facial nerve.
- Facial nerve though courses through the parotid gland, does not give any branch to the largest salivary gland.
- Buccinator is an accessory muscle of mastication, as it prevents food entering the vestibule of mouth.
- Part of the face between anterior nares and upper lip is called 'dangerous area of face' as the facial vein communicates with cavernous venous sinus situated in the cranial cavity. Any infection from this part of face can infect the intracranial venous sinus, i.e. cavernous sinus.
- Levator palpebrae superioris is supplied partly by oculomotor nerve and partly by sympathetic fibres.
- The facial muscles are subcutaneous in position and represents morphologically remnants of panniculus carnosus. Platysma helps in loosening the tight collar or tie.
- Eyelid contains Meibomian/tarsal glands, glands of Zeis, glands of Moll and glands of Wolfring and glands of Krause.

### BDC's Anatomy *e*-book

1. Surface landmarks
2. Molecular regulation of development of face
3. Further reading
4. Viva voce questions

# Right orbit seen from the front

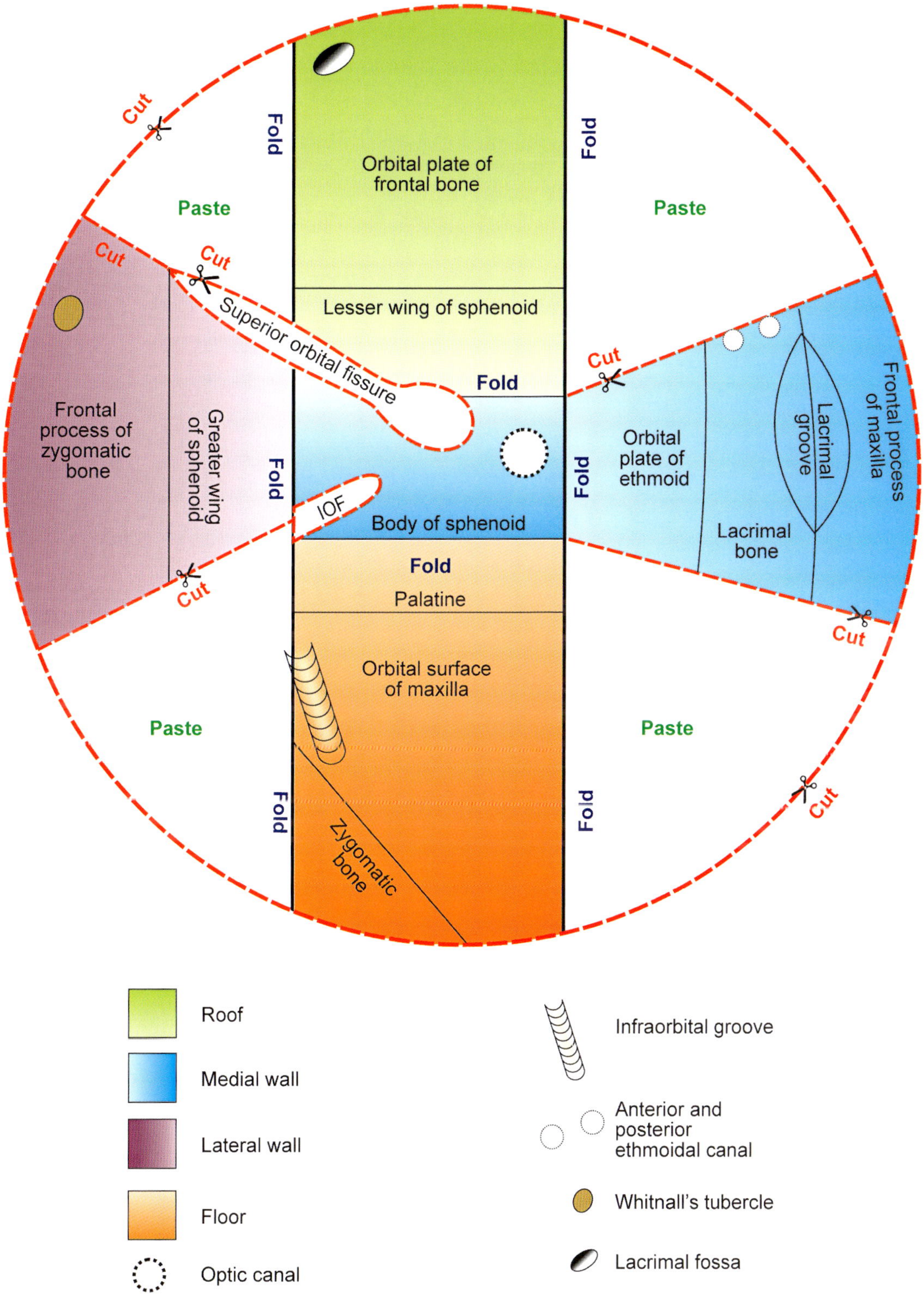

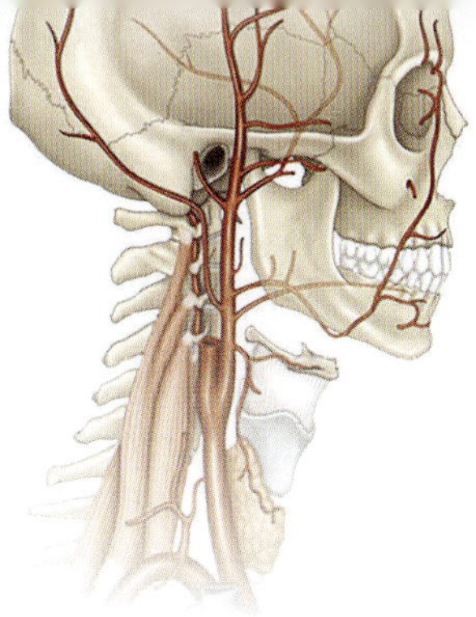

Chapter

3

# Side of the Neck

The neck extends superiorly up to external occipital protuberance, superior nuchal line, mastoid process, angle of mandible and base or inferior border of mandible. Inferiorly, the neck extends up to spine of C7 vertebra, superior border of scapula, acromion, clavicle and suprasternal notch.

On observing the neck from the lateral side, it appears quadrangular in shape. This quadrilateral area of the side of the neck is divided into two triangular areas by the sternocleidomastoid muscle as large anterior and small posterior triangles.

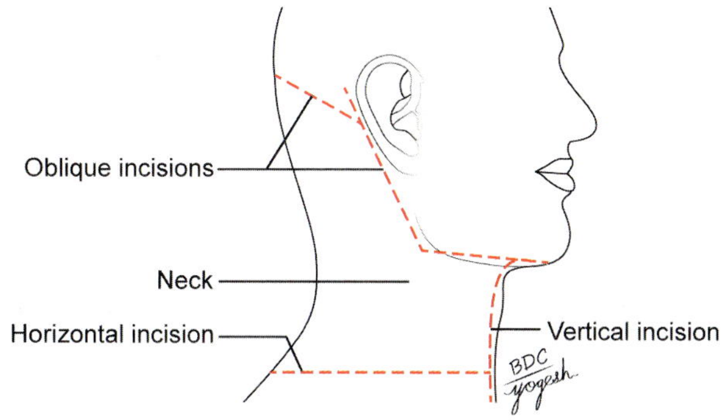


**Fig. 3.1:** Lines of dissection

## LANDMARKS

1. ***Sternocleidomastoid*** muscle is seen prominently when the neck and chin are turned to the opposite side. The ridge raised by the muscle extends from the clavicle and sternum to the mastoid process (Fig. 3.1).
2. ***External jugular vein*** crosses the sternocleidomastoid obliquely, running downwards and backwards from near the auricle to the clavicle. It is better seen in old age.
3. ***Greater supraclavicular fossa*** lies above and behind the middle one-third of the clavicle. It overlies the cervical part of the brachial plexus and the third part of the subclavian artery.
4. ***Lesser supraclavicular fossa*** is a small depression between the sternal and clavicular parts of the sternocleidomastoid. It overlies the internal jugular vein.
5. ***Mastoid process*** is a large bony projection behind the auricle.
6. ***Transverse process of the atlas vertebra*** can be felt on deep pressure midway between the angle of the mandible and the mastoid process, immediately anteroinferior to the tip of the mastoid process.
7. The ***4th cervical transverse process*** is just palpable at the level of the upper border of the thyroid cartilage; and the *6th cervical transverse process* is at the level of the cricoid cartilage.
8. The anterior tubercle of the ***transverse process of the 6th cervical vertebra*** is the largest of all such processes and is called the ***carotid tubercle*** of Chassaignac. The common carotid artery can be best pressed against this tubercle, deep to the anterior border of the sternocleidomastoid muscle.
9. The ***anterior border of the trapezius muscle*** becomes prominent on elevation of the shoulder against resistance.

## BOUNDARIES

The side of the neck is roughly quadrilateral in outline (Fig. 3.2).

It is *bounded as follows:*

*Anteriorly*: Anterior median line
*Posteriorly*: Anterior border of trapezius
*Superiorly*: Base of mandible
A line joining angle of the mandible to mastoid process
Superior nuchal line
*Inferiorly*: Clavicle.

This quadrilateral space is divided obliquely by the sternocleidomastoid muscle into the *anterior and posterior triangles* (Fig. 3.3).

## SKIN

The skin of the neck is supplied by the C2 to C4 spinal nerves.

The anterolateral part is supplied by anterior primary rami through

1. Transverse/anterior cutaneous nerve (C2, C3)
2. Great auricular nerve (C2, C3)

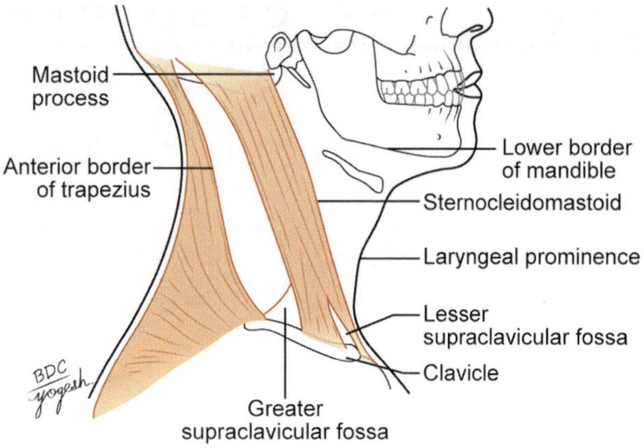


**Fig. 3.2:** Boundaries of the side of neck

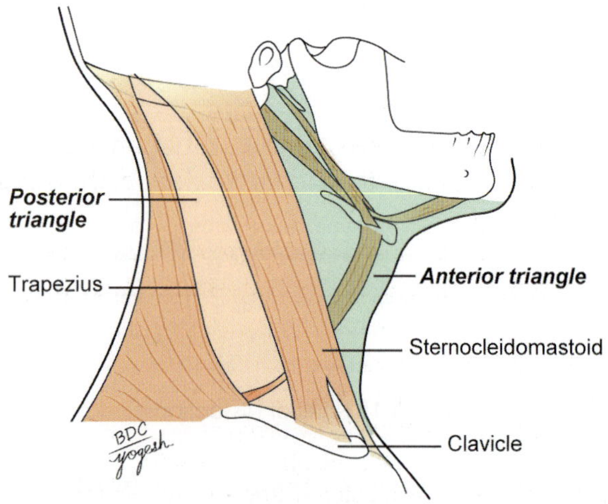


**Fig. 3.3:** Side of neck divided into anterior and posterior triangles

3. Lesser occipital nerve (C2)
4. Supraclavicular nerves (C3, C4).

A broad band of skin over the posterior part is supplied by dorsal or posterior primary rami (*see* Fig. 2.21).

*Note*: The 1st cervical spinal nerve has no cutaneous distribution. The C5, C6, C7, C8 and T1 nerves supply the upper limb through the brachial plexus; and, therefore, do not supply the neck. The territory of C4 nerve extends into the pectoral region through the supraclavicular nerves and meets T2 dermatome at the level of the 2nd costal cartilage.

## SUPERFICIAL FASCIA

Superficial fascia contains:
1. Areolar tissue
2. Platysma
3. Cutaneous nerves
4. Superficial veins
5. *Lymph vessels, lymph nodes* and small arteries.

### CLINICAL ANATOMY

The surgeon has to stitch platysma muscle separately so that skin does not adhere to deeper neck muscles, otherwise the skin will get an ugly scar.

### DISSECTION

Give a median incision from the chin downwards towards the suprasternal notch situated above the manubrium of sternum.

Make one incision in the skin of base of mandible. Continue it by oblique incision along posterior border of ramus of mandible up to mastoid process and further along the superior nuchal line till the external occipital protuberance.

One incision is given along the upper border of clavicle (Fig. 3.1). Reflect only the skin up towards the anterior border of trapezius muscle.

Platysma, a part of the subcutaneous muscle is visible. Reflect the platysma towards the mandible. Identify the anterior or transverse cutaneous nerve of the neck in the upper part of superficial fascia. Anterior jugular vein running vertically close to the median plane is also encountered. Remove the superficial fascia till the deep fascia of neck is seen (Fig. 3.1).

External jugular vein is seen above the clavicle. To open up the suprasternal space, make a horizontal incision just above the sternum. Extend this incision along the anterior border of sternocleidomastoid muscle for 3–4 cm. Reflect the superficial lamina to expose the suprasternal space and identify its contents.

Define the attachments of investing layer, pretracheal layer, prevertebral layer and carotid sheath.

*Competency:*
**AN35.1** Describe the parts, extent, attachments, modifications of deep cervical fascia.

## DEEP CERVICAL FASCIA (FASCIA COLLI)

The deep cervical fascia is the most important structure that holds the structures in the neck in place. It separates neurovascular bundles, prevents compression of vessels, trachea and oesophagus and prevents spread of infection. The deep fascia of the neck is condensed to form the following layers:
1. Investing layer
2. Pretracheal fascia
3. Prevertebral fascia
4. Carotid sheath
5. Buccopharyngeal fascia
6. Pharyngobasilar fascia.

## INVESTING LAYER

It lies deep to the platysma and surrounds the neck like a collar. It forms the roof of the posterior triangle of the neck (Figs 3.4 to 3.8).

### Attachments and Tracings

#### *Superiorly*

a. External occipital protuberance
b. Superior nuchal line

c. Mastoid process, styloid process
d. External acoustic meatus, tympanic plate
e. Base of the mandible.

*Note*: Between the angle of the mandible and the mastoid process, the fascia splits to enclose the parotid gland (Fig. 3.5).

a. The ***superficial lamina***, named ***parotid fascia***, is thick and dense and is attached to the zygomatic arch.
b. The ***deep lamina*** is thin and is attached to the styloid process, the tympanic plate and the mandible (*see* Fig. 5.2). Between the styloid process and the angle of the mandible, the deep lamina is thick and forms the ***stylomandibular ligament*** which separates the parotid gland from the submandibular gland, and is pierced by the external carotid artery.

The superficial lamina is attached to lower border of body of mandible and deep lamina to the mylohyoid line.

### *Inferiorly*

a. Spine of scapula
b. Acromion process
c. Clavicle
d. Manubrium.

*Note*: The fascia splits to enclose the suprasternal and supraclavicular spaces (Fig. 3.5).

### *Posteriorly*

a. Ligamentum nuchae and
b. Spine of C7 vertebra.

### *Anteriorly*

a. Symphysis menti
b. Hyoid bone.

Both above and below the hyoid bone, it is continuous with the fascia of the opposite side.

### Features of Investing Layer

1. The investing layer of deep cervical fascia *splits* to enclose (Figs 3.5 to 3.7):
   a. *Muscles*: Trapezius and sternocleidomastoid.
   b. *Salivary glands*: Parotid and submandibular
   c. *Spaces*: Suprasternal and supraclavicular.
2. ***Suprasternal space*** or space of Burns contains:
   a. Sternal heads of the right and left sternocleidomastoid muscles (Fig. 3.8),
   b. Jugular venous arch,
   c. Lymph node and
   d. Interclavicular ligament.
3. ***Supraclavicular space*** lying above middle 1/3rd of clavicle is traversed by (Fig. 3.6):
   a. External jugular vein,
   b. Supraclavicular nerves and
   c. Cutaneous vessels, including lymphatics.
4. It also forms *pulleys* to bind the tendons of the digastric and omohyoid muscles.
5. Forms roof of anterior and posterior triangles.
6. Forms stylomandibular ligament (Fig. 3.6) and parotidomasseteric fascia.

*Note*: ***Rule of 2*** for investing layer:
- Enclosed muscles: Trapezius, SCM
- Roofs of anterior and posterior triangles
- Enclosed glands: Submandibular and parotid
- Enclosed spaces: Suprasternal and supraclavicular
- Pullies for: Omohyoid and digastric.

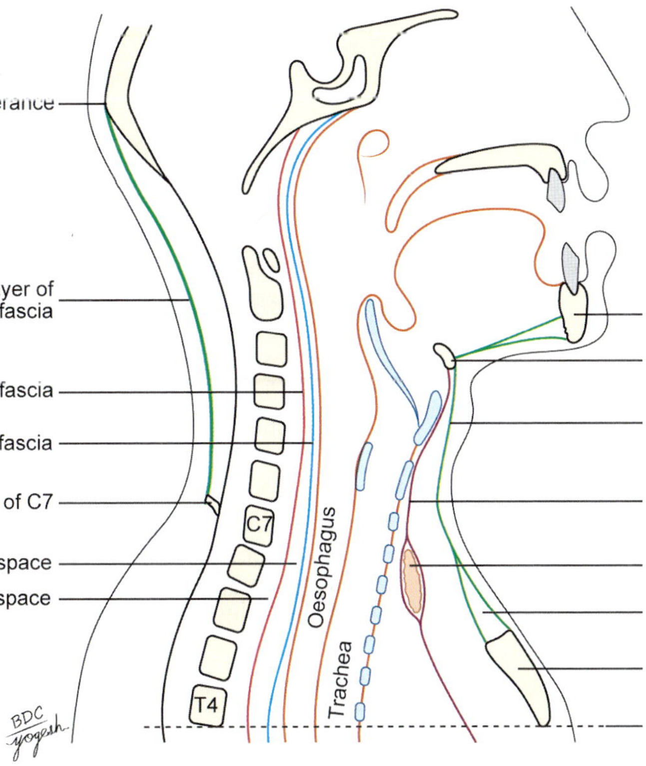


**Fig. 3.4:** Vertical extent of the first three layers of the deep cervical fascia

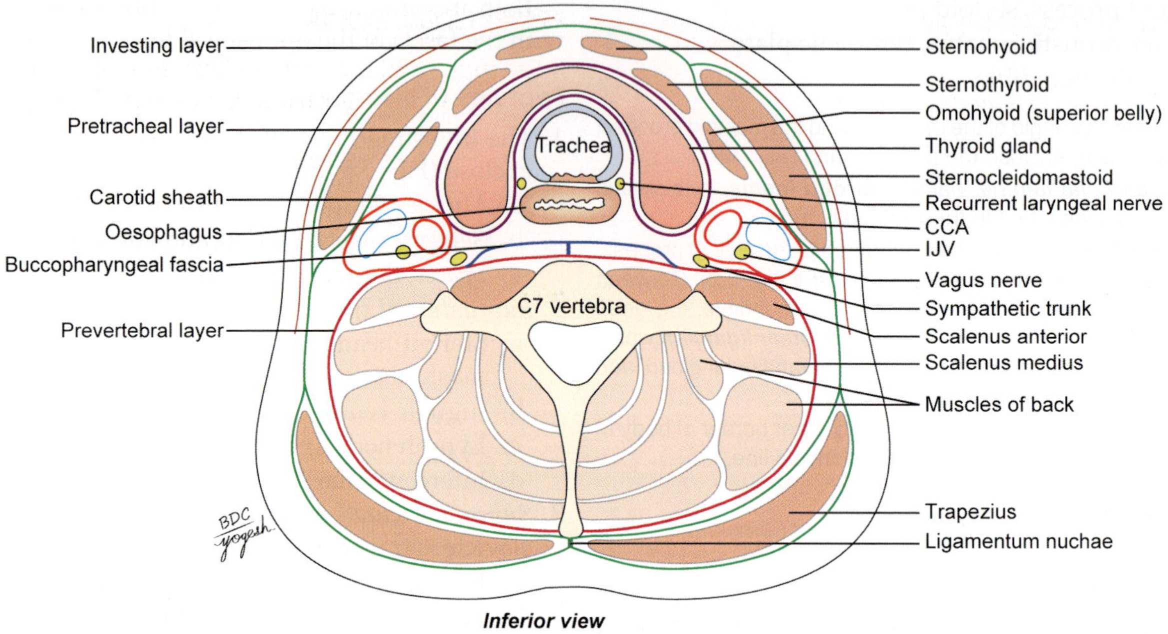


**Fig. 3.5:** Transverse section through neck at the level of the 7th cervical vertebra to show the horizontal disposition of the three layers of deep cervical fascia (CCA: Common carotid artery; IJV: Internal jugular vein)

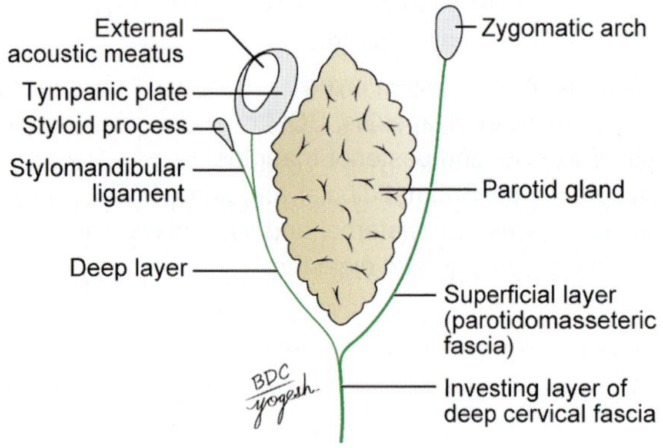


**Fig. 3.6:** Investing layer of the deep cervical fascia enclosing parotid gland (right, coronal section passing behind the ramus of mandible, posterior view)

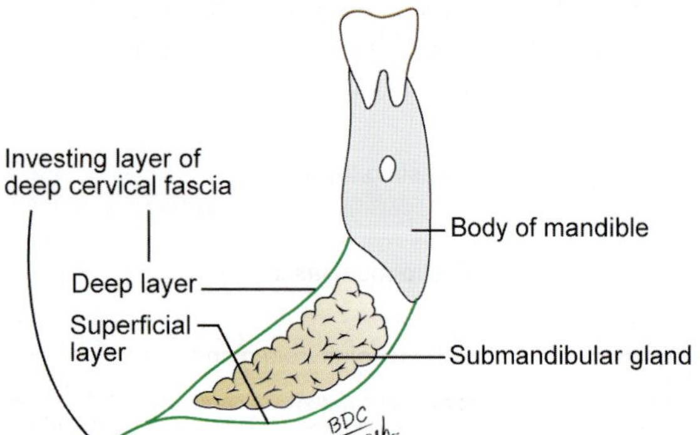


**Fig. 3.7:** Investing layer of the deep cervical fascia enclosing the submandibular gland (coronal section passing through the body of mandible, posterior view)

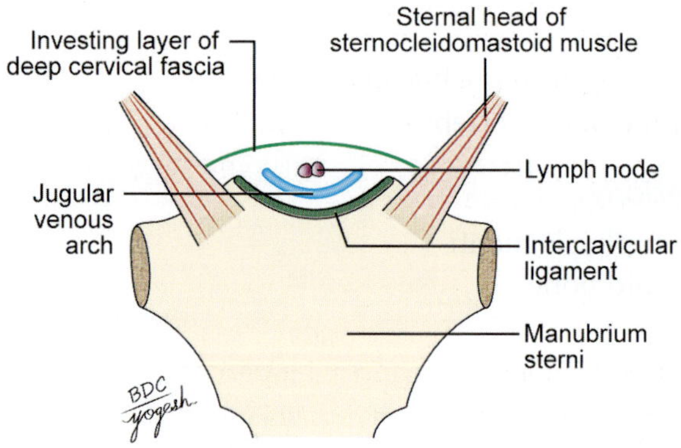


**Fig. 3.8:** Contents of suprasternal space

## CLINICAL ANATOMY

- ***Painful parotid swelling***: Parotid swellings are very painful due to the unyielding nature of parotid fascia.
- While excising the submandibular salivary gland, the external carotid artery should be secured before dividing it, otherwise it may retract through the stylomandibular ligament and cause serious bleeding. This figure also shows the superior attachment of investing layer of deep cervical fascia to tympanic plate and styloid process.
- Division of the external jugular vein in the supraclavicular space may cause air embolism and consequent death because the cut ends of the vein are prevented from contraction and closure by the fascia, attached firmly to the vein.

## PRETRACHEAL FASCIA

The importance of this fascia is that it encloses and suspends the thyroid gland and forms its false capsule (Fig. 3.2). It is continuous with buccopharyngeal fascia.

### Attachments and Tracings

#### Superiorly

1. Hyoid bone in the median plane
2. Oblique line of thyroid cartilage—laterally
3. Cricoid cartilage—more laterally.

#### Inferiorly

Below the thyroid gland, it encloses the inferior thyroid veins, passes behind the brachiocephalic veins and finally blends with the arch of the aorta and fibrous pericardium.

#### On Either Side

It forms the front of the carotid sheath and fuses with the fascia deep to the sternocleidomastoid (Fig. 3.3).

### Features of Pretracheal Fascia

1. The posterior layer of the thyroid capsule is thick. On either side, it forms a ***suspensory ligament*** for the thyroid gland known as ***ligament of Berry***. The ligaments are attached chiefly to the cricoid cartilage, and may extend to the thyroid cartilage. They support the thyroid gland and do not let it sink into the mediastinum. The capsule of the thyroid is very weak along the posterior borders of the lateral lobes.
2. Permits movement of trachea: The fascia provides a slippery surface for free movements of the trachea during swallowing.

### CLINICAL ANATOMY

- Neck infections in front of the pretracheal fascia may bulge in the suprasternal area or extend down into the anterior mediastinum.
- The thyroid gland and all thyroid swellings move with deglutition because the thyroid is attached to cartilages of the larynx by the suspensory ligaments of Berry.
- Extension of neck infection: As the pretracheal fascia extends into the superior mediastinum, a pus (infection) in front of the pretracheal fascia may extend into the superior mediastinum.

## PREVERTEBRAL FASCIA

It lies in front of the prevertebral muscles and forms the floor of the posterior triangle of the neck (Fig. 3.4).

### Attachments and Tracings

#### Superiorly

It is attached to the base of the skull.

#### Inferiorly

It extends into the superior mediastinum and blends with the anterior longitudinal ligament and body of thoracic vertebrae.

#### Anteriorly

It is separated from the pharynx and buccopharyngeal fascia by the ***retropharyngeal space***. In the lower part of neck, prevertebral and buccopharyngeal fasciae fuse. Lymph nodes lie in the retropharyngeal space.

#### Laterally

It lies deep into the trapezius and is attached to fascia of sternocleidomastoid muscle.

### Features of Prevertebral Fascia

1. The trunks of brachial plexuses lie behind the prevertebral fascia between scalenus anterior and scalenus medius muscles. The fascia is pierced by the four cutaneous branches of the cervical plexus.
2. As the trunks of the brachial plexus and the subclavian artery pass laterally through the interval between the scalenus anterior and the scalenus medius, they carry with them a covering of the prevertebral fascia known as the ***axillary sheath*** which extends into the axilla. The subclavian and axillary veins lie outside the sheath and as a result, they can dilate during increased venous return from the limb.
3. Fascia provides a fixed base for the movements of the pharynx, the oesophagus and the carotid sheaths during movements of the neck and during swallowing.

***Spaces in relation to prevertebral fascia*** (Fig. 3.9)

1. ***Retropharyngeal space*** lies between the prevertebral fascia and buccopharyngeal fascia. It allows the expansion of the pharynx during swallowing.

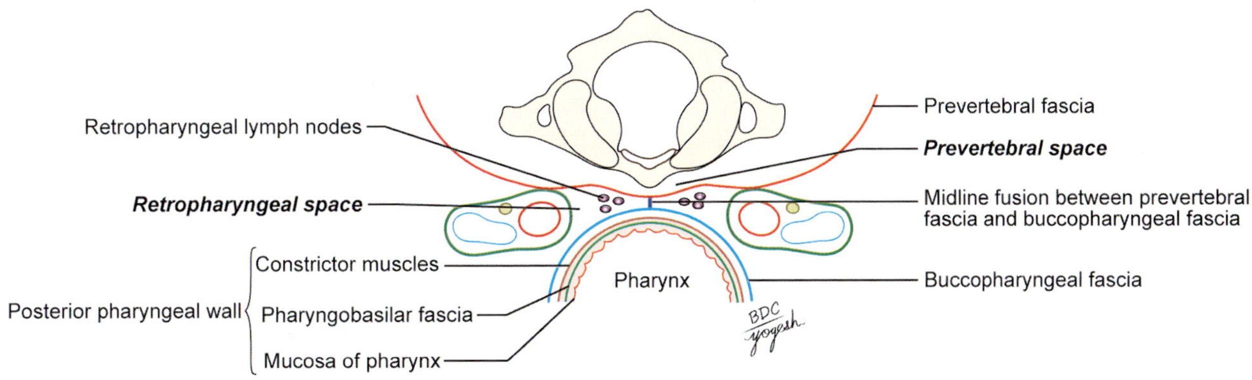


**Fig. 3.9:** Spaces in relation to prevertebral fascia

2. ***Space of Gillette*** is the right or left parts of the retropharyngeal space divided by median fibrous raphe. This space contains retropharyngeal nodes.
3. ***Prevertebral space*** lies behind the prevertebral fascia, anterior to the vertebral bodies.

## CLINICAL ANATOMY

- ***Neck infections*** behind the prevertebral fascia arise usually from tuberculosis of the cervical vertebrae or cervical caries. Pus produced as a result may extend in various directions. It may pass forwards forming a chronic retropharyngeal abscess which may form a bulging in the posterior wall of the pharynx, in the median plane. The pus may extend laterally through the axillary sheath and point in the posterior triangle, or in the lateral wall of the axilla. It may extend downwards into the superior mediastinum, where its descent is limited by fusion of the prevertebral fascia to the fourth thoracic vertebra.
- Neck infections in front of the prevertebral fascia in the retropharyngeal space usually arise from suppuration, i.e. formation of pus in the retropharyngeal lymph nodes. The pus forms an acute retropharyngeal abscess which bulges forwards in the paramedian position due to fusion of the buccopharyngeal fascia to the prevertebral fascia in the median plane. The infection may extend down through the superior mediastinum into the posterior mediastinum.

## BUCCOPHARYNGEAL FASCIA

This fascia covers all the constrictor muscles externally and extends onto the superficial aspect of the buccinator muscle.

It is attached to pharyngeal tubercle superiorly. This fascia fuses with the periosteum on the posterior part of alveolar process of maxilla. Retropharyngeal space lies posterior to buccopharyngeal fascia.

## PHARYNGOBASILAR FASCIA

This fascia is especially thickened between the upper border of superior constrictor muscle and the base of the skull. It lies deep to the pharyngeal muscles.

*Note:* ***Alar fascia*** is a layer of loose areolar tissue that lies between buccopharyngeal and prevertebral fascia. **Dangerous space** lies between alar fascia and prevertebral fascia, whereas *prevertebral space* lies between prevertebral fascia and vertebrae.

## CAROTID SHEATH

Carotid sheath is a derivative of the deep cervical fascia. It is a condensation of the fibroareolar tissue around the main vessels of the neck (Figs 3.10a and b, Flowchart 3.1)

***Formation:*** It is formed on anterior aspect by pretracheal fascia and on posterior aspect by prevertebral fascia.

***Contents:***
1. Common and internal carotid arteries
2. Internal jugular vein
3. Vagus (X) nerve
4. IX, XI, XII cranial nerves in the upper part (they pierce the carotid sheath at different points).

***Relations:***
1. The ansa cervicalis lies embedded in the anterior wall of the carotid sheath (Figs 3.10b).
2. The cervical sympathetic chain lies behind the sheath, plastered to the prevertebral fascia (Fig. 3.10b).
3. The sheath is overlapped by the anterior border of the sternocleidomastoid, and is fused to the layers of the deep cervical fascia.

## CLINICAL ANATOMY

- Carotid sheath is thick around the arteries and thin around the vein. This permits the expansion of internal jugular vein during increased venous return.
- Wall of the carotid sheath is excised to remove lymph nodes adherent to the internal jugular vein during block dissection of neck. It is usually done in cancers or tuberculosis.

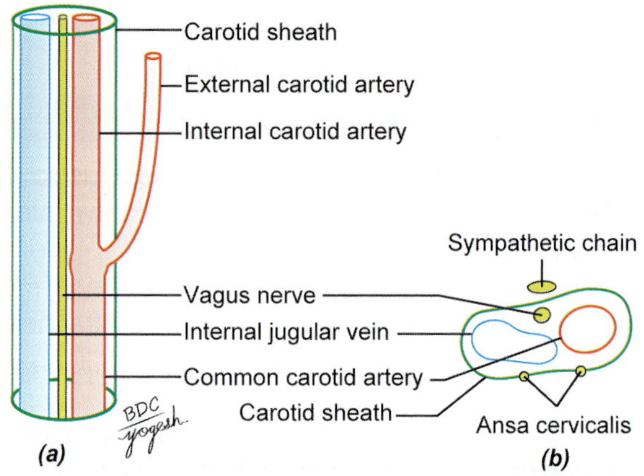


**Figs 3.10a and b:** Carotid sheath with its contents: (a) Surface view and (b) section view

**Flowchart 3.1:** Carotid sheath

***Carotid sheath***
Derivative of deep cervical fascia

| ***Formation*** | ***Extent*** | ***Content*** | ***Relations*** |
|---|---|---|---|
| Anteriorly by pretracheal fascia<br>Posteriorly by prevertebral fascia | Superiorly attached to the base of skull<br>Inferiorly blends with arch of aorta in superior mediastinum | Common and internal carotid arteries<br>Internal jugular vein<br>Vagus nerve | Anterior<br>- Ansa cervicalis<br>- SCM<br>Posterior<br>- Cervical sympathetic chain<br>- Prevertebral fascia |

***Clinical integration:*** Carotid sheath – thin around vein → Permits venous return

(SCM: Sternocleidomastoid)

***Competency:***

**AN35.10** Describe the fascial spaces of neck/pharynx.

## PHARYNGEAL SPACES

### RETROPHARYNGEAL SPACE (Flowchart 3.2)

| | |
|---|---|
| *Situation:* | Dead space behind pharynx |
| *Function:* | Acts as a bursa for expansion of pharynx during deglutition |
| *Boundaries:* | |
| *Anterior:* | Buccopharyngeal fascia |
| *Posterior:* | Prevertebral fascia. The two get fused. |
| *Sides:* | Carotid sheath |
| *Superior:* | Base of skull |
| *Inferior:* | Open and continuous with superior mediastinum. |
| *Contents:* | Retropharyngeal lymph nodes, pharyngeal plexus of vessels and nerves, loose areolar tissue. |
| *Clinical anatomy:* | Pus collection due to lymph node abscess which lies in paramedian position. It should be differentiated from cold abscess of spine of cervical vertebrae which is seen in median plane. |

### LATERAL PHARYNGEAL SPACE (Flowchart 3.2)

| | |
|---|---|
| *Situation:* | Side of pharynx |
| *Boundaries:* | |
| *Medial:* | Pharynx |
| *Posterolateral:* | Parotid gland |
| *Anterolateral:* | Medial pterygoid |
| *Posterior:* | Carotid sheath |
| *Contents:* | Branches of maxillary artery<br>Fibrofatty tissue |
| *Clinical anatomy:* | Pus collection/Ludwig's angina |

**Flowchart 3.2:** Pharyngeal spaces

***Pharyngeal spaces***
Around the constrictor of pharynx

***Retropharyngeal***
Lies behind the pharynx
Boundaries
Anterior: Buccopharyngeal fascia
Posterior: Prevertebral fascia
On each side: Carotid sheath
Superior: Base of skull
Inferior: Superior mediastinum
Contents
Retropharyngeal lymph nodes
Loose areolar tissue
Pharyngeal plexus of nerves and vessels

***Lateral pharyngeal space***
Lies on either side of pharynx
Boundaries
Medially: Pharynx, buccopharyngeal fascia
Laterally: Medial pterygoid and parotid glands
Posteriorly: Carotid sheath
Contents
Loose areolar tissue

***Clinical integration:*** Retropharyngeal abscess

***Competency:***

**AN29.2** Describe and demonstrate attachments, nerve supply, relations and actions of sternocleidomastoid.

## STERNOCLEIDOMASTOID (STERNOMASTOID) MUSCLE

It is also called sternomastoid. It is a long flat strap of muscle that extends obliquely across the side of the neck. It is enclosed within the investing layer of deep cervical fascia (Plate 3.1, Flowchart 3.3).

### Origin

***Sternal head:*** It is tendinous and arises from the superolateral part of the front of the manubrium sterni (Fig. 3.1c).

***Clavicular head:*** It is musculotendinous and arises from the medial one-third of the superior surface of the clavicle. It passes deep to the sternal head, and the two heads blend below the middle of the neck. Between the two heads, there is a small triangular depression or the lesser supraclavicular fossa, overlying the internal jugular vein.

### Insertion

It is inserted:

1. By a thick tendon into the lateral surface of *mastoid process*, from its tip to superior border.
2. By a thin aponeurosis into the lateral two-thirds of the *superior nuchal line* of the occipital bone.

### Nerve Supply

1. Spinal accessory nerve provides the motor supply. It passes through the muscle (Fig. 3.10).
2. Branches from the ventral rami of C2 and C3 are proprioceptive.

### Blood Supply

Arterial supply—one branch each from superior thyroid artery and suprascapular artery and, two branches from the occipital artery supply the big muscle. Veins follow the arteries.

**Flowchart 3.3:** Sternocleidomastoid

***Sternocleidomastoid***

***Origin***
Sternal head: Superolateral part of front of manubrium
Clavicular head: Superior surface of medial 1/3rd of clavicle

***Insertion***
Mastoid process
Superior nuchal line

***Innervation***
Spinal accessory nerve
Fibres of C2 and C3

***Actions***
Unilateral contraction
Turn chin to opposite side
Tilts head toward shoulder of same side
Bilateral contraction
Flex cervical part of vertebral column
Extends head
Draws head forward
Forced inspiration

***Clinical integration:*** Wry neck or torticollis—spasm of sternocleidomastoid muscle. It may be spasmodic, reflex, or congenital

**Plate 3.1:** Sternocleidomastoid muscle

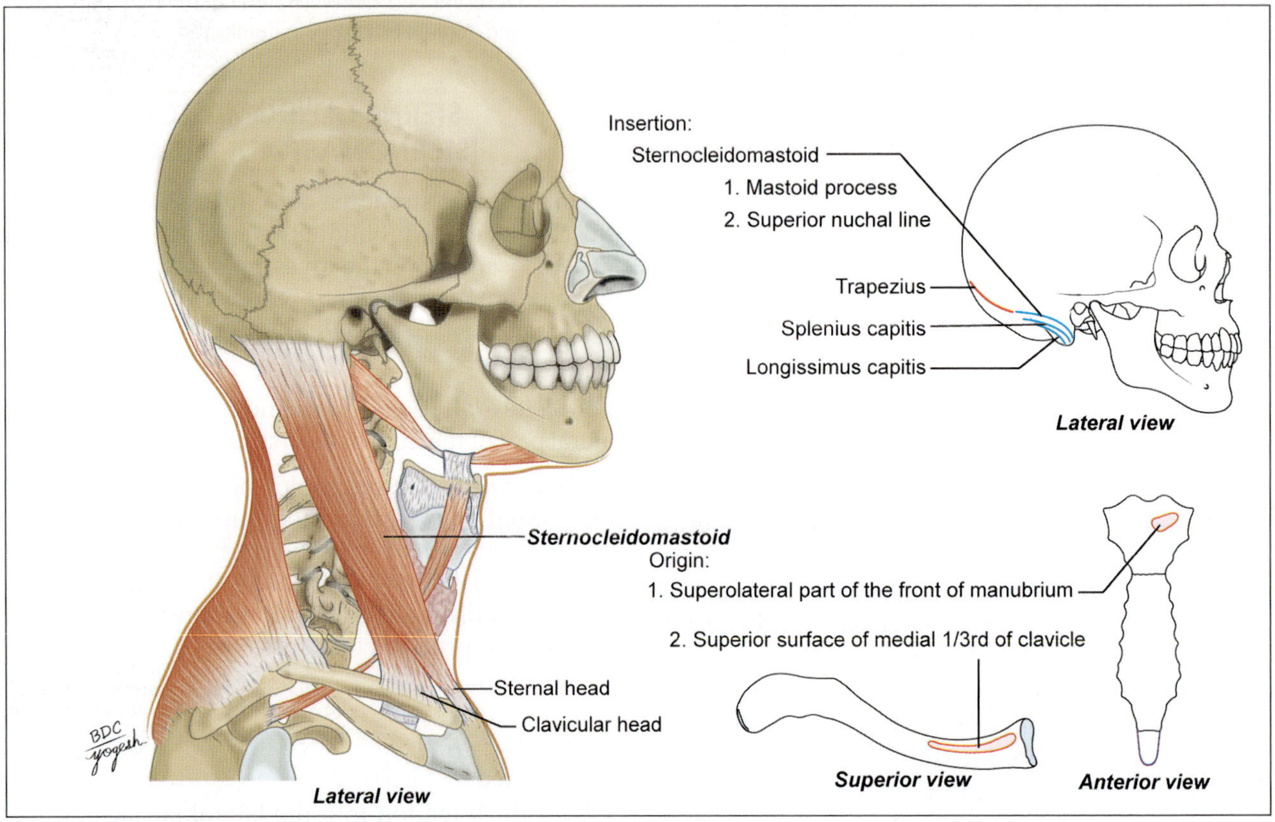


## Actions

1. When one muscle contracts:
   a. It turns the chin to the opposite side.
   b. It can also tilt the head towards the shoulder of same side.
2. When both muscles contract together:
   a. They draw the head forwards, as in eating and in lifting the head from a pillow.
   b. With the longus colli, they flex the neck against resistance.
   c. It also helps in forced inspiration.

## Relations of Sternocleidomastoid

The sternocleidomastoid is enclosed in the investing layer of deep cervical fascia. It is pierced by the accessory nerve and by the four sternocleidomastoid arteries. It has the following relations.

### Superficial

1. Skin
2. Superficial fascia, superficial lamina of the deep cervical fascia
3. Platysma
4. External jugular vein and superficial cervical lymph nodes lying along the vein
5. Great auricular, transverse or anterior cutaneous, medial supraclavicular nerves and lesser occipital nerves
6. The parotid gland overlaps the muscle.

### Deep

1. *Bones and joints*: Mastoid process and sternoclavicular joint
2. Carotid sheath
3. *Muscles*:
   a. Sternohyoid
   b. Sternothyroid
   c. Omohyoid
   d. Three scaleni
   e. Levator scapulae
   f. Splenius capitis
   g. Longissimus capitis
   h. Posterior belly of digastric.
4. *Arteries*:
   a. Common carotid
   b. Internal carotid
   c. External carotid
   d. Sternocleidomastoid arteries, two from the occipital artery, one from the superior thyroid, one from the suprascapular
   e. Occipital
   f. Subclavian
   g. Suprascapular
   h. Transverse cervical
5. *Veins*:
   a. Internal jugular
   b. Anterior jugular
   c. Facial
   d. Lingual

6. *Nerves:*
   a. Vagus/X
   b. Parts of IX, XI, XII. Spinal root of XI leaves the SCM at middle of its posterior border to lie in posterior triangle
   c. Cervical plexus
   d. Upper part of brachial plexus
   e. Phrenic
   f. Ansa cervicalis
7. Lymph nodes, superficial and deep cervical.

**Competency:**
**AN29.4** Explain anatomical basis of wry neck.

## CLINICAL ANATOMY

- Fascia of supraclavicular space is pierced by external jugular vein to drain into subclavian vein (Fig. 3.6).
- ***Torticollis*** is a deformity in which the head is bent to one side and the chin points to the other side. This is a result of spasm or contracture of the muscles supplied by the spinal accessory nerve, these being the sternocleidomastoid and trapezius. Although there are many varieties of torticollis depending on the causes; the common types are:
  a. Rheumatic torticollis due to exposure to cold or draught.
  b. Reflex torticollis due to inflamed or suppurating cervical lymph nodes which irritate the spinal accessory nerve.
  c. Congenital torticollis due to birth injury (Fig. 3.11)
- ***Wry neck:*** Shortening of the muscle fibres due to intravascular clotting of veins within the muscle. It usually occurs during difficult delivery of the baby.

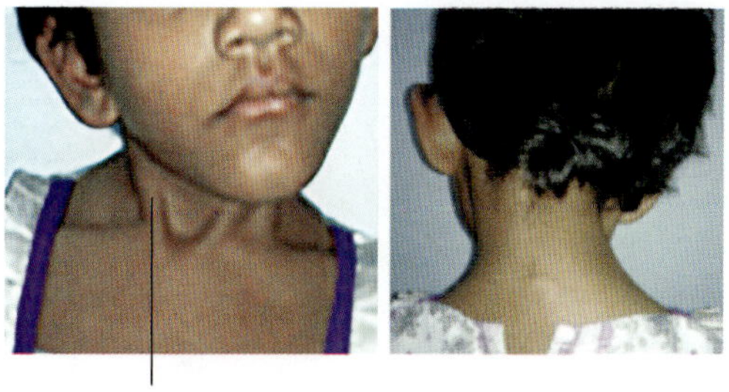


**Fig. 3.11:** Congenital torticollis

**Competency:**
**AN29.1** Describe and demonstrate the boundaries, subdivisions and contents of posterior triangle of neck.

## POSTERIOR TRIANGLE

The posterior triangle is a space on the side of the neck situated behind the sternocleidomastoid muscle (Fig. 3.12, Flowchart 3.4).

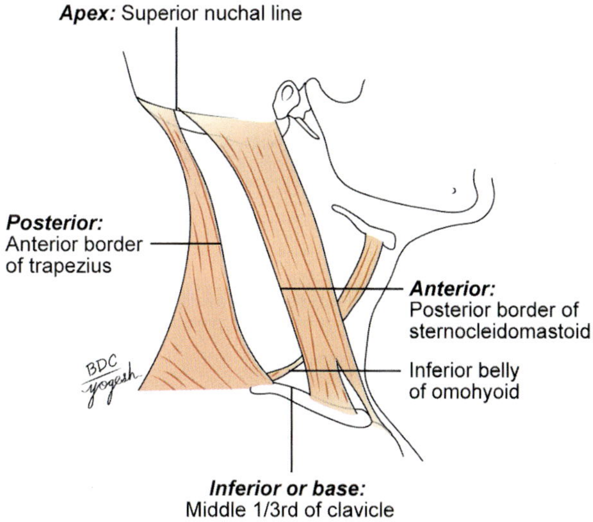


**Fig. 3.12:** Posterior triangle: Boundaries

### Boundaries

*Anterior:* Posterior border of sternocleidomastoid

*Posterior:* Anterior border of trapezius.

*Inferior or base:* Middle 1/3rd of clavicle.

*Apex:* Lies on the superior nuchal line where the trapezius and sternocleidomastoid meet.

### Roof

The roof is formed by the (Plate 3.2, Fig. 3.13)
1. *Skin*

**Flowchart 3.4:** Posterior triangle

***Posterior triangle of neck***

- ***Boundaries***
  - Anterior: Posterior border of sternocleidomastoid
  - Posterior: Anterior border of trapezius
  - Inferior: Middle 1/3rd of clavicle
  - Apex: Meeting point of sternocleidomastoid and trapezius (on superior nuchal line)
- ***Roof***
  - Skin
  - Superficial fascia
  - Platysma
  - External and posterior jugular veins
  - Great auricular, transverse cervical, supraclavicular, and lesser occipital nerves
  - Investing layer of deep cervical fascia
- ***Floor***
  - Prevertebral fascia
  - Semispinalis capitis
  - Splenius capitis
  - Levator scapulae
  - Scalenus medius
- ***Content*** — Divided by inferior belly of omohyoid into
  - ***Occipital triangle***
    - XI nerve
    - Great auricular, transverse cervical, supraclavicular and lesser occipital nerves
    - Dorsal scapular nerve
    - Branches from C3 and C4
    - Transverse cervical artery and vein
    - Occipital artery
    - Occipital nodes
  - ***Supraclavicular (subclavian triangle)***
    - Roots and trunks of brachial plexus
    - Nerve to serratus anterior
    - Nerve to subclavius
    - Suprascapular nerve
    - Third part of subclavian artery
    - Subclavian vein
    - Suprascapular artery and vein
    - Transverse cervical artery and vein
    - External jugular vein
    - Supraclavicular nodes

BDC yogesh

**Plate 3.2:** Structures piercing the roof of the posterior triangle

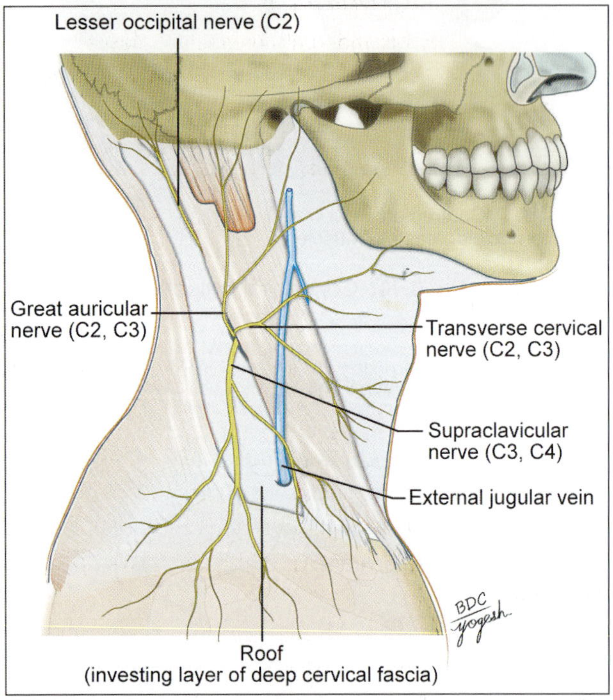


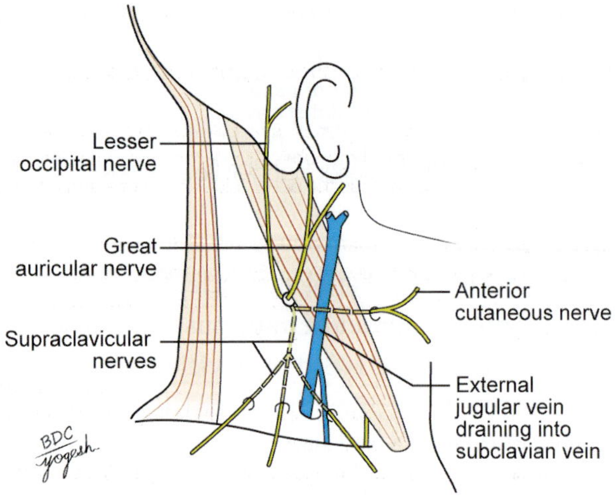


**Fig. 3.13:** Roof of the posterior triangle

2. Superficial fascia containing:
   a. Platysma
   b. External jugular and posterior external jugular veins
   c. Parts of the supraclavicular, great auricular, transverse cutaneous and lesser occipital nerves
   d. Unnamed arteries derived from the occipital, transverse cervical and suprascapular arteries.
   e. Lymph vessels which pierce the deep fascia to end in the supraclavicular nodes.
3. *Investing layer of deep cervical fascia.*

*Note:* ***External jugular vein*** lies deep to the platysma. It is formed by union of the posterior auricular vein with the posterior division of the retromandibular vein. It begins within the lower part of the parotid gland, crosses the sternocleidomastoid obliquely, pierces the anteroinferior angle of the roof of the posterior triangle, and opens into the subclavian vein.

Its tributaries are:

a. The posterior external jugular vein
b. The transverse cervical vein
c. The suprascapular vein
d. The anterior jugular vein.

The ***oblique jugular vein*** connects the external jugular vein with the internal jugular vein across the middle one-third of the anterior border of the sternocleidomastoid.

## Floor

The floor of the posterior triangle is formed by the prevertebral layer of deep cervical fascia, covering the following muscles from above downwards (Plate 3.3, Fig. 3.14):

1. Splenius capitis
2. Levator scapulae
3. Scalenus medius (Fig. 3.9b).

## Division of the Posterior Triangle

It is subdivided by the inferior belly of omohyoid into:

1. A larger upper part is called the ***occipital part.***
2. A smaller lower part is called the ***supraclavicular part*** or *subclavian part* (Fig. 3.15).

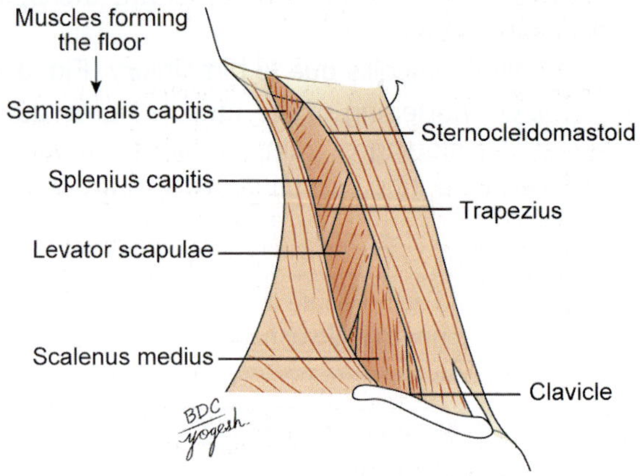


**Fig. 3.14:** Floor of the posterior triangle

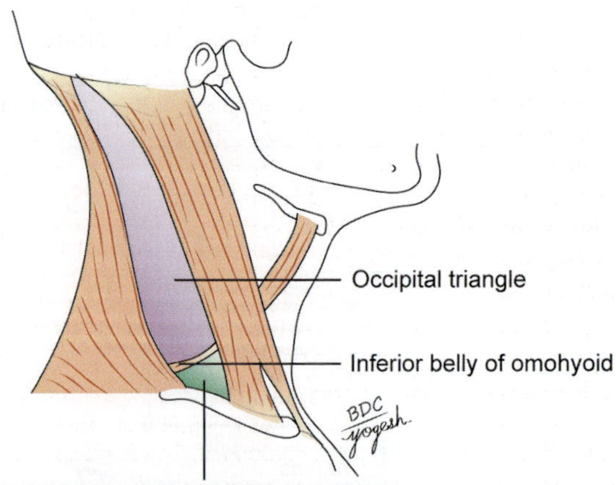


**Fig. 3.15:** Divisions of the posterior triangle of neck

**TABLE 3.1: Contents of the posterior triangle**

| *Contents* | *Occipital triangle* | *Subclavian triangle* |
|---|---|---|
| Nerves | Spinal accessory nerve<br>Four cutaneous branches of cervical plexus:<br>a. Lesser occipital (C2)<br>b. Great auricular (C2, C3)<br>c. Anterior cutaneous nerve of neck (C2, C3)<br>d. Supraclavicular nerves (C3, C4)<br>Muscular branches:<br>a. Two small branches to the levator scapulae (C3, C4)<br>b. Two small branches to the trapezius (C3, C4)<br>c. Nerve to rhomboids (proprioceptive) (C5) | Roots and trunks of brachial plexus<br>Nerve to serratus anterior (long thoracic, C5–C7)<br>Nerve to subclavius (C5, C6)<br>Suprascapular nerve (C5, C6) |
| Vessels | Transverse cervical artery and vein<br>Occipital artery | 3rd part of subclavian artery and subclavian vein<br>Suprascapular artery and vein<br>Commencement of transverse cervical artery and termination of the corresponding vein<br>Lower part of external jugular vein |
| Lymph nodes | Along the posterior border of the sternocleidomastoid, more in the lower part—the supraclavicular nodes and a few at the upper angle—the occipital nodes | A few members of the supraclavicular chain |

*Note:* **Details of the Contents of Posterior Triangle**

1. ***Spinal root of accessory nerve*** emerges a little above the middle of the posterior border of the sternocleidomastoid. It runs through a tunnel in the fascia forming the roof of the triangle, passing downwards and laterally and disappears under the anterior border of the trapezius about 5 cm above the clavicle. It is the only structure beneath the roof of triangle. It supplies both sternocleidomastoid and trapezius muscles.
2. The four ***cutaneous branches of the cervical plexus*** pierce the fascia covering the floor of the triangle, pass through the triangle and pierce the deep fascia at different points to become cutaneous (Plate 3.5, Fig. 3.6).
   a. ***Transverse cutaneous nerve***: Arises from ventral rami of C2 and C3 nerves run transversely across the sternocleidomastoid to supply skin of neck, till the sternum.
   b. ***Supraclavicular nerves***: Formed from ventral rami of C3 and C4 nerves. Emerges at posterior border of sternocleidomastoid. It descends downwards and diverges into three branches. Medial one supplies the skin over the manubrium till manubriosternal joint. Intermediate nerve crosses the clavicle to supply skin of first intercostal space to the second rib. Lateral nerve runs across the lateral side of clavicle and acromion to supply skin over the upper half of the deltoid muscle.
   c. ***Great auricular nerve***: It is the largest ascending branch of cervical plexus. Arises from ventral rami of C2 and C3 nerves. Ascends on the sternocleidomastoid muscle to reach parotid gland, where it divides into anterior and posterior branches. Anterior branch supplies lower one-third of skin on lateral surface of pinna and skin over the parotid gland and connects the gland to the auriculotemporal nerve. This cross-connection is the anatomical basis for Frey's syndrome. Posterior branch supplies lower one-third of skin on medial surface of the pinna.
   d. ***Lesser occipital***: Arises from ventral ramus of C2 segment of spinal cord. Seen at the posterior border of sternocleidomastoid muscle. It then winds around and ascends along its posterior border to supply skin of upper 2/3rd of medial surface of pinna adjoining part of the scalp.
3. *Muscular branches to the levator scapulae and the trapezius* (C3, C4) appear about the middle of the sternocleidomastoid. Those to the levator scapulae soon end in it; those to the trapezius run below and parallel to the accessory nerve across the middle of the triangle. Both nerves lie deep to the fascia of the floor.
4. Three ***trunks of the brachial plexus*** emerge between the scalenus anterior and medius and carry the axillary sheath around them (Fig. 3.17). The sheath contains the brachial plexus and the subclavian artery. These structures *lie deep* to *the floor* of posterior triangle. If prevertebral *fascia is left intact, all these structures are safe.*
5. The *nerve to the rhomboid* or ***dorsal scapular nerve*** is from C5 root, pierces the scalenus medius and passes deep to the levator scapulae to reach the back where it lies deep or anterior to the rhomboid muscles.
6. The ***nerve to the serratus anterior*** (C5–C7) arises by three roots. The roots from C5 and C6 pierce the scalenus medius and join the root from C7 over the first digitation of the serratus anterior. The nerve passes behind the brachial plexus. It descends over the serratus anterior in the medial wall of the axilla and gives branches to the digitations of the muscle.
7. The ***nerve to the subclavius*** (C5, C6) descends in front of the brachial plexus and the subclavian vessels, but behind the omohyoid, the transverse cervical and suprascapular vessels and the clavicle to reach the deep surface of the subclavius muscle. As it runs near the lateral margin of the scalenus anterior, it sometimes gives off the *accessory phrenic nerve* which joins the phrenic nerve in front of the scalenus anterior.
8. The ***suprascapular nerve*** (C5, C6) arises from the upper trunk of the brachial plexus and crosses the lower part of the posterior triangle just above and lateral to the brachial plexus, deep to the transverse cervical vessels and the omohyoid. It passes backwards over the shoulder to reach the scapula. It supplies the supraspinatus and infraspinatus muscles.
9. The ***subclavian artery*** passes behind the tendon of the scalenus anterior, over the first rib.
10. The ***transverse cervical artery*** is a branch of the thyrocervical trunk. It crosses the scalenus anterior, the phrenic nerve, the upper trunks of the brachial plexus, the nerve to the subclavius, the suprascapular nerve and the scalenus medius. At the anterior border of the levator scapulae, it divides into superficial and deep branches. The inferior belly of the omohyoid crosses the artery.
11. The ***suprascapular artery*** is also a branch of the thyrocervical trunk. It passes laterally and backwards behind the clavicle.
12. The ***occipital artery*** crosses the apex of the posterior triangle superficial to the splenius capitis.
13. The subclavian vein passes in front of the tendon of scalenus anterior muscle.

**Plate 3.3:** Muscles forming the floor of the posterior triangle

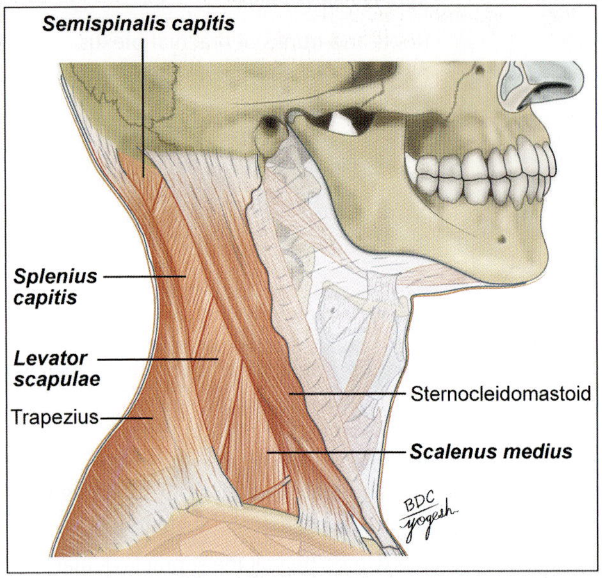


## CLINICAL ANATOMY

- ***Jugular venous pressure (JVP):*** The right external jugular vein is *examined to assess the venous pressure;* the right atrial pressure is reflected in it because there are no valves in the entire course of this vein and it is straight.
- As external jugular vein pierces the deep fascia, the margins of the vein get adherent to the fascia. So if the vein gets cut, it cannot close and air is sucked in due to negative intrathoracic pressure. That causes air embolism. To prevent this, the deep fascia has to be cut (Fig. 3.13).

*Competency:*

**AN29.5** Describe and demonstrate attachments of: (1) inferior belly of omohyoid, (2) scalenus anterior (*see* Chapter 9), (3) scalenus medius (*see* Chapter 9), and (4) levator scapulae (*see* Chapter 10).

## Contents of the Posterior Triangle

(Plate 3.4, Figs 3.16a and b)

### *Contents of Occipital Triangle*

1. Nerves:
   - Spinal accessory nerve
   - 4 cutaneous nerves: Great auricular, transverse cervical, supraclavicular and lesser occipital nerves
   - Dorsal scapular nerve for rhomboids (C5)
   - Branches from C3 and C4 root to levator scapulae and trapezius
2. Vessels:
   - Transverse cervical artery and vein
   - Occipital artery
3. Occipital nodes.

### *Contents of Subclavian or Supraclavicular Triangle*

(Plate 3.5)

1. Nerve:
   - Root and trunk of brachial plexus
   - Nerve to serratus anterior
   - Nerve to subclavius
   - Suprascapular nerve
2. Vessels
   - 3rd part of subclavian artery
   - Subclavian vein
   - Suprascapular artery and vein
   - Transverse cervical artery and vein
   - Lower part of external jugular vein
3. Supraclavicular nodes.

These are enumerated in Table 3.1.

## CLINICAL ANATOMY

- ***Supraclavicular lymphadenopathy*:** The most common swelling in the posterior triangle is due to enlargement of the supraclavicular lymph nodes. While doing biopsy of the lymph node, one must be careful in preserving the accessory nerve which may get entangled amongst enlarged lymph nodes (Fig. 3.9b).
- Supraclavicular lymph nodes are commonly enlarged in tuberculosis, Hodgkin's disease and in malignant growths of the breast, arm or chest.
- Left supraclavicular lymph nodes are also called ***Virchow's lymph nodes***. They are commonly involved in metastasis from tumours of stomach, testes and other abdominal viscera. Biopsy of supraclavicular nodes may reveal the cause of their enlargement.
- ***Block dissection of the neck*** for malignant diseases is the removal of cervical lymph nodes along with other structures involved in the growth. This procedure does not endanger those nerves of the posterior triangle which lie deep to the prevertebral fascia, i.e. the brachial and cervical plexuses and their muscular branches.
- A ***cervical rib*** may compress the 2nd part of subclavian artery. In these cases, blood supply to upper limb reaches via anastomoses around the scapula.
- Dysphagia caused by compression of the oesophagus by an abnormal subclavian artery is called ***dysphagia lusoria***.
- Elective arterial surgery of the common carotid artery is done for aneurysms, AV fistulae or arteriosclerotic occlusions. It is better to expose the common carotid artery in its upper part where it is superficial. While ligating the artery, care should be taken not to include the vagus nerve or the sympathetic chain.
- Second part of the subclavian artery may get pressed by the short scalenus anterior muscle, resulting in decreased blood supply to the upper limb. If the muscle is divided, the effects are abolished (Fig. 3.12).
- Brachial plexus block: The brachial plexus can be blocked by injecting local anaesthetic between the first rib and the skin above the clavicle. It may be required for upper limb surgeries (Fig. 3.18).

**Plate 3.4:** Contents of the right posterior triangle of the neck

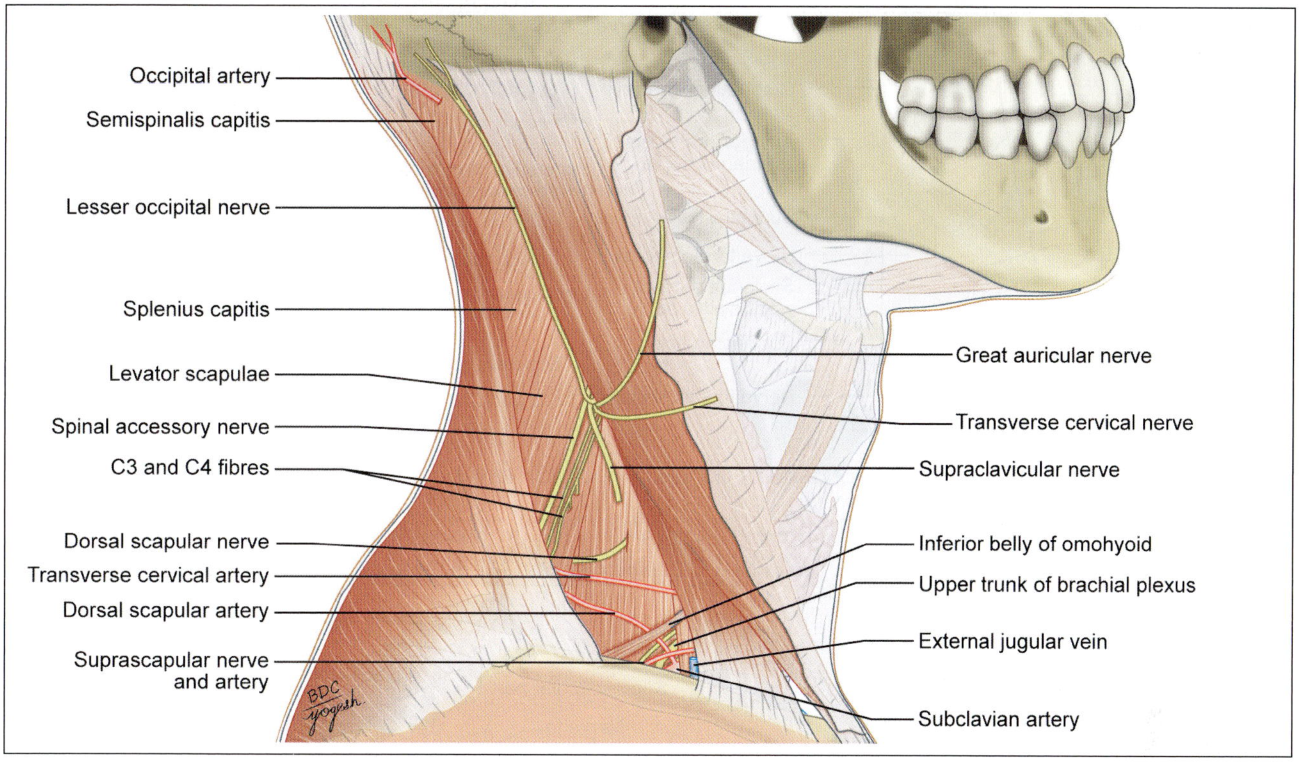


**Plate 3.5:** Structures in the supraclavicular triangle of neck

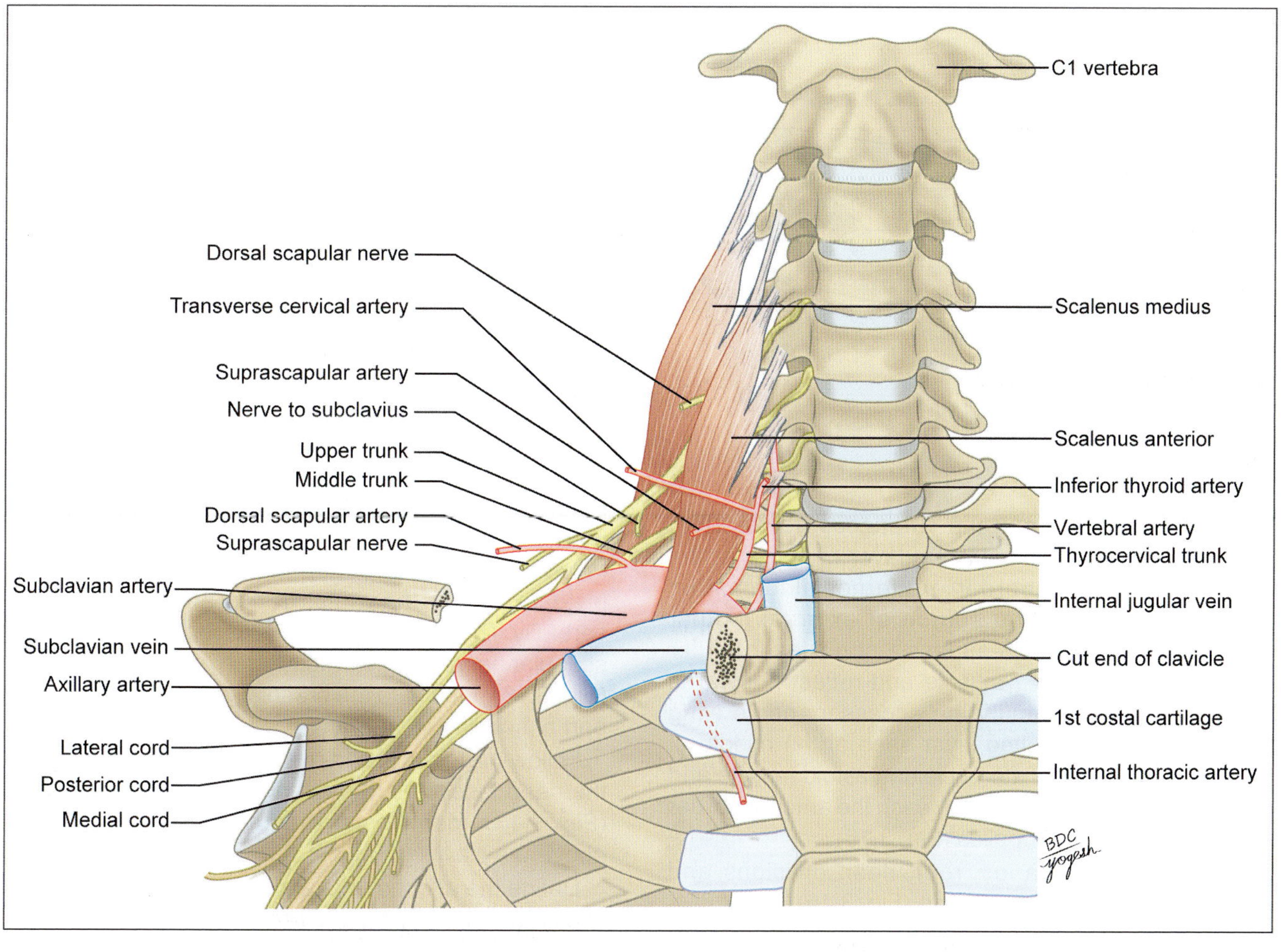

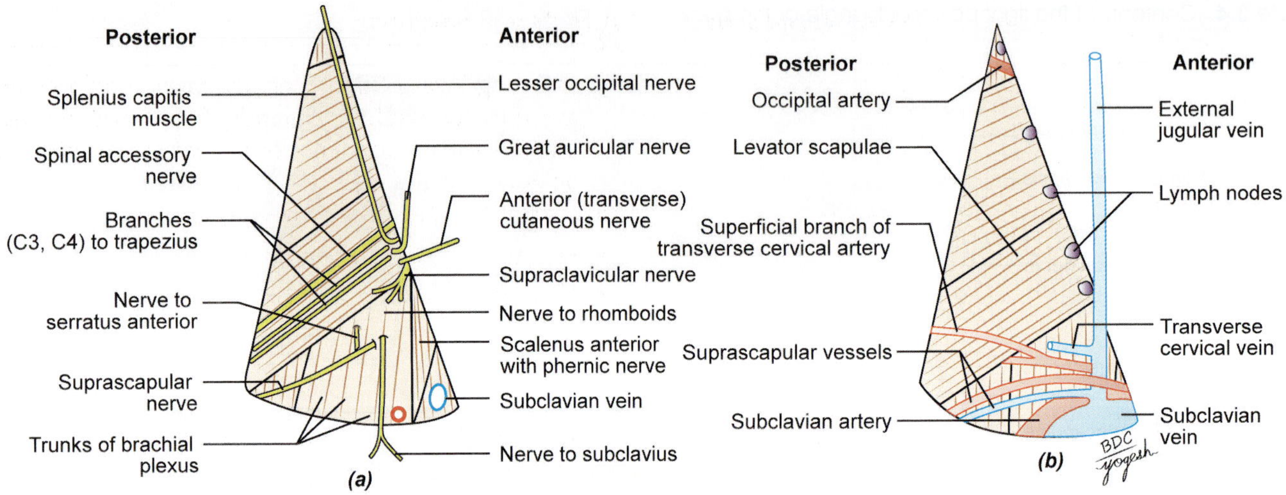


**Figs 3.16a and b:** The contents of posterior triangle of neck: (a) Nerves and (b) vessels and lymph nodes

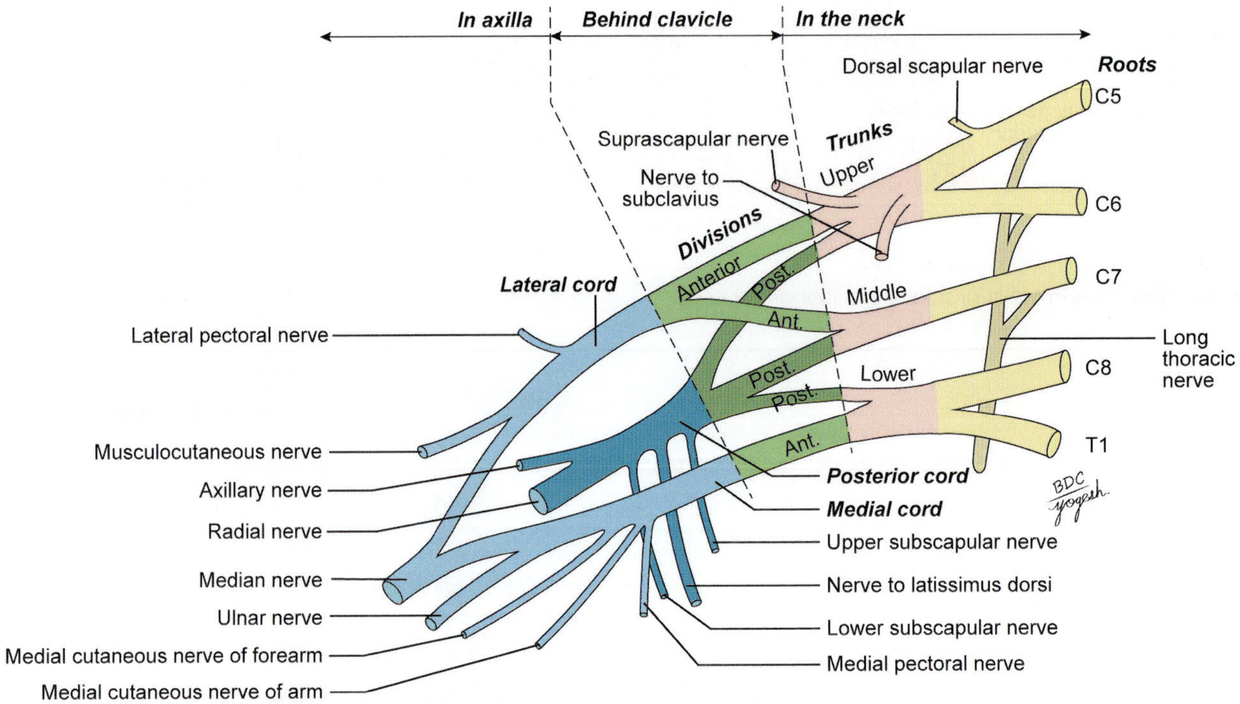


**Fig. 3.17:** Brachial plexus

## DISSECTION

Try to dissect and clean the cutaneous nerves (Fig. 3.13) which pierce the investing layer of fascia at the middle of posterior border of sternocleidomastoid muscle. Demarcate the course of external jugular vein. Cut carefully the deep fascia of posterior border of sternocleidomastoid muscle and reflect it towards trapezius muscle. Identify the accessory nerve lying just deep to the investing layer seen at the middle of the posterior border of sternocleidomastoid muscle and across the posterior triangle to reach the anterior border of trapezius which it supplies (Fig. 3.16).

Define the boundaries, roof, floor, divisions and contents of the posterior triangle (Fig. 3.16).

Identify and clean the inferior belly of omohyoid. Find the transverse cervical artery along the upper border of this muscle. Trace it both ways. Deep to this muscle is the upper or supraclavicular part of brachial plexus. Identify the roots, trunks and their branches carefully. The branches are suprascapular nerve, dorsal scapular nerve, long thoracic nerve, nerve to subclavius (Fig. 3.16). Medial to the brachial plexus locate the third part of subclavian artery.

Follow the terminal part of external jugular vein through the deep fascia into the deeply placed subclavian vein (Fig. 3.13). Identify suprascapular artery running just above the clavicle (Fig. 3.16).

Define the attachments and relations of sternocleidomastoid muscle. To expose scalenus anterior muscle, cut

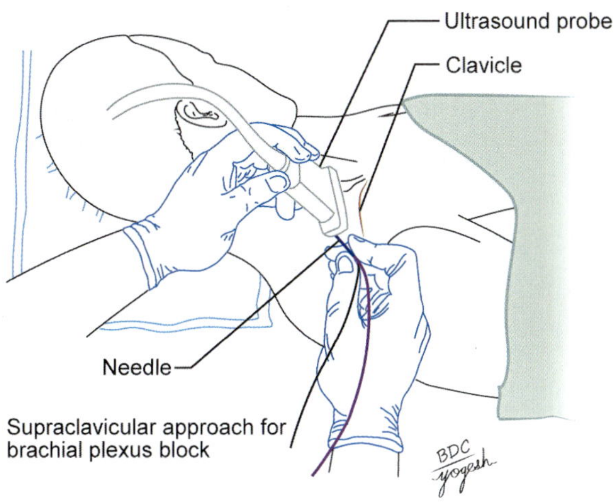


**Fig. 3.18:** Brachial plexus block

across the clavicular head of sternocleidomastoid muscle and push it medially. Scalenus anterior muscle covered by well-defined prevertebral fascia can be identified. Clean the subclavian artery and upper part of brachial plexus deep to the scalenus anterior muscle.

VIDEO

**Video 3.3 Side of the Neck:** Posterior triangle

### *Facts to Remember*

- Investing layer of deep cervical fascia encloses two muscles, two salivary glands; forms two pulleys; encloses two spaces and forms roof of posterior and anterior triangles of neck.
- Prevertebral fascia forms the axillary sheath.
- Pretracheal fascia suspends the thyroid gland.
- Ligament of Berry connects the thyroid capsule to the cricoid cartilage.
- Cold abscess of caries spine, can track down to the posterior triangle or axilla.
- Right external jugular vein is commonly used for central venous cannulation.
- Left supraclavicular nodes are called Virchow's nodes.
- Sternocleidomastoid divides the side of neck into anterior and posterior triangles.

### BDC's Anatomy *e*-book

1. Platysma
2. External jugular vein (EJV)
3. Superficial lymph node of the neck
4. Further reading
5. Viva voce questions

Chapter

# 4

# Anterior Region of the Neck

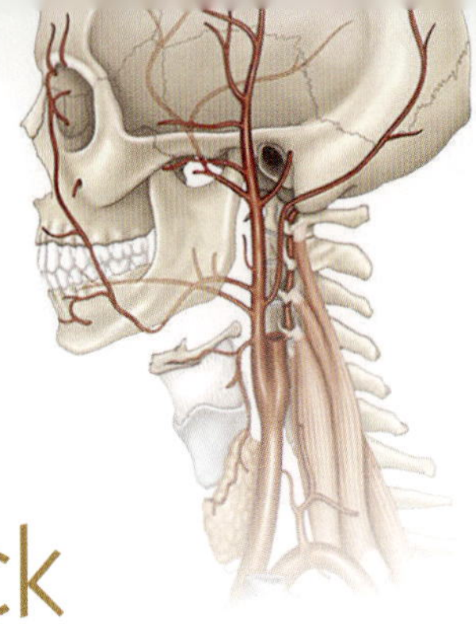

The anterior triangle of the neck lies between midline of the neck and sternocleidomastoid muscle. It is subdivided into smaller triangles.

## SURFACE LANDMARKS

1. ***Mandible*** forms the lower jaw (Fig. 4.1). The lower border of its horseshoe-shaped body is known as the *base of the mandible.* Anteriorly, this base forms the *chin*, and posteriorly it can be traced to the *angle of the mandible.*
2. The body of the U-shaped ***hyoid bone*** can be felt in the median plane just below and behind the chin, at the junction of the neck with the floor of the mouth.
3. ***Thyroid cartilage*** of the larynx forms a sharp protuberance in the median plane just below the hyoid bone. This protuberance is called the *laryngeal prominence or* ***Adam's apple***. It is prominent in males.
4. The rounded arch of the *cricoid cartilage* lies below the thyroid cartilage at the upper end of the trachea.
5. The trachea runs downwards and backwards from the cricoid cartilage. It is identified by its cartilaginous rings. However, it is partially masked by the *isthmus of the thyroid gland*, which lies against 2nd to 4th tracheal rings. The trachea is commonly palpated in the ***suprasternal notch***, which lies between the tendinous heads of origin of the right and left sternocleidomastoid muscles.

## STRUCTURES IN THE ANTERIOR MEDIAN REGION OF THE NECK

This region includes a strip 2 to 3 cm wide extending from the chin to the sternum. The structures encountered are listed below from superficial to deep (Fig. 4.2).

1. **Skin:** It is freely movable over the deeper structures due to the looseness of the superficial fascia.
2. **Superficial fascia:** It contains:
   a. Platysma
   b. Anterior jugular veins
   c. Jugular venous arch
   d. Submental lymph nodes — lying on the deep fascia below the chin
   e. Transverse or anterior cutaneous nerve of the neck.
3. **Deep fascia** (investing layer): In the upper part, it splits and encloses submandibular gland. In the lower part, it splits to enclose suprasternal space.

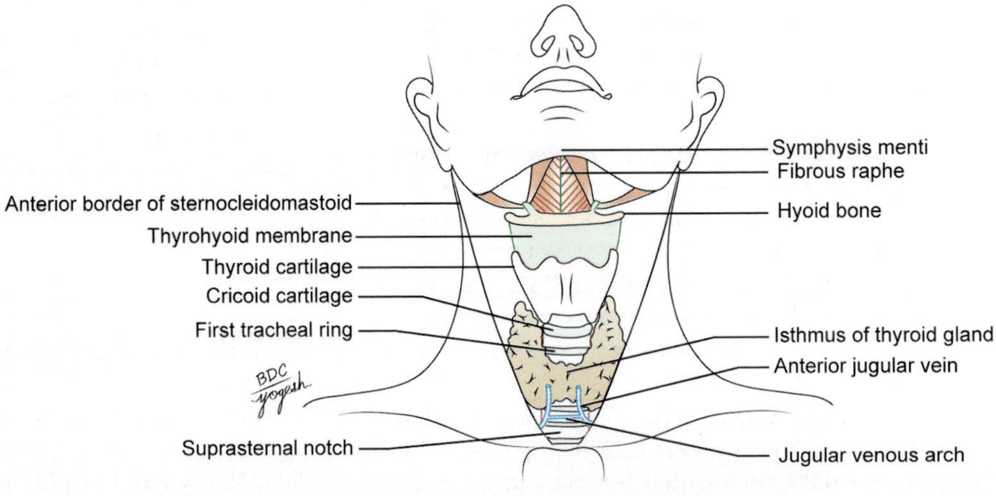


**Fig. 4.1:** Structures in the anterior median line of the neck

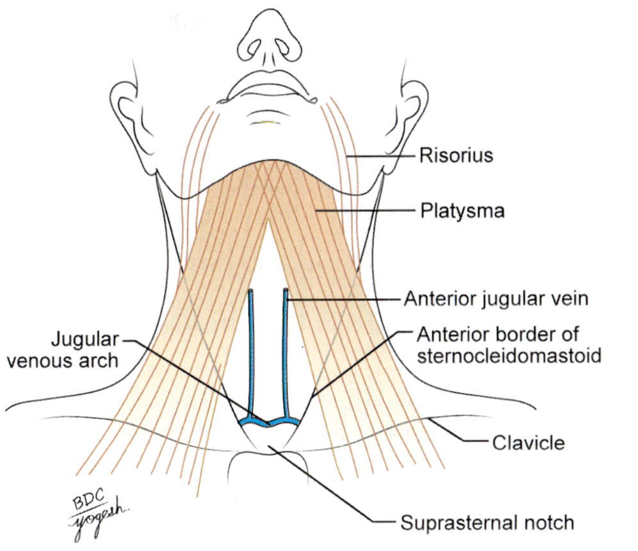


**Fig. 4.2:** Anterior region of the neck showing the platysma and the anterior jugular veins in the superficial fascia

4. **Deep structures lying above the hyoid bone**
   a. Mylohyoid muscle
   b. Anterior belly of digastric
   c. Superficial part of the submandibular salivary gland
   d. Mylohyoid nerve
   e. Submental branch of the facial artery
5. **Structures lying below the hyoid bone**
   These structures may be grouped into three planes:
   A. Superficial plane containing the infrahyoid muscles: Sternohyoid, sternothyroid, thyrohyoid and superior belly of omohyoid (Plate 4.1, Fig. 4.3 and Table 4.1).
   B. Middle plane consisting of the pretracheal fascia and the thyroid gland.
   C. Deep plane containing:
      a. Thyrohyoid membrane – pierced by the internal laryngeal nerve and the superior laryngeal vessels.

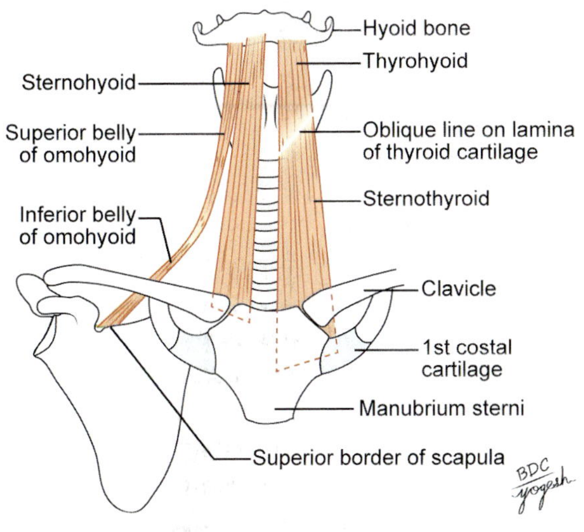


**Fig. 4.3:** The infrahyoid muscles

      b. Thyroid cartilage
      c. Cricothyroid membrane
      d. Arch of the cricoid cartilage
      e. Cricothyroid muscle
      f. Trachea, partly covered by the isthmus of the thyroid gland from the 2nd to 4th rings
      g. Carotid sheaths.

*Note*:
- ***Anterior jugular veins*** begin in the submental region below the chin. It descends in the superficial fascia about 1 cm from the median plane. About 2.5 cm above the sternum, it pierces the investing layer of deep fascia to enter the suprasternal space where it is connected to its fellow on the opposite side by a transverse channel, the *jugular venous arch* (Fig. 4.2). The vein then turns laterally, runs deep to the sternocleidomastoid just above the clavicle, and *ends in the external jugular vein* at the posterior border of the sternocleidomastoid.
- The anteroinferior part of the *hyoglossus muscle* is related to:
  a. The intermediate tendon of the *digastric* muscle with its fibrous pulley.
  b. The bifurcated tendon of the *stylohyoid* muscle embracing the digastric tendon (Fig. 4.3).
- The ***subhyoid bursa*** lies between the posterior surface of the body of the hyoid bone and the thyrohyoid membrane. It lessens friction between these two structures during the movements of swallowing.
- *Pretracheal fascia* forms the *false capsule of the thyroid gland* and the *suspensory ligaments of Berry* which attach the thyroid gland to the cricoid cartilage.

## CLINICAL ANATOMY

- The common anterior ***midline swellings*** of the neck are:
  a. Enlarged submental lymph nodes and sublingual dermoid in the submental region.
  b. Thyroglossal cyst and inflamed subhyoid bursa just below the hyoid bone.
  c. Goitre, carcinoma of larynx and enlarged lymph nodes in the suprasternal region.
- ***Tracheostomy*** is an operation in which the trachea is opened and a tube inserted into it to facilitate breathing (Fig. 4.4).
- Cut throat wounds are most commonly situated just above or just below the hyoid bone. The main vessels of the neck usually escape injury because they are pushed backwards to a deeper plane during voluntary extension of the neck.
- ***Ludwig's angina*** is the cellulitis of the floor of the mouth. The infection spreads above the mylohyoid forcing the tongue upwards. Mylohyoid is pushed downwards. There is swelling within the mouth as well as below the chin.

## DISSECTION

The skin over the anterior triangle has already been reflected following dissection in Chapter 3. Platysma is also reflected upwards. Identify the structures present in the superficial fascia and structures present in the anterior median region of neck.

**Plate 4.1:** Infrahyoid muscles

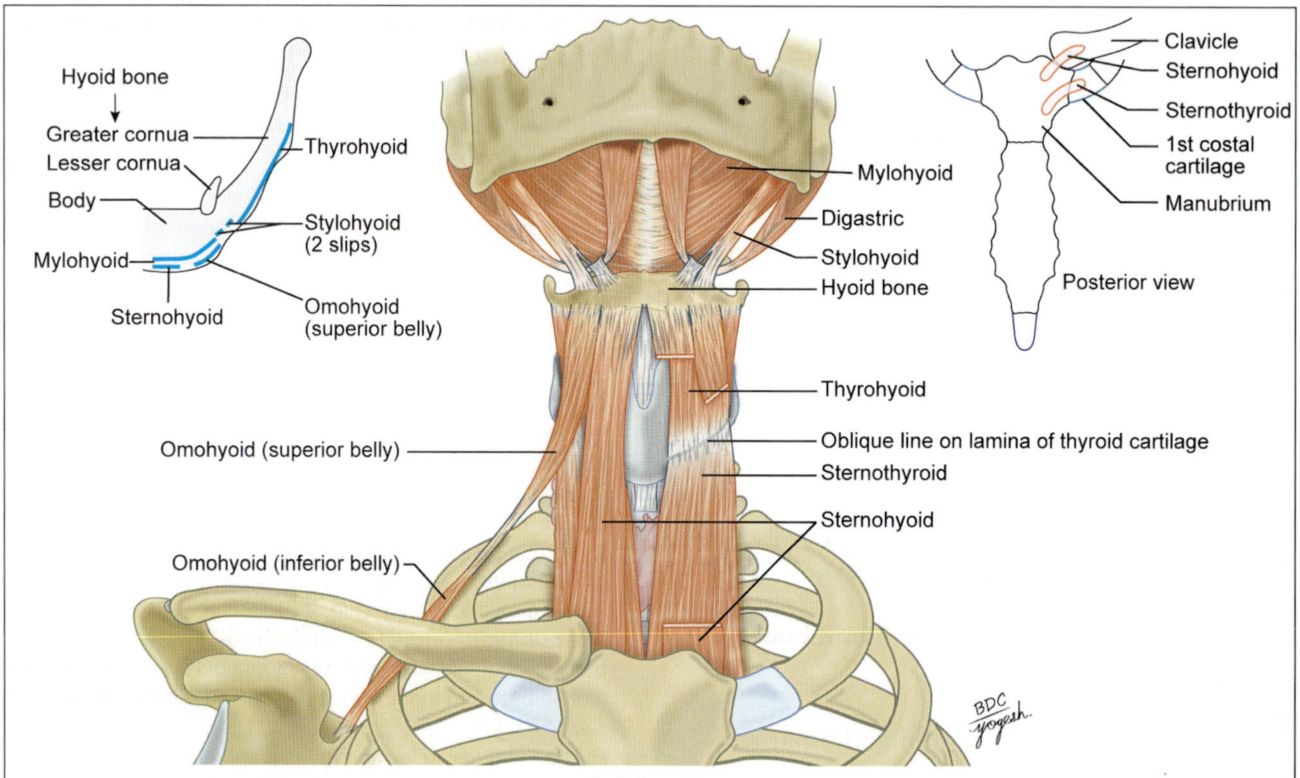


***Anterior view***

**TABLE 4.1: Infrahyoid muscles**

| *Muscle* | *Proximal attachment* | *Distal attachment* | *Nerve supply* | *Actions* |
|---|---|---|---|---|
| 1. **Sternohyoid** | a. Posterior surface of manubrium sterni<br>b. Adjoining parts of the clavicle and the posterior sternoclavicular ligament | Lower border of body of hyoid bone | Ansa cervicalis (C1–C3) | Depresses the hyoid bone following its elevation during swallowing and during vocal movements |
| 2. **Sternothyroid:** It lies deep to the sternohyoid | a. Posterior surface of manubrium sterni<br>b. Adjoining part of 1st costal cartilage | Oblique line on the lamina of the thyroid cartilage | Ansa cervicalis (C1–C3) | Depresses the larynx after it has been elevated in swallowing and in vocal movements |
| 3. **Thyrohyoid:** It lies deep to the sternohyoid | Oblique line of thyroid cartilage | Lower border of the body and the greater cornua of the hyoid bone | C1 through hypoglossal nerve | a. Depresses the hyoid bone<br>b. Elevates the larynx when the hyoid is fixed by the suprahyoid muscles |
| 4. **Omohyoid:** It has an inferior belly, a common tendon and a superior belly. It arises by the inferior belly, and is inserted through the superior belly | a. Upper border of scapula near the suprascapular notch<br>b. Adjoining part of suprascapular ligament | Lower border of body of hyoid bone lateral to the sternohyoid. The central tendon lies on the internal jugular vein at the level of the cricoid cartilage and is bound to the clavicle by a fascial pulley | Superior belly by the superior root of the ansa cervicalis, and inferior belly by inferior root of ansa cervicalis | Depresses the hyoid bone following its elevation during swallowing or in vocal movements |

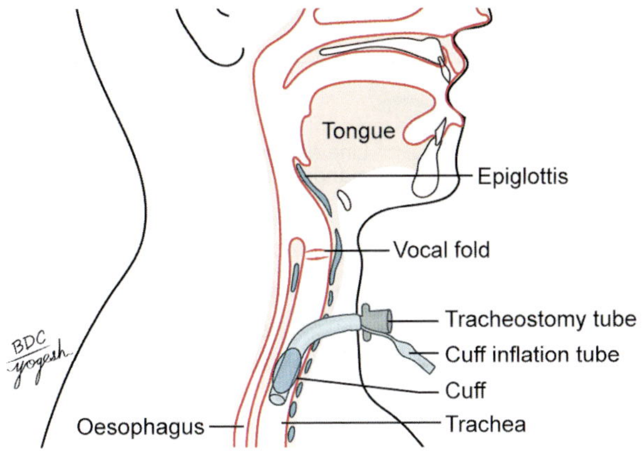


**Fig. 4.4:** Tracheostomy tube in position

*Competency:*
**AN32.1** Describe boundaries and subdivisions of anterior triangle.

## ANTERIOR TRIANGLE

The anterior triangle of the neck is a triangular area (Plate 4.2, Fig. 4.5).

### Boundaries

*Anterior*: Anterior median plane of the neck
*Posterior*: Anterior border of sternocleidomastoid
*Base*: Base of the mandible and a line joining the angle of the mandible to the mastoid process, superiorly
*Apex*: It is directed downward. It is formed by the meeting point of anterior border of sternocleidomastoid muscle and anterior median line muscle and anterior median line.

*Roof*:
1. Skin
2. Superficial fascia with platysma
3. Investing layer of deep cervical fascia

### Subdivisions

The anterior triangle is subdivided (by the digastric muscle and the superior belly of the omohyoid) into:
1. Submental,
2. Digastric,
3. Carotid, and
4. Muscular triangles (Fig. 4.5).

*Competency:*
**AN32.2** Describe and demonstrate boundaries and contents of digastric and submental triangles.

## SUBMENTAL TRIANGLE

This is a median triangle. It is bounded as follows (Plate 4.3, Fig. 4.6, Flowchart 4.1).

### Boundaries

*Apex*: Lower border of symphysis menti or chin
*Base*: Body of the hyoid bone
*On each side*: Anterior bellies of digastric muscles
*Floor*: Mylohyoid muscle and the median raphe extending from symphysis menti to the body of the hyoid bone
*Roof*: Investing layer of deep cervical fascia.

### Contents

1. Two to four small *submental lymph nodes*
2. Small submental veins join to form the anterior jugular veins.

*Note*: The ***submental lymph nodes*** are situated in the superficial fascia between the anterior bellies of the digastric muscles. They drain:
a. Superficial tissues below the chin
b. Central part of the lower lip
c. The adjoining gums
d. Anterior part of the floor of the mouth
e. The tip of the tongue.
Their efferents pass to the submandibular nodes.

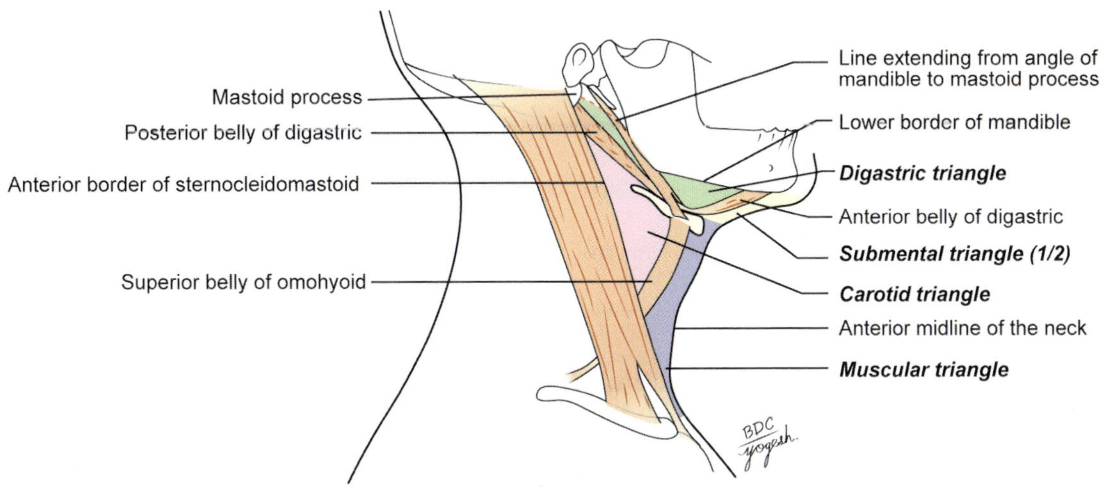


**Fig. 4.5:** The triangles of the neck. The anterior triangle is subdivided by digastric and superior belly of omohyoid. Posterior triangle is subdivided by inferior belly of omohyoid

**Plate 4.2:** Boundaries and subdivisions of the anterior triangle

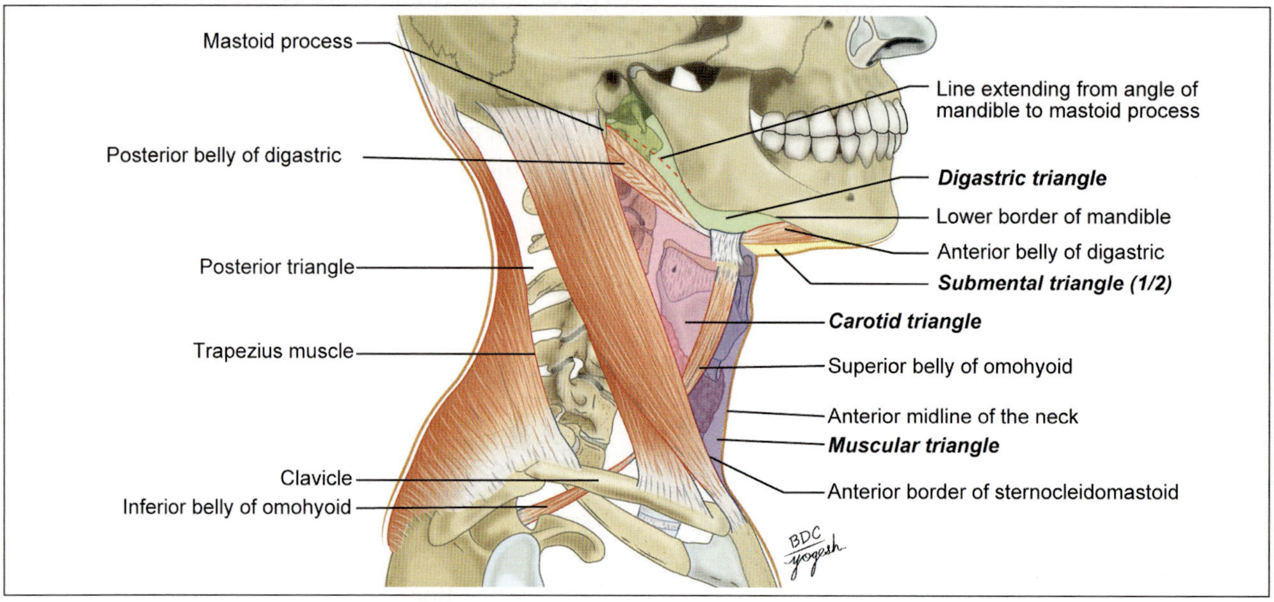


**Plate 4.3:** Boundaries and contents of the submental triangle

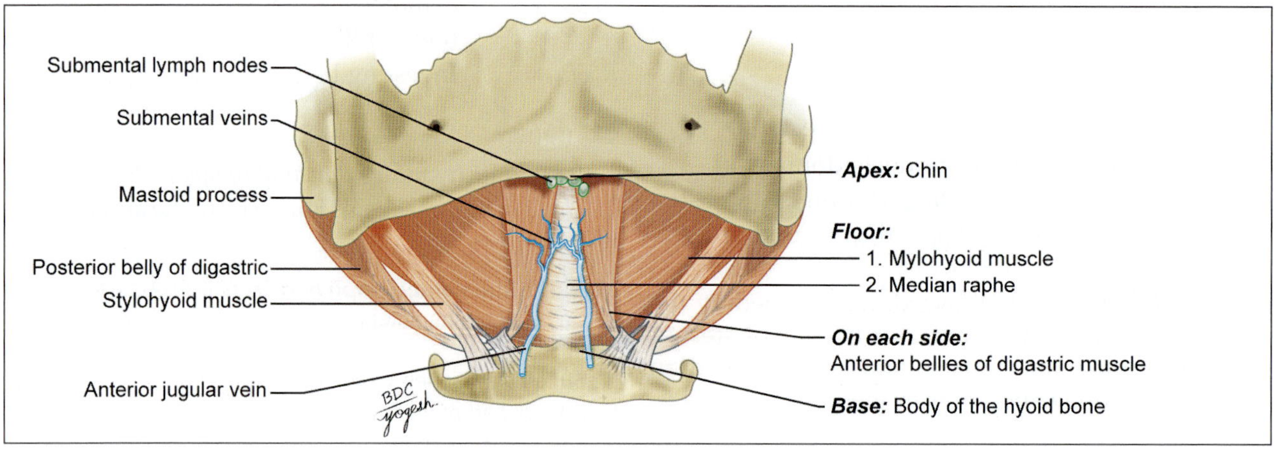


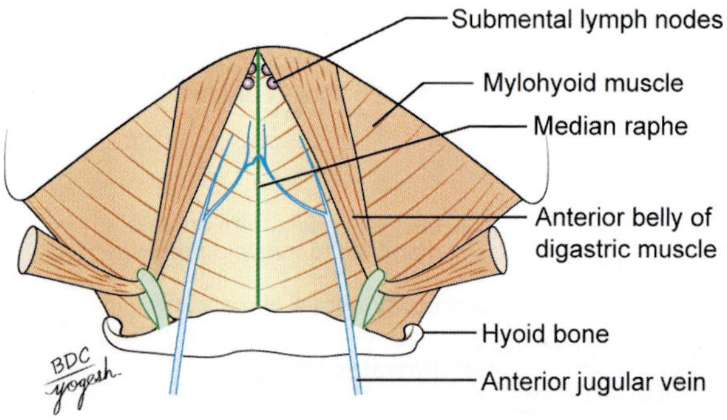


**Fig. 4.6:** Boundaries and contents of the submental triangle

**Flowchart 4.1:** Submental triangle

***Submental triangle***

Contributed by both anterior triangles of neck

***Boundaries***
- Apex: Symphysis menti
- Base: Body of hyoid bone
- On each side: Anterior bellies of digastric muscles
- Floor: Mylohyoid
- Roof: Investing layer of deep cervical fascia

***Contents***
- Submental lymph nodes
- Submental vein joins to form anterior jugular veins

## DIGASTRIC (SUBMANDIBULAR) TRIANGLE

The digastric triangle is also called submandibular triangle as it is located below the base of mandible (Figs 4.7and 4.8 and Flowchart 4.2).

*Note*: The area between the body of the mandible and the hyoid bone is known as the ***submandibular region***. The superficial structures of this region lie in the submental and digastric triangles.

### Boundaries

| | |
|---|---|
| *Anteroinferiorly:* | Anterior belly of digastric |
| *Posteroinferiorly:* | Posterior belly of digastric and the stylohyoid |
| *Superiorly or base:* | Base of the mandible and a line joining the angle of the mandible to the mastoid process. |
| *Apex:* | Intermediate tendon of digastric muscle |

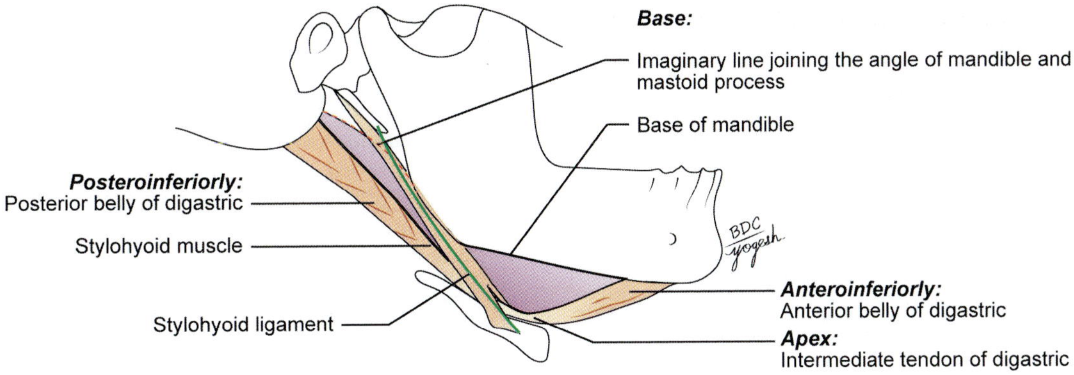


**Fig. 4.7:** Boundaries of the digastric triangle

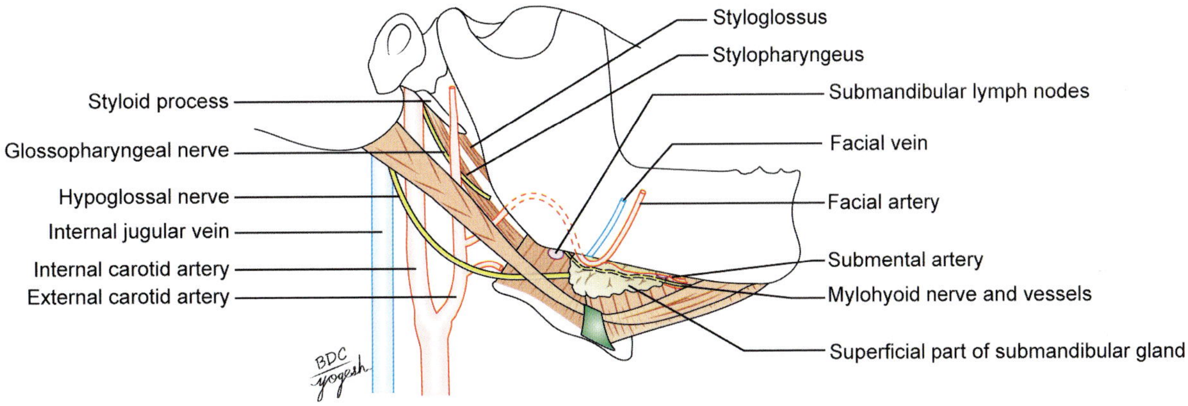


**Fig. 4.8:** Contents of the digastric triangle

**Flowchart 4.2:** Digastric or submandibular triangle

***Digastric or submandibular triangle***

| ***Boundaries*** | ***Contents*** |
|---|---|
| Anteroinferiorly:<br>Anterior belly of digastric<br>Posteroinferiorly:<br>Posterior belly of digastric<br>Stylohyoid muscle<br>Base: Base of mandible<br>Line joining angle of mandible and mastoid process<br>Apex: Intermediate tendon of digastric muscle<br>Floor: Mylohyoid<br>Hyoglossus<br>Middle constrictor | Anterior part<br>- Facial artery and vein<br>- Superficial part of submandibular gland<br>- Submandibular lymph nodes<br>- Submental artery<br>- Mylohyoid nerve and vessels<br>- Hypoglossal nerve<br>Posterior part<br>- Lower part of parotid gland<br>- External carotid artery<br>- Styloglossus, stylopharyngeus<br>- Glossopharyngeal nerve<br>- Styloid process<br>- Carotid sheath and its contents |

*Roof:* The roof of the triangle is formed by:
1. Skin
2. Superficial fascia, containing:
   a. Platysma
   b. Cervical branch of the facial nerve
   c. Ascending branch of the transverse or anterior cutaneous nerve of the neck.
3. Deep fascia, which splits to enclose the submandibular salivary gland.

*Floor*
1. Mylohyoid muscle
2. Hyoglossus
3. Middle constrictor muscle of the pharynx.

## Contents (Fig. 4.8)

The ***stylomandibular ligament*** divides the triangle into anterior and posterior parts.

### *Anterior Part of the Triangle*

Structures superficial to mylohyoid are:
1. Superficial part of the submandibular salivary gland
2. Facial vein
3. Submandibular lymph nodes
4. Facial artery is deep to it
5. Submental artery
6. Mylohyoid nerve and vessels
7. Hypoglossal nerve.

### *Posterior Part of the Triangle*

1. *Superficial structures* are:
   a. Lower part of the parotid gland
   b. External carotid artery
2. *Deep structures*, passing between the external and internal carotid arteries, are:
   a. Styloglossus
   b. Stylopharyngeus
   c. Glossopharyngeal (IX) nerve
   d. Pharyngeal branch of the vagus nerve

e. Styloid process
f. A part of the parotid gland.

3. *Deepest structures* include:
   a. Internal carotid artery
   b. Internal jugular vein
   c. Vagus nerve.

## DISSECTION

Remove the deep fascia from anterior bellies of digastric muscles to expose parts of two mylohyoid muscles. Clean the boundaries and contents of the submental triangle.

Cut the deep fascia from the mandible and reflect it downwards to expose the submandibular gland. Identify and clean anterior and posterior bellies of digastric muscles, which form the boundaries of digastric triangle. Identify the intermediate tendon of digastric after pulling the submandibular gland laterally. Clean the stylohyoid muscle, which envelops the tendon of digastric and is lying above with the posterior belly of digastric muscle (Fig. 4.7). Identify the contents of digastric triangle.

***Competency:***

**AN32.2** Describe and demonstrate boundaries and contents of muscular, carotid triangles.

## CAROTID TRIANGLE

### Boundaries

*Anterosuperiorly:* Posterior belly of the digastric muscle; and the stylohyoid (Plate 4.4, Fig. 4.9 and Flowchart 4.3).

**Flowchart 4.3:** Carotid triangle

***Carotid triangle***

***Boundaries***
Anterosuperiorly:
- Posterior belly of digastric
- Stylohyoid muscles
Anteroinferiorly:
- Superior belly of omohyoid
Posterior:
- Anterior border of sternocleidomastoid
Floor:
- Thyrohyoid
- Hyoglossus
- Inferior constrictor
- Middle constrictor
Roof:
- Investing layer of deep cervical fascia

***Contents***
Carotid arteries
Carotid sinus, carotid body
Internal jugular vein
Common facial vein
Pharyngeal vein
Lingual vein
Xth, XIth, XIIth nerves
Superior, internal and external laryngeal branches
Descendens hypoglossi
Sympathetic chain
Carotid sheath
Deep cervical nodes

*Anteroinferiorly:* Superior belly of the omohyoid.
*Posteriorly:* Anterior border of the sternocleidomastoid muscle

*Roof:*
1. Skin
2. Superficial fascia containing:
   a. Platysma
   b. Cervical branch of the facial nerve
   c. Transverse cervical nerve of the neck.
3. Investing layer of deep cervical fascia.

*Floor:*
1. Middle constrictor of pharynx
2. Inferior constrictor of the pharynx
3. Thyrohyoid membrane.

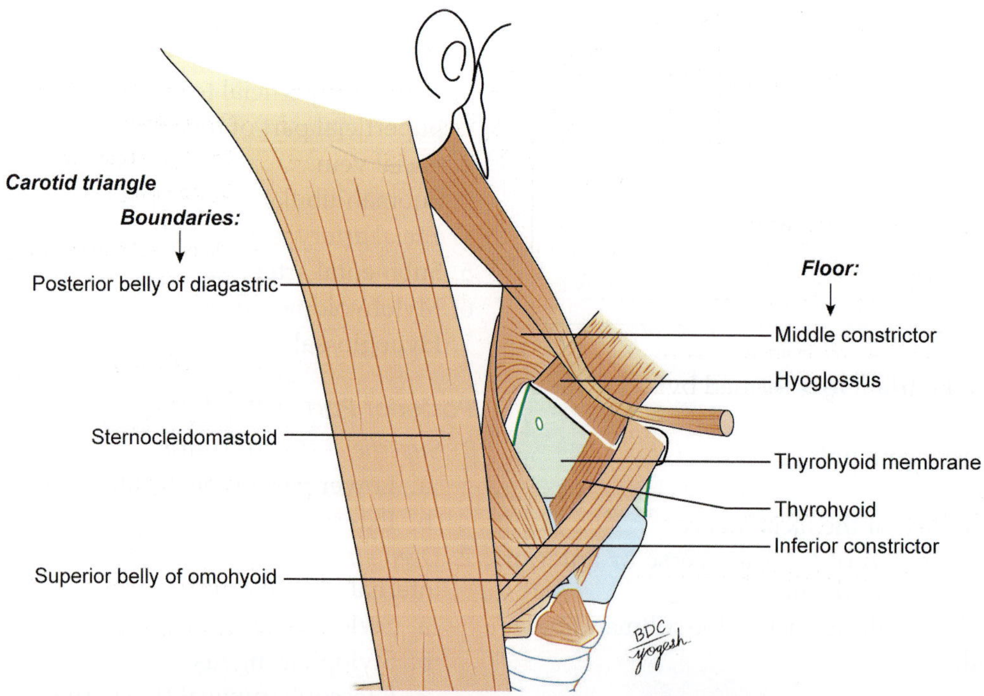


**Fig. 4.9:** Boundaries and floor of the carotid triangle

**Plate 4.4:** Carotid triangle: Boundaries and floor

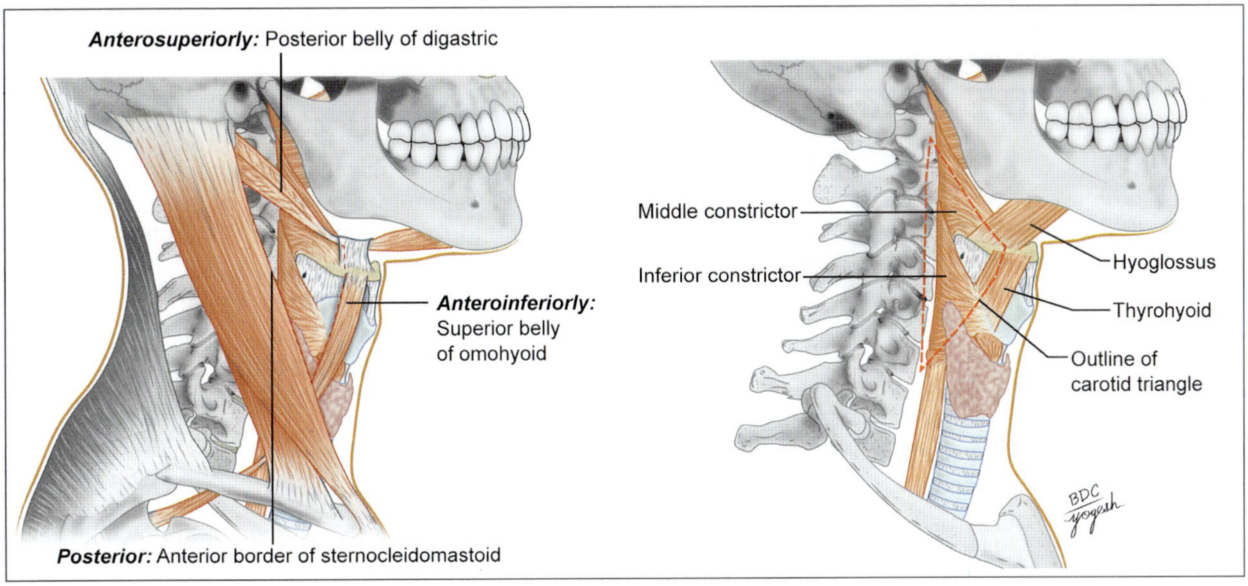


## Contents (Fig. 4.10)

### Arteries

1. Carotid arteries: Common, internal, external
2. Carotid sinus and carotid body
3. Superior thyroid, lingual, facial, ascending pharyngeal and occipital arteries.

### Veins

1. Internal jugular vein
2. Common facial vein draining into the internal jugular vein
3. Pharyngeal vein which usually ends in the internal jugular vein
4. Lingual vein which usually terminates in the internal jugular vein.

### Nerves

1. Vagus nerve
2. Spinal accessory nerve
3. Hypoglossal nerve – gives off the superior root of the ansa cervicalis or descendens hypoglossi, and another branch to the thyrohyoid.
4. Superior laryngeal branch of the vagus, dividing into the external and internal laryngeal nerves.
5. Sympathetic chain.
6. *Carotid sheath* with its contents.

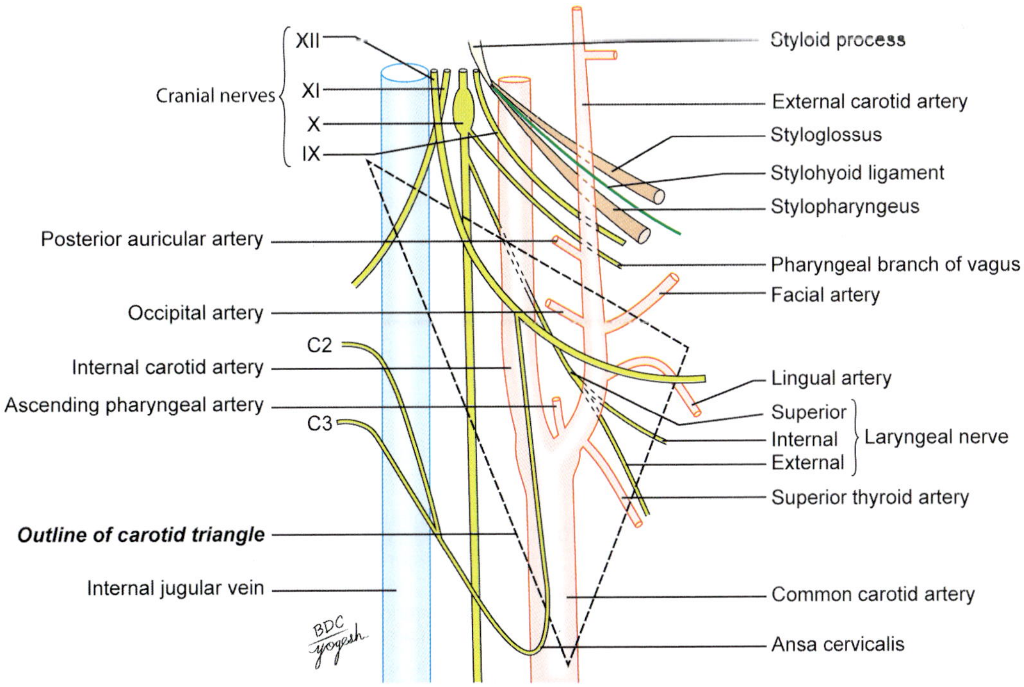


**Fig. 4.10:** The IXth, Xth, XIth and XIIth cranial nerves and their branches related to the carotid arteries and to the internal jugular vein, in and around the right carotid triangle

### Lymph Nodes

Deep cervical lymph nodes include the jugulodigastric node below the posterior belly of the digastric and the jugulo-omohyoid node above the inferior belly of the omohyoid.

#### DISSECTION

Clean the area situated between posterior belly of digastric and superior belly of omohyoid muscle, to expose the carotid arteries with internal jugular vein. Trace IX, X, XI and XII nerves in relation to these vessels.

Identify middle and inferior constrictors of pharynx and thyrohyoid membrane forming its floor.

Carefully clean and preserve superior root, the loop and inferior root of ansa cervicalis in relation to anterior aspect of carotid sheath. Locate the sympathetic trunk situated posteromedial to the carotid sheath. Dissect the branches of external carotid artery. Identify and preserve the internal laryngeal nerve in the thyrohyoid interval. Trace it posterosuperiorly till vagus. Also look for external laryngeal nerve supplying the cricothyroid muscle.

The carotid triangle provides a good view of all the large vessels and nerves of the neck, particularly when its posterior boundary is retracted slightly backwards.

## MUSCULAR TRIANGLE

### Boundaries

| | |
|---|---|
| *Anteriorly:* | Anterior median line of the neck from the hyoid bone to the sternum. |
| *Posterosuperiorly:* | Superior belly of the omohyoid muscle. |
| *Posteroinferiorly:* | Lower part of anterior border of the sternocleidomastoid muscle. |
| *Floor:* | It is formed by pretracheal fascia, thyroid and cricoid cartilages and trachea |
| *Roof:* | Investing layer of deep cervical fascia. |

### Contents

The infrahyoid muscles are the chief contents of the triangle. These muscles may also be regarded arbitrarily as forming the floor of the triangle (Fig. 4.11).

The *infrahyoid muscles* are:

a. Sternohyoid
b. Sternothyroid
c. Thyrohyoid
d. Omohyoid.

*Note*: ***Peculiarities of infrahyoid muscles***

a. Arranged in two layers – Superficial (sternohyoid and omohyoid) and deep (sternothyroid and thyrohyoid).
b. Supplied by the ventral rami of C1, C2, and C3 spinal nerves.
c. Because of their attachment to the hyoid bone and to the thyroid cartilage, they move these structures.
d. Sternohyoid, superior belly of omohyoid, and sternothyroid lie superficial to the lateral or superficial convex surface of the thyroid gland.
e. The anterior surface of isthmus of thyroid gland is covered by right and left sternothyroid and sternohyoid muscles.

The specific details of infrahyoid muscles are shown in Table 4.1.

#### DISSECTION

Identify the infrahyoid muscles on each side of the median plane. Cut through the origin of sternocleidomastoid muscle and reflect it upwards. Trace the nerve supply of infrahyoid muscles.

The superficial structures in the infrahyoid region are included in this triangle. The deeper structures (thyroid gland, trachea, oesophagus, etc.) will be studied separately at a later stage.

## ANSA CERVICALIS OR ANSA HYPOGLOSSI

*Definition*: It is also called ***ansa hypoglossi***. It is a loop of nerve fibres embedded in the anterior wall of the carotid sheath (Fig. 4.12, Flowchart 4.4).

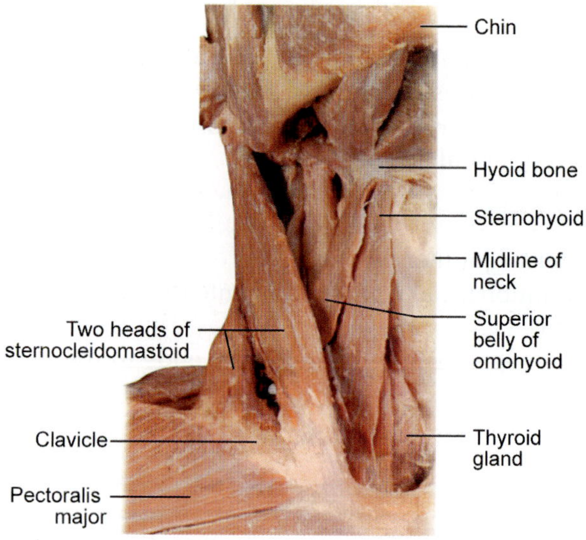


**Fig. 4.11:** Dissection of muscular triangle

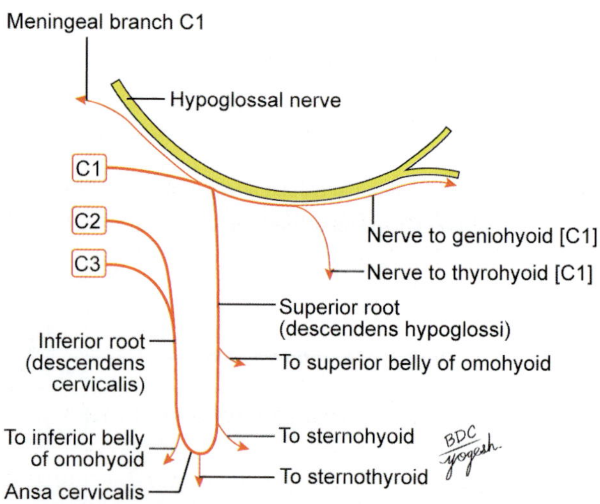


**Fig. 4.12:** Ansa cervicalis and branches of the first cervical nerve distributed through the hypoglossal nerve

**Flowchart 4.4:** Ansa cervicalis

| Ansa cervicalis | | |
|---|---|---|
| ***Definition*** | ***Formation*** | ***Distribution*** |
| Loop of nerve embeded in the anterior wall of carotid sheath | Superior root: Descendens hypoglossi C1 fibres<br>Inferior root: Descendens cervicals Fibres from C2 and C3<br>Both roots join to form loop | Superior root - Superior belly of omohyoid<br>Ansa cervicalis - Sternohyoid, sternothyroid<br>Inferior root - Inferior root of omohyoid |

### Formation

It is formed by a superior and an inferior root.

1. ***Superior root*** *or* ***descendens hypoglossi*** is the continuation of the descending branch of the hypoglossal nerve. Its fibres are derived from the C1 nerve. This root descends over the internal carotid artery and the common carotid artery.
2. ***Inferior root*** or ***descendens cervicalis*** is derived from C2 and C3 spinal nerves. As this root descends, it winds around the internal jugular vein and then continues anteroinferiorly to join the superior root in front of the common carotid artery.

### Distribution

1. *Superior root:* To the superior belly of the omohyoid.
2. *Ansa cervicalis:* To the sternohyoid, the sternothyroid.
3. *Inferior root:* To the inferior belly of the omohyoid.

*Note*: The thyrohyoid and geniohyoid are supplied by separate branches from the first cervical nerve through the hypoglossal nerve.

## COMMON CAROTID ARTERY

The right common carotid artery is a branch of the brachiocephalic artery. It begins in the neck behind the right sternoclavicular joint. The left common carotid artery is branch of the arch of the aorta.

### Carotid Sinus

The termination of the common carotid artery, or the beginning of the internal carotid artery shows a slight dilatation, known as the carotid sinus. In this region, the tunica media is thin, but the adventitia is relatively thick and receives a rich innervation from the glossopharyngeal and sympathetic nerves. The carotid sinus acts as a ***baroreceptor*** or *pressure receptor* and regulates ***blood pressure***.

### Carotid Body

Carotid body is a small, oval reddish brown structure situated behind the bifurcation of the common carotid artery. It receives a rich nerve supply mainly from the glossopharyngeal nerve, but also from the vagus and sympathetic nerves. It acts as a ***chemoreceptor*** and responds to changes in the oxygen, carbon dioxide and **pH** content of the blood.

Other *allied chemoreceptors* are found near the arch of the aorta, the ductus arteriosus and the right subclavian artery. These are supplied by the vagus nerve.

## CLINICAL ANATOMY

- ***Carotid tubercle***: It is a tubercle on the transverse process of ***C6*** vertebra. CCA can be compressed against the tubercle. It lies about 4 cm above the sternoclavicular joint.
- The carotid sinus is richly supplied by nerves. In some persons, the sinus may be hypersensitive. In such persons, sudden rotation of the head may cause slowing of heart. This condition is called '***carotid sinus syndrome***'.
- ***Potato tumour of neck*** is produced by enlargement of the carotid body. The tumour moves transversely. It is pulsating and produces attacks of fainting due to pressure on carotid sinus. The supraventricular tachycardia may be controlled by carotid sinus massage, due to inhibitory effects of vagus nerve on the heart.
- The necktie should not be tied tightly, as it may compress both the internal carotid arteries, supplying the brain.

## EXTERNAL CAROTID ARTERY

External carotid artery is one of the terminal branches of the common carotid artery. In general, it lies anterior to the internal carotid artery and supply the structures in the front of the neck and in the face (Fig. 4.13).

### Course and Relations

1. External carotid artery runs in the carotid and digastric triangles and then in the substance of parotid gland.
2. The external carotid artery begins in the carotid triangle at the level of the upper border of the thyroid cartilage opposite the disc between the 3rd and 4th cervical vertebrae. It runs upwards and slightly backwards and laterally and terminates behind the neck of the mandible by dividing into the maxillary and superficial temporal arteries.
3. The external carotid artery has a *slightly curved course* so that it is anteromedial to the internal carotid artery in its lower part and anterolateral to the internal carotid artery in its upper part.
4. *In the carotid triangle,* the external carotid artery is comparatively superficial and lies under cover of the anterior border of the sternocleidomastoid. The artery is crossed superficially by the cervical branch of the facial nerve, the hypoglossal nerve and the facial, lingual and superior thyroid veins.
   Deep to the artery, there are:
   a. Wall of the pharynx.
   b. Superior laryngeal nerve which divides into the external and internal laryngeal nerves.
   c. Ascending pharyngeal artery.

5. *Above the carotid triangle*, the external carotid artery lies deep in the substance of the parotid gland. Within the gland, it is related superficially to the retromandibular vein and the facial nerve. Deep to the external carotid artery, there are:
   a. Internal carotid artery.
   b. Structures passing between the external and internal carotid arteries; these being styloglossus, stylopharyngeus both arising from the styloid process, IX nerve, pharyngeal branch of X nerve.
   c. Two structures deep to the internal carotid artery, namely the superior laryngeal nerve and the superior cervical sympathetic ganglion.

**Branches** (Fig. 4.13, Flowchart 4.5)

*Medial*

1. Ascending pharyngeal (1st branch)

*Anterior*

2. Superior thyroid
3. Lingual
4. Facial

*Posterior*

5. Occipital
6. Posterior auricular

*Terminal*

7. Maxillary
8. Superficial temporal.

[*Mnemonics:* ***External carotid artery branches:*** **S**ome **A**natomists **L**ike **F**reaking **O**ut **P**oor **M**edical: **S**tudents; **S**uperior thyroid; **A**scending pharyngeal; **L**ingual; **F**acial; **O**ccipital; **P**osterior auricular; **M**axillary; **S**uperficial temporal]

### *Ascending Pharyngeal Artery*

This is a small branch that arises from the medial side of the external carotid artery. It arises very close to the lower end of external carotid artery. It runs vertically upwards between the side wall of the pharynx, the tonsil, medial wall of the middle ear and the auditory tube.

***Branches:*** It gives:

1. ***Pharyngeal branches*** to the pharynx, tonsil, pharyngeal ends of auditory tube, and soft palate.
2. ***Inferior tympanic branch*** to the medial wall of tympanic cavity. These branches enter the middle ear through a canaliculus for the tympanic branches of glossopharyngeal nerve.
3. ***Meningeal branches*** that enter the cranial cavity through foramen lacerum, jugular foramen and hypoglossal canal.

### *Superior Thyroid Artery*

It arises from the external carotid artery just below the level of the greater cornua of the hyoid bone.

It runs downwards and forwards parallel and just superficial to the external laryngeal nerve. It passes deep to the three long infrahyoid muscles to reach the upper pole of the lateral lobe of the thyroid gland.

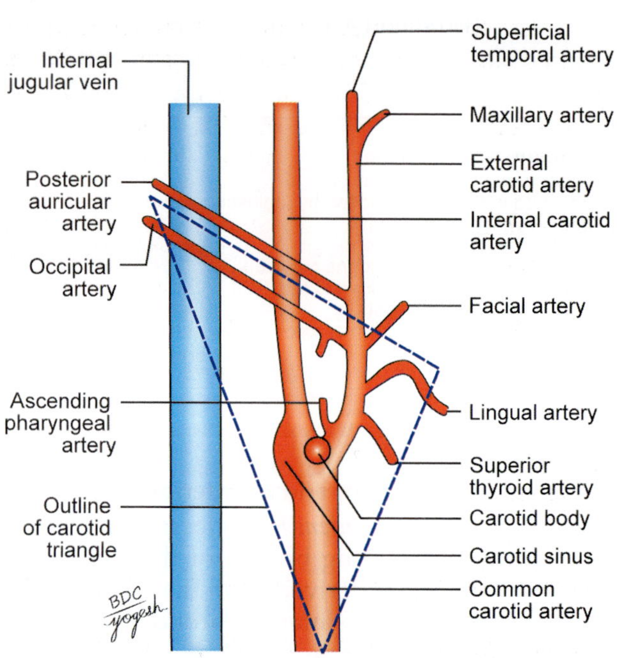


**Fig. 4.13:** Right carotid arteries including branches of the external carotid artery

**Flowchart 4.5:** External carotid artery

***External carotid artery***

| ***Beginning*** | ***Termination*** | ***Branches*** |
|---|---|---|
| Terminal branch of common carotid artery<br>Begins at the level of upper border of thyroid cartilage | Divides into maxillary and superficial temporal arteries within the parotid gland at the level of neck of mandible | Ascending pharyngeal<br>Superior thyroid<br>Lingual<br>Facial<br>Occipital<br>Posterior auricular<br>Superficial temporal<br>Maxillary |

***Branches:*** It gives:

1. *Infrahyoid branch* that runs along the lower border of hyoid bone.
2. *Superior laryngeal artery* that pierces the thyrohyoid membrane along with the internal laryngeal nerve. It supplies larynx.
3. *Cricothyroid branch* that anastomosis with similar branches of opposite sides.
4. *Sternocleidomastoid branch* to sternocleidomastoid muscle.
5. *Terminal branches*: The superior thyroid artery divides into anterior and posterior branches that supply thyroid gland.

*Note*: The superior thyroid artery and external laryngeal nerve diverge from each other as the artery approaches the thyroid gland. Hence, in thyroid gland surgeries, the superior thyroid artery is ligated near the gland to avoid injury to the nerve.

### *Lingual Artery*

The lingual artery arises from the external carotid artery opposite the tip of the greater cornua of the hyoid bone.

***Course:*** It is tortuous in its course. Its course is divided into three parts by the hyoglossus muscle, as follows:

1. ***1st part*** lies in the carotid triangle. It forms a characteristic upward loop which is crossed by the hypoglossal nerve. The lingual loop permits free movements of the hyoid bone.
2. ***2nd part*** lies deep to the hyoglossus along the upper border of hyoid bone. It is superficial to the middle constrictor of the pharynx.
3. ***3rd part*** is called the arteria profunda linguae, or the *deep lingual artery*. It runs upwards along the anterior border of the hyoglossus.
4. ***4th part:*** Finally, the artery runs horizontally forwards on the undersurface of the tongue as the ***4th part*** which is accompanied by the lingual nerve.

***Branches:*** It gives:

1. *Suprahyoid artery* which passes along the upper border of hyoid bone.
2. *Dorsal lingual artery* (3–4 in number) arises from the second part of the artery. They supply dorsal surface of tongue, palatine tonsil, and soft palate.
3. *Sublingual artery* arises from third part to supply sublingual gland and floor of the mouth.

*Note*: During surgeries of the tongue (surgical removal), the lingual artery is ligated before it gives any branch to the tongue or tonsil.

### Facial Artery

The facial artery arises from the external carotid just above the tip of the greater cornua of the hyoid bone. It runs upwards first in the neck as cervical part and then on the face as facial part. The course of the artery in both places is tortuous. The tortuosity in the neck allows free movements of the pharynx during deglutition. On the face, it allows free movements of the mandible, the lips and the cheek during mastication and during various facial expressions. The artery escapes traction and pressure during these movements.

The ***cervical part*** of the facial artery runs upwards on the superior constrictor of pharynx deep to the posterior belly of the digastric, stylohyoid and to the ramus of the mandible.

It grooves the posterior end of the submandibular salivary gland. Next, the artery makes an S bend (two loops) first winding down over the submandibular gland, and then up over the base of the mandible (*see* Fig. 7.11).

The ***facial part*** of the facial artery enters the face at anteroinferior angle of masseter muscle, runs upwards close to angle of mouth, side of nose till medial angle of eye.

***Branches:*** It gives:

*Branches from cervical part*:

1. *Ascending palatine artery*: It arises near the origin of the facial artery and ascends upward between styloglossus and stylopharyngeus. It winds around the upper border of the superior constrictor. It supplies tonsil, soft palate, pharynx, and auditory tube.
2. *Tonsillar artery*: It is the chief supply of the tonsil. It pierces the superior constrictor to reach the tonsil.
3. *Glandular branches* for submandibular gland.
4. *Submental artery* accompanies the mylohyoid nerve. It runs along the lower border of the mandible.

*Branches from facial part:*

1. Inferior labial artery
2. Superior labial artery
3. Lateral nasal artery.

### Occipital Artery

The occipital artery arises from the posterior aspect of the external carotid artery, opposite the origin of the facial artery. It is crossed by the hypoglossal nerve.

***Branches:*** It gives:

1. *Sternomastoid branches*: Upper sternomastoid branch accompanies the spinal accessory nerve. Lower sternomastoid branch loops around the hypoglossal nerve.
2. *Mastoid branch* enters the mastoid foramen to supply mastoid air cells and meninges.
3. *Meningeal branches* enter the cranial cavity through jugular foramen and condylar canals.
4. *Muscular branches*
5. *Descending branch*: It divides into
   a. *Superficial branch* which anastomoses with superficial branch of transverse cervical artery.
   b. *Deep branch* which anastomoses with deep cervical artery.
6. *Occipital branches* to scalp.

### Posterior Auricular Artery

The posterior auricular artery arises from the posterior aspect of the external carotid just above the posterior belly of the digastric. It runs upwards and backwards deep to the parotid gland, but superficial to the styloid process. It crosses the base of the mastoid process and ascends behind the auricle.

***Branches:*** It gives:

1. *Stylomastoid branch* enters the stylomastoid foramen and supplies the middle ear, mastoid antrum, air cells and facial nerve.
2. *Auricular branch* supplies the auricle.
3. *Occipital branch* supplies the scalp.

### Maxillary Artery

This is the larger terminal branch of the external carotid artery. It begins behind the neck of the mandible under cover of the parotid gland. It runs forwards deep to the neck of the mandible below the auriculotemporal nerve and enters the infratemporal fossa where it will be studied at a later stage.

### Superficial Temporal Artery

It is the smaller terminal branch of the external carotid artery. It begins, behind the neck of the mandible under cover of the parotid gland. It runs vertically upwards, crossing the root of the zygoma or preauricular point, where its *pulsations* can be easily felt. About 5 cm above the zygoma, it divides into anterior and posterior branches.

***Branches:*** It gives:

1. *Transverse facial artery* arises from the superficial temporal artery within the parotid gland. It passes forward along with the zygomatic branch of the facial nerve. It supplies parotid gland, temporomandibular joint and face.
2. *Anterior auricular branch* to the auricle and external acoustic meatus.
3. Zygomatico-orbital branch to the face.
4. *Middle temporal artery* pierces the temporal fascia to supply temporalis.
5. Anterior and posterior divisions supply temple, scalp and auricle.

## POTENTIAL TISSUE SPACES IN HEAD AND NECK

1. ***Submental space:*** Lies below inferior border of mandible. Corresponds to submental triangle. It communicates with submandibular spaces on both sides.
2. ***Submandibular space:*** Lies between anterior and posterior bellies of digastric muscle and inferior border of mandible. It communicates with sublingual and submental spaces.
3. ***Parotid space:*** Localised around parotid gland behind ramus of mandible, communicates with retropharyngeal space and even mediastinum.
4. ***Parapharyngeal space:*** Lies in suprahyoid region of neck, lateral to pharynx. It is continuous with retropharyngeal space.
5. ***Retropharyngeal space:*** Lies between anteriorly placed buccopharyngeal fascia and posteriorly placed prevertebral fascia. It communicates with peritonsillar space, submental spaces and may reach mediastinum.
6. ***Peritonsillar space:*** Lies between anterior and posterior fauces of the palatine tonsil. It communicates with sublingual space.

VIDEO

**Video 3.4** **Anterior Triangle of the Neck**

### *Facts to Remember*

- Apex of anterior triangle of neck is close to the sternum, while that of posterior triangle is close to the mastoid process.
- Submental triangle is half on each side of the midline.
- Maximum blood vessels are present in the carotid triangle.
- Superficial temporal artery can be palpated at the preauricular point.
- The necktie should not be tied tightly, as it may compress both the internal carotid arteries, supplying the brain.

### BDC's Anatomy *e*-book

1. Subhyoid bursa
2. Lingual artery
3. Further reading
4. Viva voce questions

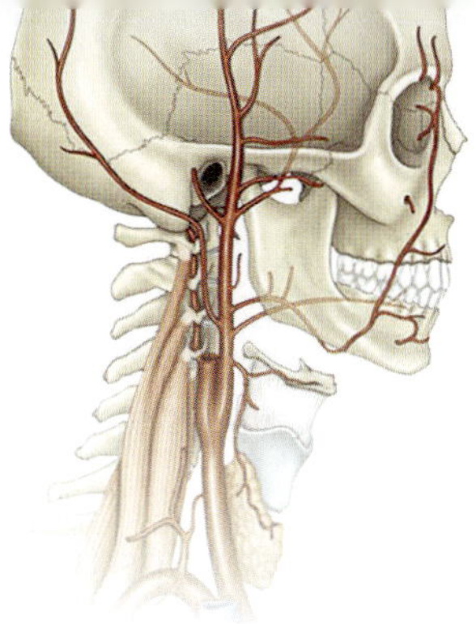

Chapter

5

# Parotid Region

The parotid region is a region located on the posterolateral side of the face. It contains the parotid gland and facial nerve. The boundaries of the parotid region are as follows:

*Anteriorly*: Posterior border of ramus of mandible masseter and medial pterygoid muscles

*Posteriorly*: Mastoid process
Sternocleidomastoid muscle

*Superiorly*: External acoustic meatus
Posterior part of temporomandibular joint

*Medially*: Styloid process
Styloid group of muscles.

Facial nerve is described in detail in Chapter 6, *BD Chaurasia's Human Anatomy, Volume 4*. Its extracranial course is given in this chapter.

## SALIVARY GLANDS

There are three pairs of large salivary glands—the parotid, submandibular and sublingual. In addition, there are numerous small glands in the tongue, the palate, the cheeks and the lips. These glands produce saliva which keeps the oral cavity moist and helps in chewing and swallowing. The saliva also contains enzymes that aid digestion.

**Competency:**

**AN28.9** Describe and demonstrate the parts, borders, surfaces, contents, relations and nerve supply of parotid gland with course of its duct and surgical importance.

## PAROTID GLAND

The parotid gland is the largest of the salivary glands (*Para* = around; *otic* = ear). It weighs about 25 g.

### Location

The parotid glands are situated in the pyramidal *retromandibular fossa* or ***parotid bed*** (Fig. 5.1). The boundaries of the parotid bed are as follows:

*Anteriorly*: Ramus of mandible with medial pterygoid and masseter

*Posteriorly*: Mastoid process with sternocleidomastoid and posterior belly of digastric

*Superiorly*: External acoustic meatus and temporomandibular joint

*Medially*: Styloid apparatus

The gland overlaps these structures. Skin over the gland is supplied by great auricular nerve (C2, C3).

### Capsule of Parotid Gland

The investing layer of the deep cervical fascia forms a capsule or ***parotid sheath*** (Fig. 5.2). It is supplied by great auricular nerve.

The parotid sheath has two laminae:

a. *Superficial lamina* is thick, strong, unyielding and adherent to the glands. Superiorly, it is attached to the inferior border of the zygomatic arch. Anteriorly, it blends with the epimysium of masseter to form *parotidomasseteric fascia*.
b. *Deep lamina* is thin. It is attached to the tympanic plate and styloid process. *Stylomandibular ligament* is a thickened part of deep lamina that extends from the tip of styloid process to the angle of mandible.

*Note*: Recent concept:

The ***superficial Musculo-aponeurotic system*** (SMAS) is a single tissue plane in the face. It is composed of muscle fibres and fibrous or fibroaponeurotic tissue. It is not directly attached to bone.

Inferiorly, it becomes continuous with platysma in the neck. The superficial layer of the parotid capsule is a component of the SMAS, and not from the investing layer of deep cervical fascia [*Reference*: Gray's Anatomy, 42nd ed].

## CLINICAL ANATOMY

- ***Parotid swellings*** are very painful due to the unyielding nature of the parotid fascia.
- ***Mumps*** is an infectious disease of the salivary glands (usually the parotid) caused by a specific virus. Viral parotitis or mumps characteristically does not suppurate. Its complications are orchitis and pancreatitis (Fig. 5.3).
- ***Accessory parotid gland*** is a detached part of the parotid gland that lies between the zygomatic arch and the parotid duct. It drains into the main parotid duct.

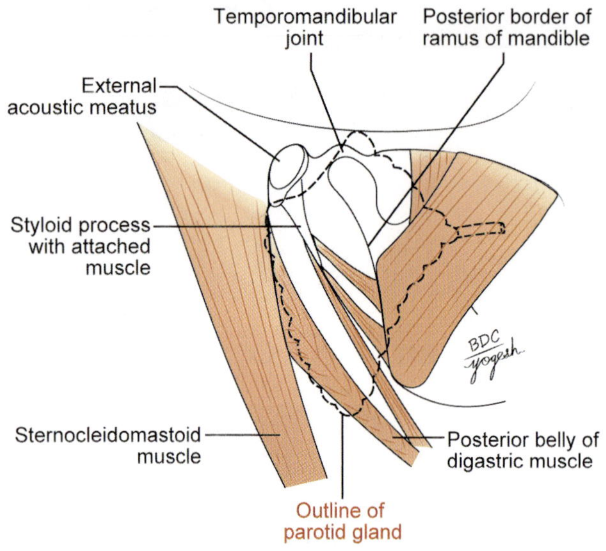


**Fig. 5.1:** Location of parotid gland

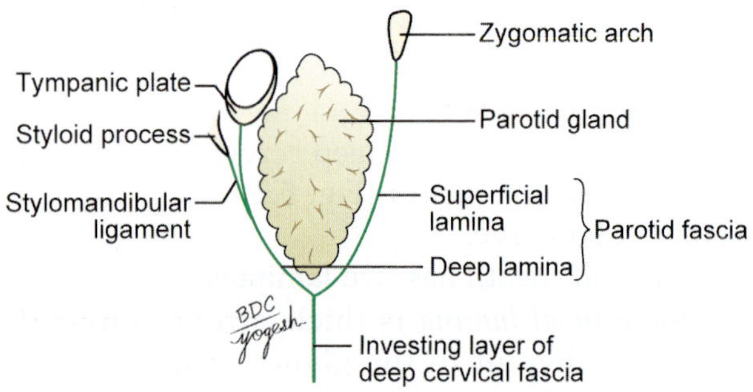


**Fig. 5.2:** Parotid capsule (coronal section)

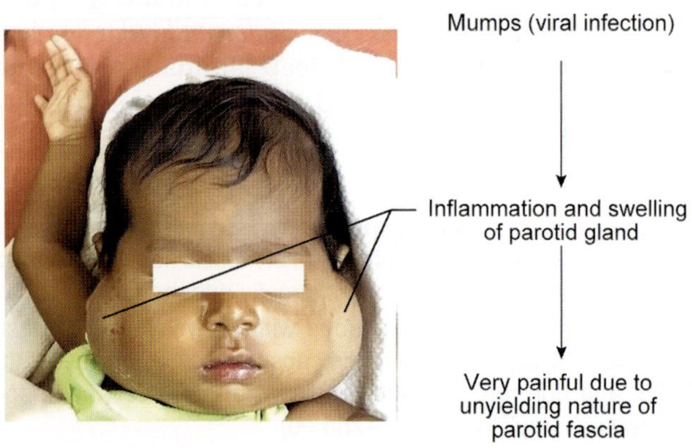


**Fig. 5.3:** Mumps (*Image courtesy*: Dr Jaikumar GR)

## External Features

The parotid gland resembles an inverted pyramid with apex directed downward (Figs 5.4a and b, Flowchart 5.1). The gland presents:

- Apex
- *Four surfaces*:
  1. Superior surface (base)
  2. Superficial
  3. Anteromedial
  4. Posteromedial
- *Three borders*:
  1. Anterior
  2. Posterior
  3. Medial.

## Relations (Plate 5.1, Figs 5.5 to 5.7, Flowchart 5.2)

### *Apex*

The apex is directed downwards. It overlaps the posterior belly of the digastric.

Structures emerging through apex:

1. Cervical branch of the facial nerve
2. Anterior and posterior divisions of the retromandibular vein.

### *Superior Surface or Base*

It forms the upper end of the gland which is small and concave.

It is related to:

1. External acoustic meatus
2. Posterior surface of the temporomandibular joint.

Structures emerging through the superior surface:

1. Superficial temporal vessels.
2. Auriculotemporal nerve.

### *Superficial Surface*

It is the largest of the four surfaces. It is covered with:

1. Skin
2. Superficial fascia containing the anterior branches of the great auricular nerve, the preauricular or superficial parotid lymph nodes and the posterior fibres of the platysma and risorius
3. Superficial lamina of the parotid fascia
4. A few deep parotid lymph nodes embedded in the gland.

### *Anteromedial Surface*

It is grooved by the posterior border of the ramus of the mandible. It is related to:

1. Masseter
2. Lateral surface of the temporomandibular joint
3. Posterior border of the ramus of the mandible
4. Medial pterygoid
5. Emerging branches of the facial nerve and maxillary artery.

### *Posteromedial Surface*

It is moulded to the mastoid and the styloid processes and the structures attached to them. Thus, it is related to:

1. Mastoid process, with the sternocleidomastoid and the posterior belly of the digastric.
2. Styloid process, with structures attached to it.
3. Deep to styloid apparatus: Internal carotid artery, internal jugular vein, last 4 cranial nerves.

Structures entering through posteromedial surface:

1. Facial nerve
2. External carotid artery

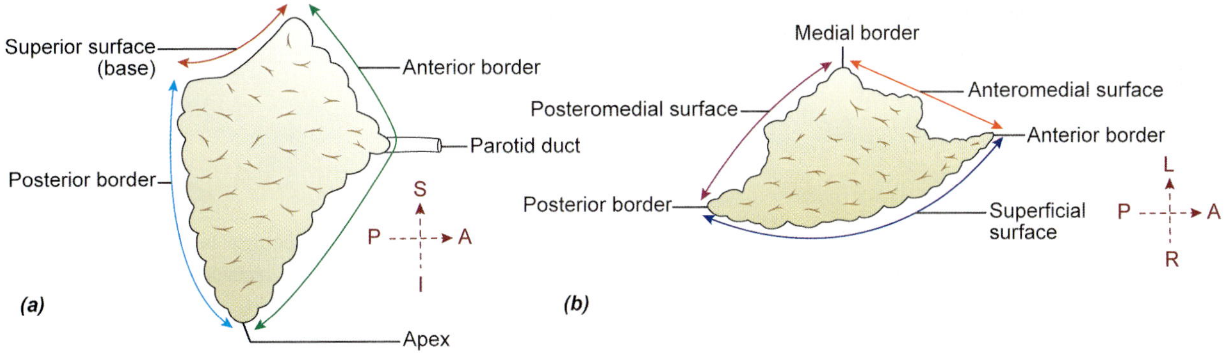


**Figs 5.4a and b:** External features of parotid gland: (a) Lateral view and (b) horizontal section through parotid gland

**Flowchart 5.1:** Parotid gland: External features

***External features of parotid gland***

- ***Apex***
  - Directed downward
  - Related to posterior belly of digastric
- ***Base***
  - Superior surface
  - Relations:
    1. External acoustic meatus
    2. TMJ
- ***Surfaces***
  - ***Superficial***
    - Relations:
    - Skin
    - Superficial fascia with great auricular nerve
    - Platysma
    - Superficial lamina of parotid fascia
  - ***Anteromedial***
    - Relations:
    - Masseter
    - Ramus of mandible
    - Medial pterygoid
    - Temporomandibular joint
    - Emerging branches of facial nerve
    - Emerging maxillary artery
  - ***Posteromedial***
    - Relations:
    - Mastoid process
    - Sternocleidomastoid
    - Posterior belly of digastric
    - Styloid apparatus
    - Internal carotid artery
    - Internal jugular vein
    - Last four cranial nerves
- ***Borders***
  - Anterior
  - Posterior
  - Medial

(TMJ: Temporomandibular joint)

**Flowchart 5.2:** Structures emerging from the parotid gland

***Structures emerging from the parotid gland***

- ***Apex***
  - Cervical branch of facial nerve
  - Anterior and posterior divisions of retromandibular vein
- ***Base***
  - Superficial temporal vessels
  - Auriculotemporal nerve
- ***Posteromedial surface***
  - Facial nerve
  - External carotid artery
- ***Anterior border***
  - Temporal branch of 7th nerve
  - Zygomatic branch of 7th nerve
  - Transverse facial vessels
  - Upper buccal branch of 7th nerve
  - Parotid duct
  - Lower buccal branch of 7th nerve
  - Marginal mandibular branch of 7th nerve
- ***Posterior border***
  - Posterior auricular vessels
  - Posterior auricular branch of facial nerve

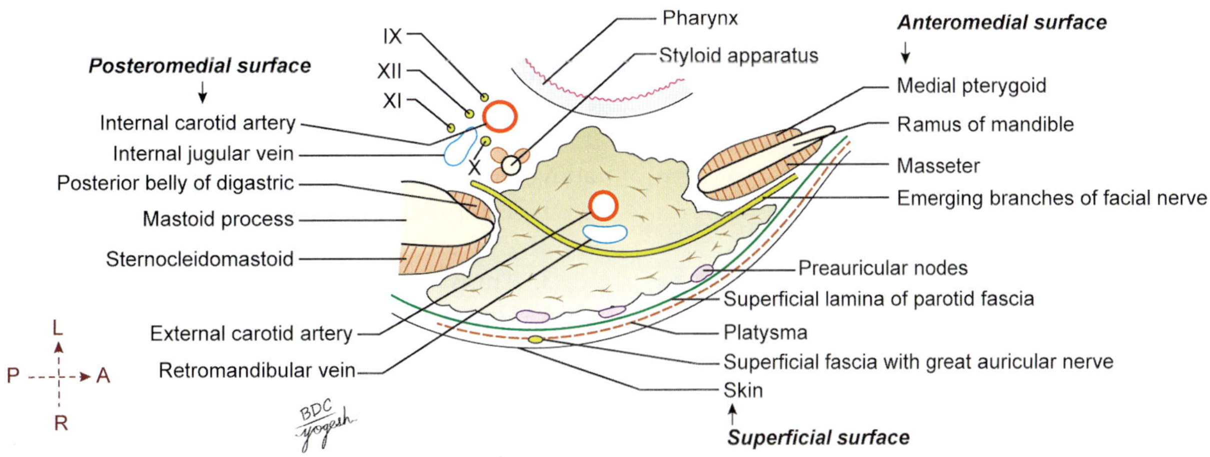


**Fig. 5.5:** Relations of the parotid gland

**Plate 5.1:** The structures emerging at the periphery of the parotid gland

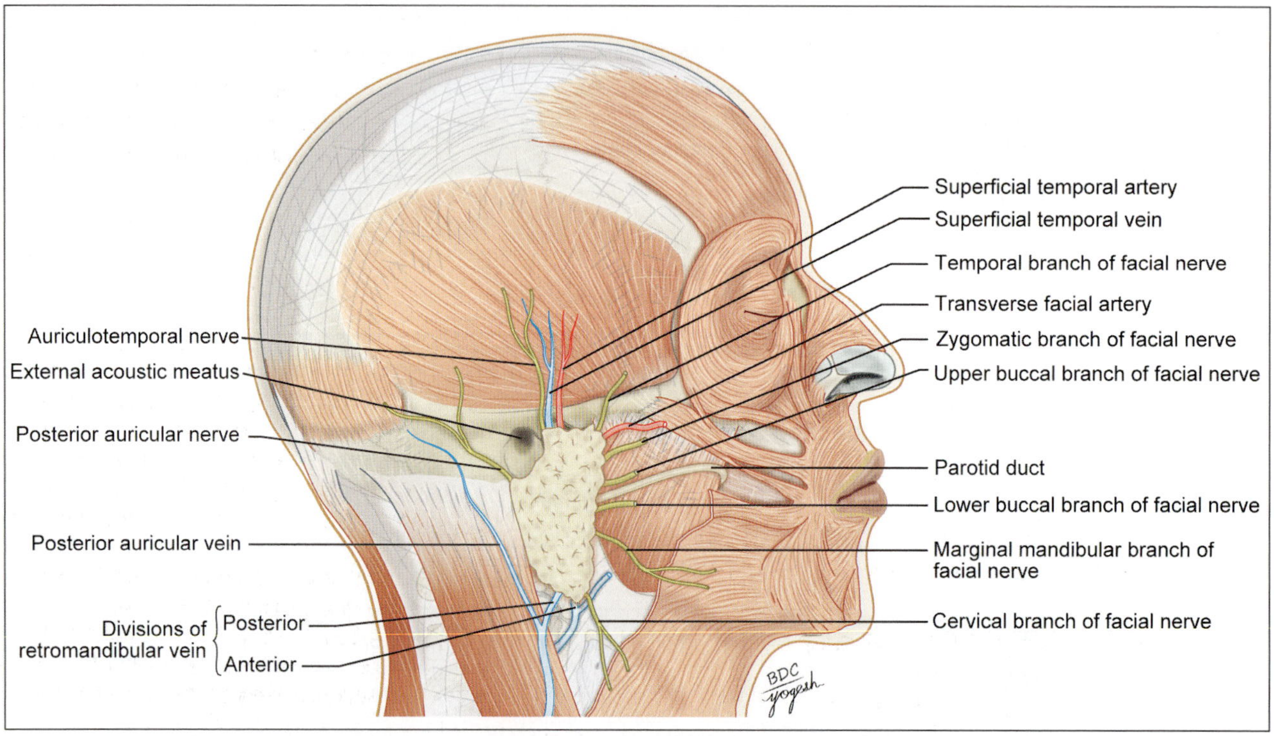


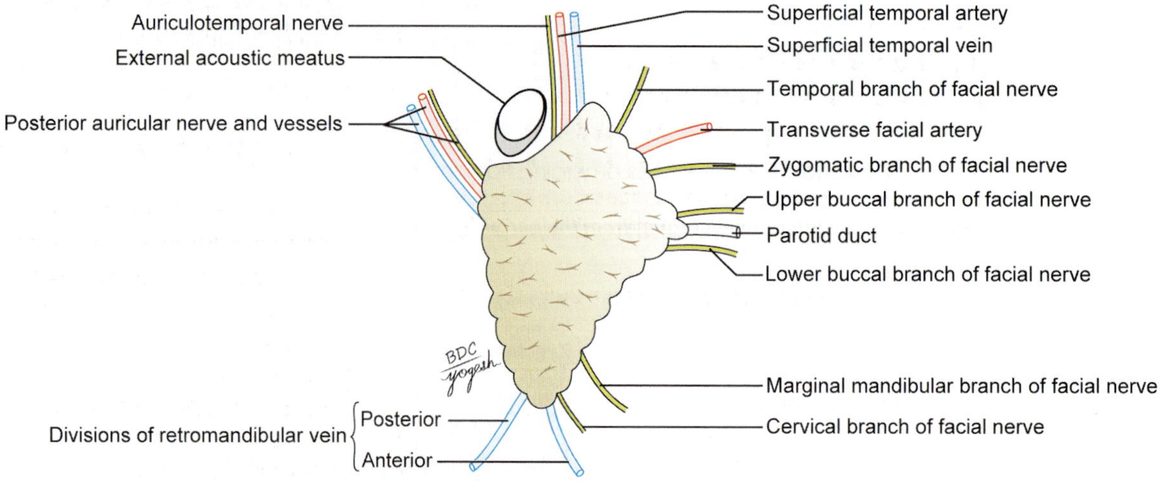


**Fig. 5.6:** Structures emerging at the periphery of the parotid gland

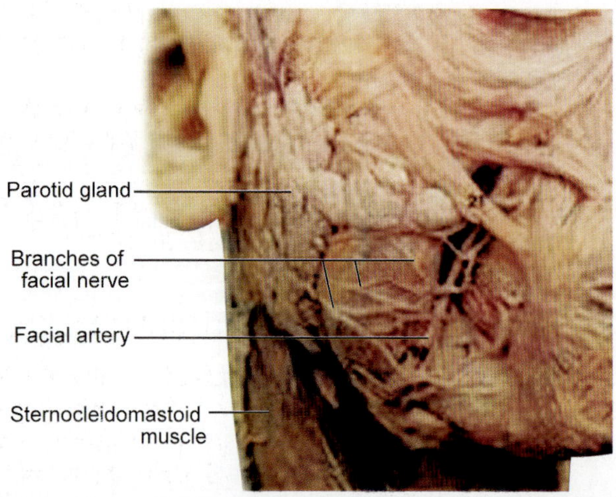


**Fig. 5.7:** Parotid gland

### *Anterior Border*

It separates the superficial surface from the anteromedial surface. It extends from the anterior part of the superior surface to the apex.

Structures emerging from the anterior border from above downward:

1. Temporal branch of facial nerve
2. Zygomatic branch of facial nerve
3. Transverse facial vessels
4. Upper buccal branch of facial nerve
5. Parotid duct
6. Lower buccal branch of facial nerve
7. Marginal mandibular branch of facial nerve.

In addition, the accessory parotid glands' facial process lies on the parotid duct close to this border.

### Posterior Border

It separates the superficial surface from the posteromedial surface. It overlaps the sternocleidomastoid.

Structures emerging deep to posterior border:
1. Posterior auricular vessels.
2. Posterior auricular branch of facial nerve.

### Medial Edge or Pharyngeal Border

It separates the anteromedial surface from the posteromedial surface. It is related to the lateral wall of the pharynx.

## Structures within the Parotid Gland

Three main structures are present within the parotid gland. From superficial to deep, they are as follows (Figs 5.8a to c, Flowchart 5.2):
1. Facial nerve and its branches
2. Retromandibular vein
3. External carotid artery.

### Facial Nerve

The facial nerve enters the posteromedial surface of the parotid gland, and runs forward through the gland crossing the retromandibular vein and the external carotid artery. Behind the neck of the mandible, the divides into two branches – temporofacial and cervicofacial. These form a plexus called *pes anserinus*, which gives 5 terminal branches, e.g. temporal, zygomatic, buccal, marginal mandibular and cervical which emerge along the anterior border and apex of the parotid gland (Fig. 5.8a).

### Arteries

The ***external carotid artery*** enters the gland through its posteromedial surface (Fig. 5.5c). The ***maxillary artery*** leaves the gland through its anteromedial surface. The ***superficial temporal artery*** gives transverse facial artery and emerges at the anterior part of the superior surface.

### Veins

The ***retromandibular vein*** is formed within the gland by the union of the ***superficial temporal*** and ***maxillary veins***. In the lower part of the gland, the vein divides into *anterior and posterior divisions* which emerge close to the apex (lower pole) of the gland (Fig. 5.5b).

## Accessory Processes of Parotid Gland

- Facial process—along parotid duct. It lies between zygomatic arch and the parotid duct.
- Pterygoid process—between mandibular ramus and medial pterygoid.
- Glenoid process—between external acoustic meatus and temporomandibular joint.
- Poststyloid process.

## Blood Supply

The parotid gland is supplied by the external carotid artery and its branches that arise within the gland. The veins drain into the external jugular vein and internal jugular vein.

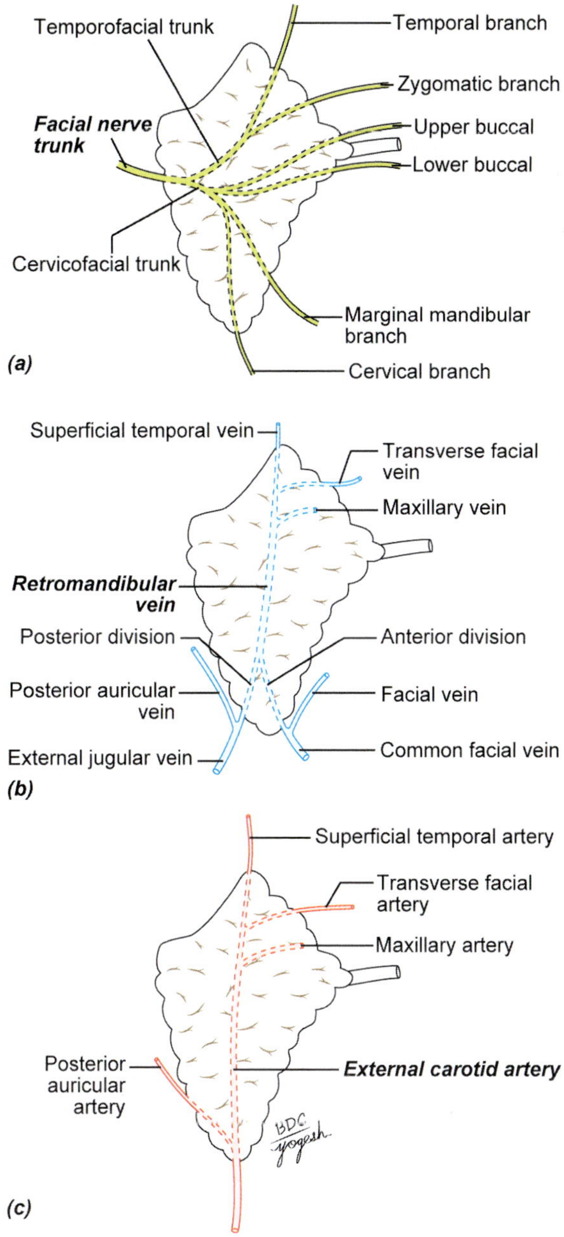


**Figs 5.8a to c:** The structures traversing the parotid gland: (a) Facial nerve (pes anserinus branching pattern), (b) retromandibular vein, and (c) external carotid artery

## Lymphatic Drainage

Lymph drains first to the parotid nodes and from there to the upper deep cervical nodes.

## Nerve Supply (Fig. 5.9, Flowchart 5.3)

1. ***Parasympathetic nerves*** are secretomotor. They reach the gland through the auriculotemporal nerve.

   The *preganglionic fibres* begin in the inferior salivatory nucleus; pass through the glossopharyngeal nerve, its tympanic branch, the tympanic plexus and the lesser petrosal nerve; and relay in the otic ganglion.

   The *postganglionic fibres* pass through the auriculotemporal nerve and reach the gland.
2. ***Sympathetic nerves*** are postganglionic, vasomotor, and are derived from the plexus around the middle

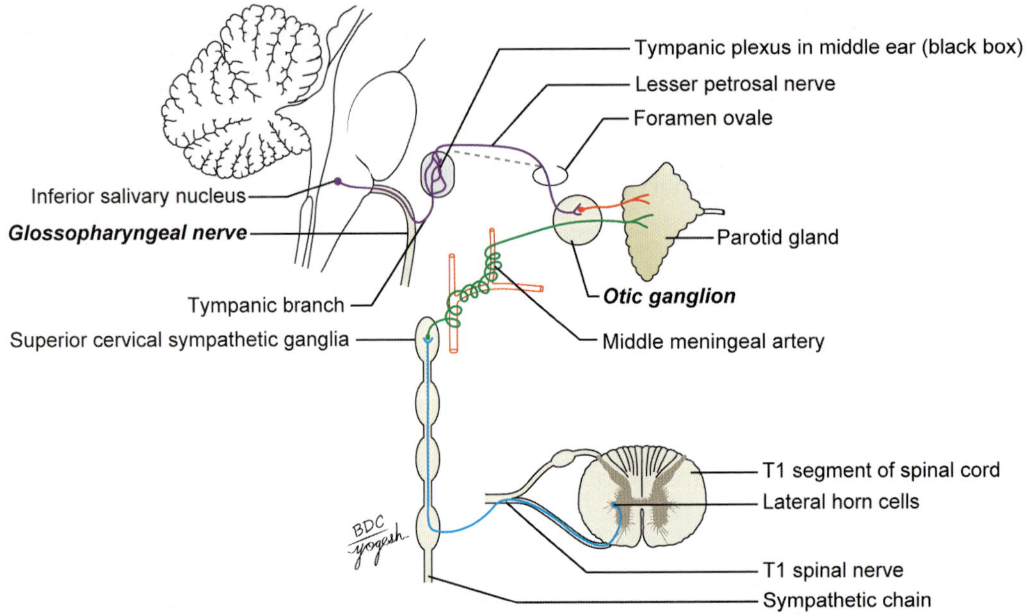


**Fig. 5.9:** Innervation of parotid gland (schematic representation, Purple line): Preganglionic parasympathetic fibres, Red line: Postganglionic parasympathetic fibres, Blue line: Preganglionic sympathetic fibres, Green line: Postganglionic sympathetic fibres, *Note*: Lesser petrosal nerve enter the middle cranial fossa and exit through the foramen ovale. Middle cranial fossa shown by grey dotted line

**Flowchart 5.3:** Nerve supply of parotid gland

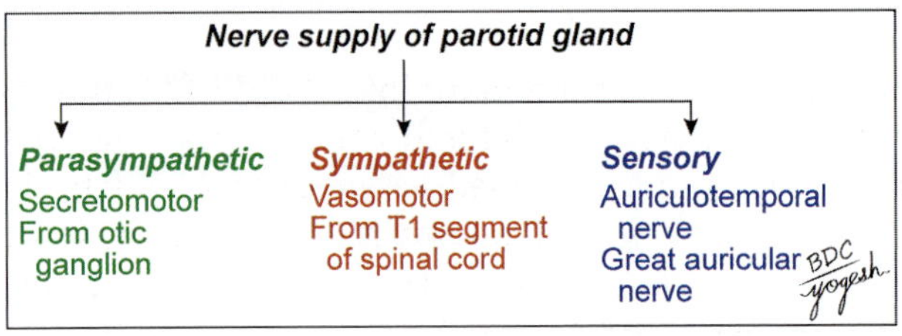


meningeal artery. These fibres start from lateral horn of T1 segment of spinal cord. These synapse in superior cervical ganglion. Postganglionic fibres travel along branches of external carotid, maxillary arteries and their branches, e.g. middle meningeal artery.

3. *Sensory nerves* to the gland come from the auriculotemporal nerve, but the parotid fascia is innervated by the sensory fibres of the great auricular nerve (C2, C3).

## PAROTID LYMPH NODES

The parotid lymph nodes lie partly in the superficial fascia and partly deep to the deep fascia over the parotid gland. They drain:

1. Temple
2. Side of the scalp
3. Lateral surface of the auricle
4. External acoustic meatus
5. Middle ear
6. Parotid gland
7. Upper part of the cheek
8. Parts of the eyelids and orbit.

Efferents from these nodes pass to the upper group of deep cervical nodes.

## PAROTID DUCT/STENSON'S DUCT

(Figs 5.10 and 5.11, Flowchart 5.4)

Parotid or Stenson's duct is thick-walled and is about 5 cm long [Nicolaus Steno, Dutch Anatomist, 1638–86].

### Course

It emerges from the middle of the anterior border of the gland. It runs forwards and slightly downwards on the masseter.

After emerging from the parotid gland, the duct runs forward on the masseter, between the upper and lower buccal nerves. Then, it runs medially along the anterior border of masseter and pierces:

1. Buccal pad of fat
2. Buccopharyngeal fascia
3. Buccinator
4. Oral mucosa.

Before piercing the mucosa, the duct runs obliquely forward and opens into the vestibule of mouth opposite the crown of upper 2nd molar tooth.

*Note*: This typical course of the duct prevents air entry in the duct during blowing of mouth (as in trumpet blowing).

**Flowchart 5.4:** Parotid duct

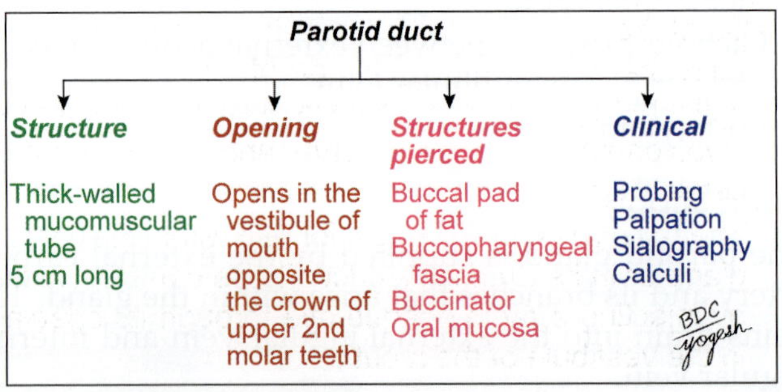

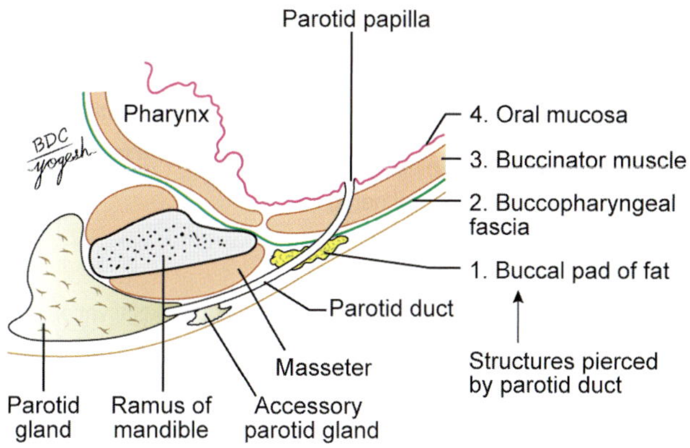


**Fig. 5.10:** Structures pierced by parotid duct

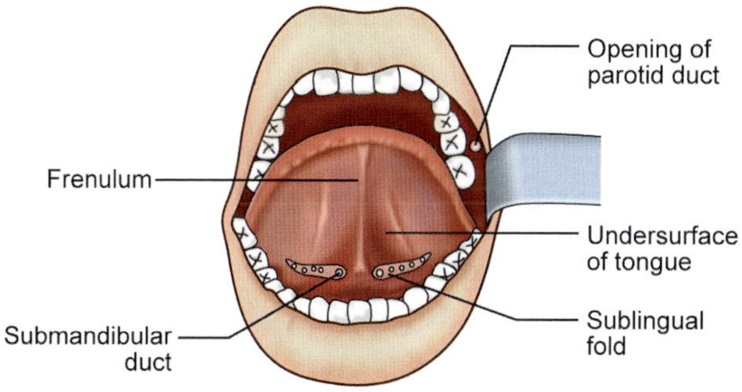


**Fig. 5.11:** Openings of salivary glands

***Competency:***
**AN28.10** Explain the anatomical basis of Frey's syndrome.

## CLINICAL ANATOMY

- Probing the parotid duct is difficult due to its tortuous course.
- ***Palpation of parotid duct:*** The parotid duct can be rolled up and down against the tense-masseter on clinching of teeth. The duct lies about one fingerbreadth below the zygomatic arch.
- ***Parotid sialography*** is a radiological visualisation of the parotid duct and its tributaries by injecting radio-opaque into the parotid duct through its oral opening.
- A *parotid abscess* may be caused by spread of infection from the opening of parotid duct in the mouth cavity (Fig. 5.12).
- ***Parotid abscess*** can be drained by horizontal incision/making many small holes known as Hilton's method (Fig. 5.12) below the angle of mandible.
- **Parotidectomy** is the removal of the parotid gland.
- ***Mixed parotid tumour*** is a slow growing lobulated painless tumour without any involvement of the facial nerve. Malignant change of such a tumour is indicated by pain, rapid growth, fixity with hardness, involvement of the facial nerve, and enlargement of cervical lymph nodes.
- The ***parotid calculi*** may get formed within the parotid gland or in its Stenson's duct. These can be located by injecting a radio-opaque dye through its opening in the vestibule of the mouth.

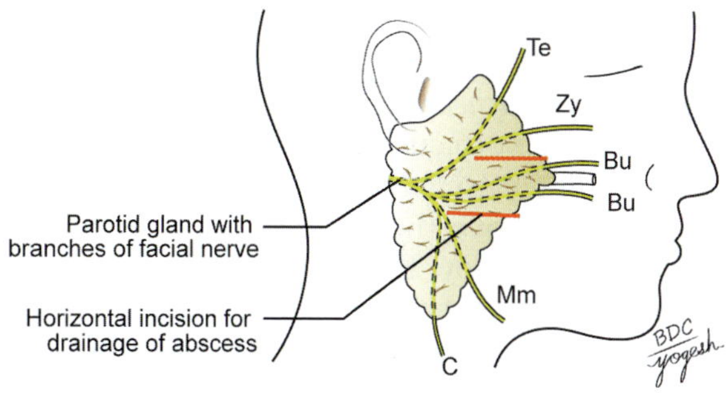


**Fig. 5.12:** Horizontal incision for draining parotid abscess. Branches of facial nerve also seen. Te—temporal; Zy—zygomatic, Bu—upper and lower buccal; Mm—marginal mandibular; C—cervical

## FACIAL NERVE: EXTRACRANIAL COURSE

It is the nerve of the 2nd branchial arch. The facial nerve leaves the skull by passing through the stylomastoid foramen.

**In its extracranial course,** the facial nerve crosses the lateral side of the base of the styloid process. Then the nerve enters the posteromedial surface of the parotid gland, runs forwards through the gland crossing the retromandibular vein and the external carotid artery.

### Branches

Behind the neck of the mandible, the divides into two branches – temporofacial and cervicofacial (Fig. 5.8a). These form a plexus called *pes anserinus,* which gives 5 terminal branches, e.g. temporal, zygomatic, buccal, marginal mandibular and cervical which emerge along the anterior border and apex of the parotid gland.

#### *Branches of Facial Nerve at its Exit from the Stylomastoid Foramen*

1. Communicating branches with adjacent cranial and spinal nerves.
2. ***Posterior auricular nerve*** arises just below the stylomastoid foramen. It ascends between the mastoid process and the external acoustic meatus, and supplies:
   a. Auricularis posterior
   b. Occipitalis
   c. Intrinsic muscles on the back of auricle.
3. ***Digastric branch*** arises close to the previous nerve. It is short and supplies the posterior belly of the digastric.
4. ***Stylohyoid branch*** arises with the digastric branch, is long and supplies the stylohyoid muscle.

#### *Terminal Branches*

1. ***Temporal branches*** cross the zygomatic arch and supply:
   a. Auricularis anterior
   b. Auricularis superior
   c. Intrinsic muscles on the lateral side of the ear
   d. Frontalis

e. Orbicularis oculi
f. Corrugator supercilii.

2. ***Zygomatic** branches* run across the zygomatic bone and supply the orbicularis oculi.
3. ***Buccal** branches* are two in number. The upper buccal branch runs above the parotid duct and the lower buccal branch below the duct. They supply muscles in that vicinity, especially the buccinator.
4. ***Marginal mandibular** branch* runs below the angle of the mandible deep to the platysma. It crosses the body of the mandible and supplies muscles of the lower lip and chin.
5. ***Cervical** branch* emerges from the apex of the parotid gland and runs downwards and forwards in the neck to supply the platysma.

## CLINICAL ANATOMY

- ***Bell's palsy:*** Sudden paralysis of facial nerve at the stylomastoid foramen, results in asymmetry of corner of mouth, inability to close the eye, disappearance of nasolabial fold and loss of wrinkling of skin of forehead on the same side.
- ***Patey's faciovenous plane:*** It is a plane that divides the parotid glands into large superficial and small deep parts or lobes. Isthmus is a part of glandular tissue present in the Patey's faciovenous plane and it connects superficial and deep parts. This plane is traversed by facial nerve and its branches and retromandibular vein. In the surgical removal of parotid gland, care should be taken along this plane (Fig. 5.13).

## FREY'S SYNDROME

It is also called auriculotemporal syndrome, Frey-Baillarger syndrome [Lucja Frey, Polish neurologist, 1889–1942], or Dupuy's syndrome (Fig. 5.14).

It is a rare neurological disorder resulting in gustatory sweating.

*Cause:* Damage to auriculotemporal and great auricular nerves in the parotid gland injuries or surgeries.

*Anatomical basis:* Parasympathetic fibres of auriculotemporal nerve stimulate the parotid gland to enhance its secretion and sympathetic fibres of the great auricular nerve stimulate sweat glands in the facial skin. After damage to both nerves, during regeneration, the parasympathetic fibres of auriculotemporal nerve grow and join the sympathetic fibres of the great auricular nerve. This results in sweating rather than salivation during eating. Hence, it is called *gustatory sweating* or *Frey's syndrome.*

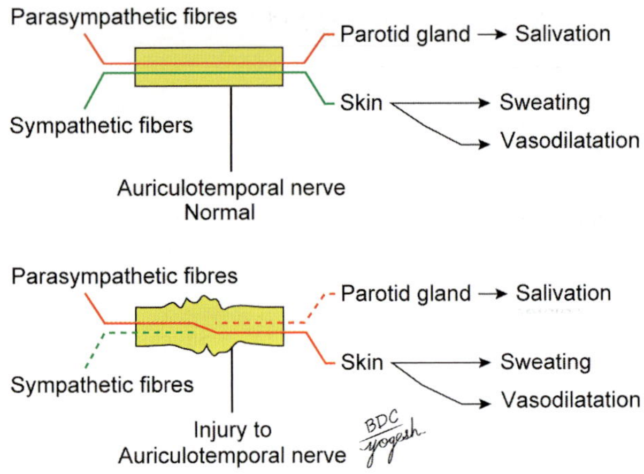


**Fig. 5.14:** Anatomical basis of Frey's syndrome

### Histology of Parotid Gland

1. It is a large serous gland. It is a compound tubuloacinar gland. It is covered by thick capsule and divided into number of lobes and lobules (Plate 5.2).
2. *Acini*: Parotid gland consists of serous acini. These acini are surrounded by myoepithelial cells.
3. *Ducts*: Parotid gland has number of intralobular (intercalated and striated) ducts and interlobular and lobar ducts. Intercalated ducts are lined by low cuboidal epithelium. Striated ducts are lined by simple columnar epithelium with basal infoldings. These ducts are large and conspicuous in parotid gland. Other ducts are lined by stratified cuboidal to stratified squamous epithelium.
4. Large amounts of adipose tissue often occur in the parotid gland; this is one of its distinguishing features.

### Development

The parotid gland is ectodermal in origin. It develops from the buccal epithelium just lateral to the angle of mouth. The outgrowth branches repeatedly to form the duct system and acini. The mesoderm forms the intervening connective tissue septa.

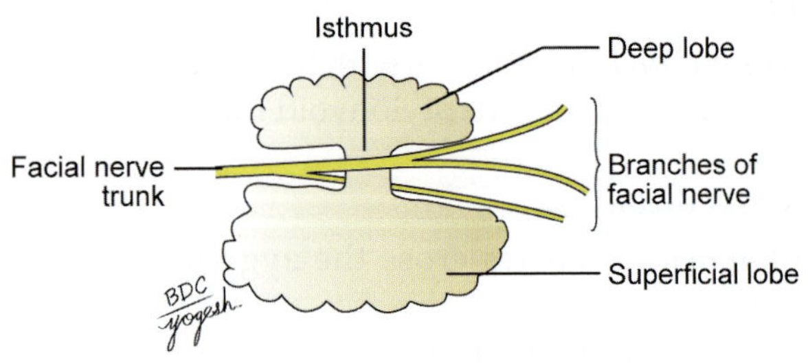


**Fig. 5.13:** Patey's faciovenous (neurovenous) plane in the parotid gland (Transverse section through the parotid gland, retromandibular vein is not shown for clarity)

## DISSECTION

Carefully cut through the fascial covering of the parotid gland from the zygomatic arch above to the angle of mandible below. While removing tough fascia, dissect the structures emerging at the periphery of the gland.

Trace the duct of the parotid gland anteriorly till the buccinator muscle. Trace one or more of the branches of facial nerve till its trunk in the posterior part of the gland. The trunk can be followed till the stylomastoid foramen. Trace its posterior auricular branch. Trace the course of

**Plate 5.2:** Histology of parotid gland

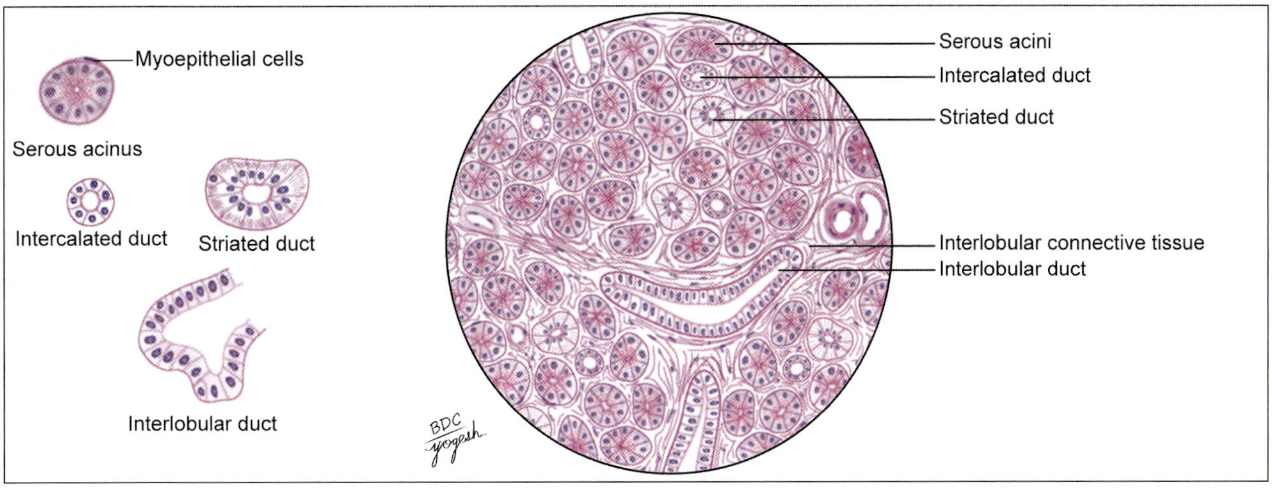


retromandibular vein and external carotid artery in the gland, removing the glands in pieces. Clean the facial nerve already dissected. Study the extracranial course of facial nerve.

VIDEO

**Video 3.5 Parotid Gland**

### *Facts to Remember*

- Facial nerve courses through the parotid gland, *without supplying any structure in it*.
- Skin over the parotid gland is supplied by great auricular nerve C2, C3.
- The deepest structure in the substance of parotid gland is the external carotid artery.
- Otic ganglion is the only parasympathetic ganglion with four roots, including a motor root.
- Facial nerve divides into temporofacial and cervicofacial branches. The former gives temporal and zygomatic branches. The latter gives buccal, marginal mandibular and cervical branches.
- Parotid gland is the largest salivary gland in the body.
- Mumps is the commonest infection of the parotid gland.
- Parotid duct opens into the vestibule of mouth opposite the crown of upper 2nd molar tooth.
- Hilton's horizontal incision prevents injury to the facial nerve in parotid surgeries.

### BDC's Anatomy *e*-book

1. Extent of parotid gland
2. Further reading
3. Viva voce questions

Chapter

# 6

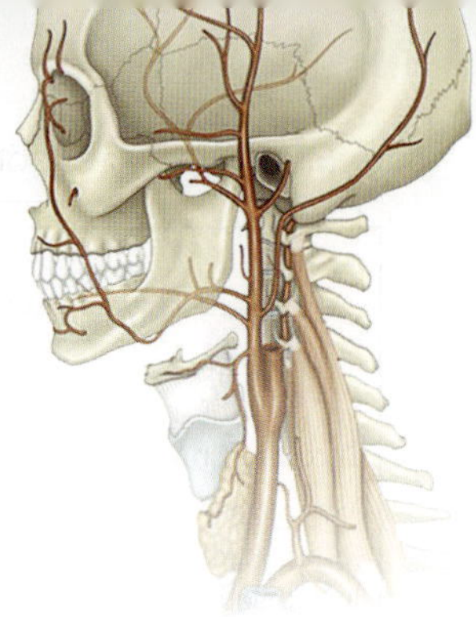

# Temporal and Infratemporal Regions

Temporal and infratemporal regions include the following:

1. Muscles of mastication
2. Mandibular branch of trigeminal nerve
3. Temporomandibular joint (TMJ) that allows movements during speech and mastication
4. Otic ganglion
5. Maxillary artery.

***Competency:***
**AN33.1** Describe and demonstrate extent, boundaries and contents of temporal and infratemporal fossae.

## TEMPORAL FOSSA

In order to understand these regions, the osteology of the temporal fossa and the infratemporal fossa should be studied. The *temporal fossa* lies on the side of the skull and is bounded by the superior temporal line and the zygomatic arch.

### Boundaries (Plate 6.1)

*Anterior:* Zygomatic and frontal bones
*Posterior:* Inferior temporal line and supramastoid crest
*Superior:* Superior temporal line
*Inferior:* Zygomatic arch (zygoma)
*Inferomedial:* It communicates with infratemporal fossa
*Floor:* Parts of frontal, parietal, temporal and greater wing of sphenoid
*Lateral:* Temporal fascia

### Contents

1. Temporalis muscle
2. Middle temporal artery (branch of superficial temporal artery)
3. Zygomaticotemporal nerve and artery
4. Deep temporal nerves for supplying temporalis muscle
5. Deep temporal artery, branch of maxillary artery

## INFRATEMPORAL FOSSA

It is an irregular space under the base of the skull, below the level of zygomatic arch.

### Boundaries (Plate 6.2)

*Anterior:* Posterior surface of body of maxilla
*Posterior:* Styloid process
*Roof:* Infratemporal surface of greater wing of sphenoid
*Medial:* Lateral pterygoid plate and pyramidal process of palatine bone, pterygomaxillary fissure with mandibular canal.
*Lateral:* Ramus of mandible.

### Communications (Fig. 6.1)

The communications of the infratemporal fossa are as follows:

*Superiorly:*

1. Foramen ovale—to communicate with cranial cavity
2. Foramen spinosum—to communicate with cranial cavity
3. Gap deep to the zygomatic arch—to communicate with temporal fossa.

*Inferiorly:* Opens and continues with parapharyngeal space
*Anteriorly:* Inferior orbital fissure—to communicate with orbit
*Medially:* Pterygomaxillary fissure—to communicate with pterygopalatine fossa

### Major Contents

1. *Muscles:* Lateral pterygoid, medial pterygoid and tendon of temporalis
2. *Blood vessels:* Maxillary artery, maxillary vein and pterygoid venous plexus
3. *Nerves:*
   - Mandibular nerve and its branches
   - Chorda tympani nerve (branch of facial nerve)
   - Otic ganglion
4. Sphenomandibular ligament.

**Plate 6.1:** Boundaries of temporal fossa

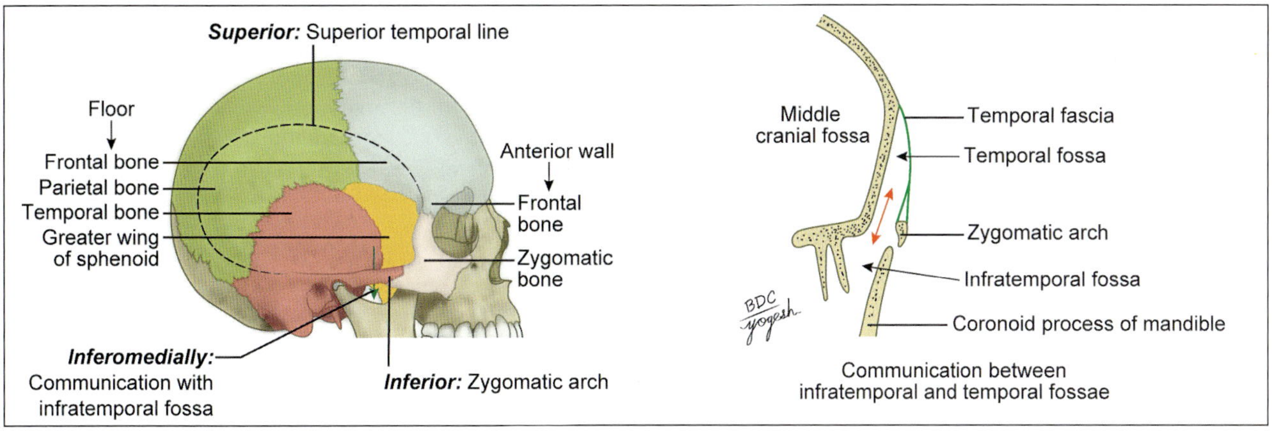


**Plate 6.2:** Location of infratemporal fossa (inferior view)

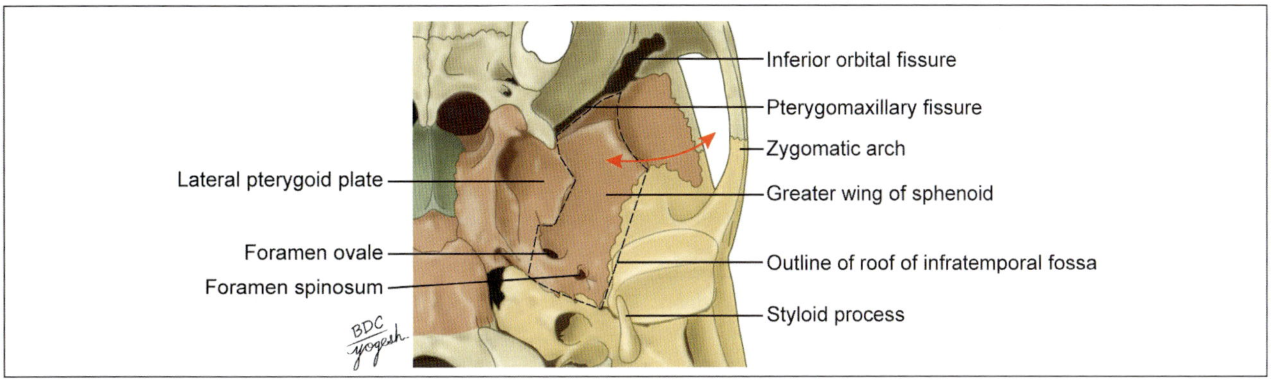


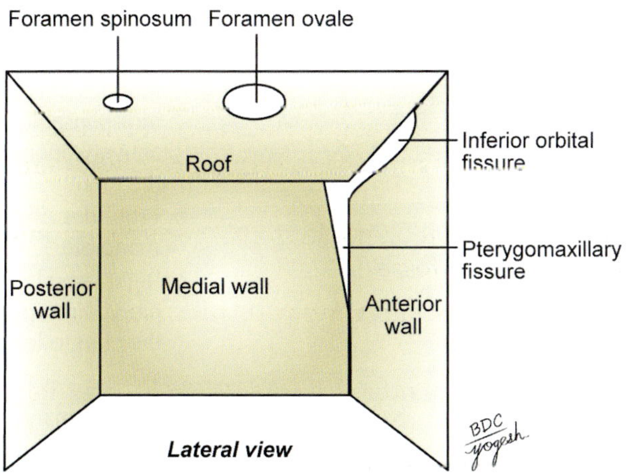


**Fig. 6.1:** Communications of infratemporal fossa

## TEMPORAL FASCIA

The temporal fascia is a thick aponeurotic sheet that roofs over the temporal fossa and covers the temporalis muscle. The fascia is extremely dense. In some species (e.g. tortoise), the temporal fascia is replaced by bone.

### *Attachments*

1. *Superiorly*, the fascia is single layered and is attached to the superior temporal line.
2. *Inferiorly*, it splits into two layers which are attached to the inner and outer lips of the upper border of the zygomatic arch. The small gap between the two layers contains fat, a branch from the superficial temporal artery and the zygomaticotemporal nerve.

### *Surfaces*

1. The *superficial surface* of the temporal fascia receives an expansion from the epicranial aponeurosis. This surface gives origin to the auricularis anterior and superior and is related to the superficial temporal vessels, the auriculotemporal nerve, and the temporal branch of the facial nerve.
2. The *deep surface* of the temporal fascia gives origin to some fibres of the temporalis muscle.

*Competency:*
**AN33.2** Describe and demonstrate attachments, direction of fibres, nerve supply and actions of muscles of mastication.

## MUSCLES OF MASTICATION

The principal muscles of the mastication are as follows (Table 6.1, Plate 6.3, Figs 6.2 to 6.5):

1. Masseter
2. Temporalis
3. Lateral pterygoid
4. Medial pterygoid.

**TABLE 6.1: Major muscles of mastication** (Figs 6.2 to 6.5)

| *Muscle* | *Origin* | *Fibres* | *Insertion* | *Nerve supply* | *Actions* |
|---|---|---|---|---|---|
| 1. **Masseter** Quadrilateral, covers lateral surface of ramus of mandible has three layers (Fig. 6.3) | **Zygomatic arch maxillary process of the zygomatic bone**<br>a. *Superficial layer* (largest): From anterior 2/3rd of lower border of zygomatic arch and adjoining zygomatic process of maxilla<br>b. *Middle layer:* From lower border of posterior 1/3rd of zygomatic arch<br>c. *Deep layer:* From deep surface of zygomatic arch | a. Superficial fibres pass downwards and backwards at 45°<br>b. Middle fibres pass vertically downwards<br>c. Deep fibres pass vertically downwards | **Lateral surface of ramus of mandible**<br>a. *Superficial layer* into the lower part of the lateral surface of ramus of mandible<br>b. *Middle layer* into the central part of ramus of the mandible<br>c. *Deep layer* into rest of the ramus of the mandible | Masseteric nerve, a branch of anterior division of mandibular nerve | a. Elevates mandible to close the mouth to bite<br>b. Superficial fibres cause protrusion |
| 2. **Temporalis** Fan-shaped, fills the temporal fossa (Fig. 6.4) | a. **Temporal fossa**, excluding zygomatic bone<br>b. Temporal fascia | Anterior fibres run vertically, middle obliquely and posterior horizontally. All converge and pass through a gap deep to zygomatic arch | a. Margins and deep surface of **coronoid process**<br>b. Anterior border of **ramus of the mandible** | Two deep temporal branches from anterior division of mandibular nerve | a. Elevates mandible<br>b. Helps in side-to-side grinding movement<br>c. Posterior fibres retract the protruded mandible |
| 3. **Lateral pterygoid** Short, conical, has upper and lower heads (Fig. 6.5) | a. ***Upper head*** (small): From infratemporal surface and crest of greater wing of sphenoid bone<br>b. ***Lower head*** (larger): From lateral surface of lateral pterygoid plate. Origin is medial to insertion | Fibres run backwards and laterally and converge for insertion | a. **Pterygoid fovea** on the anterior surface of neck of mandible<br>b. Anterior margin of articular disc and capsule of temporomandibular joint. Insertion is posterolateral and at a slightly higher level than origin | A branch from anterior division of mandibular nerve | a. Depresses mandible to open mouth, with suprahyoid muscles. It is indispensable for actively opening the mouth<br>b. Protrudes mandible<br>c. Right lateral pterygoid turns the chin to left side |
| 4. **Medial pterygoid** Quadrilateral, has a small superficial and a large deep head (Fig. 6.5) | a. ***Superficial head*** (small slip): From tuberosity of maxilla and adjoining bone<br>b. ***Deep head*** (quite large): From medial surface of lateral pterygoid plate and adjoining process of palatine bone | Fibres run downwards, backwards and laterally. The two heads embrace part of the lower head of lateral pterygoid (Fig. 6.5) | Roughened area on the medial surface of angle and adjoining **ramus of mandible**, below and behind the mandibular foramen and mylohyoid groove | Nerve to medial pterygoid, branch of the main trunk of mandibular nerve | a. Elevates mandible<br>b. Helps protrude mandible<br>c. Right medial pterygoid with right lateral pterygoid turn the chin to left side as part of grinding movements |

[*Mnemonics: **Function of Lateral (La) vs. Medial (Me) pterygoid muscles:*** **"La"**: Jaw is open, so lateral pterygoid opens mouth. **"Me"**: Jaw is closed, so medial pterygoid closes the mouth]

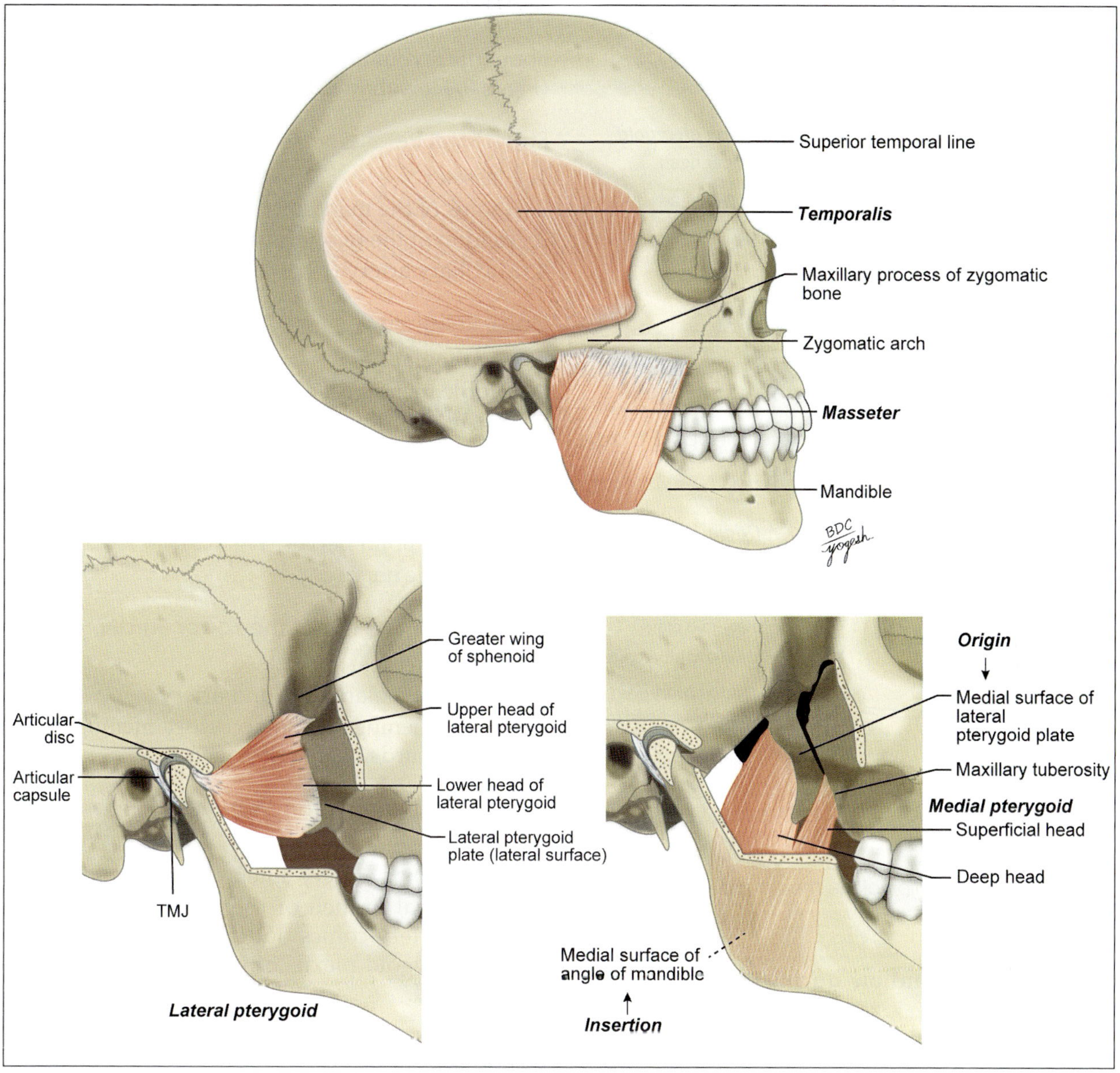


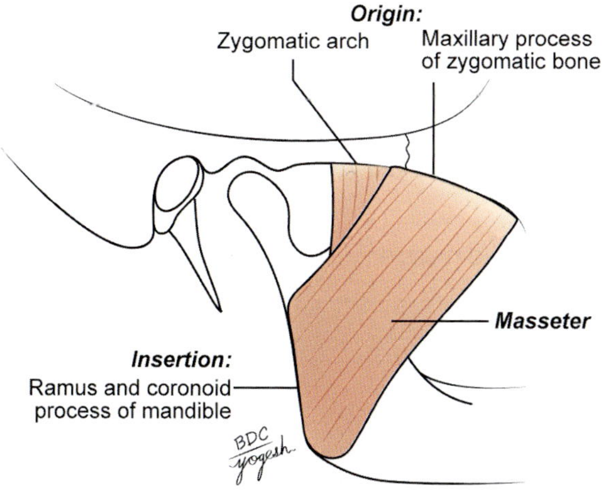


**Fig. 6.2:** Origin and insertion of the masseter muscle

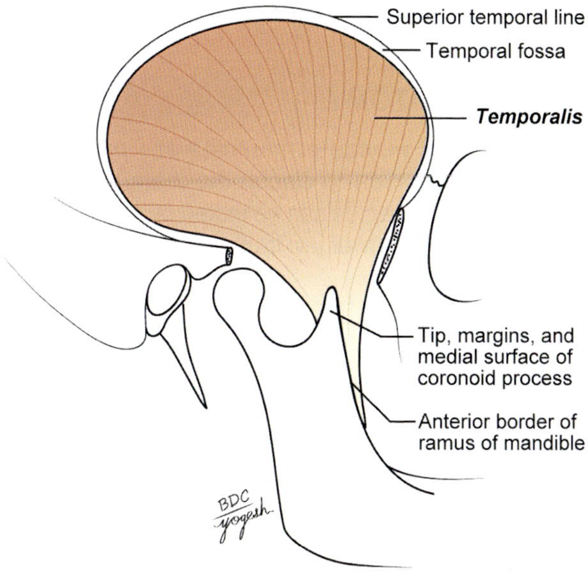


**Fig. 6.3:** Origin and insertion of the temporalis muscle

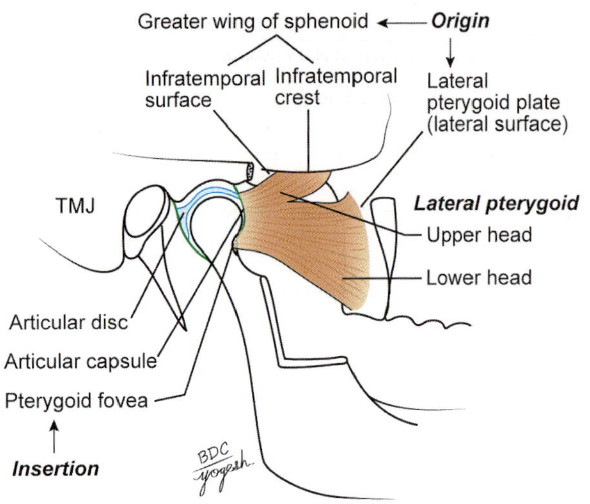


**Fig. 6.4:** Origin and insertion of the lateral pterygoid muscle (TMJ: Temporomandibular joint)

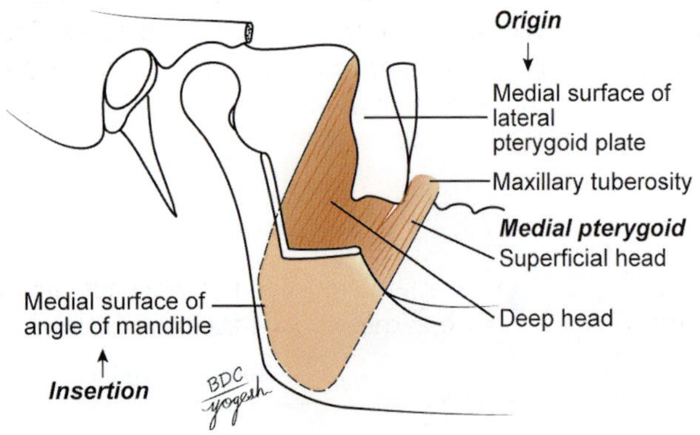


**Fig. 6.5:** Origin and insertion of the medial pterygoid muscle

### Peculiarities

1. They move the mandible during mastication and speech.
2. These develop from the mesoderm of the 1st branchial arch.
3. They are supplied by the mandibular nerve which is the nerve of the 1st arch.

## CLINICAL ANATOMY

Temporalis and masseter muscles are palpated by requesting the person to clench the teeth. Medial and lateral pterygoid muscles can be tested by requesting the person to move the lower jaw from one side to other side.

## RELATIONS OF LATERAL PTERYGOID

The lateral pterygoid may be regarded as the key muscle of this region because its relations provide a fair idea about the layout of structures in the infratemporal fossa (Fig. 6.6, Flowchart 6.1). The relations are as follows:

### Superficial Relations

1. Masseter
2. Ramus of the mandible
3. Tendon of the temporalis
4. Maxillary artery (Fig. 6.6).

### Deep Relations

1. Mandibular nerve
2. Middle meningeal artery (Fig. 6.6)
3. Sphenomandibular ligament
4. Deep head of the medial pterygoid

### Structures Emerging at the Upper Border

1. Deep temporal nerves (Fig. 6.6)
2. Masseteric nerve

### Structures Emerging at the Lower Border

1. Lingual nerve
2. Inferior alveolar nerve and artery
3. Middle meningeal and accessory meningeal arteries pass upwards deep to it (Fig. 6.6).

### Structures Passing through the Gap Between the Two Heads

1. The maxillary artery enters the gap
2. The buccal branch of the mandibular nerve with buccal artery comes out through the gap (Fig. 6.6). The pterygoid plexus of veins surrounds the lateral pterygoid.

## RELATIONS OF MEDIAL PTERYGOID

The superficial and deep heads of medial pterygoid enclose the lower head of lateral pterygoid muscle.

### Superficial Relations (Fig. 6.7)

The upper part of the muscle is separated from the lateral pterygoid muscle by:

1. Lateral pterygoid plate
2. Lingual nerve
3. Inferior alveolar nerve.

**Flowchart 6.1:** Relations of lateral pterygoid muscle

***Relations of lateral pterygoid muscle***

| *Superficial* | *Deep* | *Upper border* | *Lower border* | *Between two heads* |
|---|---|---|---|---|
| Masseter | Mandibular nerve | Deep temporal nerve | Lingual nerve | Maxillary artery |
| Ramus of mandible | Middle meningeal artery | Masseteric nerve | Inferior alveolar artery and nerve | Buccal branch of mandibular nerve |
| Tendon of temporalis | Sphenomandibular ligament | | Middle meningeal artery | |
| Maxillary artery | Deep head of medial pterygoid muscle | | Accessory meningeal artery | |

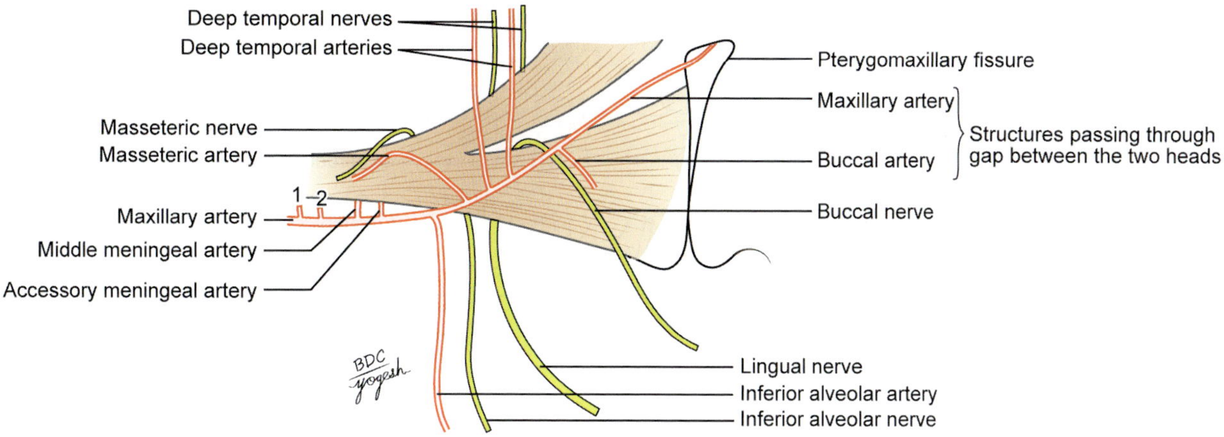


**Fig. 6.6:** Some relations of the lateral pterygoid muscle and branches of maxillary artery

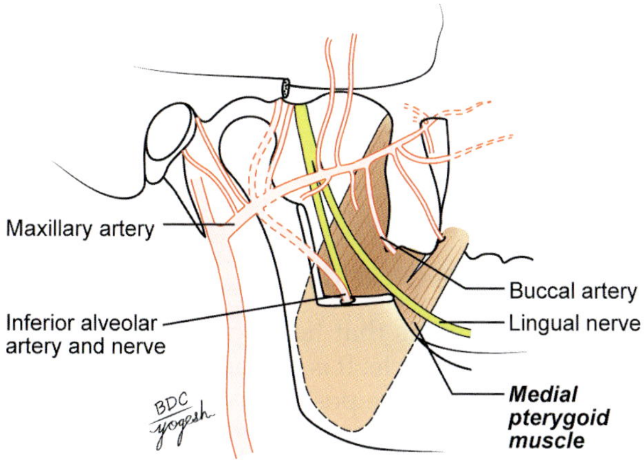


**Fig. 6.7:** Superficial relations of the medial pterygoid muscle

Lower down the muscle is separated from the ramus of the mandible by the lingual and inferior alveolar nerves, the maxillary artery, and the sphenomandibular ligament.

### Deep Relations

The relations are:
1. Tensor veli palatini
2. Superior constrictor of pharynx
3. Styloglossus
4. Stylopharyngeus attached to the styloid process.

### DISSECTION

Identify the masseter muscle extending from the zygomatic arch to the ramus of the mandible (Plate 6.3). Cut the zygomatic arch in front of and behind the attachment of masseter muscle and reflect it downwards. Divide the nerve and blood vessels to the muscle. Clean the ramus of mandible by stripping off the masseter muscle from it.

Give an oblique cut from the centre of mandibular notch to the lower end of anterior border of ramus of mandible. Turn this part of the bone including the insertion of temporalis muscle upwards. Strip the muscle from the skull and identify deep temporal nerves and vessels.

Make one cut through the neck of the mandible. Give another cut through the ramus at a distance of 4 cm from the neck. Remove the bone carefully in between these two cuts, avoiding injury to the underlying structures. The lateral pterygoid is exposed in the upper part and medial pterygoid in the lower part of the dissection (Fig. 6.5).

## MAXILLARY ARTERY

This is the larger terminal branch of the external carotid artery, given off behind the neck of the mandible.

### Course and Relations

The maxillary artery is divided into three parts (Fig. 6.8, Flowchart 6.2 and Table 6.2).

1. **First (mandibular) part** runs horizontally forwards, first between the neck of the mandible and the sphenomandibular ligament, below the auriculotemporal nerve, and then along the lower border of the lateral pterygoid.
2. **Second (pterygoid) part** runs upwards and forwards superficial to the lower head of the lateral pterygoid.
3. **Third (pterygopalatine) part** passes between the two heads of the lateral pterygoid and through the pterygomaxillary fissure, to enter the pterygopalatine fossa.

**Flowchart 6.2:** Maxillary artery

***Maxillary artery***
Divided into 3 parts by lateral pterygoid

- ***Beginning and termination***
  - Terminal branch of ECA
  - Begins at neck of mandible
  - Continues as sphenopalatine artery
- ***Branches***
  - ***1st part***: Deep auricular, Anterior tympanic, Middle meningeal, Accessory meningeal, Inferior alveolar
  - ***2nd part***: Masseteric, Deep temporal, Pterygoid, Buccal
  - ***3rd part***: Posterior superior alveolar, Infraorbital, Greater palatine, Pharyngeal, Artery to pterygoid canal, Sphenopalatine

BDC yogesh

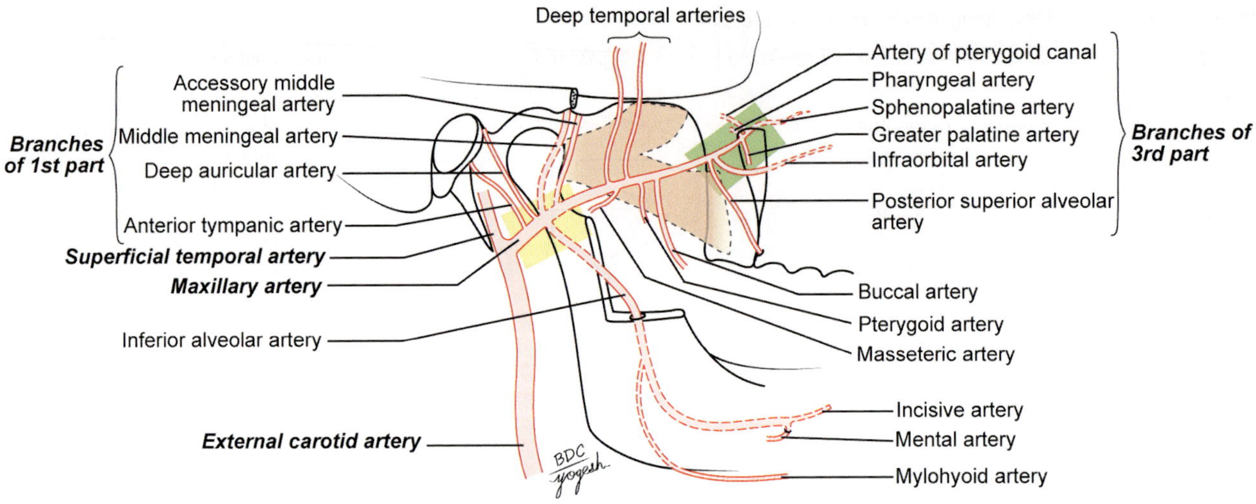


**Fig. 6.8:** Branches of three parts of the maxillary artery

### Branches

*From the first part*
1. Deep auricular
2. Anterior tympanic
3. Middle meningeal
4. Accessory meningeal
5. Inferior alveolar.

*From the second part*
1. Masseteric
2. Deep temporal
3. Pterygoid
4. Buccal.

*From third part*
1. Posterior superior alveolar
2. Infraorbital
3. Greater palatine
4. Pharyngeal
5. Artery to pterygoid canal
6. Sphenopalatine (terminal branch or continuation).

### CLINICAL ANATOMY

- The anterior branch of middle meningeal artery is likely to be injured at the pterion in roadside accidents. It leads to ***extradural haemorrhage*** (*see* Fig. 1.9). The clot must be sucked out at the earliest, otherwise it may compress the motor area of brain.
- Bleeding from lower teeth is from branches of inferior alveolar artery (1st part of maxillary artery) and from upper teeth is from branches of 3rd part of maxillary artery. These are posterior-superior alveolar and infraorbital arteries.
- Sphenopalatine is the terminal branch of 3rd part of maxillary artery. It anastomoses with neighbouring vessels to form large capillary plexus called ***Kiesselbach's plexus*** at the anteroinferior angle of the nasal septum. It is a common site of bleeding from nose or ***epistaxis*** and is known as ***Little's area***. So sphenopalatine artery is called '***the artery of epistaxis***'.

***Competency:***
**AN33.4** Explain the clinical significance of pterygoid venous plexus.

## PTERYGOID PLEXUS OF VEINS

It is a plexus of veins that lies around and within the lateral pterygoid muscle. It is drained into the maxillary vein which begins at the posterior end of the plexus.

### Communications

1. With the inferior ophthalmic vein through the inferior orbital fissure.
2. With the cavernous sinus through the emissary veins.
3. With the facial vein through the deep facial vein.

### Significance

1. *Blood pump*: The contraction of the lateral pterygoid muscle pumps the blood from the pterygoid plexus of veins into cavernous sinus and maxillary vein.
2. *Spread of infection or emboli*: The infection or thromboemboli coming from facial vein or inferior ophthalmic vein may spread to cavernous sinus through the communications with pterygoid plexus of veins.

### DISSECTION

External carotid artery divides into its two terminal branches, maxillary and superficial temporal on the anteromedial surface of the parotid gland. The maxillary artery, appears in this region. Identify some of its branches. Most important to be identified is the middle meningeal artery. Learn its course and branches given in *see* Chapter 12. Accompanying these branches are the veins and pterygoid venous plexus and the superficial content of infratemporal fossa. Remove these veins. Try to see its communication with the cavernous sinus and facial vein.

**TABLE 6.2: Branches of maxillary artery** (Figs 6.6 and 6.8)

| *Branches* | *Foramina transmitting* | *Enters in* | *Distribution* |
|---|---|---|---|
| **A. Of first part** | | | |
| 1. Deep auricular | Enters the external acoustic meatus through foramina at its floor | External acoustic meatus | Skin of external acoustic meatus, and outer surface of tympanic membrane |
| 2. Anterior tympanic | Petrotympanic fissure | Tympanic cavity | Inner surface of tympanic membrane |
| 3. Middle meningeal | Foramen spinosum | Middle cranial fossa | Supplies more of bone and less of meninges; also 5th and 7th nerves, middle ear and tensor tympani |
| 4. Accessory meningeal | Foramen ovale | Middle cranial fossa | Main distribution is extracranial to pterygoids |
| 5. Inferior alveolar | Mandibular foramen | Mandibular canal | Lower 8 teeth and mylohyoid muscle |
| **B. Of second part** | | | |
| 1. Masseteric | — | — | Masseter |
| 2. Deep temporal | — | — | Temporalis (two branches) |
| 3. Pterygoid | — | — | Lateral and medial pterygoids |
| 4. Buccal | — | — | Skin of the cheek |
| **C. Of third part** | | | |
| 1. Posterior superior alveolar | Alveolar canals in body of maxilla | Body of maxilla | Upper molar and premolar teeth and gums; maxillary sinus |
| 2. Infraorbital | Inferior orbital fissure | Inferior orbital groove or canal | Lower orbital muscles; lacrimal sac; maxillary sinus; upper incisor and canine teeth |
| 3. Greater palatine | Greater palatine canal | Greater palatine canal to hard palate | Soft palate; tonsil; palatine glands and mucosa of upper gums |
| 4. Pharyngeal | Pharyngeal (palatinovaginal) canal | Nasopharynx | Roof of nose and pharynx; auditory tube; sphenoidal sinus |
| 5. Artery of pterygoid canal | Pterygoid canal | Pterygoid canal | Auditory tube; upper pharynx and middle ear |
| 6. Sphenopalatine (terminal part) | Sphenopalatine foramen | Nasal cavity | Lateral and medial walls of nose and various air sinuses (artery of epistaxis) |

*Note:* ***Details of branches of the maxillary artery***

1. ***Deep auricular artery*** supplies the external acoustic meatus, the tympanic membrane and the temporomandibular joint.
2. ***Anterior tympanic*** **branch** supplies the middle ear including the medial surface of the tympanic membrane.
3. ***Middle meningeal artery*** lies between lateral pterygoid and sphenomandibular ligaments, then between two roots of auriculotemporal nerve, enters the skull through foramen spinosum to reach middle cranial fossa. It divides into a large frontal branch which courses towards the *pterion* and a smaller parietal branch.
4. ***Accessory meningeal artery*** enters the cranial cavity through the foramen ovale. Apart from the meninges, it supplies structures in the infratemporal fossa.
5. ***Inferior alveolar artery*** runs downwards and forwards medial to the ramus of the mandible to reach the mandibular foramen. Passing through this foramen, the artery enters the mandibular canal (within the body of the mandible) in which it runs downwards and then forwards. Before entering the mandibular canal, the artery gives off a ***lingual branch*** to the tongue; and a ***mylohyoid branch*** that descends in the mylohyoid groove (on the medial aspect of the mandible) and runs forwards above the mylohyoid muscle. Within the mandibular canal, the artery gives branches to the mandible and to the roots of each tooth attached to the bone. It also gives off a ***mental branch*** that passes through the mental foramen to supply the chin.
6. ***Posterior superior alveolar artery*** arises just before the maxillary artery enters the pterygomaxillary fissure. It descends on the posterior surface of the maxilla and gives branches that enter canals in the bone to supply the molar and premolar teeth and the maxillary air sinus.
7. ***Infraorbital artery*** also arises just before the maxillary artery enters the pterygomaxillary fissure. It enters the orbit through the *inferior orbital fissure*. It then runs forwards in relation to the floor of the orbit, first in the infraorbital groove and then in the infraorbital canal to emerge on the face through the infraorbital foramen. It gives off some ***orbital branches***, for structures in the orbit; ***middle superior alveolar branch*** for premolar teeth and the ***anterior superior alveolar*** **branches** that enter apertures in the maxilla to reach the incisor and canine teeth attached to the bone.

   After emerging on the face, the infraorbital artery gives branches to the lacrimal sac, the nose and the upper lip.
8. ***Greater palatine artery*** runs downwards in the greater palatine canal to emerge on the posterolateral part of the hard palate through the greater palatine foramen. It then runs forwards near the lateral margin of the palate to reach the incisive canal (near the midline) through which some terminal branches enter the nasal cavity. Branches of the artery supply the palate and gums. While still within the greater palatine canal, it gives off the ***lesser palatine arteries*** that emerge on the palate through the lesser palatine foramina and run backwards into the soft palate and tonsil.
9. ***Pharyngeal branch*** runs backwards through a canal related to the inferior aspect of the body of the sphenoid bone (pharyngeal or palatinovaginal canal). It supplies part of the nasopharynx, the auditory tube and the sphenoidal air sinus.
10. ***Artery of the pterygoid canal*** runs backwards in the canal of the same name and helps to supply the pharynx, the auditory tube and the tympanic cavity.
11. ***Sphenopalatine artery*** passes medially through the sphenopalatine foramen to enter the cavity of the nose. It gives off ***posterolateral nasal branches*** to the lateral wall of the nose and to the paranasal sinuses; and ***posteromedial branches*** to the nasal septum. Sphenopalatine artery is the artery of 'epistaxis'.

*Competency:*
AN33.3 Describe and demonstrate articulating surface, type and movements of temporomandibular joint.

## TEMPOROMANDIBULAR JOINT

### Type of Joint

This is a complex, bicondylar synovial joint (Fig. 6.9, Flowchart 6.3).

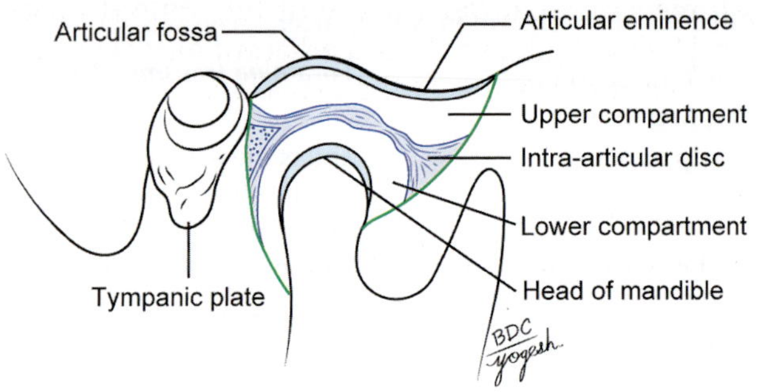


Fig. 6.9: Articular surfaces of right temporomandibular joint

### Articular Surfaces

***Superior articular surface*** is formed by the following parts of the temporal bone:

1. Tubercle of root of zygoma (zygomatic arch) and its anterior root.
2. Anterior part of mandibular fossa.
3. Posterior non-articular part formed by the tympanic plate.

***Inferior articular surface*** is formed by the head of the mandible.

The articular surfaces are covered with *fibrocartilage*. The joint cavity is divided into upper and lower parts by an intra-articular disc.

*Note*: Usually, the synovial joint has articular surface covered by hyaline cartilage.

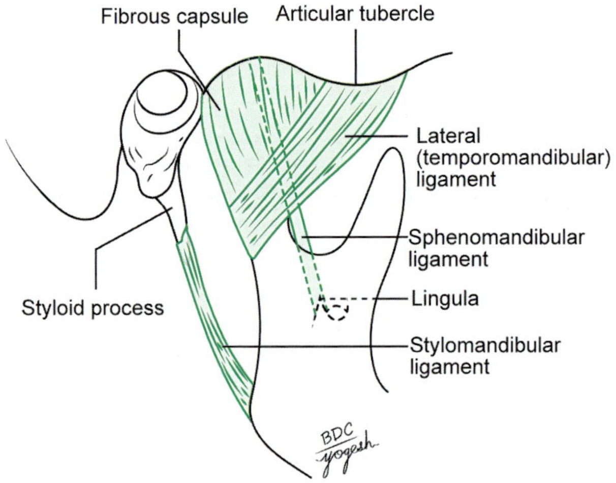


Fig. 6.10: Ligaments of the temporomandibular joint

### Ligaments (Fig. 6.10)

1. ***Fibrous capsule*** is attached *above* to the articular eminence, the circumference of the mandibular fossa in front and the squamotympanic fissure behind, and *below* to the neck of the mandible. The capsule is loose above the intra-articular disc, and tight below it. The ***synovial membrane*** lines the fibrous capsule and the neck of the mandible.
2. ***Lateral temporomandibular ligament*** reinforces and strengthens the lateral part of the capsular ligament. Its fibres are directed downwards and backwards. It is attached above to the tubercle of root of zygoma and its anterior root, and below to the posterolateral aspect of the neck of the mandible.
3. ***Sphenomandibular ligament*** is an accessory ligament, that lies on a deep plane away from the fibrous capsule. It is attached superiorly to the spine of the sphenoid, and inferiorly to the lingula of the mandibular foramen. It is a remnant of the dorsal part of Meckel's cartilage.
   The ligament is related *laterally* to:
   a. Lateral pterygoid muscle
   b. Auriculotemporal nerve
   c. Maxillary artery.
   The ligament is related *medially* to:
   a. Chorda tympani nerve
   b. Wall of the pharynx.
   Near its lower end, it is pierced by the mylohyoid nerve and vessels.
4. ***Stylomandibular ligament*** is another accessory ligament of the joint. It represents a thickened part of the *deep cervical fascia* which separates the parotid and submandibular salivary glands. It is attached

Flowchart 6.3: Temporomandibular joint

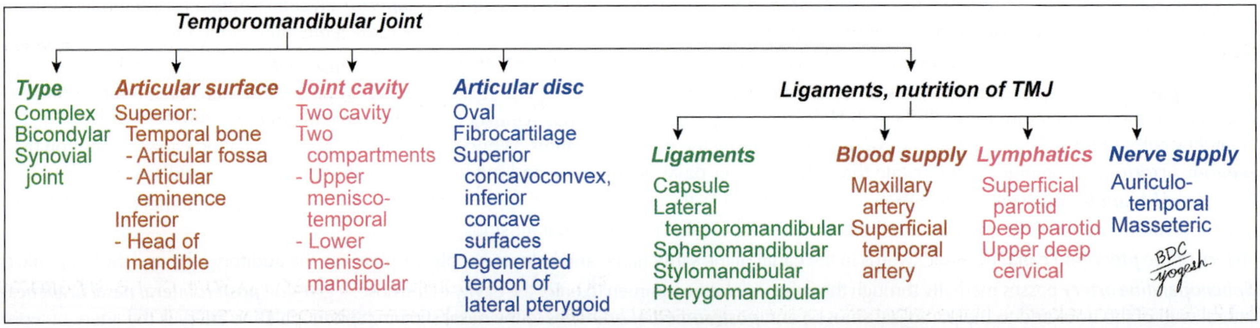

above to the lateral surface of the styloid process, and below to the angle and adjacent part of posterior border of the ramus of the mandible.

## Joint Cavity and Articular Disc

The temporomandibular joint has an oval intra-articular disc. This intra-articular disc divides the joint cavity into:

1. Upper ***menisco-temporal compartment*:** It permits gliding movements.
2. Lower ***menisco-mandibular compartment*:** It permits gliding and rotational movements.

### *Articular Disc* (Fig. 6.11)

The disc has a concavoconvex superior surface and a concave inferior surface. The periphery of the disc is attached to the fibrous capsule.

The disc is composed of an anterior region, anterior thick band, intermediate thin region, posterior thick band and bilaminar region containing venous plexus. The disc represents the degenerated primitive insertion of lateral pterygoid.

*Functions*

1. The disc prevents friction between the articulating surfaces.
2. It acts as a cushion and helps in shock absorption. It stabilises the condyle by filling up the space between articulating surfaces.
3. The proprioceptive fibres present in the disc help to regulate movements of the joint.
4. The disc helps in distribution of weight across the TMJ by increasing the area of contact.

## Relations of Temporomandibular Joint

(Figs 6.12 and 6.13)

### *Lateral*

1. Skin and fasciae
2. Parotid gland
3. Temporal branches of the facial nerve.

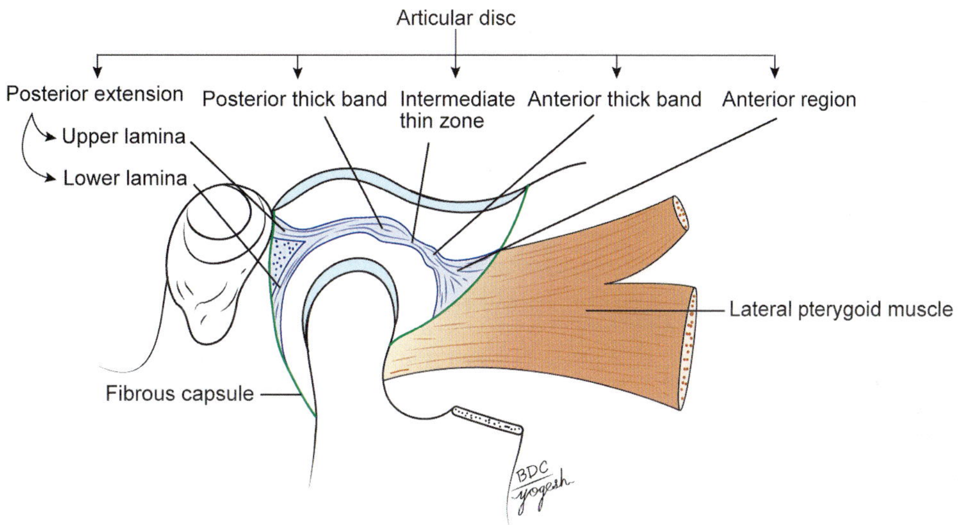


**Fig. 6.11:** Articular disc of temporomandibular joint

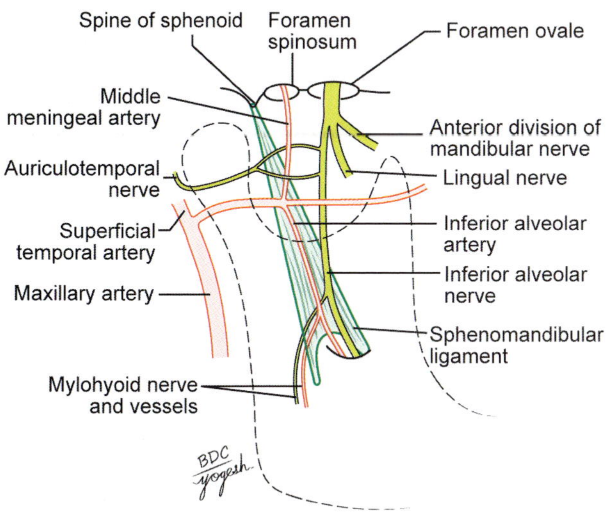


**Fig. 6.12:** Superficial relations of the sphenomandibular ligament

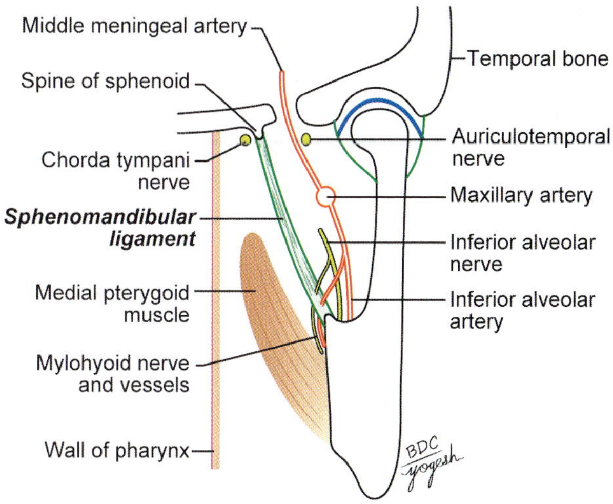


**Fig. 6.13:** Superficial and deep relations of the sphenomandibular ligament (coronal section, posterior view)

### Medial

1. Tympanic plate separates the joint from the internal carotid artery
2. Spine of the sphenoid, with upper end of the spheno-mandibular ligament attached to it
3. Auriculotemporal and chorda tympani nerves
4. Middle meningeal artery.

### Anterior

1. Lateral pterygoid
2. Masseteric nerve and artery.

### Posterior

1. Parotid gland separates the joint from the external auditory meatus
2. Superficial temporal vessels
3. Auriculotemporal nerve

### Superior

1. Middle cranial fossa
2. Middle meningeal vessels

### Inferior

Maxillary artery and vein.

## Blood Supply

Branches from superficial temporal and maxillary arteries. Veins follow the arteries.

## Nerve Supply

Auriculotemporal nerve and masseteric nerve.

## Movements (Figs 6.14a to d and 6.15)

1. Depression (open mouth)
2. Elevation (closed mouth)
3. Protrusion (protraction of chin)
4. Retrusion (retraction of chin)
5. Lateral or side-to-side movements during chewing or grinding.

The muscles producing these movements are listed in Table 6.3.

**TABLE 6.3: Movements of TMJ and the responsible muscles**

| *Movement* | *Muscles and factors* |
|---|---|
| Depression | Lateral pterygoid<br>Gravity<br>Digastric<br>Geniohyoid<br>Mylohyoid |
| Elevation | Masseter<br>Medial pterygoid<br>Temporalis |
| Protrusion | Medial and lateral pterygoid |
| Retraction | Posterior fibres of temporalis |
| Side-by-side or chewing movements | Medial and lateral pterygoids of one side contracting alternately with that of contralateral side muscles |

### Mechanism of TMJ Movements

The movement of the TMJ occurs into two compartments as follows:

1. *Meniscotemporal compartment*—permits gliding movement that mostly occurs in protrusion, retraction, and chewing.
2. *Meniscomandibular compartment*—permits the rotational movement.

The ***rotational movements*** take place around two axes:

1. *Transverse axis* passing mediolaterally through the centre of neck of mandible.
2. *Vertical axis* passing through the posterior border of ramus of mandible.

Rotational movement around transverse axis takes place during depression and elevation. Rotational movement around the vertical axis takes place during side-to-side movements.

***Depression*** occurs in three phases:

1. *Initial phase*: The depression is initiated in the lower compartment by ***forward rotation of mandibular*** head below the disc. Here, the transverse axis passing through the mandibular neck remains fixed and head moves forward and downward in the lower fixed compartments.
2. *Middle phase*: Then the movement takes place in the upper or meniscotemporal compartments by ***forward gliding of the disc*** carrying the mandibular heads with it. In this phase, the transverse axis moves itself and allows the head to move forward below the disc. Here, the disc and the head glide forward together until further movement is prevented by tension of the posterior fibres of temporalis and upper lamella of articular disc.
3. *Final phase*: In this phase, the transverse axis becomes fixed at one place and the ***head rotates around this axis*** to induce further forward and downward movements in the lower meniscomadibular compartments until the head reaches the summit of the articular tubercle.

Movement of the ***elevation*** takes place in a reverse order to that of depression.

***Side-by-side movement***: In this movement, the mandibular head of one side glides forward in the upper meniscotemporal compartments and rotates below the disc around the vertical axis passing through the posterior border of opposite ramus of the mandible. This is followed by reverse movement and rotation of opposite head of mandible to produce side-by-side movement.

***Range of mandibular movements***

- Maximal depression: 50 mm
- Routine depression: 40 mm
- It includes the rotational components of 25 mm and anterior translatory gliding of 15 mm
- Maximal range of protrusion: 10 mm
- Maximal lateral movement: 10 mm

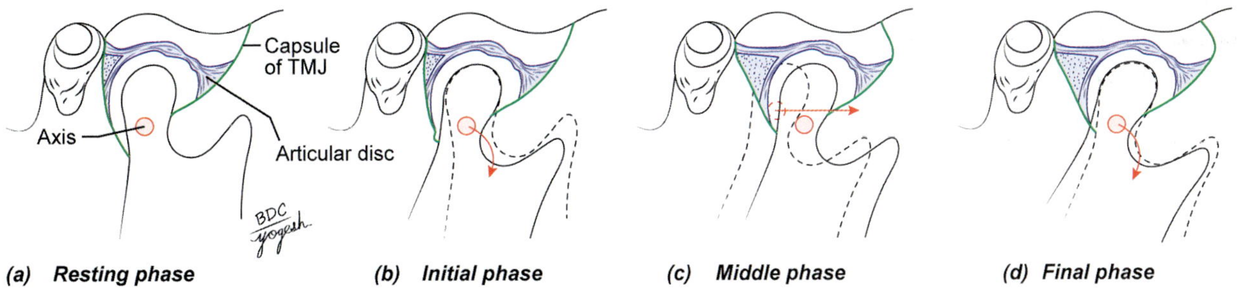


**Figs 6.14a to d:** Movements in lower and upper compartments during opening of the mouth

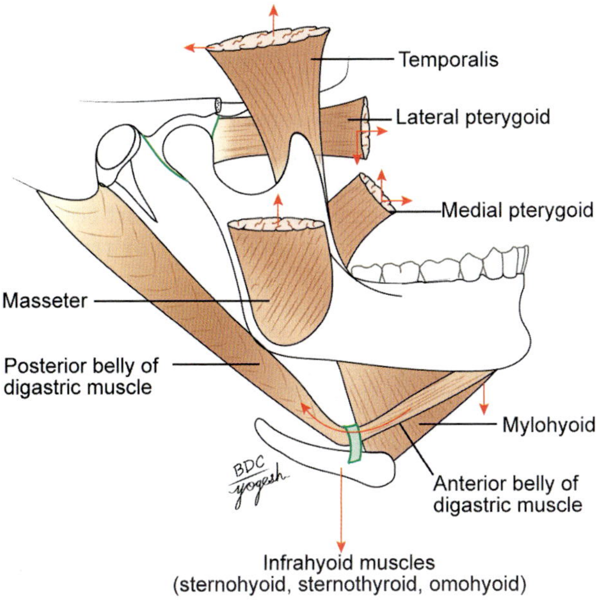


**Fig. 6.15:** Movements of temporomandibular joint (arrows) by muscles of mastication

### Factors Maintaining Stability of TMJ

The TMJ is supported by the following factors that maintain the stability of TMJ:

1. *Bones:* Articular tubercles prevent the anterior dislocation and postglenoid tubercles prevent the posterior dislocation of TMJ.
2. *Ligaments:* Lateral temporomandibular ligament prevents the backward dislocation of TMJ.
3. *Muscles:* Tension of the posterior fibres of temporalis prevents the anterior dislocation and tension of lateral pterygoid prevents the posterior dislocation.
4. *Position of mandible:* The TMJ is more stable in occlusion position, that is, when the mouth is closed.

***Competency:***

**AN33.5** Describe the features of dislocation of temporomandibular joint.

## CLINICAL ANATOMY

- ***Palpation of TMJ:*** To palpate the TMJ, ask the patient to open and close the mouth several times and then move the opened jaw side-by-side and finally forward and backward. During these movements, the TMJ is palpated by placing a finger into the anterior wall of outer portion of external auditory meatus, and the moving condyle of mandible can be felt. The TMJ can also be palpated by placing a finger about 1.5 cm medial to the tragus of ear.
- ***Dislocation of mandible:*** The mandible is commonly dislocated anteriorly (Fig. 6.16).
- During excessive opening of mouth, the head of mandible dislocates anteriorly as it slips forward underneath the articular eminence in the infratemporal fossa. The patient cannot close the mouth.
- ***Reduction of dislocated TMJ:*** To reduce the dislocated TMJ, the condyle of mandible must be brought back behind the articular eminence. For this, lower down the ramus of mandible by placing the thumbs on the last molar teeth and simultaneously elevating the chin with other fingers (Figs 6.17a and b).
- ***TMJ syndrome:*** The TMJ syndrome includes symptoms that are due to TMJ disorder or those that are associated with muscle involvement including fractures. These are as follows:
  1. Facial pain due to spasm of masseter
  2. Headache due to spasm of temporalis
  3. Jaw pain due to spasm of lateral pterygoid.
- ***Clicking sound at TMJ:*** The movement of TMJ may produce clicking sound or jaw popping. It may occur due to joint function or disorder such as arthritis, broken or dislocated mandibular head, muscular spasm, malocclusion of teeth and infection of parotid glands.
- Damage to VII nerve or auriculotemporal nerve may occur during TMJ surgeries (Fig. 6.18)

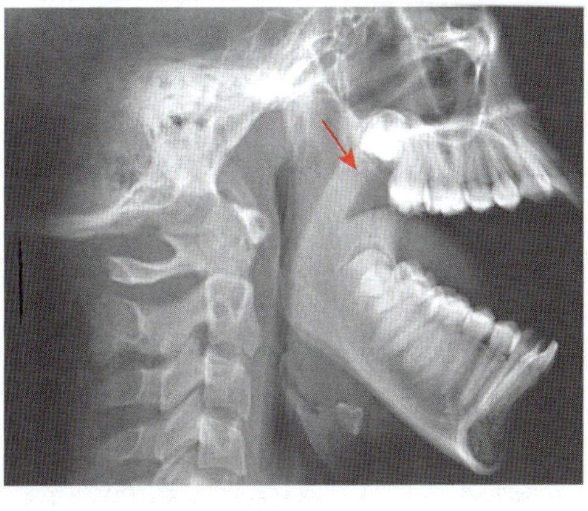

**Fig. 6.16:** Dislocation of the head of mandible

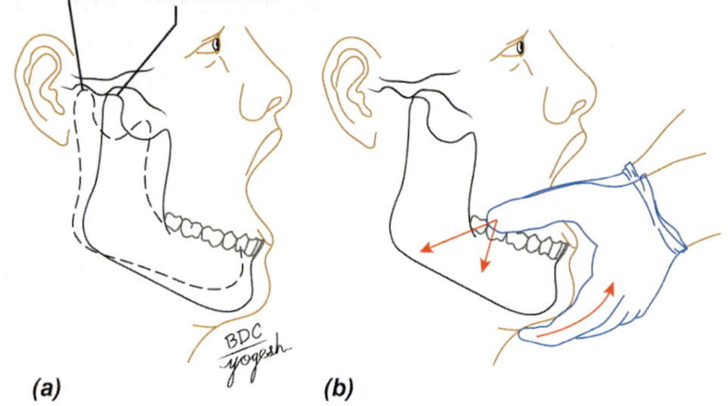


**Figs 6.17a and b:** Dislocation of temporomandibular joint: (a) Anterior dislocation and (b) reduction of dislocated TMJ

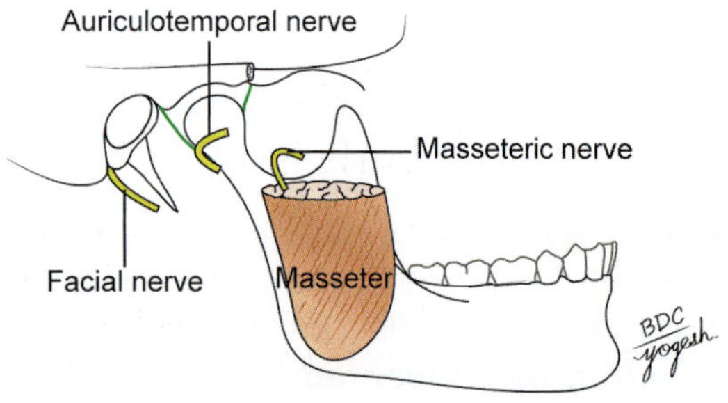


**Fig. 6.18:** Nerves related to temporomandibular joint

**DISSECTION**

Cut the lateral pterygoid muscle close to its insertion. Dislodge the head of mandible from the articular disc. Locate the articular cartilages covering the head of the mandible and the mandibular fossa. Take out the articular disc as well and study its shape and its role in increasing the varieties of movements.

## MANDIBULAR NERVE

This is the largest mixed branch of the trigeminal nerve. It is the nerve of the 1st branchial arch and supplies all structures derived from that arch. Otic and submandibular ganglia are associated with this nerve (Fig. 6.19).

### Course and Relations

Mandibular nerve begins in the middle cranial fossa through a large sensory root and a small motor root. The ***sensory root*** arises from the lateral part of the trigeminal ganglion and leaves the cranial cavity through the foramen ovale.

The ***motor root*** lies deep to the trigeminal ganglion and to the sensory root. It also passes through the foramen ovale to join the sensory root just below the foramen thus forming the main trunk. The ***main trunk*** lies in the infratemporal fossa, on the tensor veli palatini, deep to the lateral pterygoid. After a short course, the main trunk divides into a small ***anterior trunk*** and a large ***posterior trunk***.

### Branches (Table 6.4)

*From the main trunk:*

1. Meningeal branch
2. Nerve to the medial pterygoid.

*From the anterior trunk:*

1. A sensory branch—Buccal nerve
2. Motor branches—Masseteric and deep temporal nerves and the nerve to the lateral pterygoid.

*From the posterior trunk:*

1. Auriculotemporal nerve
2. Lingual nerve
3. Inferior alveolar nerve.

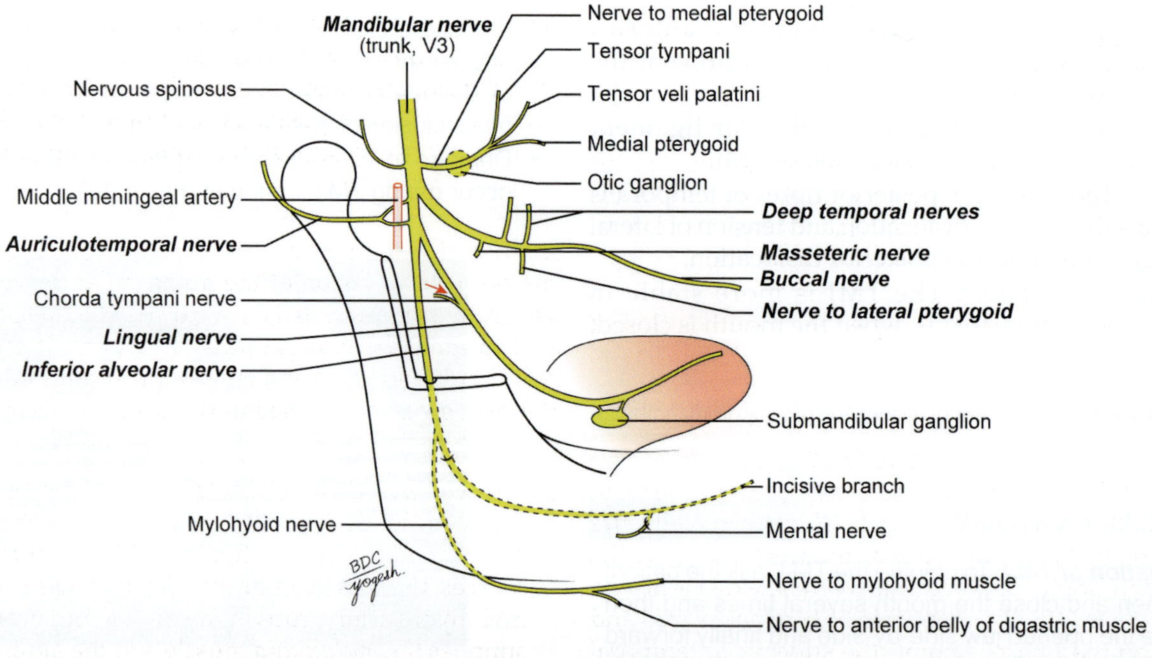


**Fig. 6.19:** Distribution of mandibular nerve (V3)

| TABLE 6.4: Branches of the mandibular nerve (CN V3) | | |
|---|---|---|
| **Muscular** | **Sensory** | **Others** |
| Temporalis and masseter | Meningeal Auriculotemporal | Carries taste fibres |
| Medial and lateral pterygoids | Inferior alveolar and mental | Carries secretomotor fibres |
| Tensor veli palatini and tensor tympani | Lingual | Articular |
| Mylohyoid and digastric (anterior belly) | Buccal | — |

## Distribution of Mandibular Nerve

### Meningeal Branch or Nervus Spinosus

Meningeal branch enters the skull through the *foramen spinosum* with the middle meningeal artery and supplies the dura mater of the middle cranial fossa.

### Nerve to Medial Pterygoid

Nerve to medial pterygoid arises close to the otic ganglion and supplies the ***medial pterygoid*** from its deep surface. This nerve gives a motor root to the otic ganglion which does not relay and supplies the ***tensor veli palatini***, and the ***tensor tympani muscles***.

### Buccal Nerve

Buccal nerve is the only ***sensory*** branch of the anterior division of the mandibular nerve. It passes between the two heads of the lateral pterygoid, runs downwards and forwards, and supplies the skin of cheek and mucous membrane related to the buccinator. It also supplies the labial aspect of gums of molar and premolar teeth.

### Masseteric Nerve

Masseteric nerve emerges at the upper border of the lateral pterygoid just in front of the temporomandibular joint, passes laterally through the mandibular notch in company with the masseteric vessels, and enters the deep surface of the ***masseter***. It also supplies the temporomandibular joint.

### Deep Temporal Nerves

Deep temporal nerves are two nerves—anterior and posterior. They pass between the skull and the lateral pterygoid and enter the deep surface of the ***temporalis***.

### Nerve to Lateral Pterygoid

Nerve to lateral pterygoid enters the deep surface of the muscle.

### Auriculotemporal Nerve

Auriculotemporal nerve arises by two roots that run backwards, encircle the middle meningeal artery, and unite to form a single trunk. The nerve continues backwards between the neck of the mandible and the sphenomandibular ligament, above the maxillary artery. Behind the neck of the mandible, it turns upwards and ascends on the temple behind the superficial temporal vessels.

#### *Distribution*

1. ***Auricular part*** of the nerve supplies the skin of the tragus; and the upper parts of the pinna, the external acoustic meatus and the tympanic membrane. (Note that the lower parts of these regions are supplied by the great auricular nerve and the auricular branch of the vagus nerve.)
2. ***Temporal part*** supplies the skin of the temple. *In addition,* the auriculotemporal nerve also supplies the parotid gland (secretomotor and sensory) and the temporomandibular joint.

### Lingual Nerve

Lingual nerve is a branch of the posterior division of the mandibular nerve.

***Course:*** Lingual nerve begins 1 cm below the skull. About 2 cm below skull, it is joined by chorda tympani nerve at an acute angle. Then it lies in contact with mandible medial to 3rd *molar tooth*. Finally, it lies on surface of hyoglossus and genioglossus to reach the tongue.

***Relations:*** It begins 1 cm below the skull. It runs first between the tensor veli palatini and the lateral pterygoid, and then between the lateral and medial pterygoids.

About 2 cm below the skull, it is joined by the chorda tympani nerve.

Emerging at the lower border of the lateral pterygoid, the nerve runs downwards and forwards between the ramus of the mandible and the medial pterygoid. Next, it lies in direct contact with the mandible, medial to the third molar tooth between the origins of the superior constrictor and the mylohyoid muscles.

It soon leaves the gum and runs over the hyoglossus deep to the mylohyoid. Finally, it lies on the surface of the genioglossus deep to the mylohyoid. Here it winds around the submandibular duct and divides into its terminal branches.

***Distribution:*** It is sensory to the anterior 2/3rd of the tongue and to the floor of the mouth. However, the fibres of the chorda tympani (branch of facial nerve) which is secretomotor to the submandibular and sublingual salivary glands and gustatory to the anterior 2/3rd of the tongue, are also distributed through the lingual nerve.

### Inferior Alveolar Nerve (Fig. 6.20)

Inferior alveolar nerve is the larger terminal branch of the posterior division of the mandibular nerve. It runs vertically downwards lateral to the medial pterygoid and to the sphenomandibular ligament. It enters the mandibular foramen and runs in the mandibular canal. It is accompanied by the inferior alveolar artery.

#### *Branches*

1. The ***mylohyoid branch*** contains all the motor fibres of the posterior division. It arises just before the inferior alveolar nerve enters the mandibular foramen. It pierces the sphenomandibular ligament with the mylohyoid artery, runs in the mylohyoid groove, and supplies the ***mylohyoid*** muscle and the ***anterior belly of the digastric***.

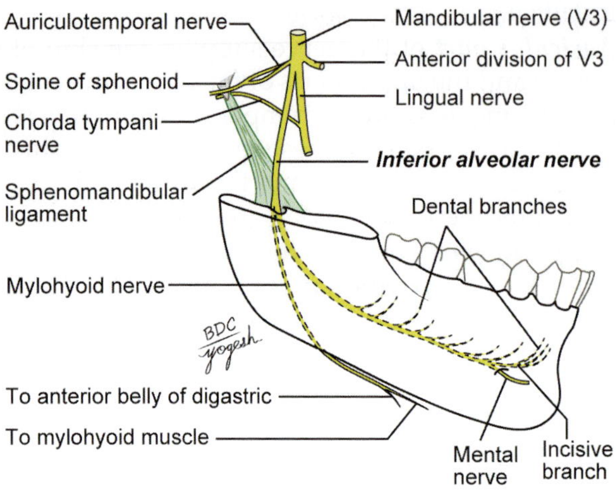


**Fig. 6.20:** Inferior alveolar nerve

2. While running in the mandibular canal, the inferior alveolar nerve gives branches that supply the lower teeth and gums.
3. ***Mental nerve*** emerges at the mental foramen and supplies the skin of the chin, and the skin and mucous membrane of the lower lip.
4. ***Incisive branch*** supplies the labial aspect of gums of canine and incisor teeth.

**DISSECTION**

Identify middle meningeal artery arising from the maxillary artery and trace it till the foramen spinosum. Note the two roots of auriculotemporal nerve surrounding the artery. Trace the origin of the auriculotemporal nerve from mandibular nerve (Fig. 6.11). Dissect all the other branches of the nerve. Identify the chorda tympani nerve joining the lingual branch of mandibular nerve. Lift the trunk of mandibular nerve laterally and locate the otic ganglion.

Trace all connections of the otic ganglion.

## OTIC GANGLION

The otic ganglion is a small, oval peripheral parasympathetic ganglion (Fig. 6.21, Flowchart 6.4).

*Size*: 2–3 mm (pinhead)

### *Neurological relationship:*

*Topographic relation:* It is connected with mandibular nerve.

*Functional relation:* It is related functionally to glossopharyngeal nerve.

***Location:*** It is situated in the infratemporal fossa, immediately below the foramen ovale.

### *Relations*

*Lateral:* Main trunk of mandibular nerve

*Medial:* Tensor veli palatini

*Anterior:* Middle meningeal artery

*Posterior:* Medial pterygoid muscle.

### *Roots (connections and distribution)*

It has four roots as follows:

1. ***Parasympathetic or secretomotor root:*** It consists of pre- and post-ganglionic fibres:

   *Preganglionic fibres* begin in the inferior salivatory nucleus in the medulla and pass through glossopharyngeal and then its tympanic branch. This branch forms lesser petrosal nerve. This lesser petrosal nerve enters the middle cranial fossa and further traverses through foramen ovale. Finally, fibres from lesser petrosal nerve relay in the otic ganglion.

   *Post-ganglionic fibres* from the cells of otic ganglion join auriculotemporal nerve and supply the parotid gland.
2. ***Sympathetic root:*** The lateral horn cells of T1 segment of spinal cord give rise to the preganglionic sympathetic fibres. They traverse to T1 nerve, sympathetic chain, and relay in superior cervical sympathetic ganglion. Post-ganglionic fibres reach the parotid gland through a plexus around middle meningeal artery and auriculotemporal nerve. These fibres pass through the otic ganglion without relaying.
3. ***Sensory root:*** These are the fibres of auriculotemporal nerve that pass through the otic ganglion without relaying and supplying parotid gland.
4. ***Motor root:*** Fibres from the nerve to medial pterygoid pass through the otic ganglion without relay. They supply tensor veli palatini and tensor tympani muscles.

### *Functions*

Fibres from the otic ganglion supply parotid gland as follows:

1. Parasympathetic fibres—secretomotor
2. Sympathetic fibres—vasomotor
3. Sensory fibres—carry sensation.

*Note*: Motor fibres supply tensor veli palatini and tensor tympani.

**CLINICAL ANATOMY**

- ***Frey's syndrome:*** It is a rare neurological disorder resulting in gustatory sweating (Fig. 11.11). It may result due to damage to auriculotemporal and great auricular nerves in the parotid gland injuries or surgeries. The parasympathetic fibres of auriculotemporal nerve stimulate the parotid gland to enhance its secretion and sympathetic fibres of the great auricular nerve stimulate sweat glands in the facial skin. After damage to these both nerves, during regeneration, the parasympathetic fibres of auriculotemporal nerve grow and join the sympathetic fibres of the great auricular nerve. This results in sweating rather than salivation during eating. Hence, it is called *gustatory sweating* or *Frey's syndrome*.
- ***Clinical testing of mandibular nerve:*** The motor part of the mandibular nerve is tested clinically by asking the patient to clench her/his teeth and then feeling for the contracting masseter and temporalis muscles on the two sides. If one masseter is paralysed, the jaw

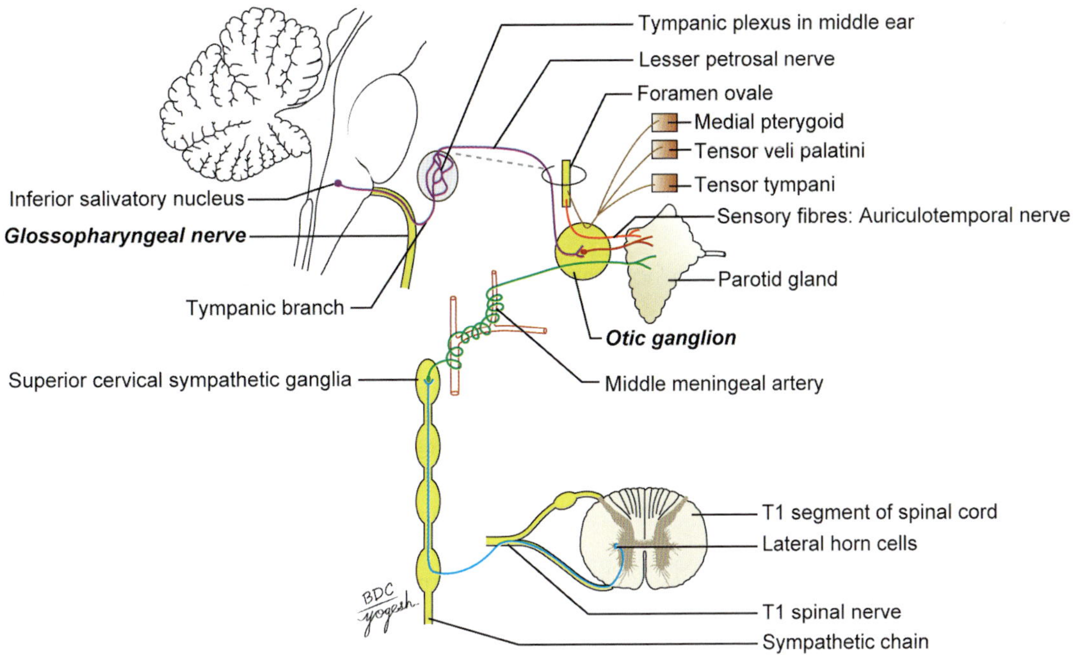


**Fig. 6.21:** Innervation of parotid gland (schematic representation, Purple line: Preganglionic parasympathetic fibres, Red line: Post-ganglionic parasympathetic fibres, Blue line: Preganglionic sympathetic fibres, Green line: Post-ganglionic sympathetic fibres, *Note*: Lesser petrosal nerve enter the middle cranial fossa and exit through the foramen ovale. Middle cranial fossa shown by grey dotted line)

**Flowchart 6.4:** Otic ganglion

***Otic ganglion***

- ***Parasympathetic fibres***
  - ***Preganglionic fibres***
    - Inferior salivatory nucleus → Glossopharyngeal nerve → Tympanic nerve → Tympanic plexus → Lesser petrosal nerve → Relay in otic ganglion
  - ***Postganglion fibres***
    - Otic ganglion → Join auriculotemporal nerve → Parotid gland
- ***Sympathetic fibres***
  - ***Preganglionic***
    - Lateral horn cells → T1 segment → Sympathetic chain → Relay in superior cervical sympathetic ganglion
  - ***Postganglionic***
    - Plexus around external carotid and middle meningeal artery → Fibres join auriculotemporal nerve → Parotid gland
- ***Sensory fibres***
  - Through auriculotemporal nerve

deviates to the paralysed side, on opening the mouth by the action of the normal lateral pterygoid of the opposite side. The activity of the pterygoid muscles is tested by asking the patient to move the chin from side-to-side.

- ***Referred pain:*** In cases with cancer of the tongue, pain radiates to the ear and to the temporal fossa, over the distribution of the auriculotemporal nerve as both lingual and auriculotemporal nerves are branches of mandibular nerve. Sometimes the lingual nerve is divided to relieve intractable pain of this kind. This may be done where the nerve lies in contact with the mandible below and behind the last molar tooth, covered only by mucous membrane.
- ***Mandibular neuralgia:*** Trigeminal neuralgia of the mandibular division is often difficult to treat. In such cases, the sensory root of the nerve may be divided behind the ganglion, and this is now the operation of choice when pain is confined to the distribution of the maxillary and mandibular nerves. During division, the ophthalmic fibres that lie in the superomedial part of the root are spared, to preserve the corneal reflex thus avoiding damage to the cornea (Fig. 6.22).
- ***Lingual nerve injury:*** Lingual nerve lies in contact with mandible, medial to the 3rd molar tooth. In extraction of malplaced 'wisdom' tooth, care must be taken not to injure the lingual nerve. Its injury results in loss of general and taste sensations from anterior two-thirds of the tongue oral mucosa, gingivae, chin and lower lip.
- ***Jaw-jerk reflex:*** The mandibular nerve supplies both the efferent and afferent loops of the jaw-jerk reflex, as it is a mixed nerve. Tapping the chin causes contraction of the pterygoid muscles. A lesion at the foramen ovale leads to paraesthesia along the mandible, tongue, temporal region and paralysis of

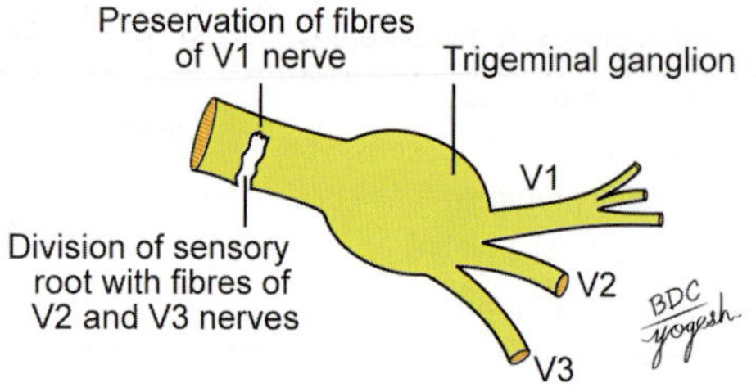


**Fig. 6.22:** Partial cutting of the sensory root of trigeminal nerve

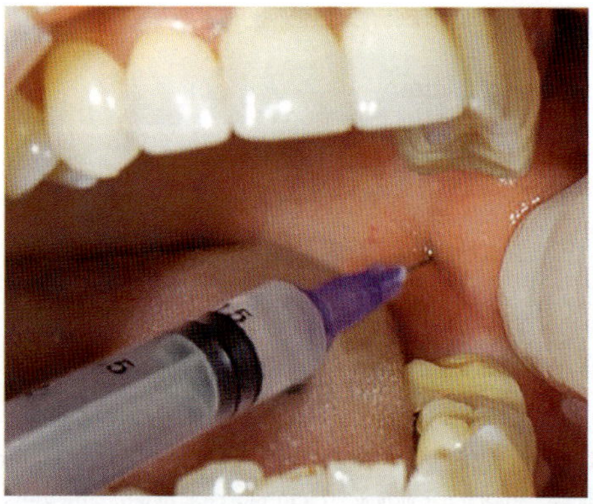

**Fig. 6.23:** Injection given in mandibular foramen for anaesthetising the inferior alveolar nerve before extraction of last molar tooth

the muscles of mastication. This also leads to loss of jaw-jerk reflex.

- ***Inferior alveolar nerve block:*** In extraction of mandibular teeth, inferior alveolar nerve needs to be anaesthetised. The drug is given into the nerve before it enters the mandibular canal (Fig. 6.20).
- During extraction of the 3rd molar, the buccal nerve may get involved by the local anaesthesia causing temporary numbness of the cheek (Fig. 6.23).

VIDEO

**Video 3.6 Infratemporal Fossa:** Muscles of mastication, Mandibular nerve

### *Facts to Remember*

- Mandibular nerve is associated with two parasympathetic ganglia, i.e. otic and submandibular ganglia.
- Only muscle of mastication which depresses the TMJ is the lateral pterygoid muscle.
- Masseter is the chief elevator of the mandible.
- Spine of sphenoid is related medially to chorda tympani and laterally to auriculotemporal nerves.
- Auriculotemporal nerve and branches of facial nerve are related to temporomandibular joint.
- The most common dislocation of the TMJ is anterior.
- Inferior alveolar nerve block is given for dental procedures of the lower jaw.
- Trismus or locked jaw occurs due to spasm of both the masseters. It is typically seen in tetanus.
- The course of the maxillary artery is divided into three parts by a lateral pterygoid.
- Middle meningeal artery is encircled by two roots of auriculotemporal nerve.

### BDC's Anatomy *e*-book

1. Landmarks on the lateral side of the head
2. Maxillary artery: Territory of distribution
3. Further reading
4. Viva voce questions

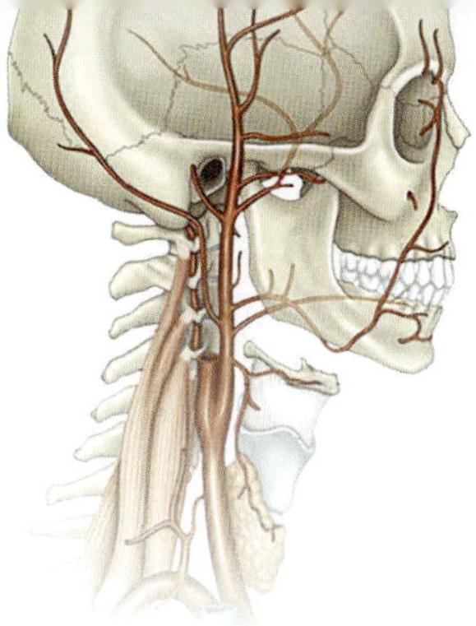

Chapter

7

# Submandibular Region

*Competency:*

**AN34.1** Describe and demonstrate the superficial and deep structures, muscles, nerves, vessels, and glands in the submandibular region.

Submandibular region includes deeper structures in the area between the mandible and hyoid bone, including the floor of the mouth and the root of the tongue.

***Contents of submandibular region:***

1. Suprahyoid muscles
2. Submandibular and sublingual salivary glands
3. *Nerves*: Lingual, hypoglossal and glossopharyngeal nerves, and submandibular ganglion
4. *Vessels*: Lingual and facial arteries
5. Root of tongue and floor of mouth.

## SUPRAHYOID MUSCLES

The suprahyoid muscles are the digastric, the stylohyoid, the mylohyoid and the geniohyoid. The muscles are in following layers (Figs 7.1 to 7.5, Tables 7.1 and 7.2, Plate 7.1):

1. *First layer*: Digastric (Greek *two bellies*) and stylohyoid
2. *Second layer*: Mylohyoid (Greek *pertaining to hyoid bone*)
3. *Third layer*: Geniohyoid and hyoglossus
4. *Fourth layer*: Genioglossus.

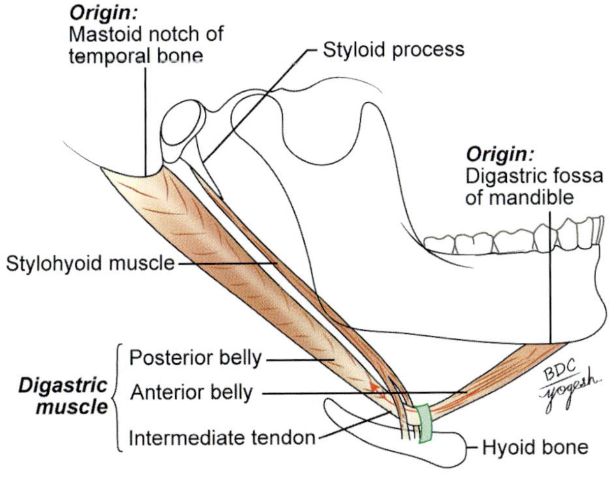


**Fig. 7.1:** Digastric muscle

### DISSECTION

Cut the facial artery and vein present at the anteroinferior angle of masseter muscle. Separate the origin of anterior belly of digastric muscle from the digastric fossa near the symphysis menti. Push the mandible upwards. Clean and expose the posterior belly of digastric muscle and its accompanying stylohyoid muscle. Identify the digastrics, stylohyoid, mylohyoid, geniohyoid and hyoglossus.

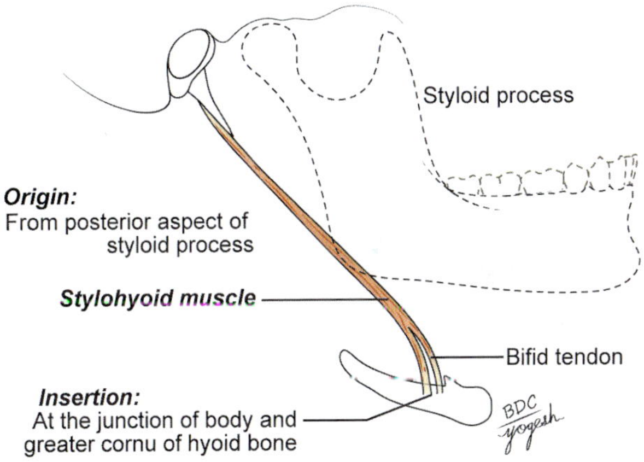


**Fig. 7.2:** Stylohyoid muscle

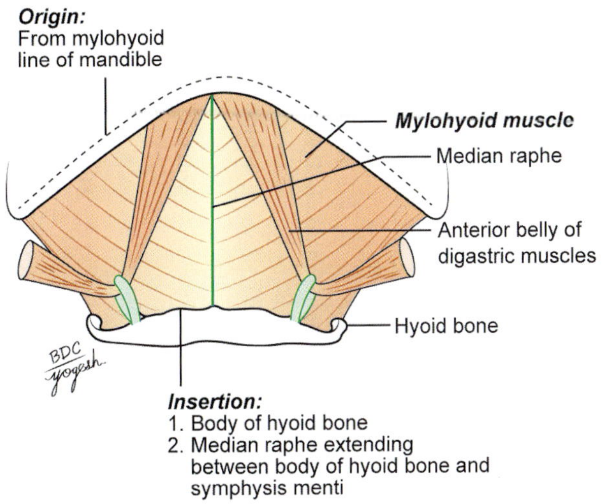


**Fig. 7.3:** Mylohyoid muscle

**TABLE 7.1: Suprahyoid muscles** (Figs 7.1 to 7.5)

| *Muscle* | *Origin* | *Fibres* | *Insertion* | *Nerve supply* | *Actions* |
|---|---|---|---|---|---|
| 1. **Digastric** (DG): It has two bellies united by an intermediate tendon. Anterior belly is unipennate and posterior belly is bipennate (Table 7.2) | a. Anterior belly (DGA): From digastric fossa of **mandible**<br>b. Posterior belly (DGP): From mastoid notch of **temporal bone** | a. Anterior belly runs downwards and backwards<br>b. Posterior belly runs downwards and forwards | Both heads meet at the **intermediate tendon** which perforates stylohyoid and is held by a fibrous pulley to the hyoid bone | a. Anterior belly by nerve to mylohyoid (V3)<br>b. Posterior belly by facial nerve (VII) | a. Depresses mandible when mouth is opened widely or against resistance; it is secondary to lateral pterygoid<br>b. Elevates hyoid bone |
| 2. **Stylohyoid** (SH): Small muscle, lies on upper border of DGP | Posterior surface of **styloid process** | Tendon is perforated by DGP tendon | Junction of body and greater cornua of **hyoid bone** | Facial nerve (VII) | a. Pulls hyoid bone upwards and backwards<br>b. With other hyoid muscles, it fixes the hyoid bone |
| 3. **Mylohyoid** (MH): Flat, triangular muscle; two mylohyoids form floor of mouth cavity, deep to DGA | **Mylohyoid line** of mandible | Fibres run medially and slightly downwards | a. Posterior fibres: Body of **hyoid bone**<br>b. Middle and anterior fibres; **median raphe**, between mandible and hyoid bone | Nerve to mylohyoid (V3) | a. Elevates floor of mouth in first stage of deglutition<br>b. Helps in depression of mandible, and elevation of hyoid bone |
| 4. **Geniohyoid** (GH): Short and narrow muscle; lies above medial part of MH | **Inferior genial tubercle** of mandible | Runs backwards and downwards | Anterior surface of body of **hyoid bone** | C1 through hypoglossal nerve | a. Elevates hyoid bone<br>b. May depress mandible when hyoid is fixed |
| 5. **Hyoglossus:** It is a muscle of tongue. It forms important landmark in this region | Whole length of greater cornua and lateral part of body of **hyoid bone** | Fibres run upwards and forwards | Side of **tongue** between styloglossus and inferior longitudinal muscle of tongue | Hypoglossal (XII) nerve | Depresses tongue makes dorsum convex, retracts the protruded tongue |
| 6. **Genioglossus:** It is the bulkiest muscle of tongue. It is fan-shaped | **Superior genial tubercle** of mandible | Fibres radiate | Upper fibres pass upwards and forwards to tip of **tongue**. Middle fibres along whole length of dorsum. Lower fibres into body of **hyoid** | Hypoglossal (XII) | Pulls posterior part of tongue forwards, i.e. protrudes tongue. It is a life-saving muscle |

**Plate 7.1:** Suprahyoid muscles

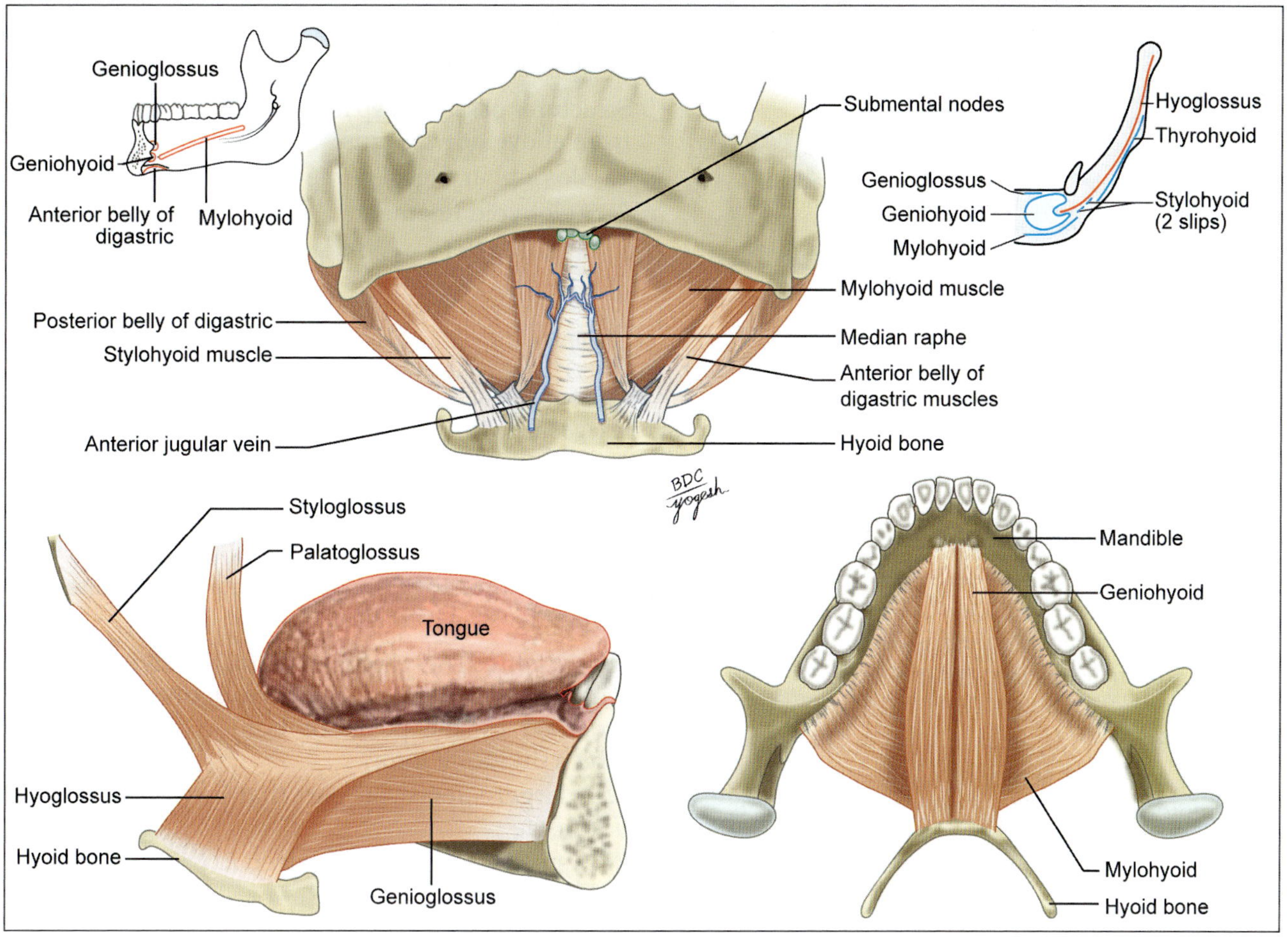


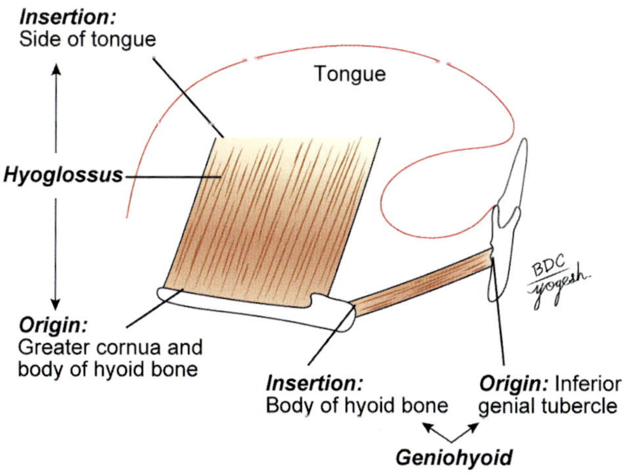


**Fig. 7.4:** Geniohyoid and hyoglossus muscles

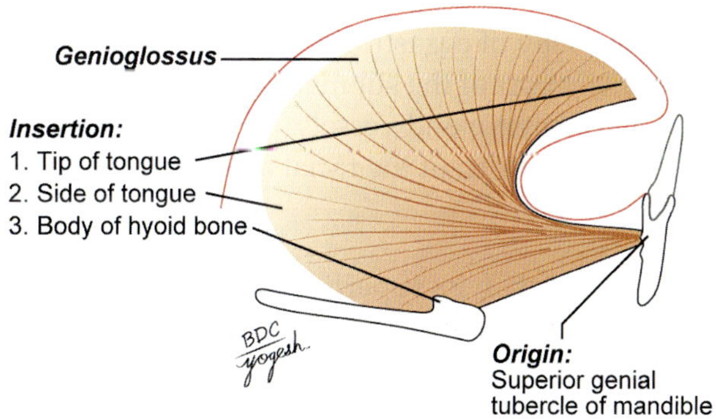


**Fig. 7.5:** Genioglossus muscle

| TABLE 7.2: Differences between the anterior and posterior bellies of digastric | | |
|---|---|---|
| ***Feature*** | ***Anterior belly*** | ***Posterior belly*** |
| Structure | Unipennate | Bipennate |
| Development | 1st pharyngeal arch | 2nd pharyngeal arch |
| Innervation | Mylohyoid branch of inferior alveolar nerve (mandibular nerve) | Facial nerve |

## Relations of Posterior Belly of Digastric (Fig. 7.6)

### *Superficial*

1. Mastoid process with the sternocleidomastoid, splenius capitis and the longissimus capitis
2. Stylohyoid
3. Parotid gland with retromandibular vein
4. Submandibular salivary gland and lymph nodes
5. Angle of the mandible with medial pterygoid

### *Deep*

1. Transverse process of the atlas with superior oblique and the rectus capitis lateralis

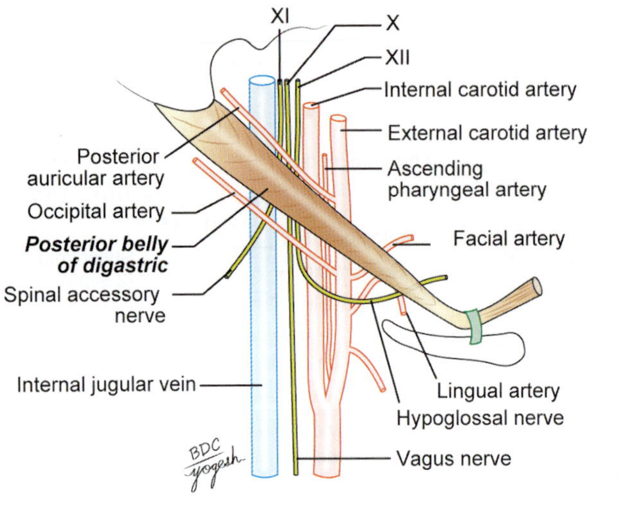


**Fig. 7.6:** Relations of the posterior belly of the digastric muscle

2. Internal carotid, external carotid, lingual, facial and occipital arteries
3. Internal jugular vein
4. Vagus, accessory and hypoglossal cranial nerves
5. The hyoglossus muscle.

### *Upper Border*

1. Posterior auricular artery
2. Stylohyoid muscle.

### *Lower Border*

Lower border is related to occipital artery.

### Relations of Mylohyoid (Fig. 7.7)

#### *Superficial*

1. Anterior belly of digastric
2. Superficial part of the submandibular salivary gland
3. Mylohyoid nerve and vessels
4. Submental branch of the facial artery.

#### *Deep*

1. Hyoglossus with its superficial relations, namely the styloglossus, the lingual nerve, the submandibular ganglion, the deep part of the submandibular salivary gland, the submandibular duct, the hypoglossal nerve and the venae comitantes hypoglossi.
2. The genioglossus with its superficial relations, namely the sublingual salivary gland, the lingual nerve, submandibular duct, the lingual artery, and the hypoglossal nerve.

### Relations of Hyoglossus

#### *Superficial*

Styloglossus, lingual nerve, submandibular ganglion, deep part of the submandibular gland, submandibular duct, hypoglossal nerve and veins accompanying it.

#### *Deep*

1. Inferior longitudinal muscle of the tongue
2. Genioglossus
3. Middle constrictor of the pharynx
4. Glossopharyngeal nerve
5. Stylohyoid ligament
6. Lingual artery.

Structures passing deep to posterior border of hyoglossus from above downwards:
1. Glossopharyngeal nerve
2. Stylohyoid ligament
3. Lingual artery.

*Competency:*
**AN34.2** Describe and demonstrate the morphology, relations and nerve supply of submandibular salivary gland and submandibular ganglion.

## SUBMANDIBULAR SALIVARY GLAND

This is a large salivary gland, situated in the anterior part of the digastric triangle.

***Dimensions:*** The gland is about the size of a walnut weighing about 15 to 20 g. It is roughly J-shaped, being indented by the posterior border of the mylohyoid which divides it into:
1. A larger superficial part that lies superficial to the muscle
2. A small deep part lying deep to the muscle (Fig. 7.8, Flowchart 7.1).

### Superficial Part

This part of the gland fills the digastric triangle. It extends superiorly deep to the mandible up to the mylohyoid line. Inferiorly: It overlaps stylohyoid and the posterior belly of digastric (Fig. 7.8). It has three surfaces:
1. Inferior
2. Lateral
3. Medial.

### *Coverings of Superficial Part*

It is partially enclosed between two layers of deep cervical fascia. The superficial (Fig. 7.6) layer of fascia covers the inferior surface of the gland and is attached to the base of the mandible. The deep layer covers the medial surface of the gland and is attached superiorly to the mylohyoid line of the mandible (Fig. 7.9).

**Flowchart 7.1:** Submandibular gland

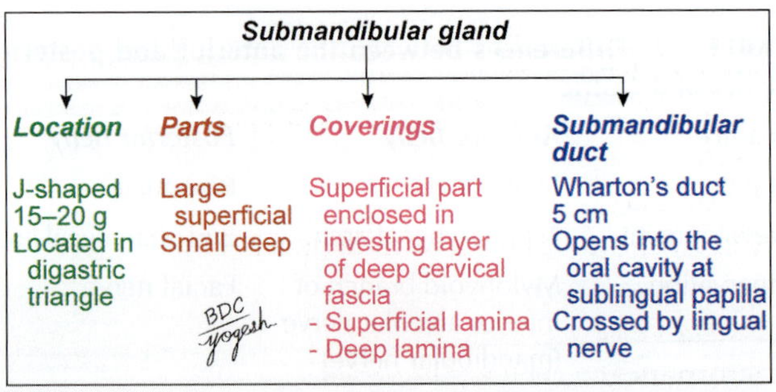

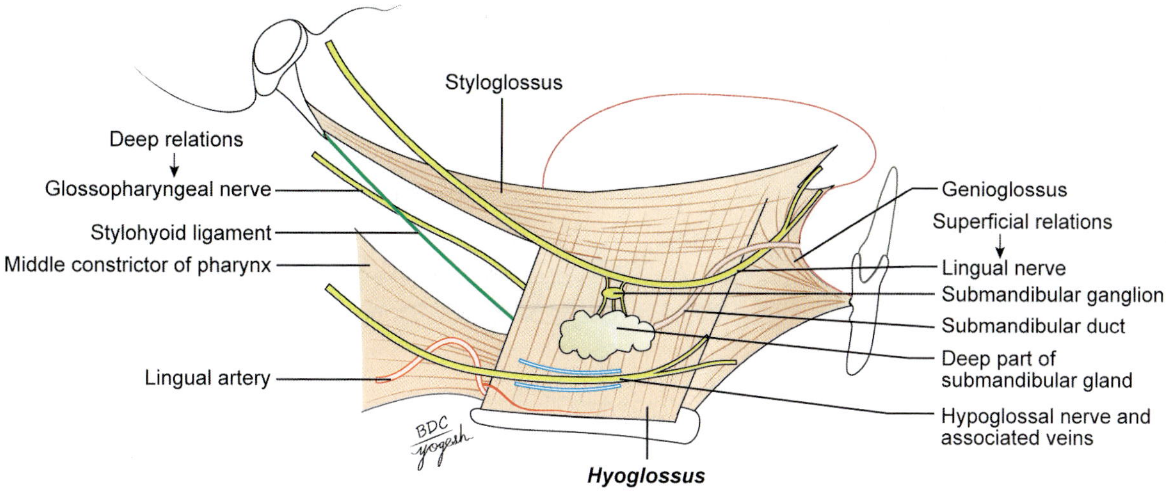


**Fig. 7.7:** Relations of the hyoglossus and genioglossus muscles

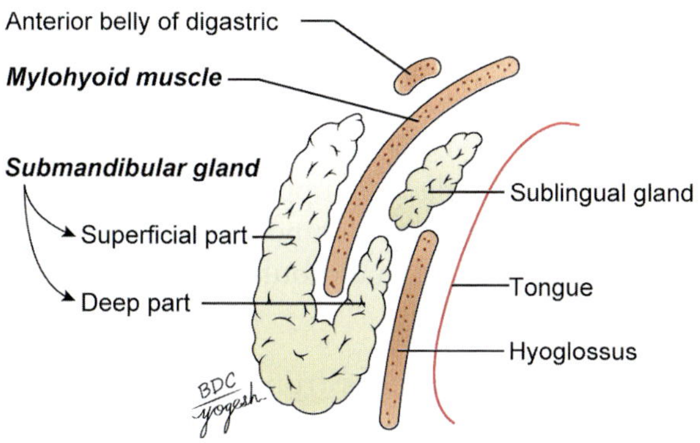


**Fig. 7.8:** Horizontal section through the submandibular region showing the location of the submandibular and sublingual glands

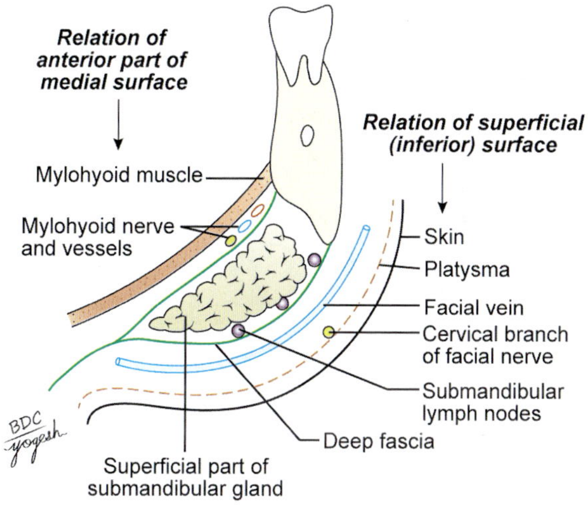


**Fig. 7.10:** Relationship of the inferior and medial surfaces of the submandibular gland

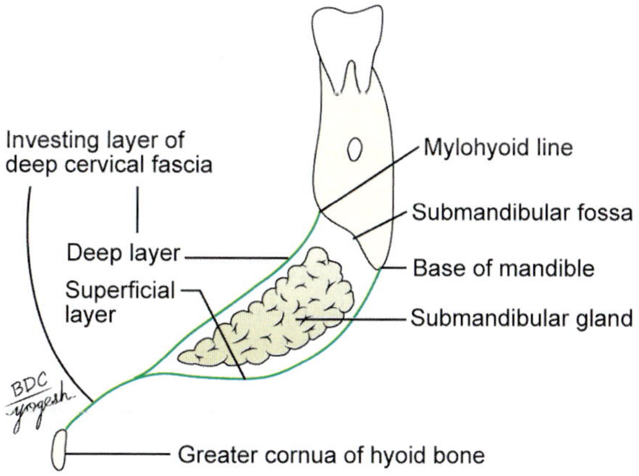


**Fig. 7.9:** Fascial coverings of the superficial part of the submandibular salivary gland

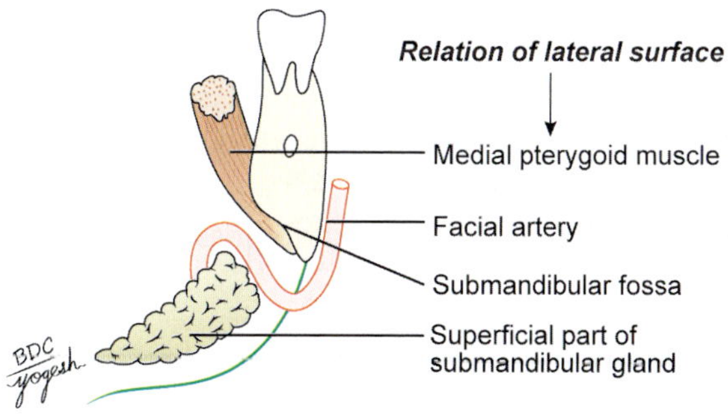


**Fig. 7.11:** Relationship of the lateral surface of the submandibular gland

**Relations** (Figs 7.10 to 7.12)

***Inferior or superficial surface:*** It is covered by:

1. Skin
2. Platysma
3. Cervical branch of the facial nerve
4. Investing fascia
5. Facial vein
6. Submandibular lymph nodes.

***Lateral surface:*** It is related to:

1. The submandibular fossa on the mandible
2. Insertion of the medial pterygoid
3. The facial artery.

***Medial surface:*** It is divided into three parts which are related to:

1. *Anterior part:* Mylohyoid, submental branch of facial artery, mylohyoid nerve and vessels

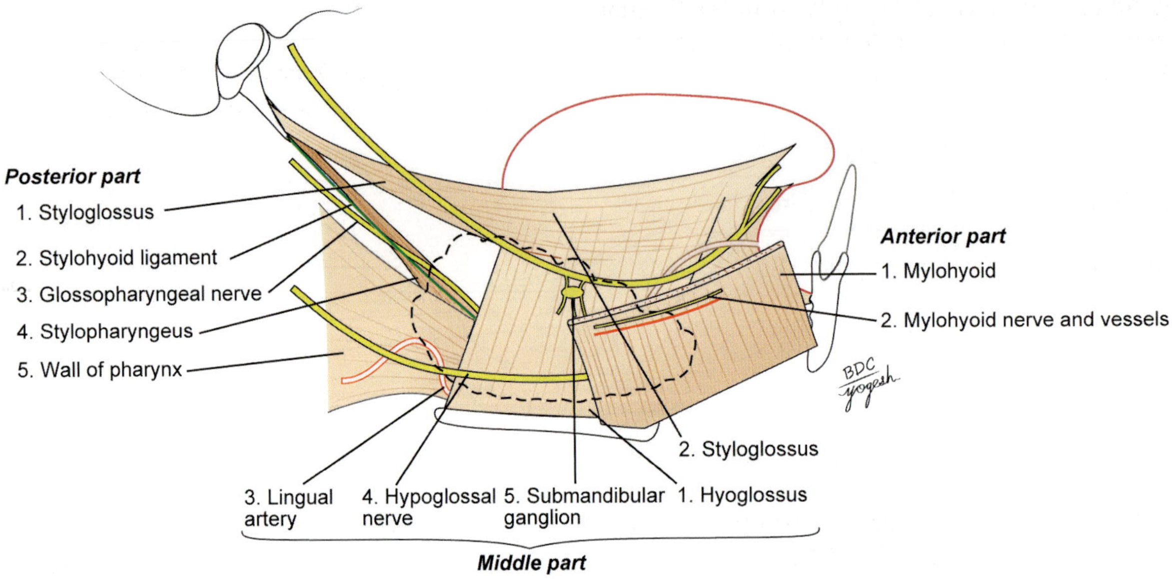


**Fig. 7.12:** Relations of the medial surface of submandibular gland

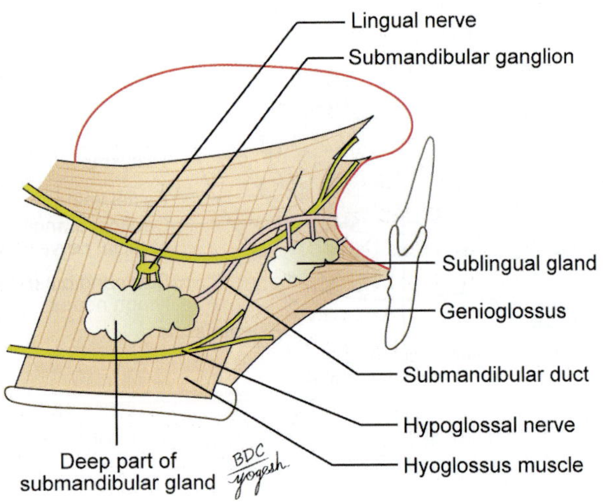


**Fig. 7.13:** Deep part of submandibular gland and sublingual gland

2. *Middle part:* Hyoglossus, styloglossus, lingual artery, XII nerve
3. *Posterior part:* Stylohyoid, styloglossus, IX nerve.

## Deep Part

This part is small in size. It lies deep to the mylohyoid and superficial to the hyoglossus and the styloglossus (Fig. 7.13). Posteriorly, it is continuous with the superficial part around the posterior border of the mylohyoid. Anteriorly, it extends up to the posterior end of the sublingual gland.

### Relations

Present in between mylohyoid and hyoglossus.

*Laterally:* Mylohyoid (removed)
*Medially:* Hyoglossus
*Above:* Lingual nerve with submandibular ganglion
*Below:* Hypoglossal nerve.

## Blood Supply and Lymphatic Drainage

The submandibular gland is supplied by the facial artery.

The veins drain into the common facial or lingual vein.

Lymph passes to submandibular lymph nodes.

## Nerve Supply (Fig. 7.14)

It is supplied by branches from the submandibular ganglion. These branches convey:

1. Secretomotor fibres
2. Sensory fibres from the lingual nerve
3. Vasomotor sympathetic fibres from the plexus on the facial artery.

The secretomotor pathway is shown in Flowchart 7.2.

## SUBMANDIBULAR DUCT/WHARTON'S DUCT

It is thin walled, and is about 5 cm long [Thomas Wharton, English anatomist, 1614–73. He also discovered Wharton's jelly of the umbilical cord].

It emerges at the anterior end of the deep part of the gland and runs upwards and forwards on the hyoglossus, between the lingual and hypoglossal nerves. At the anterior border of the hyoglossus, the duct is crossed by the lingual nerve (Fig. 7.2). It opens on the floor of the mouth, on the summit of the sublingual papilla, at the side of the frenulum of the tongue.

# SUBLINGUAL SALIVARY GLAND

This is the smallest of the three salivary glands. It is almond-shaped and weighs about 3 to 4 g. It lies above the mylohyoid, below the mucosa of the floor of the mouth, medial to the sublingual fossa of the mandible and lateral to the genioglossus (Fig. 7.13).

***Ducts:*** About 15 ducts emerge from the gland. Most of them open directly into the floor of the mouth on the summit of the sublingual fold. A few of them join the submandibular duct (*see* Fig. 17.2).

The gland receives its blood supply from the lingual and submental arteries. The nerve supply is similar to that of the submandibular gland.

**DISSECTION**

Submandibular gland is seen in the digastric triangle. On pushing the superficial part of the gland posteriorly, the entire mylohyoid muscle is exposed. The deep part of the gland lies on the superior surface of the muscle. Separate the facial artery from the deep surface of gland and identify its branches in neck. The hyoglossus muscle is recognised as a quadrilateral muscle lying on deeper plane than mylohyoid muscle. Identify lingual nerve with submandibular ganglion, and hypoglossal nerve running on the hyoglossus muscle from lateral to the medial side. Deep part of gland and its duct are also visible on this surface of hyoglossus muscle (Fig. 7.4).

Carefully release the hyoglossus muscle from the hyoid bone and reflect it towards the tongue. Note the structures deep to the muscle, e.g. genioglossus muscle, lingual artery, vein and middle constrictor of the pharynx.

## SUBMANDIBULAR GANGLION

The submandibular ganglion is a peripheral parasympathetic ganglion [Langley's ganglion].

Neurological relationship (Fig. 7.14, Flowchart 7.2):

- *Topographic relation*: It is connected with the lingual branch of mandibular division of trigeminal nerve.
- *Functional relation*: Functionally, it is related to the facial nerve.

***Size:*** Size of pinhead.

***Location:*** It is located on the outer surface of the hyoglossus muscle. It is suspended from the lingual nerve by two roots. It lies deep to mylohyoid muscle.

### Relations

*Superior:* Lingual nerve
*Inferior:* Deep part of submandibular gland
*Superficial:* Mylohyoid muscle
*Deep:* Hyoglossus muscle

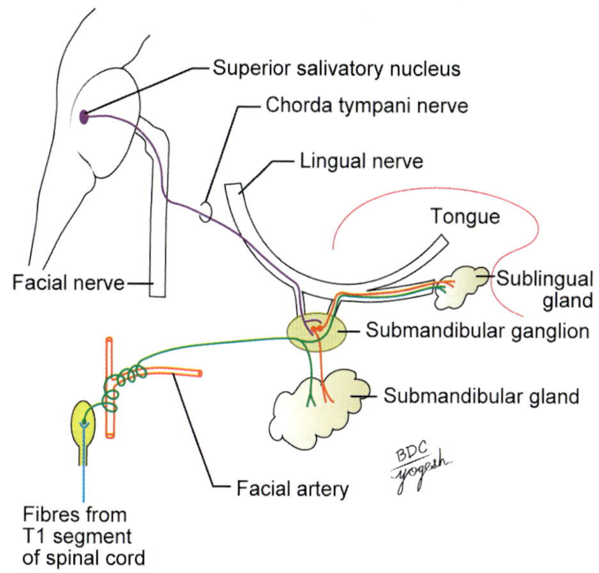


**Fig. 7.14:** Connection of the submandibular ganglion

***Roots*** *(connection and distribution)*

It has three roots as follows:

1. *Parasympathetic* or *secretomotor root*: It consists of pre- and postganglionic fibres as follows:
   a. *Preganglionic fibres* begin from the *superior salivatory nucleus* in the *pons* and pass through *facial nerve*. In the facial canal, these fibres join the *chorda tympani* branch of facial nerve, which traverses through middle ear and joins the *lingual nerve* in the infratemporal fossa. Further, these fibres reach the *submandibular ganglion* through the lingual nerve, and they relay in the ganglion.
   b. *Postganglionic fibres* from the cells of submandibular ganglion join the *lingual nerve* supply sublingual gland. Few fibres from the ganglion directly supply the submandibular gland.
2. *Sympathetic root*: The lateral horn cells of *T1 segment* of spinal cord give rise to the preganglionic sympathetic fibres. They traverse through T1 nerve, sympathetic chain and relay in *superior cervical sympathetic ganglion*. Postganglionic fibres reach the submandibular ganglion through a plexus around the facial artery and pass through this ganglion without relaying. They supply submandibular and sublingual glands.

**Flowchart 7.2:** Submandibular ganglion

***Submandibular ganglion***
Peripheral parasympathetic ganglion

***Neurological relation***
Topographic:
Lingual nerve
Functional:
Facial nerve
Pinhead size
Lies on hyoglossus muscle

***Roots***

***Parasympathetic***
Superior salivatory nucleus
→ Facial nerve → Chorda tympani
→ Lingual nerve → s/m ganglion
→ Postganglionic fibres
→ Submandibular and sublingual glands

***Sympathetic***
Lateral horn cells of T1
→ Superior cervical ganglion
→ Relay
→ Plexus around facial artery
→ Submandibular ganglion
→ Submandibular and sublingual glands

***Sensory***
Fibres from lingual nerve

3. *Sensory root*: The sensory fibres from the lingual nerve pass through the submandibular ganglion without relaying.

### Function

The fibres from the submandibular ganglion supply the submandibular and sublingual glands as follows:

1. Parasympathetic fibres — secretomotor
2. Sympathetic fibres — vasomotor
3. Sensory fibres — carry sensation.

## HISTOLOGY

### Histology of Submandibular Gland

1. Submandibular gland is mixed salivary gland. It has a well-defined capsule. Septa arising from capsule divide the gland into number of lobes and lobules (Plate 7.2).
2. *Acini*: Gland shows presence of both serous and mucous acini. Few mucous acini also show serous demilunes.
3. *Ducts*: Gland has lobar, interlobular, and intralobular (striated and intercalated) ducts. Intercalated ducts are less in number than in the parotid gland.

### Histology of Sublingual Gland

1. Sublingual gland is not surrounded by well-defined capsule. Intercalated ducts are less in number than in the parotid gland (Plate 7.3).
2. *Acini*: Sublingual gland predominantly has *mucous acini*. Few serous and seromucous acini are also present. Mucous secretory units are tubular (not purely acinar).
3. *Ducts*: Sublingual gland do not have intercalated duct (rarely present), and striated ducts are also very few. Interlobular and lobar ducts are present.

Comparison of the three salivary glands is given in Table 7.3.

## DEVELOPMENT

1. The submandibular and sublingual glands develop as an endodermal outgrowth from the floor of the mouth at alveologingival sulcus.
2. The submandibular gland arises as a single large bud which branches and develops to form submandibular duct and gland.
3. The sublingual gland arises as multiple small buds that form the gland with multiple ducts.

*Competency:*
AN34.3 Describe the basis of formation of submandibular stones.

## CLINICAL ANATOMY

- ***Ranula*** is a cystic swelling in the floor of mouth due to obstruction of sublingual salivary gland. It results in mucus retention. It looks like the belly of frog (Rana hexadactyla), hence called ranula. It is a soft, bluish swelling.
- ***Injury to spine of sphenoid*** may involve both chorda tympani and auriculotemporal nerves and results into loss of secretion from all three salivary glands.
- Submandibular lymph nodes lie both within and outside the submandibular salivary gland. The gland is to be removed, if lymph nodes are affected in many diseases especially carcinoma of tongue. Cancer of the tongue or of the gland may metastasise into the mandible also.
- ***Palpation of submandibular gland***: It can be palpated bimanually by putting one finger within the mouth and one outside (Fig. 7.15).
- ***Calculi or stones in submandibular duct***: The stone is more common in the submandibular duct than the parotid duct because of:
  1. The thick secretions of submandibular gland

**TABLE 7.3: Comparison of the three salivary glands**

| | *Parotid* | *Submandibular* | *Sublingual* |
|---|---|---|---|
| Location | In relation to external ear, angle of mandible, mastoid process | Lies in submandibular fossa close to angle of mandible | Lies in sublingual fossa on the base of the mandible |
| Size | Largest | Medium sized | Smallest |
| Relation to fascia | Enclosed by investing layer of cervical fascia | Enclosed by investing layer of cervical fascia | Not enclosed |
| Type of gland | Purely serous secreting | Mixed, both serous and mucus secreting | Purely mucus secreting |
| Gross features | Comprises 3 surfaces, 3 borders, apex and base, 1 artery, 1 vein, 1 nerve and lymph nodes lie within the gland | Comprises 3 surfaces, inferior, lateral and medial. 1 artery indents the posterior end of the gland. Only lymph nodes lie within it | Related closely to lingual nerve and submandibular duct |
| Secretomotor root | From IX cranial nerve | From VII cranial nerve | From VII cranial nerve |
| Sympathetic root | Plexus around middle meningeal artery | Plexus around facial artery | Same as submandibular gland |
| Sensory | Auriculotemporal nerve | Lingual nerve | Lingual nerve |
| Development | Ectoderm | Endoderm | Endoderm |
| Opening of the duct | Vestibule of mouth opposite 2nd upper molar tooth | Papilla on sublingual fold in the floor of the mouth | 10–12 ducts open on sublingual fold in the floor of the mouth |

**Plate 7.2:** Histology of submandibular gland

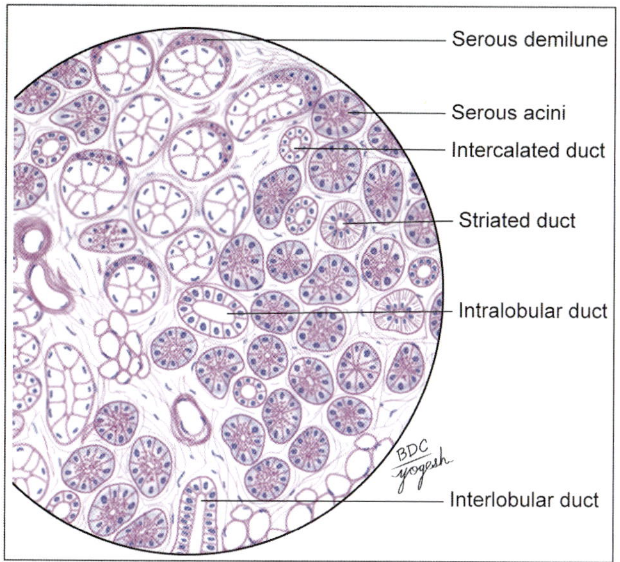


**Plate 7.3:** Histology of sublingual gland

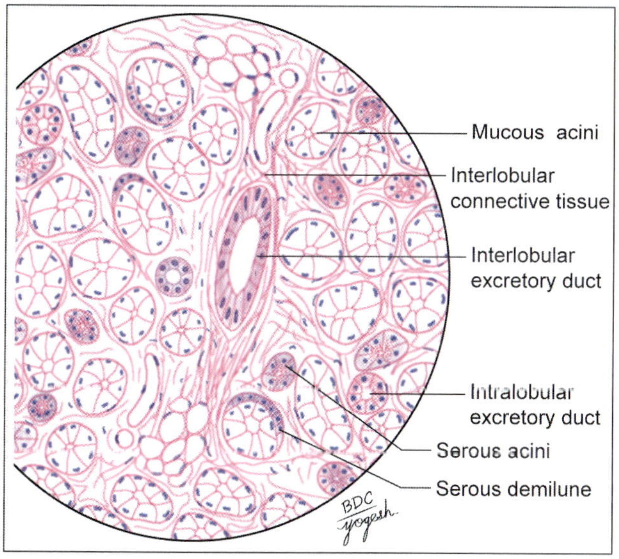


2. Tortuous and antigravity (upwards) course of the submandibular duct.

- The stone of the submandibular gland can be palpated or detected radiologically. It may require surgical removal.

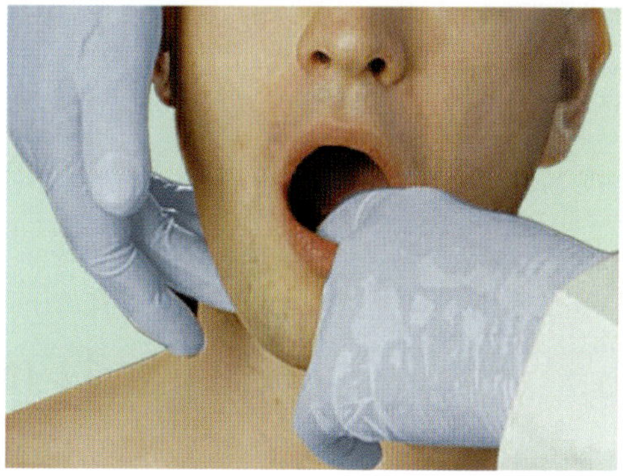

**Fig. 7.15:** Bimanual palpation of submandibular gland and lymph nodes

VIDEO

**Video 3.7 Submandibular Salivary Gland**

### *Facts to Remember*

- Chorda tympani nerve carries secretomotor fibres to the submandibular ganglion. It also carries taste from most of the anterior two-thirds of the tongue.
- The submandibular lymph nodes are also present in the submandibular gland. In cancer of the tongue, this gland is also excised to get rid off the lymph nodes with secondaries from the tongue.
- Facial artery is tortuous to accommodate to the movements of pharynx. It is the chief artery of the palatine tonsil. Its course is S-shaped.
- Suprahyoid muscles are disposed in four layers:
  - 1st layer: Digastric and stylohyoid
  - 2nd layer: Mylohyoid
  - 3rd layer: Geniohyoid and hyoglossus
  - 4th layer: Genioglossus

### BDC's Anatomy *e*-book

1. Relation of marginal mandibular branch of facial nerve
2. Relations of sublingual gland
3. Further reading
4. Viva voce questions

Chapter

# 8

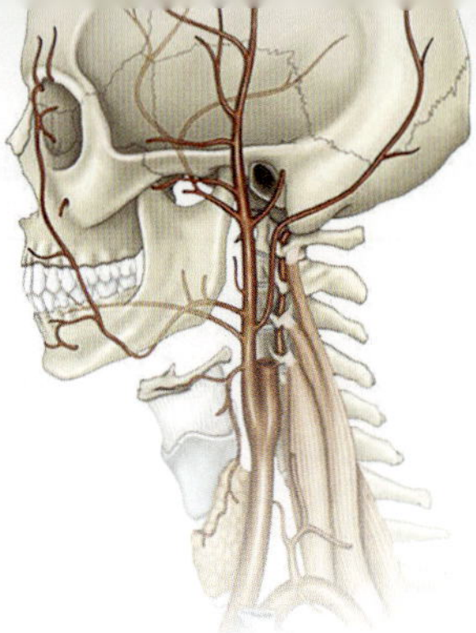

# Structures in the Neck

There are numerous structures in the neck. For convenience, they may be grouped as follows:

1. *Glands:* Thyroid and parathyroid
2. *Thymus:* Involutes at puberty
3. *Arteries:* Subclavian and carotid
4. *Veins:* Subclavian, internal jugular and brachiocephalic
5. *Nerves:* Glossopharyngeal, vagus, accessory and hypoglossal
6. *Sympathetic trunk:* It has three cervical ganglia
7. Lymph nodes and thoracic duct
8. Styloid apparatus.

***Competency:***
**AN35.2** Describe and demonstrate location, parts, borders, surfaces, relations and blood supply and applied anatomy of thyroid gland. Also describe the parathyroid glands in brief.

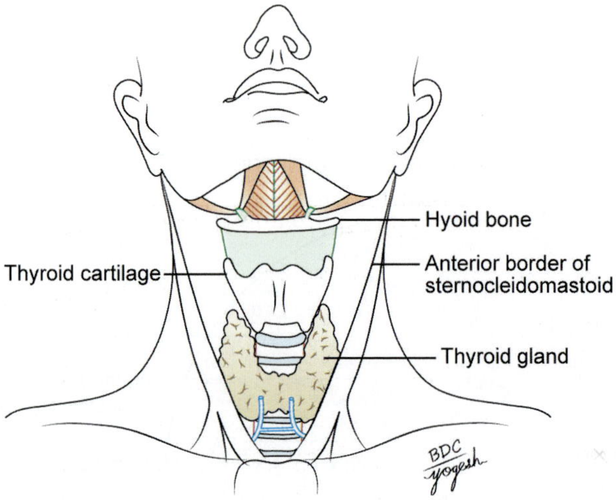


**Fig. 8.1:** Position of thyroid gland

## THYROID GLAND

The thyroid (shield-like, Greek) is an endocrine gland with a rich blood supply situated in the lower part of the front and sides of the neck. Since, it is placed superficially, it can easily be examined (Figs 8.1 and 8.2, Flowchart 8.1).

### Functions

1. It secretes tri-iodothyronine (T3), tetra-iodothyronine (T4), or thyroxine and calcitonin.
2. It regulates the basal metabolic rate.
3. It promotes the psychosomatic growth of the body.
4. It modulates the calcium metabolism.

### Parts of Thyroid Gland (Fig. 8.2)

The gland is H-shaped and consists of the following parts:

1. Two lobes — right and left
2. *Isthmus* — connects both lobes
3. Pyramidal lobe — may project upwards from the isthmus (or from one of the lobes).

*Note:* ***Levator glandulae thyroideae*** is a fibrous or fibromuscular band that is sometimes present and connects the pyramidal lobe to the body of the hyoid bone.

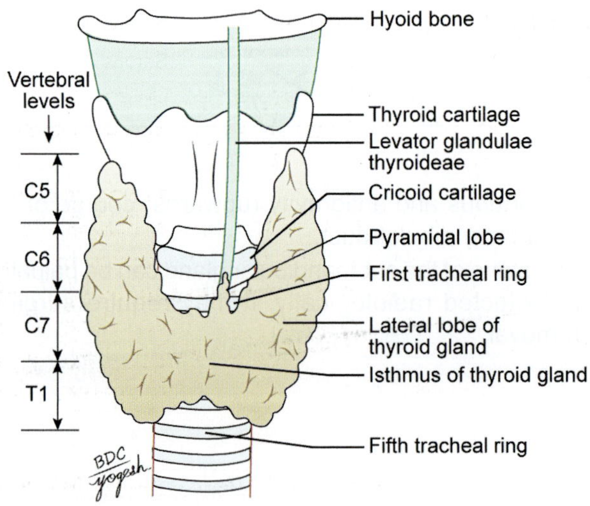


**Fig. 8.2:** Parts and extent of the thyroid gland

### Location and Extent (Fig. 8.1)

1. The gland lies against vertebrae C5–C7 and T1, embracing the upper part of the trachea (Fig. 8.1).
2. Each *lobe* extends from the middle of thyroid cartilage to the 4th or 5th tracheal rings. The lobe is prevented

**Flowchart 8.1:** Thyroid gland

***Features of thyroid gland***

- ***Parts***: Two lobes; Isthmus; Pyramidal lobe
- ***Location***: In neck: C5–C7, T1 level; Extent: From oblique line of thyroid cartilage to 5th tracheal ring
- ***Dimensions***: Weight: 25 g; Lobe 5 x 2 x 2 cm; Isthmus: 1.25 x 1.25 cm
- ***Capsules***: Inner true capsule; Outer false capsule; Capillary plexus lies deep to true capsule

***Blood supply of thyroid gland***

- ***Arteries***: Superior thyroid; Inferior thyroid; Thyroidea ima artery; Accessory thyroid arteries
- ***Venous drainage***: Superior thyroid → IJV; Middle thyroid → IJV; Inferior thyroid → Brachiocephalic vein; Fourth thyroid (Kocher's) → IJV

***Lobe of thyroid gland***

- ***Apex***: Directed upward; Lies between sternothyroid and inferior constrictor
- ***Base***: Extends up to 5th tracheal ring; Closely related to inferior thyroid artery and recurrent laryngeal nerve
- ***Surfaces***
  - ***Lateral***: Convex; Covered by SCM; Sternohyoid; Superior belly of omohyoid; Sternothyroid
  - ***Medial***: Related to: Trachea, oesophagus; Inferior constrictor; Cricothyroid; Cricoid and thyroid cartilages; External laryngeal and recurrent laryngeal nerves
  - ***Posterolateral***: Related to: Carotid sheath
- ***Borders***
  - ***Anterior***: Thin; Related to: Anterior branches of superior thyroid artery
  - ***Posterior***: Rounded; Related to: Inferior thyroid artery; Arterial anastomosis; Parathyroid glands; Thoracic duct (on left)

(IJV: Internal jugular vein, SCM: Sternocleidomastoid)

from ascending by thyrohyoid muscle. It is prevented from descending down by *ligament of Berry*.

3. The *isthmus* extends from the 2nd to the 4th tracheal ring.

## Dimensions and Weight

Each lobe measures about 5 × 2.5 × 2.5 cm and the isthmus 1.2 × 1.2 cm. On average, the gland weighs about 25 g.

*Note*: The thyroid gland is larger in females than in males, and further increases in size during menstruation and pregnancy.

## Capsules of Thyroid (Figs 8.3a and b)

The thyroid gland has two capsules: Inner true capsule and outer false capsule:

1. ***True capsule:*** It is the peripheral condensation of the connective tissue of the gland.
2. ***False capsule:*** It is derived from the pretracheal layer of the deep cervical fascia.

   ***Features of false capsule***

   a. It is thin along the posterior border of the lateral lobe.

   b. It is thicker on the medial surface of the lateral lobe.

   c. *Suspensory ligament of Berry*: It is a thickened part of pretracheal fascia (false capsule) that connects the lobes of thyroid gland with the cricoid cartilage.

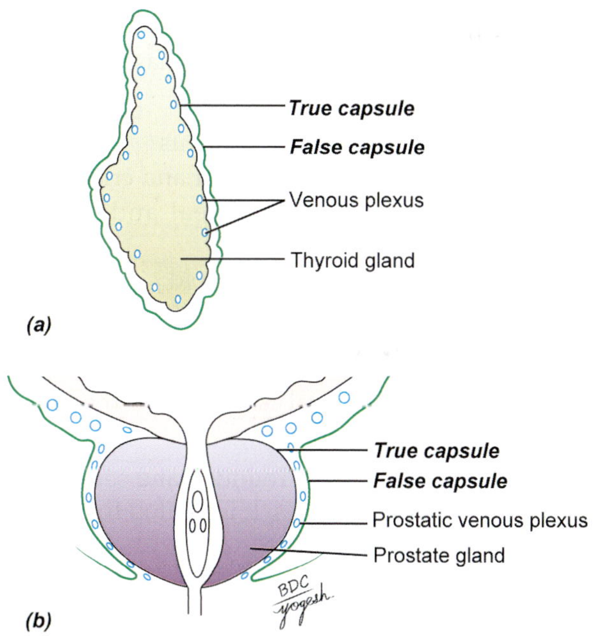


**Figs 8.3a and b:** Schemes of comparing the relationship of the venous plexuses related to (a) The thyroid gland and (b) the prostate, with the true and false capsules around these organs. Note the plane of cleavage along which the organ is separated from neighbouring structures during surgical removal

## CLINICAL ANATOMY

- A dense capillary plexus is present deep to the true capsule. To avoid haemorrhage during operations, the thyroid is removed along with the true capsule. It can be compared with the prostate in which the venous plexus lies between the two capsules of the gland, and therefore, during prostatectomy, both capsules are left behind (Figs 8.3a and b).
- In prostatic surgeries, the venous plexus lies between two capsules. Hence, the prostate should be removed, leaving behind both capsules.
- As the capsule of the thyroid gland is thin along the posterior border, its swelling more commonly extends backward rather than forming a visible swelling in the neck.
- ***Swallowing and thyroid movements***: The thyroid moves up and down during swallowing as it is attached to the cricoid cartilage by the ligament of Berry.

### Parts and Relations of Lobes

The lobes are conical in shape having (Figs 8.4 and 8.5):

a. Apex
b. Base
c. Three surfaces: Lateral, medial and posterolateral
d. Two borders: Anterior and posterior.

***Apex***

It is directed upwards and slightly laterally.

It is limited superiorly by the attachment of the sternothyroid muscle to the oblique line of thyroid cartilage which is medial to the apex. Thus it lies between inferior constrictor and sternothyroid muscles. The apex is related to superior thyroid artery and the external laryngeal nerve.

***Base***

It is at level with the 4th or 5th tracheal ring.

It is related to inferior thyroid artery and recurrent laryngeal nerve.

***Lateral or superficial surface*** is convex, and is covered by:

a. Sternohyoid
b. Superior belly of omohyoid
c. Sternothyroid
d. Anterior border of the sternocleidomastoid.

***Medial surface*** is related to:

a. Two tubes—trachea and oesophagus
b. Two muscles—inferior constrictor and cricothyroid
c. Two nerves—external laryngeal and recurrent laryngeal
d. Two cartilages—thyroid and cricoid.

***Posterolateral surface*** is related to the carotid sheath and overlaps the common carotid artery.

***Anterior border*** is thin and is related to the anterior branch of superior thyroid artery

***Posterior border*** is thick and rounded and separates the medial and posterior surfaces. It is related to:

a. Inferior thyroid artery
b. Anastomosis between the posterior branch of superior and ascending branch of inferior thyroid arteries
c. Parathyroid glands
d. Thoracic duct only on the left side.

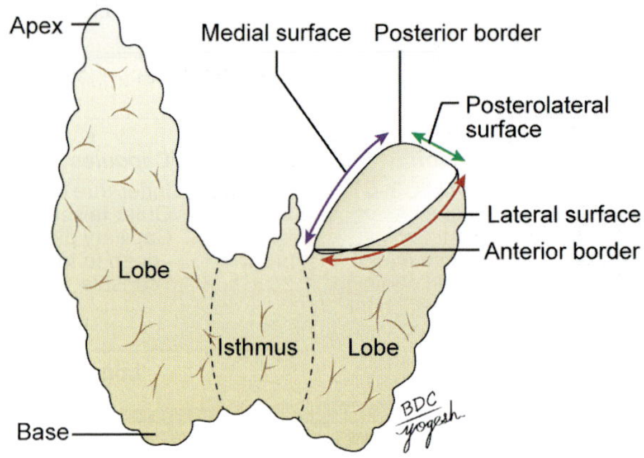


**Fig. 8.4:** Parts of lobes of the thyroid gland

### Parts and Relations of Isthmus

*Isthmus* connects the lower parts of the two lobes (Figs 8.5 and 8.6).

It has:

*Two surfaces*: Anterior and posterior

*Two borders*: Superior and inferior.

- *Anterior surface* is covered by:
  a. Right and left sternothyroid and sternohyoid muscles
  b. Anterior jugular veins
  c. Fascia and skin.
- *Posterior surface* is related to the 2nd to 4th tracheal rings.
- *Upper border* is related to anterior branches of the right and left superior thyroid arteries which anastomose here.
- *Lower border:* Inferior thyroid veins leave the gland at this border.

### Arterial Supply

The thyroid gland is supplied by the superior and inferior thyroid arteries (Figs 8.6 to 8.8).

1. ***Superior thyroid artery*** is the 1st anterior branch of the external carotid artery. It runs downwards and forwards in intimate relation to the external laryngeal nerve. After giving branches to adjacent structures, the artery pierces the pretracheal fascia to reach the apex of the lobe where the nerve deviates medially.

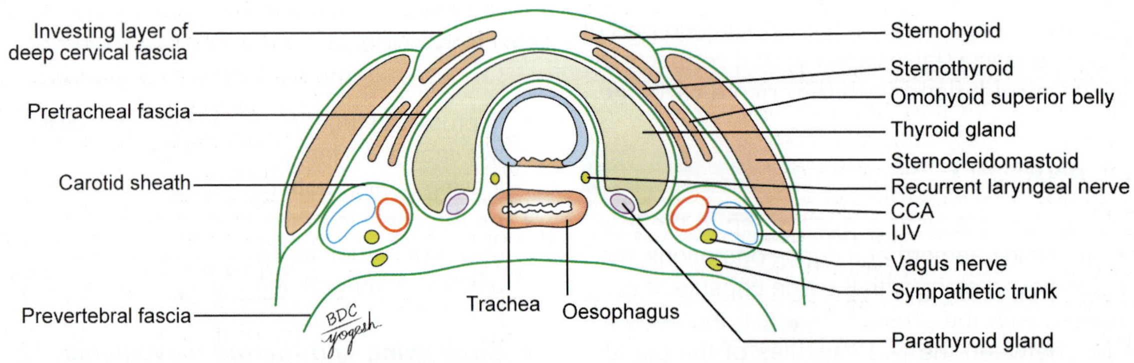


**Fig. 8.5:** Relations of thyroid gland (transverse section of the anterior part of the neck at the level of thyroid isthmus, inferior view. CCA: Common carotid artery, IJV: Internal jugular vein)

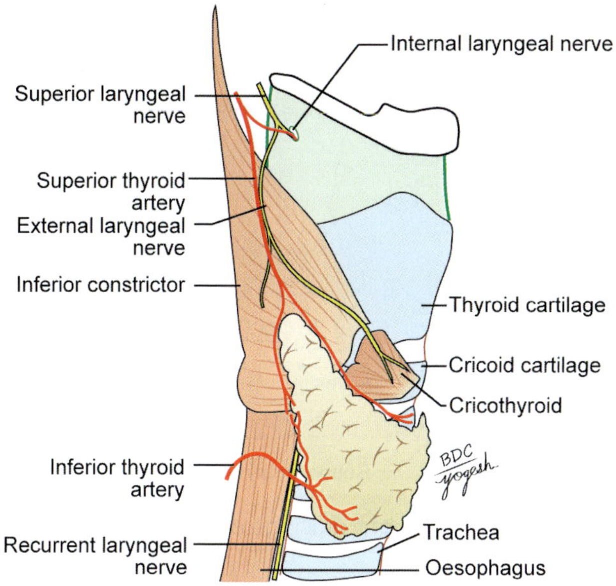


**Fig. 8.6:** Deep relations of the thyroid gland

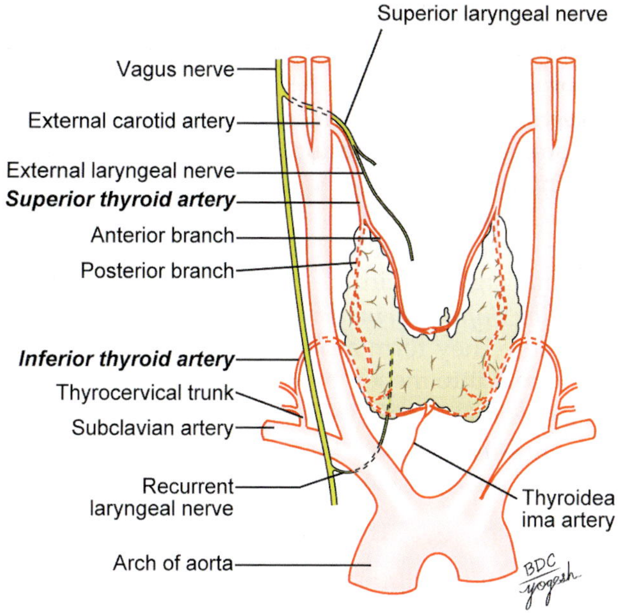


**Fig. 8.7:** Arterial supply of anterior aspect of thyroid gland

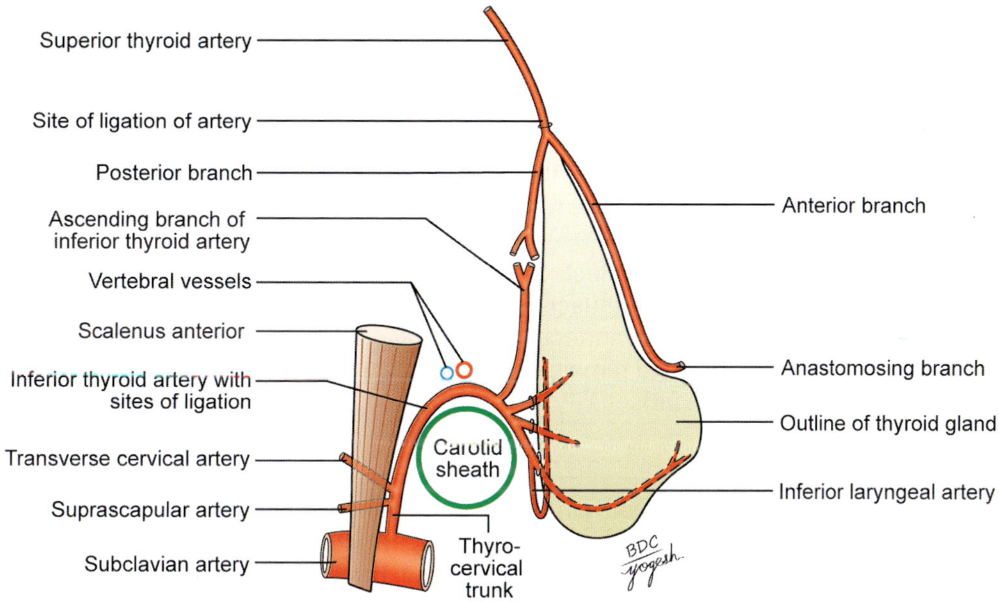


**Fig. 8.8:** Arterial supply of the surfaces of thyroid gland. Sites of ligatures of the superior and inferior thyroid arteries are shown

At the upper pole, the artery divides into anterior and posterior branches.

a. The ***anterior branch*** descends on the anterior border of the lobe and continues along the upper border of the isthmus to anastomose with its counterpart on the opposite side.
b. The ***posterior branch*** descends on the posterior border of the lobe and anastomoses with the ascending branch of inferior thyroid artery.

2. ***Inferior thyroid artery*** is a branch of thyrocervical trunk (which arises from the subclavian artery). It runs first upwards, then medially, and finally downwards to reach the base of the gland. It gives off branches to adjacent structures. Its terminal part is intimately related to the recurrent laryngeal nerve, while proximal part is away from the nerve.

   The artery divides into ***4 to 5 glandular branches*** which pierce the fascia separately to reach the lower part of the gland. One ***ascending branch*** anastomoses with the posterior branch of the superior thyroid artery and supplies the parathyroid glands.
3. Sometimes (in 3% of individuals), the thyroid is also supplied by the ***lowest thyroid artery (thyroidea ima artery)*** which arises from the brachiocephalic trunk or directly from the arch of the aorta. It enters the lower part of the isthmus.
4. ***Accessory thyroid arteries*** arising from tracheal and oesophageal arteries also supply the thyroid.

### Venous Drainage

The thyroid is drained by the superior, middle and inferior thyroid veins (Fig. 8.9).

1. ***Superior thyroid vein*** emerges at the upper pole and accompanies the superior thyroid artery. It ends in the internal jugular vein.
2. ***Middle thyroid vein*** is a short, wide channel that emerges at the middle of the lobe and soon enters the internal jugular vein.
3. ***Inferior thyroid veins*** emerge at the lower border of isthmus. They form a plexus in front of the trachea and drain into the left brachiocephalic vein.
4. ***Fourth thyroid vein*** **(Kocher)** may emerge between the middle and inferior veins, and drain into the internal jugular vein.

### Lymphatic Drainage

Lymph from the upper part of the gland reaches the upper deep cervical lymph nodes either directly or through the prelaryngeal nodes. Lymph from the lower part of the gland drains to the lower deep cervical nodes directly, and also through the pretracheal and paratracheal nodes (Fig. 8.10).

### Nerve Supply

Nerves are derived mainly from the middle cervical ganglion and partly from the superior and inferior cervical ganglia. These are vasoconstrictor.

#### DISSECTION

Sternocleidomastoid muscle has already been reflected laterally from its origin. Cut the sternothyroid muscle near its origin and reflect it upwards. Clean the surface of trachea and identify inferior thyroid vein and remains of the thymus gland (darker in colour than fat).

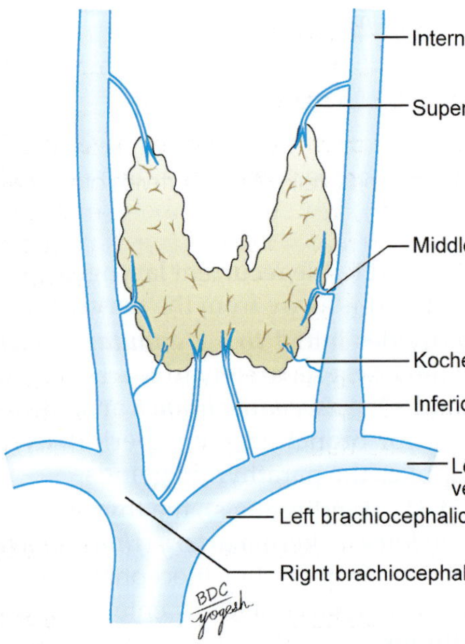


**Fig. 8.9:** Venous drainage and lymphatic drainage of the thyroid gland. Deep cervical lymph nodes are also shown

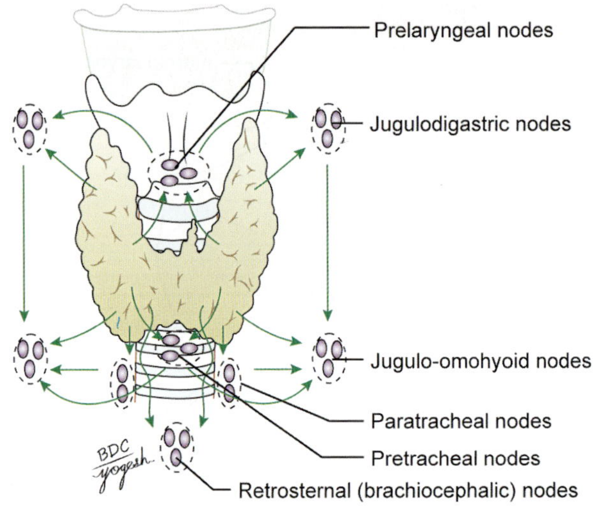


**Fig. 8.10:** Lymphatic drainage of the thyroid gland

Isthmus of the thyroid gland lies on the 2nd–4th tracheal rings. Pyramidal lobe, if present, projects from the upper border of the isthmus. On each side of isthmus is the lateral lobe of the gland. Clean the lobes and identify the vessels of thyroid gland. Identify the recurrent laryngeal nerves tucked between the lateral surfaces of trachea and oesophagus. Look for beaded thoracic duct present on the left of oesophagus. Trace the superior and inferior thyroid arteries. Identify cricothyroid and inferior constrictor muscles lying medial to the lobes of thyroid gland (Figs 8.1 to 8.6).

***Thyroid gland (butterfly shaped)***

Cut the isthmus of the thyroid gland and turn one of the lobes laterally. Locate an anastomosis between the posterior branch of superior thyroid and ascending branch of inferior thyroid arteries supplying the gland. Identify the two parathyroid glands on the sides of this anastomotic vessel (Figs 8.7 and 8.12).

*Competency:*

**AN35.8** Describe the anatomically relevant clinical features of thyroid swellings.

#### CLINICAL ANATOMY

- Any swelling of the thyroid gland (***goitre)*** should be palpated from behind (Figs 8.11 and 8.12).
- Removal of the thyroid (***thyroidectomy***) with true capsule may be necessary in hyperthyroidism.
- In subtotal thyroidectomy, the posterior parts of both lobes are left behind. This avoids the risk of simultaneous removal of the parathyroids and also of postoperative myxoedema (caused by deficiency of thyroid hormones).
- During thyroidectomy, the superior thyroid artery is ligated near the gland to save the external laryngeal nerve. The stem of inferior thyroid artery is not ligated (Fig. 8.7). Its glandular branches are ligated

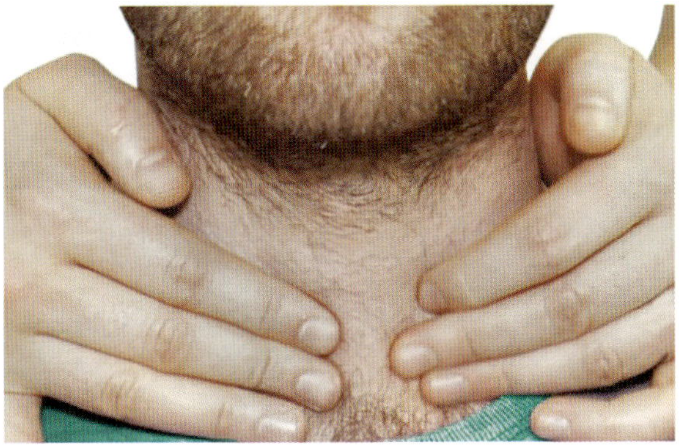

Fig. 8.11: Palpation of thyroid gland from behind

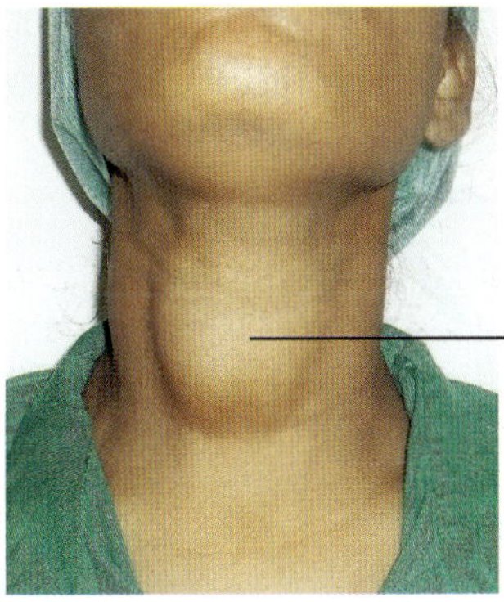


Fig. 8.12: Goitre (*Image Courtesy*: Dr Uday Kumbhar)

separately. In this way, blood supply to parathyroid glands is maintained.

- ***Hypothyroidism*** causes cretinism in infants and myxoedema in adults.
- Benign ***tumours*** of the gland may displace and even compress neighbouring structures such as:
  a. Trachea — causing dyspnoea (difficulty in breathing)
  b. Oesophagus — causing dysphagia (difficulty in swallowing)
  c. Recurrent laryngeal nerve — dysphonia (hoarseness of voice).

***Competency:***

**AN43.2** Identify, describe and draw the microanatomy of pituitary gland, thyroid, parathyroid gland, tongue, salivary glands, tonsil, cornea, retina.

Microanatomy of thyroid and parathyroid glands is described in this chapter. Rest of the tissues/glands are described in appropriate chapters.

## Histology of Thyroid Gland (Plate 8.1)

- Thyroid gland is covered by thin connective tissue capsule. Septa arising from capsule divide the gland into number of lobules.
- Thyroid gland is made up of ***follicles*** lined by simple cuboidal epithelium (ranges from squamous to low columnar) with rounded nuclei.
- Lumen of follicle contains pink homogeneous ***colloid*** material that consists of thyroglobulin.

**Plate 8.1:** Histology of thyroid gland

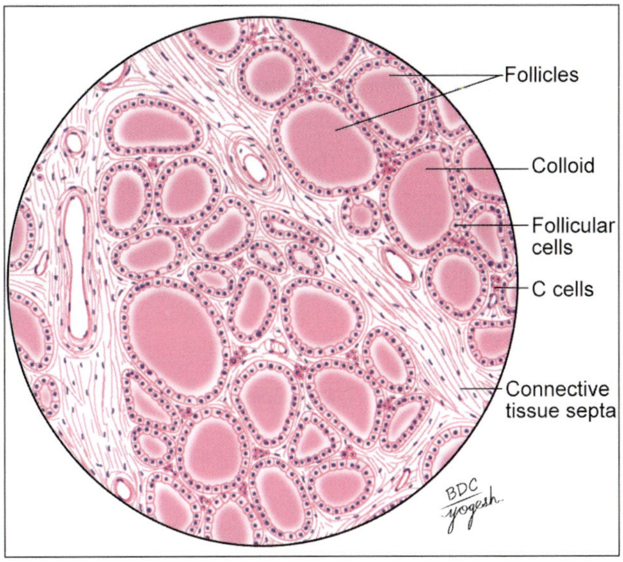


- Few ***parafollicular/C-cells*** are present in relation to follicles. C-cells secrete calcitonin that reduces blood calcium levels.
- In between follicles, rich vascular connective tissue is present.

***Competency:***

**AN43.4** Describe the development and developmental basis of congenital anomalies of face, palate, tongue, branchial apparatus, pituitary gland, thyroid gland and eye.

Development of thyroid gland is described in this chapter. For development of rest of the organs, please refer to appropriate chapters.

## Development of Thyroid Gland

Thyroid gland develops from the following two sources (Fig 8.13):

A. Follicles from thyroglossal duct.
B. Parafollicular cells from ultimobranchial body (a part of caudal pharyngeal complex).

On the floor of the primitive pharynx, over the first arch in the midline, there is a swelling called *tuberculum impar*. By the 24th day, just behind tuberculum impar, pharyngeal epithelium forms a depression (endodermal diverticulum) called *thyroglossal duct*. The opening of thyroglossal duct in the pharynx is represented by the *foramen caecum*.

By the end of the third month (12th week), follicular cells start producing thyroid hormones. The thyroid gland is the first gland that develops after fertilisation.

### *Anomalies of Thyroid Gland*

1. Sometimes, isthmus or one lobe of the thyroid gland may be absent or small.
2. *Anomalies of location*: The thyroid gland may lie at any position at the passage of thyroglossal duct. It may be lingual, intralingual, suprahyoid, or infrahyoid thyroid gland (Fig. 8.14).

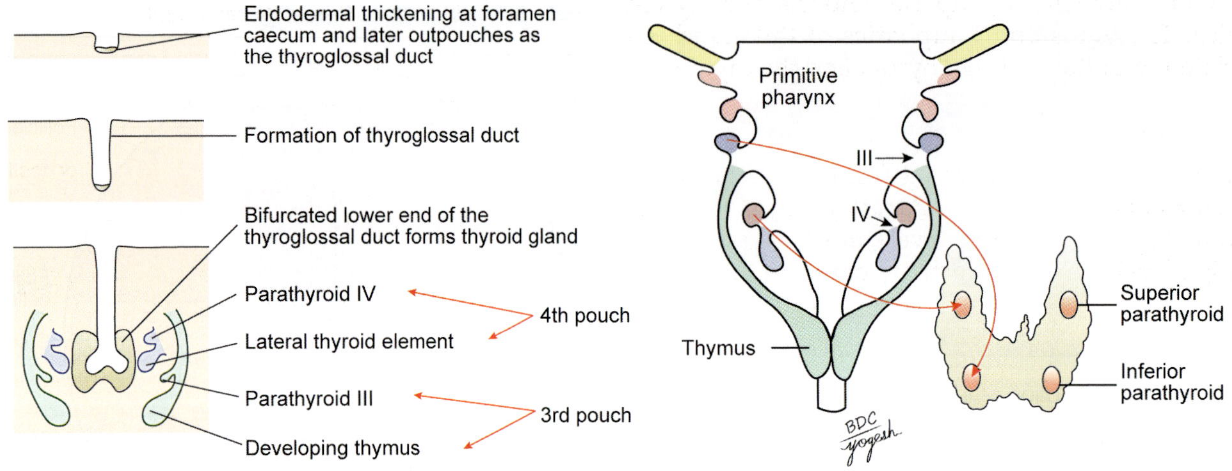


**Fig. 8.13:** Development of thyroid, parathyroid and thymus glands. Parathyroids are placed posteriorly

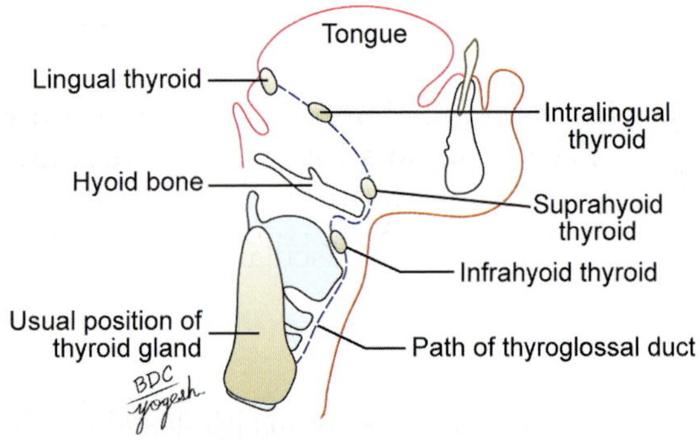


**Fig. 8.14:** Anomalies of the position of the thyroid gland and locations of the thyroglossal cyst

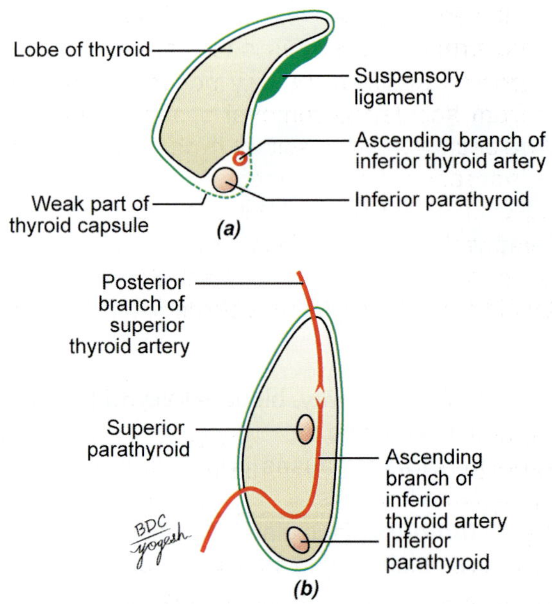


**Figs 8.15a and b:** Schemes to show the location of the parathyroid glands: (a) The left lobe of the thyroid gland and (b) posterior view of the left lobe of the thyroid gland

3. *Ectopic thyroid tissue*: Ectopic thyroid is the presence of thyroid tissue in locations other than usual (normal) thyroid gland locations. It is mostly found in larynx, trachea, oesophagus, pericardium and ovaries.

## PARATHYROID GLANDS

Parathyroid glands are two pairs (superior and inferior) of small endocrine glands, that usually lie on the posterior border of the thyroid gland, within the false capsule (Figs 8.15a and b).

1. The *superior parathyroids* are also referred to as *parathyroid IV* because they develop from the endoderm of the *4th pharyngeal pouch.*
2. The *inferior parathyroids*, similarly, are also called *parathyroid III* because they develop from the *3rd pouch.*

The parathyroids secrete the hormone *parathormone* which controls the metabolism of calcium and phosphorus along with thyrocalcitonin.

Each parathyroid gland is oval or lentiform in shape, measuring 6 × 4 × 2 mm (the size of a split pea). Each gland weighs about 50 mg.

### Position

The *superior parathyroid* is more constant in position and usually lies in the middle of the posterior border of the lobe of the thyroid gland. It is usually dorsal to the recurrent laryngeal nerve.

The *inferior parathyroid* is more variable in position. It may lie:

1. Within the thyroid capsule, below the inferior thyroid artery and near the lower pole of the thyroid lobe.
2. Behind and outside the thyroid capsule, immediately below the inferior thyroid artery.
3. Within the substance of the lobe near its posterior border. It is usually ventral to the recurrent laryngeal nerve.

*Note*: The anastomosis between the branches of superior and inferior thyroid arteries is usually a good guide to the glands because they usually lie close to it.

### Vascular Supply

The parathyroid glands receive a rich blood supply from the inferior thyroid artery and from the anastomosis between the branches of superior and inferior thyroid arteries. The veins and lymphatics of the gland are associated with those of the thyroid and the thymus.

### Nerve Supply

Vasomotor nerves are derived from the middle and superior cervical ganglia. Parathyroid activity is controlled by blood calcium levels; low levels stimulate and high levels inhibit the activity of the glands.

## CLINICAL ANATOMY

- ***Tumours*** of the parathyroid glands lead to excessive secretion of parathormone (hyperparathyroidism). This leads to increased removal of calcium from bone, making them weak and liable to fracture. Calcium levels in blood increase (hypercalcaemia) and increased urinary excretion of calcium can lead to the formation of stones in the urinary tract.
- ***Hypoparathyroidism*** may occur spontaneously or from accidental removal of the glands during thyroidectomy. This results in hypocalcaemia leading to increased neuromuscular irritability causing muscular spasm and convulsions (tetany) (Fig. 8.16).
- Parathyroid glands are tough glands and will continue to function, if these are transplanted from an excised thyroid gland into the sternocleidomastoid muscle.

### Histology of Parathyroid Gland (Plate 8.2)

Parathyroid gland shows cords or sheets of cells separated by numerous capillaries.

- It shows two types of cells: (1) chief, and (2) oxyphil cells.
- *Chief cells* are more in number, small in size, and consist of a spherical nucleus with small amount of cytoplasm. They secrete PTH hormone.

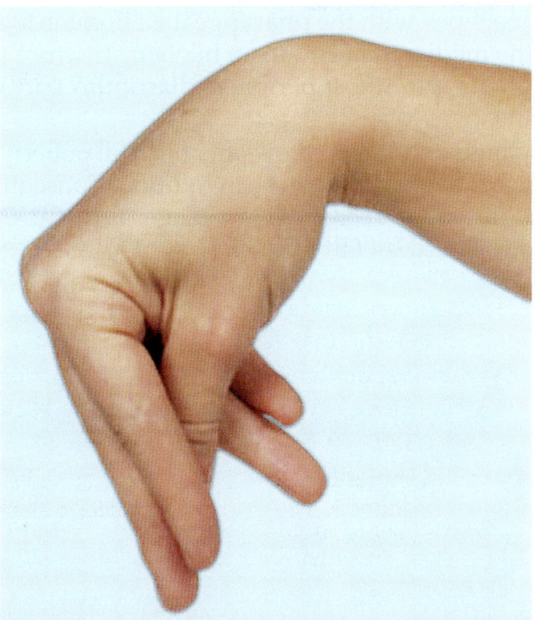

**Fig. 8.16:** Spasm in the hand due to tetany

**Plate 8.2:** Histology of the parathyroid gland

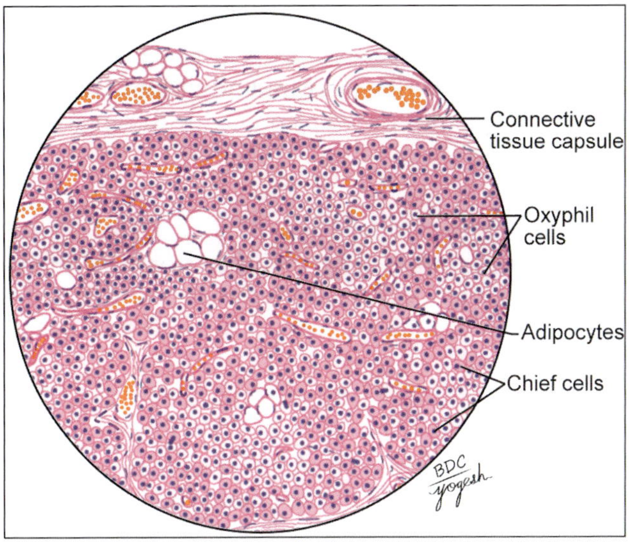


- *Oxyphil (eosinophilic) cells* are less in number, larger in size, and small intense-staining nucleus with eosinophilic cytoplasm. They do not secrete any hormones. Oxyphilic cells appear just before puberty.

### Development of Parathyroid Glands

***Inferior parathyroid glands:*** They are derived from the dorsal wing of the 3rd pharyngeal pouch.

- Primordia of the inferior parathyroids along with primordia of thymus lose their connection with the pharyngeal wall.
- The downward migrating thymus also pulls the inferior parathyroids with it, which finally come to rest on the inferior part of dorsal surface of the thyroid gland.

***Superior parathyroid glands:*** They are derived from the endoderm of 4th pharyngeal pouch.

- The primordia of superior parathyroid glands, after losing connection with the pharyngeal wall, come to rest on the superior part of dorsal surface of the thyroid gland.
- As mentioned above, because of downwards migration with the thymus, the parathyroid glands derived from 3rd pouch become inferiorly located as compared to those derived from the 4th pouch.

## THYMUS

The thymus (Greek *thyme leaf*) is an important lymphoid organ, situated in the anterior and superior mediastina of the thorax, extending above into the lower part of the neck. It is well developed at birth, continues to grow up to puberty, and thereafter, undergoes gradual atrophy and replacement by fat.

The thymus is a bilobed structure, made up of two pyramidal lobes of unequal size which are connected together by areolar tissue.

*Each lobe develops from the endoderm of the 3rd pharyngeal pouch.* It lies on the pericardium, the great vessels of the superior mediastinum, and the trachea.

The thymus weighs 10–15 g at birth, 30–40 g at puberty, and only 10 g after mid-adult life. Thus, after puberty, it becomes inconspicuous due to replacement by fat.

### Blood Supply

The thymus is supplied by branches from the internal thoracic and inferior thyroid arteries. Its veins drain into the left brachiocephalic, internal thoracic and inferior thyroid veins.

### Nerve Supply

Vasomotor nerves are derived from the stellate ganglion. The capsule is supplied by the phrenic nerve and by the descendens cervicalis.

### Functions

1. The thymus controls lymphopoiesis and maintains an effective pool of circulating lymphocytes, competent to react to innumerable antigenic stimuli.
2. It controls development of the peripheral lymphoid tissues of the body during the neonatal period. By puberty, the main lymphoid tissues are fully developed.
3. The cortical lymphocytes of the thymus arise from stem cells of bone marrow origin. Most (95%) of the lymphocytes (T lymphocytes) produced are autoallergic (act against the host or 'self' antigens), short-lived (3–5 days) and never move out of the organ. They are destroyed within the thymus by phagocytes. Their remnants are seen as Hassall's corpuscles.
4. The remaining 5% of the T lymphocytes are longlived (3 months or more), and move out of the thymus to join the circulating pool of lymphocytes where they act as immunologically competent but uncommitted cells, i.e. they can react to any unfamiliar, new antigen. On the other hand, the other circulating lymphocytes (from lymph nodes, spleen, etc.) are committed cells, i.e. they can mount an immune response only when exposed to a particular antigen. Thymic lymphopoiesis, lympholysis and involution are all intrinsically controlled.
5. The medullary epithelial cells of the thymus are thought to secrete:
   a. *Lymphopoietin,* which stimulates lymphocyte production both in the cortex of the thymus and in peripheral lymphoid organs.
   b. The *competence-inducing factor,* which may be responsible for making new lymphocytes competent to react to antigenic stimuli.
6. Normally, there are no germinal centres in the thymic cortex. Such centres appear in autoimmune diseases. This may indicate a defect in the normal function of the thymus.

## CLINICAL ANATOMY

- ***Involution*** of the thymus is enhanced by hypertrophy of the adrenal cortex, injection of cortisone or of androgenic hormone. The involution is delayed by castration and adrenalectomy.
- ***Thymic tumours*** may press on the trachea, oesophagus and the large veins of the neck, causing hoarseness, cough, dysphagia and cyanosis.
- ***Myasthenia gravis:*** It is a rare autoimmune disease. It is associated in 70% cases of thymoma (tumour of epithelioreticular cells). In myasthenia gravis, antibodies slowly destroy cholinergic receptors from skeletal muscle and cause weakness of muscles. It results in double vision (eye muscles), drooping of eyelid, dysarthria (muscles of throat), and so on (Fig. 8.17).

### Histology of Thymus (Plate 8.3)

1. The thymus is surrounded by a thin connective tissue capsule. Thymus is divided into number of incomplete lobules by septa arising from capsule.
2. The thymus has outer darkly stained ***cortex*** and inner lightly stained ***medulla***. Medulla of adjacent lobules is continuous with each other.
3. Medulla shows ***Hassall's corpuscles***: A central pink hyalinised material surrounded by type VI epithelioreticular cells.
4. Epithelioreticular cells (type I-VI): Form meshwork, form blood–thymic barrier, and secrete thymosin and thymopoietin.

### Development of Thymus

- Thymus develops from the endoderm of the ventral wing of the third pharyngeal pouch and from the mesenchyme into which the epithelial tubes grow.
- The bilateral primordia of the thymus lose their connections with the pharyngeal wall, come together in the median plane to form bilobed structure which migrates into the superior mediastinum part of the thoracic cavity.
- Thymus continues to grow after birth till puberty, after which it begins to undergo involution. Consequently, it is difficult to recognise in old age, as it is atrophied and replaced by fatty tissue.

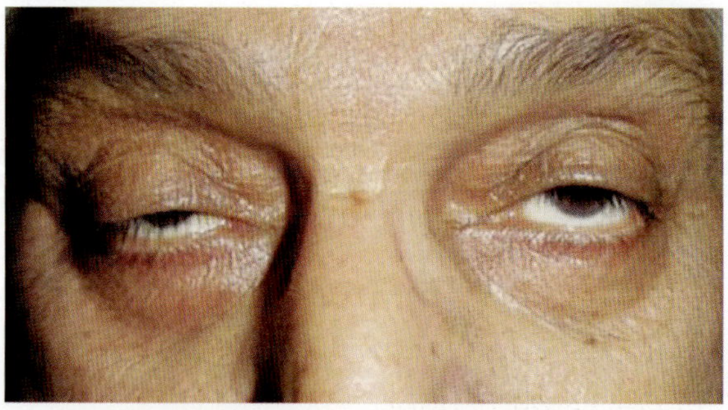

**Fig. 8.17:** Myasthenia gravis

**Plate 8.3:** Histology of thymus

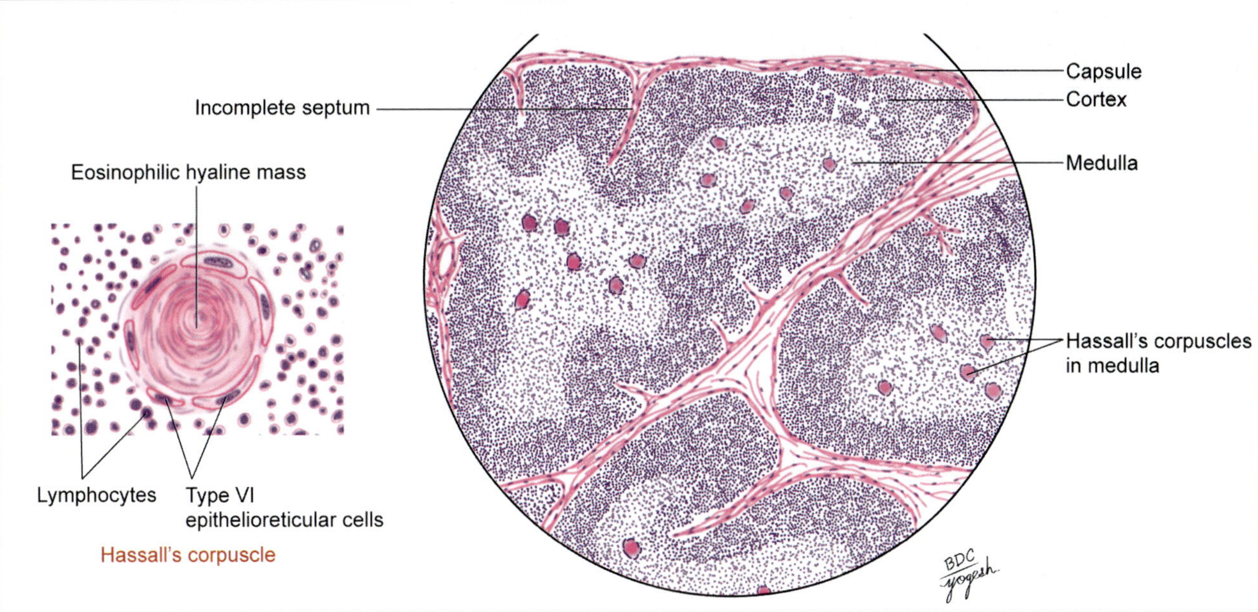


## BLOOD VESSELS OF THE NECK

*Competency:*
AN35.3 Demonstrate and describe the origin, parts, course and branches of subclavian artery.

### SUBCLAVIAN ARTERY

This is the principal artery which continues as axillary artery for the upper limb. It also supplies a considerable part of the neck and brain through its branches (Fig. 8.18, Flowchart 8.2).

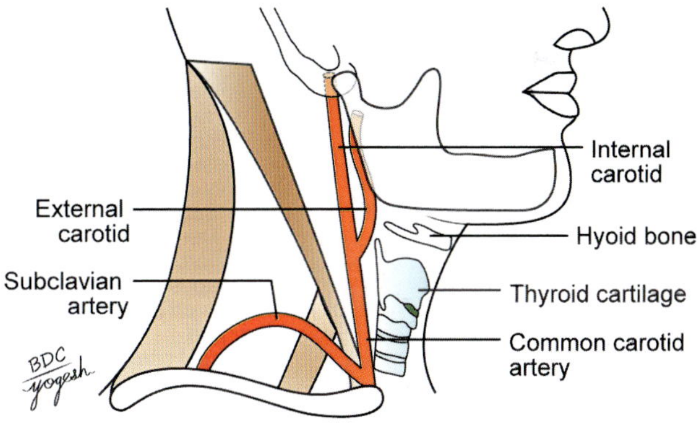


**Fig. 8.18:** Origin and course of the subclavian arteries

**Beginning** (Fig. 8.18)

On the *right side*, it is a branch of the brachiocephalic artery. It arises posterior to the sternoclavicular joint.
On the *left side*, it is a branch of the arch of the aorta. It ascends and enters the neck posterior to the left sternoclavicular joint. Both arteries pursue a similar course in the neck.

**Course** (Figs 8.18 and 8.19)

1. Each artery arches laterally from the sternoclavicular joint to the outer border of the first rib where it ends by becoming continuous with the axillary artery.
2. The scalenus anterior muscle crosses the artery anteriorly and divides it into three parts. The first part is medial, the second part posterior, and the third part lateral to scalenus anterior.

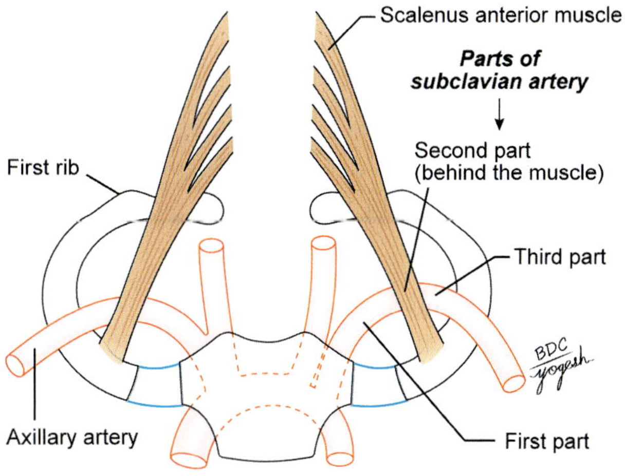


**Fig. 8.19:** Course of subclavian and carotid arteries

**Relations of the First Part** (Fig. 8.20)

***Anterior***

Immediate relations from medial to lateral side are:
1. Common carotid artery
2. Vagus
3. Internal jugular vein
4. The sternothyroid and the sternohyoid muscles
5. Sternocleidomastoid

Structures in the Neck 8

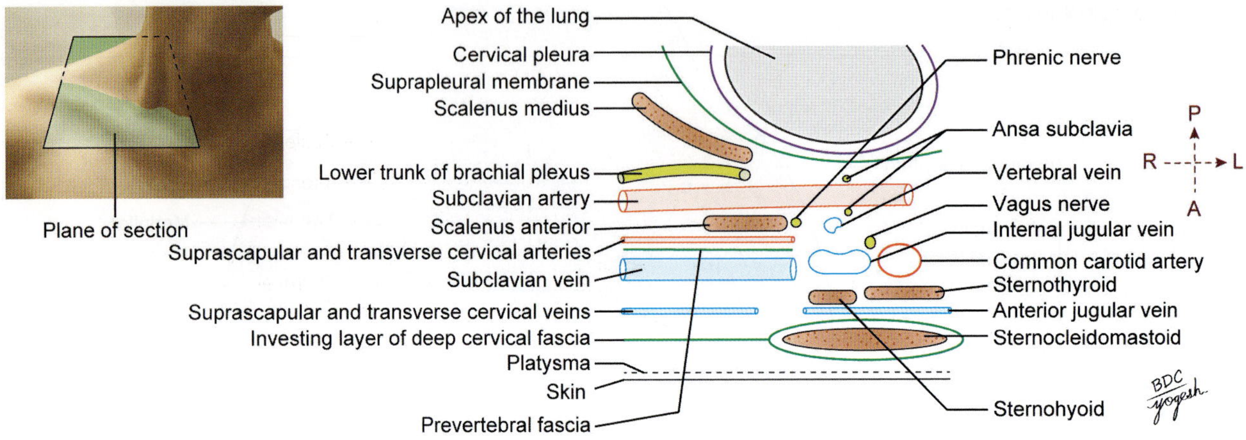


**Fig. 8.20:** Schematic diagram to show the relations of right subclavian artery

**Flowchart 8.2:** Subclavian artery (SA)

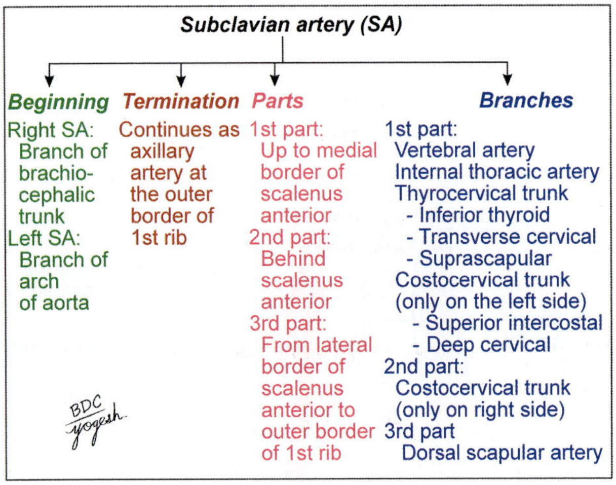


#### *Posterior* (*Posteroinferior*)

1. Suprapleural membrane
2. Cervical pleura
3. Apex of lung

### Relations of the Second Part

#### *Anterior*

1. Scalenus anterior
2. Right phrenic nerve deep to the prevertebral fascia
3. Sternocleidomastoid

#### *Posterior* (*Posteroinferior*)

1. Suprapleural membrane
2. Cervical pleura
3. Apex of lung

#### *Superior*

Upper and middle trunks of the brachial plexus.

### Relations of the Third Part

#### *Anterior*

1. Middle 1/3rd of the clavicle
2. The posterior border of the sternocleidomastoid

#### *Posterior* (*Posteroinferior*)

1. Scalenus medius
2. Lower trunk of brachial plexus
3. Suprapleural membrane
4. Cervical pleura
5. Apex of lung.

#### *Superior*

Upper and middle trunks of brachial plexus.

#### *Inferior*

First rib.

### Branches (Figs 8.21 and 8.22)

#### *From the first part*

1. Vertebral artery
2. Internal thoracic artery
3. Thyrocervical trunk, which divides into three branches (Flowchart 8.3):
   a. Inferior thyroid
   b. Suprascapular
   c. Transverse cervical arteries.
4. Costocervical trunk, which divides into two branches (Flowchart 8.3):
   a. Superior intercostal
   b. Deep cervical arteries.

   This artery comes *from second part* on the right side.

***From the third part:*** Dorsal scapular artery—occasionally.

#### *Vertebral Artery*

Vertebral artery is the 1st and largest branch of the 1st part of the subclavian artery. It runs a long course and ends in the cranial cavity by supplying the brain. It is divided into four parts. Its details are described in *see* Chapter 9, page 163.

#### *Internal Thoracic Artery*

Internal thoracic artery arises from the inferior aspect of the 1st part of the subclavian artery opposite the origin of the thyrocervical trunk. The origin lies near the medial border of the scalenus anterior. The artery

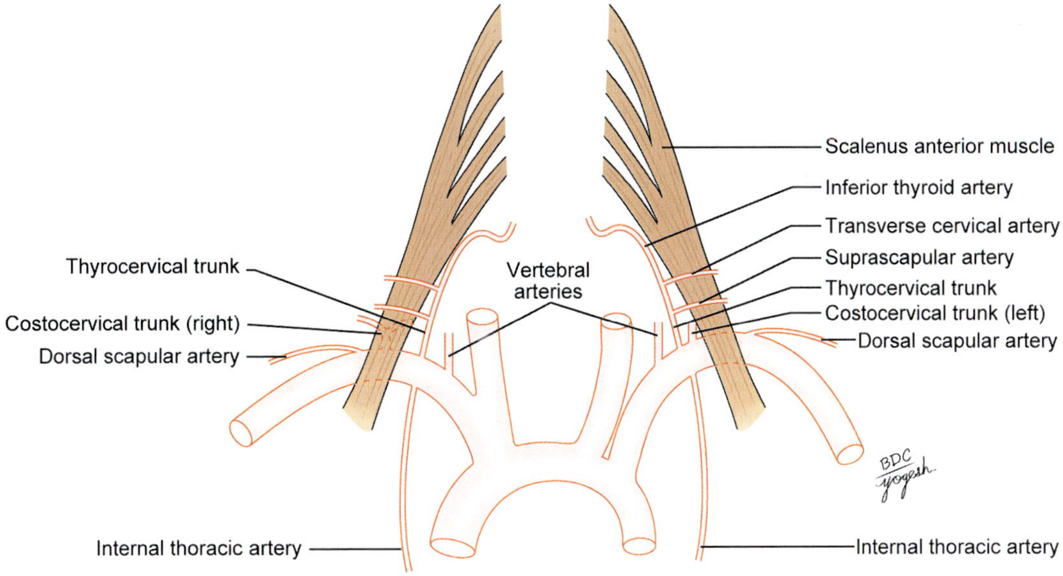


**Fig. 8.21:** Branches of the subclavian artery

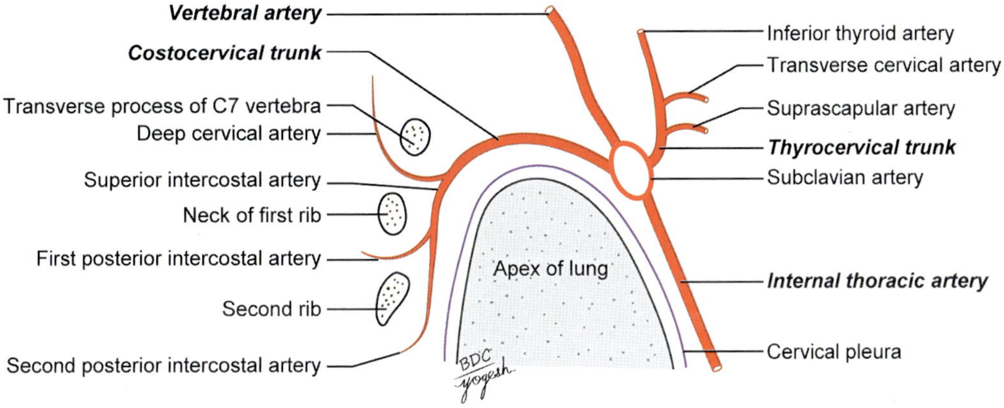


**Fig. 8.22:** Branches of the subclavian artery. Note that the branches actually arise at different levels, but are shown at same level schematically

**Flowchart 8.3:** Thyrocervical and costocervical trunks

***Thyrocervical and costocervical trunks***

| | ***Thyrocervical trunk*** | ***Costocervical trunk*** |
|---|---|---|
| Beginning | From 1st part of subclavian artery (SA) | On left: From 1st part of SA<br>On right: From 2nd part of SA |
| Termination | Divides into three branches | Divides into two branches |
| Branches | Inferior thyroid artery<br>- Ascending cervical<br>- Inferior laryngeal<br>- Tracheal, oesophageal, and pharyngeal branches<br>Transverse cervical artery<br>- Superficial and deep cervical branches<br>Suprascapular artery | Deep cervical artery<br>Superior (highest) intercostal artery<br>- First two posterior intercostal arteries |

runs downwards and medially in front of the cervical pleura. The artery enters the thorax by passing behind the 1st costal cartilage and runs till 6th intercostal space where it ends by dividing into superior epigastric and musculophrenic arteries (For details, *see* Chapter 14, *BD Chaurasia's Human Anatomy, Volume 1*).

### Thyrocervical Trunk

Thyrocervical trunk is a short, wide vessel that arises from the front of the 1st part of the subclavian artery (Flowchart 8.3). It almost immediately divides into the inferior thyroid, suprascapular and transverse cervical arteries.

***Inferior thyroid artery:*** In addition to glandular branches to the thyroid, it gives:

1. ***Ascending cervical artery*** which runs upwards in front of the transverse processes of cervical vertebrae.
2. ***Inferior laryngeal artery*** which accompanies the recurrent laryngeal nerve, and enters the larynx deep to the lower border of the inferior constrictor.
3. Other branches which supply the pharynx, the trachea, the oesophagus and surrounding muscles.

***Suprascapular artery:*** It runs laterally and downwards, and crosses the scalenus anterior and the phrenic nerve.

It lies behind the internal jugular vein and the sternocleidomastoid. It then crosses the trunks of the brachial plexus and runs in the posterior triangle, behind and parallel with the clavicle, to reach the superior border of the scapula (*see* Fig. 3.16b).

It crosses above the suprascapular ligament and takes part in the anastomoses around the scapula (*see* Chapter 6, *BD Chaurasia's Human Anatomy, Volume 1*).

***Transverse cervical artery:*** It runs laterally above the suprascapular artery (*see* Fig. 3.16b).

It crosses the scalenus anterior and the sternocleidomastoid. It then crosses the brachial plexus and the floor of the posterior triangle to reach the anterior border of trapezius, where it divides into superficial and deep branches. The ***superficial branch*** accompanies the spinal root of accessory nerve till the lower end of the muscle.

The ***deep branch*** passes deep to levator scapulae and takes part in the anastomoses around the scapula.

*Note*: Sometimes the two branches may arise separately; the superficial from thyrocervical trunk and the deep from the third part of subclavian artery. Then these are named ***superficial cervical*** and ***dorsal scapular arteries***.

### Dorsal Scapular Artery

This artery occasionally arises from the 3rd part of subclavian artery.

*Note*: If transverse cervical does not divide into superficial and deep branches but continues as superficial branch, the distribution of deep branch is taken over by dorsal scapular artery.

### Costocervical Trunk

Costocervical trunk arises from the posterior surface of the 2nd part of the subclavian artery on the right side; but from the 1st part of the artery on the left side. It arches backwards over the cervical pleura and divides into the descending superior intercostal and ascending deep cervical arteries at the neck of the 1st rib (Flowchart 8.3).

***Superior intercostal artery:*** It descends in front of the neck of the 1st rib, and divides into the 1st and 2nd posterior intercostal arteries.

***Deep cervical artery:*** It is analogous to the posterior branch of a posterior intercostal artery. It passes backwards between the transverse process of the 7th cervical vertebra and the neck of the 1st rib. It then ascends between the semispinalis capitis and cervicis up to the axis vertebra. It anastomoses with the occipital and vertebral arteries.

***Competency:***
**AN35.9** Describe the clinical features of compression of subclavian artery and lower trunk of brachial plexus by cervical rib.

## CLINICAL ANATOMY

- The 3rd part of the subclavian artery can be effectively compressed against the 1st rib after depressing the shoulder. The pressure is applied downwards, backwards, and medially in the angle between the sternocleidomastoid and the clavicle.
- A ***cervical rib*** may compress the subclavian artery, diminishing the radial pulse (Fig. 8.23).
- The right subclavian artery may arise from the descending thoracic aorta. In that case, it passes posterior to the oesophagus which may be compressed and the condition is known as ***dysphagia lusoria***.
- An aneurysm may form in the third part of the subclavian artery. Its pressure on the brachial plexus causes pain, weakness, and numbness in the upper limb.
- Obstruction to the subclavian artery proximal to the origin of vertebral artery may lead to 'stealing of blood from the brain through the opposite vertebral artery'. This may provide necessary blood to the affected side. The nervous symptoms incurred are called '***subclavian steal syndrome***' (Fig. 8.24).

## DISSECTION

Identify scalenus anterior muscle in the anteroinferior part of the neck. Subclavian artery gets divided into three parts by this muscle. Identify vertebral, internal thoracic artery and the thyrocervical trunk with its branches arising from the first part of the artery, costocervical arising from 2nd part and either dorsal scapular or none from the third part.

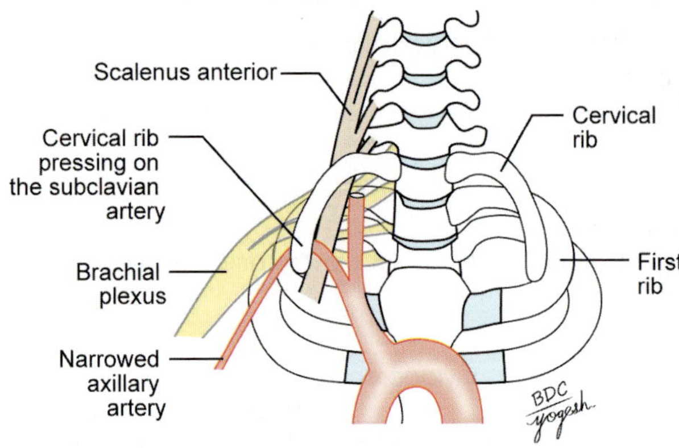


**Fig. 8.23:** The cervical rib pressing on the subclavian artery narrowing the axillary artery and diminishing the radial pulse

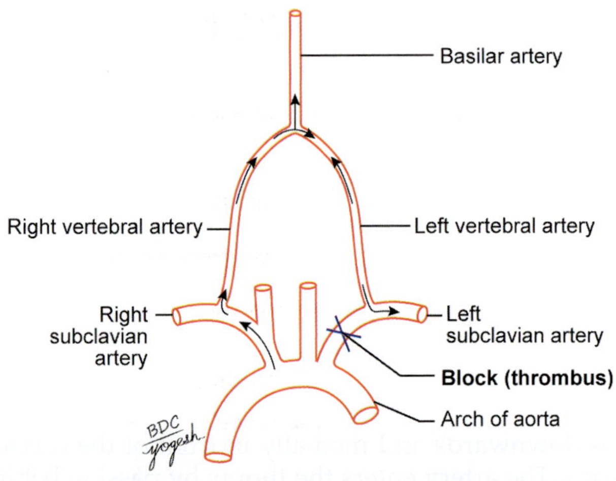


**Fig. 8.24:** Subclavian steal syndrome

## COMMON CAROTID ARTERY

The right common carotid artery arises from the brachiocephalic artery behind the right sternoclavicular joint. The left common carotid artery arises from the arch of aorta in the thoracic cavity. It ascends toward the left sternoclavicular joint to the neck. The common carotid artery is enclosed in the *carotid sheath.*

### Course

Common carotid artery begins in the thorax in front of the trachea opposite a point a little to the left of the centre of the manubrium. It ascends to the back of left sternoclavicular joint and enters the neck.

In the neck, both arteries have a similar course. Each artery runs upwards within the carotid sheath, under cover of the anterior border of the sternocleidomastoid. It lies in front of the lower four cervical transverse processes. At the level of the upper border of the thyroid cartilage, the artery ends by dividing into the external and internal carotid arteries.

### Relations of the Artery in the Neck (Fig. 8.25)

#### *Anterior Relations*

1. The common carotid artery is crossed by the superior belly of omohyoid at the level of cricoid cartilage.
2. Below the omohyoid, the artery is deeply situated, and is covered by:
   a. Sternocleidomastoid
   b. Anterior jugular vein
   c. Sternohyoid
   d. Sternothyroid and the middle thyroid vein.

#### *Posterior Relations*

1. Transverse process of vertebrae C4–C7, and the muscles attached to their anterior tubercles (longus colli, longus capitis and scalenus anterior)
2. The inferior thyroid artery crosses medially at the level of the cricoid cartilage
3. Vertebral artery
4. On the left side, the thoracic duct crosses laterally behind the artery at the level of vertebra C7, in front of the vertebral vessels.

#### *Medial Relations*

1. Thyroid gland
2. Larynx and pharynx; trachea, oesophagus and recurrent laryngeal nerve.

#### *Lateral Relation*

Internal jugular vein.

#### *Posterolateral Relation*

Vagus nerve.

### CLINICAL ANATOMY

The pulsation of common carotid artery can be felt by compressing against the carotid tubercle, i.e. the anterior tubercle of the transverse process of vertebra C6 which lies at the level of the cricoid cartilage.

### DISSECTION

The common carotid artery has been exposed in the carotid triangle. Clean it in its entire course. Identify the internal carotid artery and trace it till it leaves the neck.

***Veins***

Identify the tributaries of subclavian, internal jugular and brachiocephalic veins.

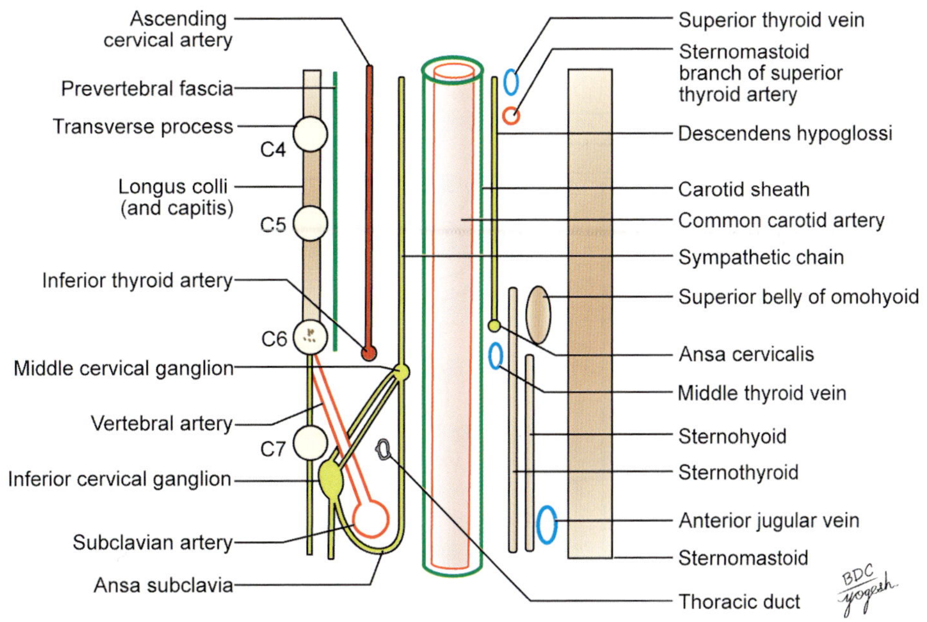


**Fig. 8.25:** Schematic sagittal section showing posterior relations of the common carotid artery

## INTERNAL CAROTID ARTERY

The internal carotid artery is one of the two terminal branches of the common carotid artery. It begins at the level of the upper border of the thyroid cartilage opposite the disc between the 3rd and 4th cervical vertebrae and ends inside the cranial cavity by supplying the brain. This is the principal artery of the brain and the eye. It also supplies the related bones and meninges.

For convenience of description, the course of the artery is divided into four parts:

1. Cervical part, in the neck
2. Petrous part, within the petrous temporal bone
3. Cavernous part, within the cavernous sinus
4. Cerebral part in relation to base of the brain.

### Cervical Part

1. It ascends vertically in the neck from its origin to the base of the skull to reach the lower end of the carotid canal. This part is enclosed in the carotid sheath (with the internal jugular vein and the vagus nerve)
2. No branches arise from the internal carotid artery in the neck
3. Its initial part usually shows a dilatation, the *carotid sinus* which acts as a baroreceptor
4. The lower part of the artery (in the carotid triangle) is comparatively superficial. The upper part, above the posterior belly of digastric, is deep into the parotid gland, the styloid apparatus, and many other structures.

### *Relations* (Fig. 8.26)

#### *Anterior or superficial*

1. In the carotid triangle:
   a. Anterior border of sternocleidomastoid
   b. External carotid artery is anteromedial to it.
2. Above the carotid triangle:
   a. Posterior belly of digastric
   b. Stylohyoid
   c. Stylopharyngeus
   d. Styloid process
   e. Parotid gland with structures within it.

#### *Posterior*

1. Superior cervical ganglion
2. Carotid sheath
3. The glossopharyngeal, vagus, accessory and hypoglossal nerves at the base of the skull.

#### *Medial*

1. Pharynx
2. The external carotid is anteromedial to it below the parotid.

#### *Lateral*

1. Internal jugular vein
2. Temporomandibular joint (at the base of the skull).

### Petrous Part

In the carotid canal, the artery first runs upwards and then turns forwards and medially at right angles. It emerges at the apex of the petrous temporal bone, in the posterior wall of the foramen lacerum where it turns upwards and medially.

### Cavernous and Cerebral Parts

Cavernous part runs in the cavernous sinus. Cerebral part lies at base of skull and gives ophthalmic, anterior cerebral, middle cerebral, posterior communicating and anterior choroidal arteries.

### Branches (Fig. 8.27, Flowchart 8.4)

*Cervical part*

No branch.

*Petrous part*

1. Caroticotympanic branches
2. Pterygoid branch.

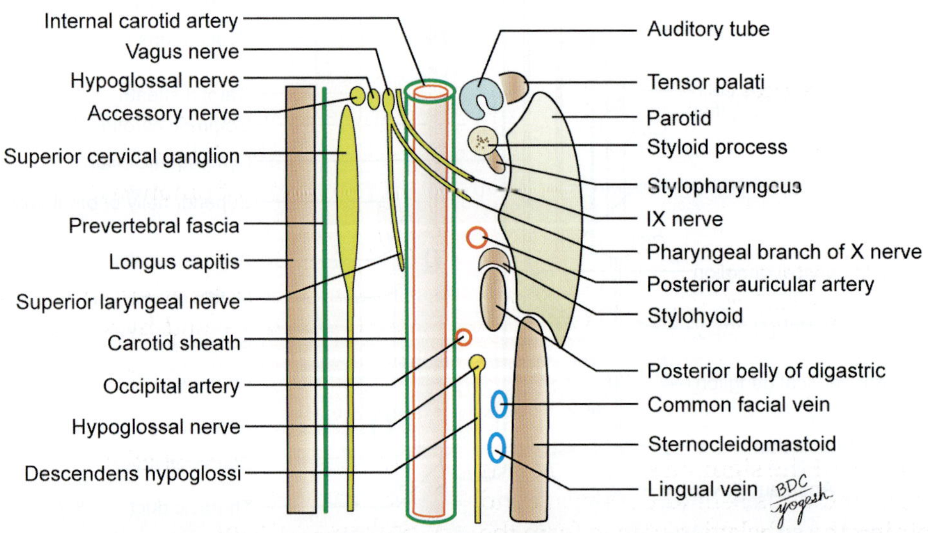


**Fig. 8.26:** Schematic sagittal section showing the anterior and posterior relations of the internal carotid artery

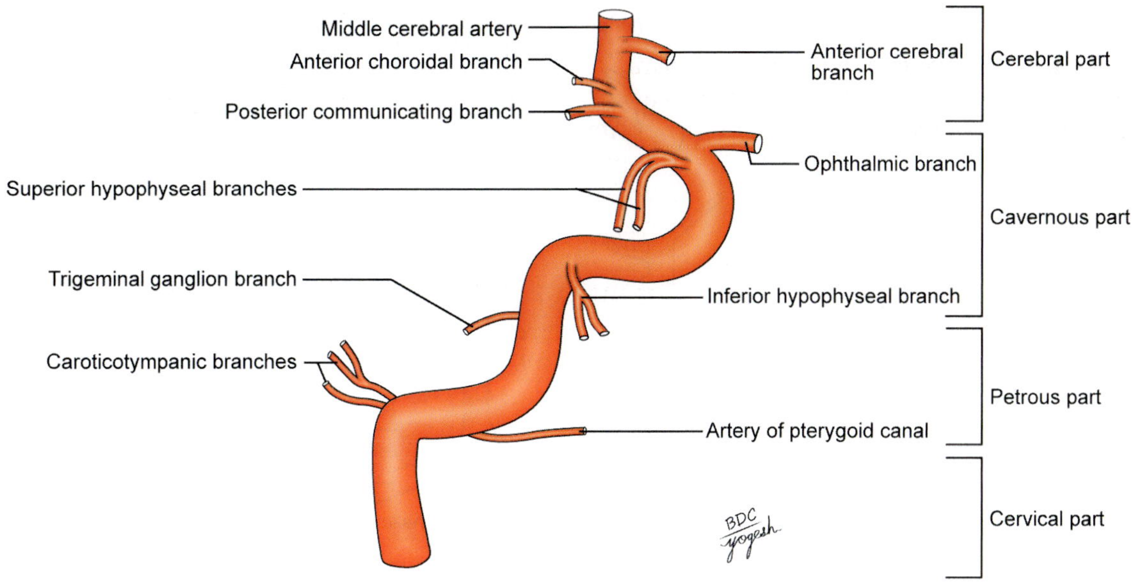


**Fig. 8.27:** Branches and parts of the right internal carotid artery

**Flowchart 8.4:** Internal carotid artery

***Internal carotid artery***

- ***Beginning***
  - Terminal branch of CCA at the level of upper border of lamina of thyroid cartilage
- ***Termination***
  - Divides into anterior and middle cerebral arteries
- ***Parts and branches***
  - Cervical part: No branch
  - Petrous part
    1. Caroticotympanic branch
    2. Pterygoid branch
  - Cavernous part
    1. Cavernous branches
    2. Superior and inferior hypophyseal arteries
  - Cerebral part: Ophthalmic, anterior choroidal, posterior communicating, anterior cerebral, middle cerebral

(CCA: Common carotid artery)

*Cavernous part*

1. Cavernous branches
2. Superior and inferior hypophyseal arteries.

*Cerebral part*

1. Ophthalmic artery
2. Anterior choroidal artery
3. Posterior communicating artery
4. Anterior cerebral artery
5. Middle cerebral artery.

***Competency:***

**AN35.4** Describe and demonstrate origin, course, relations, tributaries and termination of internal jugular and brachiocephalic veins.

## INTERNAL JUGULAR VEIN

It is a direct continuation of the sigmoid sinus. It begins at the jugular foramen and ends behind the sternal end of the clavicle by joining the subclavian vein to form the brachiocephalic vein (Fig. 8.28, Flowchart 8.5).

### Features

1. *Superior bulb:* It is a dilatation at the beginning of the internal jugular vein. It lies in the *jugular fossa* of the temporal bone.
2. *Inferior bulb:* It is a dilation near the termination of the internal jugular vein. It lies in the lesser supraclavicular fossa.
3. *Larger right internal jugular vein*: The right IJV is larger than the left as it is a direct continuation of larger right sigmoid sinus (larger superior sagittal sinus). The left IJV is a continuation of smaller left sigmoid sinus (smaller inferior sagittal sinus).
4. *Enclosed within the carotid sheath*: IJV, carotid arteries, and vagus nerve are enclosed with the carotid sheath which is thinner around the vein.
5. *Lymph nodes*: The deep cervical nodes lie along the entire course of IJV.
6. *Lymphatic duct*: At *jugulo-subclavian angle* on the left, the thoracic duct opens, whereas, on the right, the *right lymphatic duct* opens.

### Relations

#### *Superficial*

1. Sternocleidomastoid
2. Posterior belly of digastric
3. Superior belly of omohyoid
4. Parotid gland
5. Styloid process
6. The internal carotid artery, and the glossopharyngeal, vagus, accessory and hypoglossal cranial nerves (at the base of skull).

#### *Posterior*

1. Transverse process of atlas
2. Cervical plexus
3. Scalenus anterior
4. First part of subclavian artery.

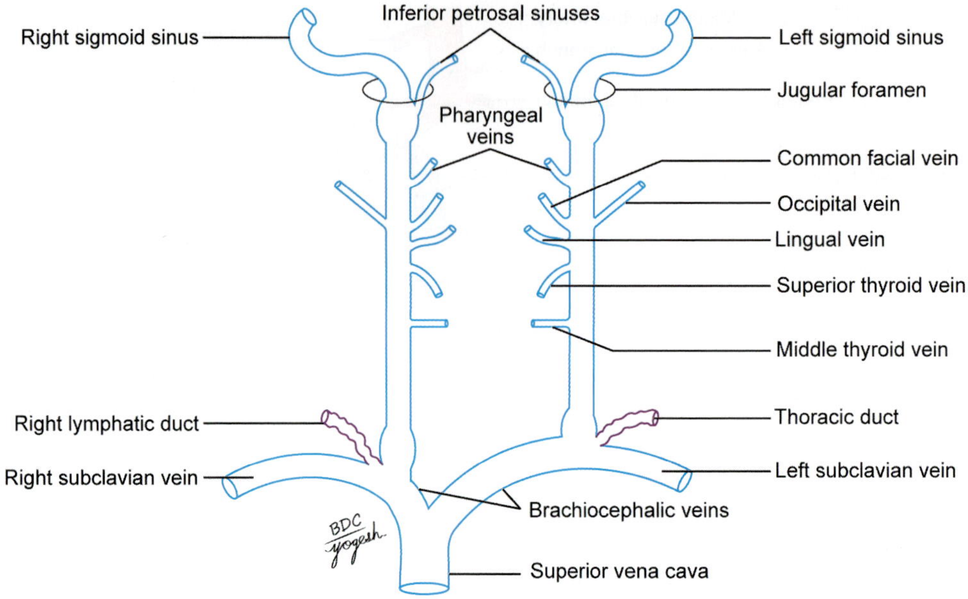


**Fig. 8.28:** Internal jugular veins

**Flowchart 8.5:** Internal jugular vein (IJV)

***Internal jugular vein***

***Beginning and termination***

Beginning: As a continuation of sigmoid sinus

Termination: Joins subclavian vein to form brachiocephalic vein

***Tributaries***

Inferior petrosal sinus
Common facial, lingual veins
Pharyngeal vein
Superior and middle thyroid veins, occipital vein
Thoracic duct on the left
Right lymphatic duct on right
Communicating oblique vein

***Clinical integration:*** Cannulation of IJV, thrill in mitral stenosis, Queckenstedt's test, cervical lymphadenopathy along with IJV

### Medial

1. Internal carotid artery
2. Common carotid artery
3. Vagus nerve.

### Tributaries

1. Inferior petrosal sinus
2. Common facial vein
3. Lingual vein
4. Pharyngeal veins
5. Superior thyroid vein
6. Middle thyroid vein.

*Note*: In the middle of the neck, the internal jugular vein may communicate with the external jugular vein through the oblique jugular vein which runs across the anterior border of the sternocleidomastoid.

[*Mnemonics: **Tributaries of Internal Jugular Vein:*** "**M**edical **S**chools **L**et **C**onfident **P**eople **I**n" From inferior to superior: **M**iddle thyroid; **C**ommon facial; **S**uperior thyroid; **P**haryngeal; **L**ingual **I**nferior petrosal sinus]

## CLINICAL ANATOMY

- ***Cannulation of IJV:*** It can be cannulation through the apex of the lesser supraclavicular triangle that lies between the two heads of the sternocleidomastoid muscle. The needle should be directed backward and upward to avoid the puncture of cervical pleura. If it is punctured, it will lead to pneumothorax.
- ***Thrill*** can be felt sometimes at the lesser supraclavicular triangle during atrial systole, especially in cases of mitral stenosis.
- ***Queckenstedt's test:*** Compression of the internal jugular veins increases the rate of CSF flow during lumbar puncture. Block in the spinal subarachnoid space result in the failure of this increase of CSF flow.
- ***Cervical lymphadenopathy and IJV:*** The IJV is a surgical guide for removal of cervical lymph nodes. In malignant and tubercular lymphadenopathy, the lymph nodes often adhere to IJV and resection of such lymph nodes becomes difficult. It may require the removal of a segment of IJV.

## SUBCLAVIAN VEIN

### Course

It is a continuation of the axillary vein. It begins at the outer border of the first rib, and ends at the medial border of the scalenus anterior by joining the internal jugular vein to form the brachiocephalic vein (Fig. 8.29).

It lies:

1. In front of the subclavian artery, the scalenus anterior and the right phrenic nerve.
2. Behind the clavicle and the subclavius.
3. Above the first rib and pleura.

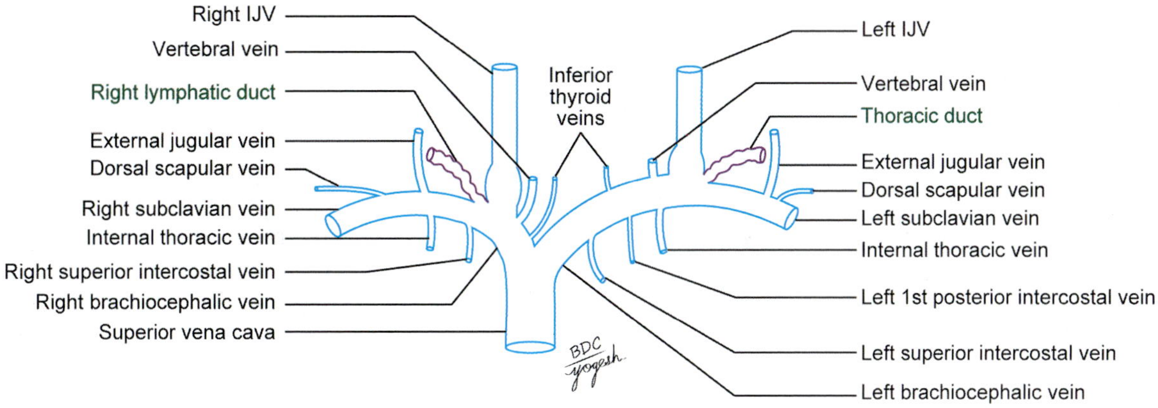


**Fig. 8.29:** Subclavian and brachiocephalic veins

Its tributaries are:

1. External jugular vein
2. Dorsal scapular vein
3. Thoracic duct on the left side
4. Right lymphatic duct on the right side.

## BRACHIOCEPHALIC VEIN

1. The right brachiocephalic vein (2.5 cm long) is shorter than the left (6 cm long) (Fig. 8.29).
2. Each vein is formed behind the sternoclavicular joint, by the union of the internal jugular vein and the subclavian vein.
3. The right vein runs vertically downwards. The left vein runs obliquely downwards and to the right behind the upper half of the manubrium sterni. The two brachiocephalic veins unite at the lower border of the right first costal cartilage to form the superior vena cava.

### Tributaries

The *tributaries* correspond to the branches of the 1st part of the subclavian artery. These are as follows:

***Right brachiocephalic:***

1. Vertebral
2. Internal thoracic
3. First posterior intercostal
4. Right lymphatic duct.

***Left brachiocephalic:***

1. Vertebral
2. Internal thoracic
3. Inferior thyroid on both sides
4. First posterior intercostal
5. Left superior intercostal
6. Thymic and pericardial veins
7. Thoracic duct.

*Competency:*
**AN35.7** Describe the course and branches of IX, X, XI and XII nerve in the neck.

# NERVES OF THE NECK

## GLOSSOPHARYNGEAL NERVE—IX NERVE

Glossopharyngeal nerve exits the cranial cavity via anterior part of jugular foramen.

### Course (Fig. 8.30)

1. It runs between internal carotid artery and internal jugular vein, lying deep to the styloid process and muscles attached to the process.
2. Then it courses between internal carotid and external carotid arteries, where it curves around the lateral border of stylopharyngeus muscle.
3. As it reaches submandibular region, it passes deep to hyoglossus muscle to reach the area of palatine tonsil and base of the tongue.

### Branches (Figs 8.31a and b)

1. Tympanic branch courses through middle ear and gives secretomotor root to otic ganglion.
2. Carotid branch for carotid body and carotid sinus.
3. Muscular for stylopharyngeus muscle.
4. Carries taste from vallate papillae of tongue.
5. Carries general sensations from posterior one-third of tongue and palatine tonsil.
6. Branch to pharyngeal plexus.

## VAGUS NERVE—X NERVE

Vagus leaves the cranial cavity through jugular foramen lying posterior to IX nerve. Soon it is joined course by cranial root of XI nerve. In the neck, the nerve lies in the carotid sheath, medial to internal jugular vein and posterior to internal carotid and common carotid arteries.

Then it passes through thorax and abdomen.

### Branches in Neck

1. Meningeal
2. Auricular
3. Pharyngeal for most muscles of soft palate 4 out of 5 and pharynx 5 out 6, carotid for carotid body

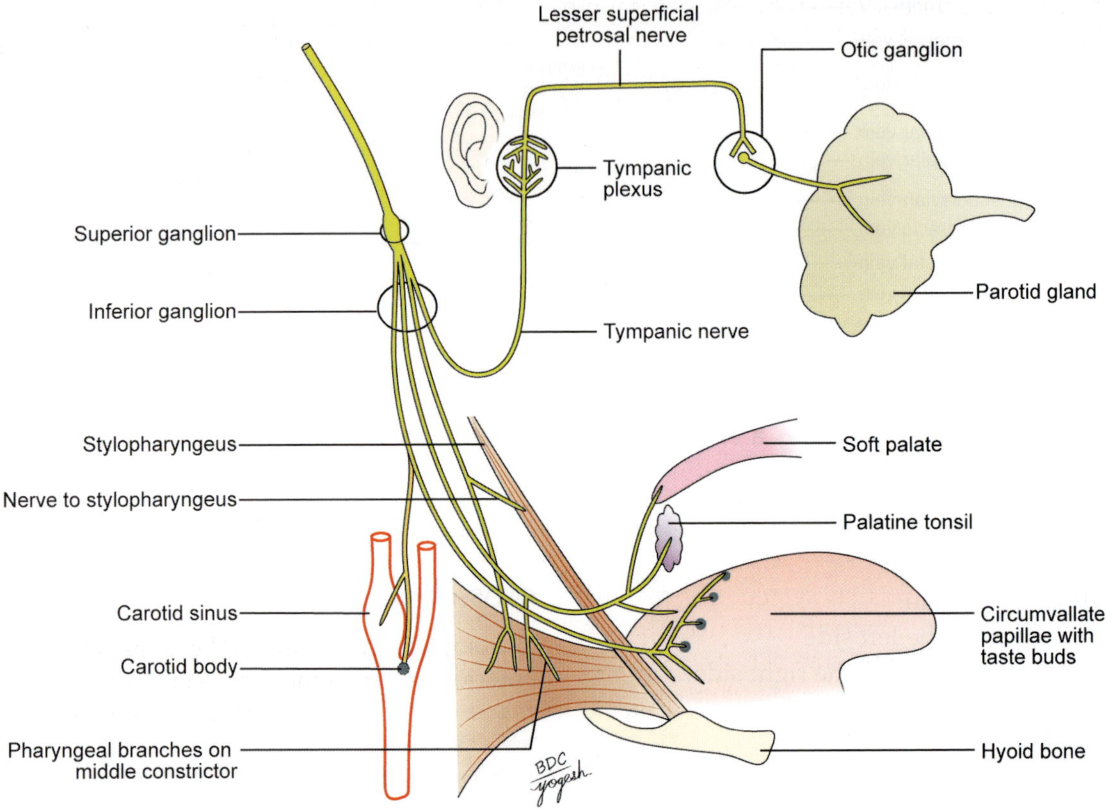


**Fig. 8.30:** Distribution of glossopharyngeal nerve

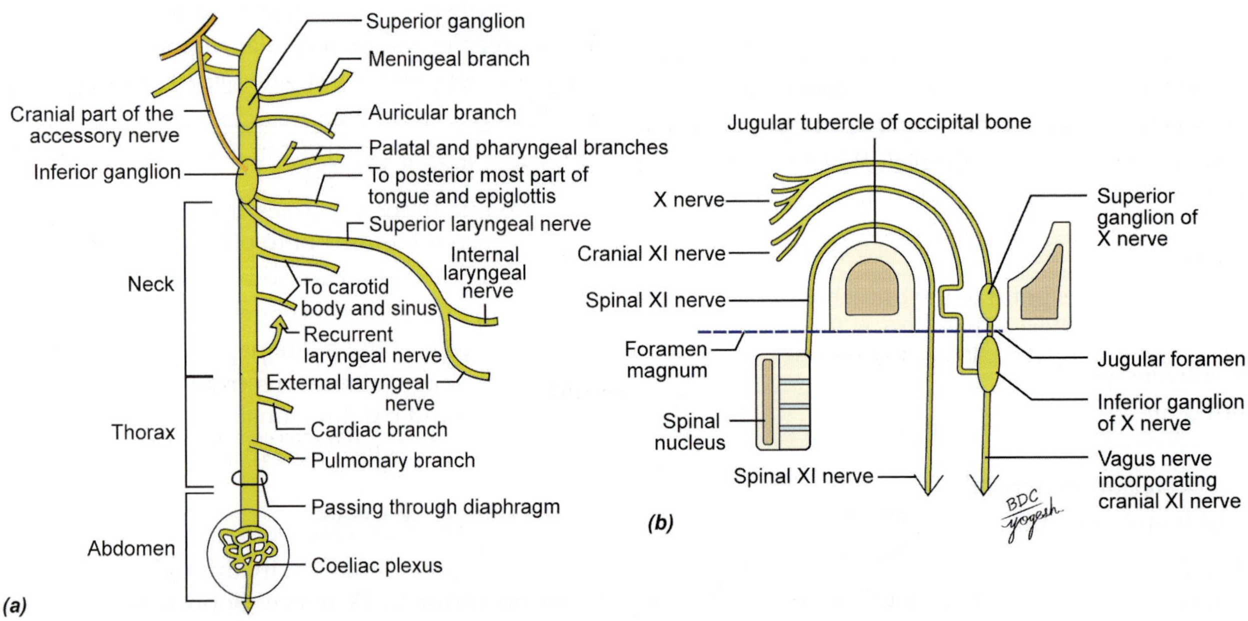


**Figs 8.31a and b:** (a) Branches of vagus nerve and (b) course of accessory nerve

and carotid sinus, superior laryngeal gives internal laryngeal for mucous membrane of larynx and external laryngeal for cricothyroid muscle.

4. Right recurrent laryngeal is given off in neck while left one is given off in thorax. The nerves supply all intrinsic muscles of larynx and sensory branches to mucous membrane of larynx below vocal cords.
5. Cardiac branches for deep cardiac plexus.

## ACCESSORY NERVE—XI NERVE

This nerve also leaves the cranial cavity through the jugular foramen. It is made up of a cranial root and a spinal root. The two roots join in jugular foramen, but again separate as it pass out of the foramen. Cranial root joins X nerve and gets distributed with it for 4 out of 5 palatal muscles, 5 out of 6 pharyngeal muscles and all laryngeal muscles. The spinal root descends between internal jugular vein and internal carotid artery for some distance. It then lies superficial to internal jugular vein to reach anterior border of sternocleidomastoid muscle. It enters the muscle, supplies it and leaves the muscle at its posterior border a little above its middle.

Then it passes downwards and backwards in the posterior triangle of neck. Finally, it leaves posterior triangle by passing deep to trapezius.

Thus the spinal root of XI nerve supplies: Sternocleidomastoid and trapezius muscles.

Details can be read from Chapter 6, *BD Chaurasia's Human Anatomy, Volume 4.*

### DISSECTION

The course of IX–XI cranial nerves has been seen in different chapters. Now trace these nerves and their branches.

The sympathetic trunk has been identified as lying posteromedial to the carotid sheath. Trace it upwards and downwards and locate the three cervical ganglia.

Dissect the formation and branches of the cervical plexus. Identify the phrenic nerve on the surface of scalenus anterior muscle behind the prevertebral fascia.

***Competency:***

**AN35.6** Describe and demonstrate the extent, formation, relation and branches of cervical sympathetic chain.

## CERVICAL PART OF SYMPATHETIC TRUNK

The cervical parts of the right and left sympathetic trunks are situated one on each side of the cervical part of the vertebral column, behind the carotid sheath (common carotid and internal carotid arteries) and in front of the prevertebral fascia (Fig. 8.32).

### Formation

There are *no white rami communicantes* (i.e. incoming root) in the neck and this part of the trunk is formed by fibres that emerge from segments T1 to T4 of the spinal cord, and then ascend into the neck. Grey rami communicantes (i.e. outgoing roots) are present.

### Relations

#### *Anterior*

1. Internal carotid artery
2. Common carotid artery
3. Carotid sheath
4. Inferior thyroid artery.

#### *Posterior*

1. Prevertebral fascia
2. Longus capitis and cervicis muscles
3. Transverse processes of the lower six cervical vertebrae.

## GANGLIA

Theoretically, there should be eight sympathetic ganglia corresponding to the eight cervical nerves, but due to fusion, there are only three ganglia—superior, middle and inferior.

### Superior Cervical Ganglion

#### *Size and Shape*

This is the largest of the three ganglia. It is spindle-shaped, and about 2.5 cm long.

#### *Situation and Formation*

It lies just below the skull, opposite the second and third cervical vertebrae, behind the carotid sheath and in front of the prevertebral fascia (longus capitis). It is formed by fusion of the upper 4 cervical ganglia.

***Communications:*** With cranial nerves IX, X and XII, and with the external and recurrent laryngeal nerves.

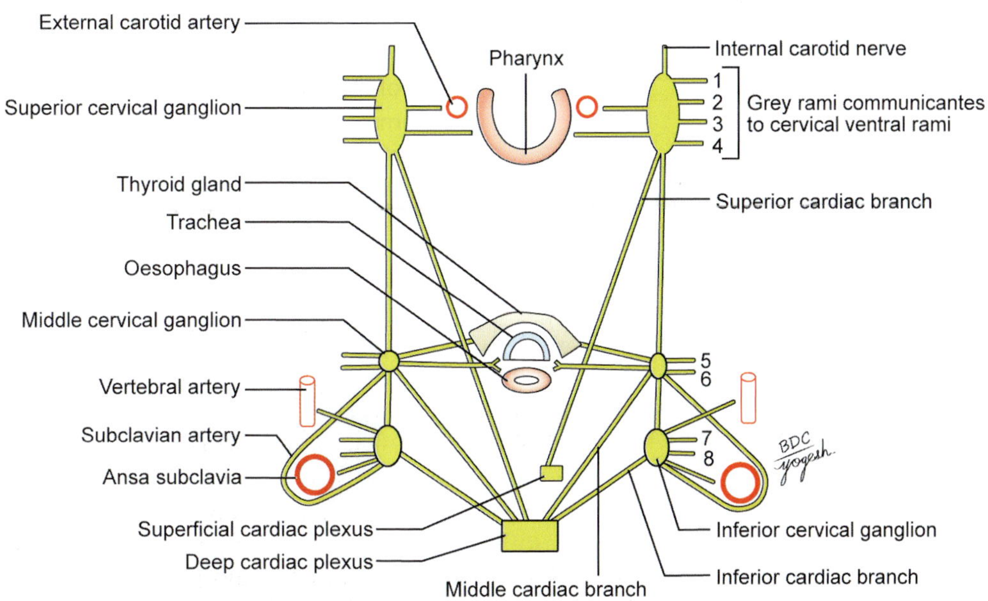


**Fig. 8.32:** The cervical sympathetic trunks and their branches

#### Branches

1. *Grey rami communicantes* to ventral primary rami of upper four cervical nerves.
2. *Pharyngeal branches* to carotid body and pharyngeal plexus.
3. *Cardiac branches*: Right cardiac branches join the deep cardiac plexus, whereas left cardiac branches join the superficial cardiac plexus.
4. External carotid branches form plexus around the external carotid artery. Some of these fibres pass through the otic and submandibular ganglia.
5. Ascending fibres form the internal carotid nerve or plexus around the internal carotid artery. This plexus gives rise to:
   a. *Caroticotympanic nerve* that enters middle ear and forms tympanic plexus along with the branch of glossopharyngeal nerve.
   b. *Deep petrosal nerve* joins the greater petrosal nerve to form *nerve to pterygoid canal*. Some of these fibres supply dilator pupillae through ciliary ganglion and Müller's muscle.
   c. *Nervus conarii* pass through the tentorium cerebelli to supply the pineal glands.
   d. Terminal branches accompany the branches of internal carotid artery.

### Middle Cervical Ganglion

#### Size and Shape

This ganglion is very small. It may be divided into 2 to 3 smaller parts or may be absent.

#### Situation

It lies in the lower part of the neck, in front of vertebra C6 just above the inferior thyroid artery, behind the carotid sheath.

#### Formation

It is formed by fusion of the fifth and sixth cervical ganglia connections. It is connected with the inferior cervical ganglion directly, and also through a loop that winds around the subclavian artery. This loop is called the ansa subclavia.

#### Branches

1. Grey rami communicantes are given to the ventral rami of the 5th and 6th cervical nerves.
2. *Thyroid branches* accompany the inferior thyroid artery to the thyroid gland. They also supply the parathyroid glands.
3. Tracheal and oesophageal branches.
4. The *middle cervical cardiac branch* is the largest of the sympathetic cardiac branches. It goes to the deep cardiac plexus.

### Inferior Cervical Ganglion

#### Size, Shape and Formation

It is formed by fusion of 7th and 8th cervical ganglia. This is often fused with the first thoracic ganglion and is then known as the *cervicothoracic ganglion* or *stellate ganglion* because it is star-shaped.

It is situated between the transverse process of vertebra C7 and the neck of the first rib. It lies behind the vertebral artery, and in front of ramus of spinal nerve C8. *A cervicothoracic ganglion extends in front of the neck of the first rib.*

#### Branches

1. *Grey rami communicantes* are given to the ventral rami of nerves C7 and C8.
2. *Vertebral branches* form a plexus around the vertebral artery.
3. *Subclavian branches* form a plexus around the subclavian artery. This plexus is joined by branches from the ansa subclavia.
4. An *inferior cervical cardiac branch* goes to the deep cardiac plexus.

The branches of the cervical sympathetic ganglia are listed in Table 8.1.

***Competency:***
**AN31.3** Describe anatomical basis of Horner's syndrome.

### CLINICAL ANATOMY

- The head and neck are supplied by sympathetic nerves arising from the upper four thoracic segments of the spinal cord. Most of these preganglionic fibres pass through the stellate ganglion to relay in the superior cervical ganglion.
- Injury to cervical sympathetic trunk produces Horner's syndrome. It is characterized by:
  a. Ptosis—drooping of the upper eyelid.
  b. Miosis—constriction of the pupil.
  c. Anhydrosis—loss of sweating on that side of the face.
  d. Enophthalmos—retraction of the eyeball.
  e. Loss of the ciliospinal reflex—pinching the skin on the nape of the neck does not produce dilatation of the pupil (which normally takes place).
- Horner's syndrome can also be caused by a lesion within the central nervous system anywhere at or above the first thoracic segment of the spinal cord involving sympathetic fibres (Fig. 8.33).

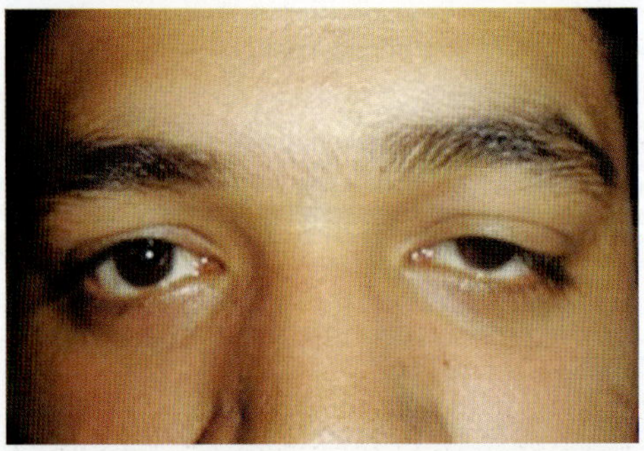

**Fig. 8.33:** Horner's syndrome on left side

**TABLE 8.1: Branches of cervical sympathetic ganglia**

| | *Superior cervical ganglion* | *Middle cervical ganglion* | *Inferior cervical ganglion* |
|---|---|---|---|
| Arterial branches | • Along internal carotid artery is internal carotid nerve which gives deep petrosal, nerve to Müller's muscle, to dilator pupillae, to pineal gland<br>• Along common carotid and external carotid arteries for all 3 salivary glands | Along inferior thyroid artery | Along subclavian and vertebral arteries |
| Grey rami communicantes | Along 1–4 cervical nerves | Along 5 and 6 cervical nerves | Along 7 and 8 cervical nerves |
| Along cranial nerves | Along cranial nerves IX, X, XI and XII | — | — |
| Visceral branches | Pharynx, cardiac | Thyroid, cardiac | Cardiac |

*Competencies:*

**AN28.5** Describe cervical lymph nodes and lymphatic drainage of head, face and neck.

**AN35.5** Describe and demonstrate extent, drainage and applied anatomy of cervical lymph nodes.

## LYMPHATIC DRAINAGE OF HEAD AND NECK

Lymph nodes in head and neck are as follows:
1. Superficial group
2. Deep group
3. Deepest group.

### Superficial Group (Fig. 8.34)

#### *Buccal and Mandibular Nodes*

The buccal node lies on the buccinator, and the mandibular node at the lower border of the mandible near the anteroinferior angle of the masseter, in close relation to the marginal mandibular branch of the facial nerve. They drain part of the cheek and the lower eyelid. Their efferents pass to the anterosuperior group of deep cervical nodes.

#### *Preauricular Nodes*

Drain parotid gland, temporal region, middle ear, etc.

#### *Postauricular (Mastoid) Nodes*

The postauricular nodes lie on the mastoid process, superficial to the sternocleidomastoid and deep to the auricularis posterior. They drain a strip of scalp just above and behind the auricle, the upper half of the medial surface and margin of the auricle, and the posterior wall of the external acoustic meatus. Their efferents pass to the posterosuperior group of deep cervical nodes.

#### *Occipital Nodes*

The occipital nodes lie at the apex of the posterior triangle superficial to the attachment of the trapezius. They drain the occipital region of the scalp. Their efferents pass to the supraclavicular members of the posteroinferior group of deep cervical nodes.

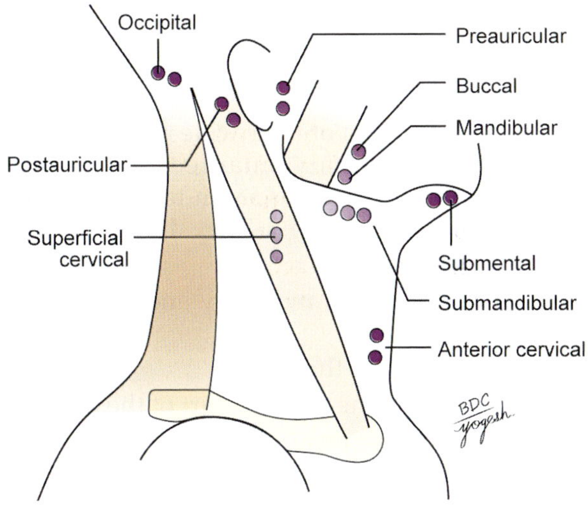


**Fig. 8.34:** Superficial lymph nodes of the neck

#### *Anterior Superficial Cervical Nodes*

The anterior cervical nodes lie along the *anterior jugular vein* and are unimportant. The suprasternal lymph node is a member of this group. They drain the skin of the anterior part of the neck below the hyoid bone. Their efferents pass to the deep cervical nodes of both sides.

#### *Lateral Superficial Cervical Nodes*

The superficial cervical nodes lie along the *external jugular vein* superficial to the sternocleidomastoid. They drain the lobule of the auricle, the floor of the external acoustic meatus, and the skin over the lower parotid region and the angle of the jaw. Their efferents pass around both borders of the muscle to reach the upper and lower deep cervical nodes.

### Deep Group

It comprises five levels of lymph nodes (Fig. 8.35).

#### *Submental and Submandibular Nodes*

Submental nodes lie deep to the chin. These drain the lymph from tip of tongue and anterior part of floor of mouth. The submandibular nodes drain lateral surface of tongue, lower gums and teeth and central area of forehead. The *submandibular lymph nodes* are clinically

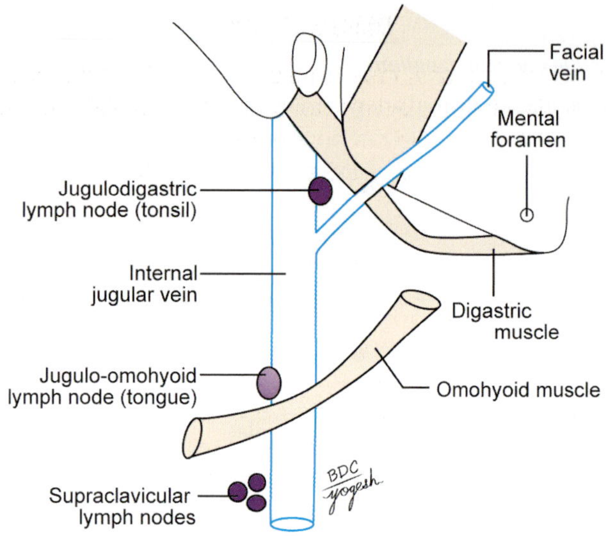


**Fig. 8.35:** Deep groups of lymph nodes in the neck

very important because of their wide area of drainage. They are very commonly enlarged. The nodes lie beneath the deep cervical fascia on the surface of the submandibular salivary gland. They drain:

1. Centre of the forehead.
2. Nose with the frontal, maxillary and ethmoidal air sinuses.
3. The inner canthus of the eye.
4. The upper lip and the anterior part of the cheek with the underlying gum and teeth.
5. The outer part of the lower lip with the lower gums and teeth excluding the incisors.
6. The anterior two-thirds of the tongue excluding the tip, and the floor of the mouth. They also receive efferents from the submental lymph nodes.

The *efferents* from the submandibular nodes pass mostly to the jugulo-omohyoid node and partly to the jugulodigastric node. These nodes are situated along the internal jugular vein and are members of the deep cervical chain.

### Upper Lateral Nodes around Internal Jugular Vein

The *jugulodigastric node* is a member of this group. It lies below the posterior belly of digastric, between the angle of the mandible and anterior border of the sternocleidomastoid, in the triangle bounded by the posterior belly of digastric, the facial vein and the internal jugular vein. It is the main node draining the *tonsil*.

### Middle Lateral Nodes around Internal Jugular Vein

These drain thyroid and parathyroid glands. They receive efferents from prelaryngeal, pretracheal and paratracheal lymph nodes.

### Lower Lateral Nodes around Internal Jugular Vein

The *jugulo-omohyoid node* is a group of nodes. It lies just above the intermediate tendon of the omohyoid, under cover of the posterior border of the sternocleidomastoid. It is the main lymph node of the *tongue*.

### Lymph Nodes in Posterior Triangle

The lymph nodes are present around the spinal root of accessory nerve.

***Efferents*** of the deep cervical lymph nodes join together to form the *jugular lymph trunks*, one on each side. The left jugular trunk opens into the thoracic duct. The right trunk may open either into the right lymphatic duct, or directly into the angle of junction between the internal jugular and subclavian veins.

## Deepest Group

### Prelaryngeal and Pretracheal Nodes

The prelaryngeal and pretracheal nodes lie deep to the investing fascia, the prelaryngeal nodes on the cricothyroid membrane, and the pretracheal in front of the trachea below the isthmus of the thyroid gland. They drain the larynx, the trachea and the isthmus of the thyroid. They also receive afferents from the anterior cervical nodes. Their efferents pass to the nearby deep cervical nodes.

### Paratracheal Nodes

The paratracheal nodes lie on the sides of the trachea and oesophagus along the recurrent laryngeal nerves. They receive lymph from the oesophagus, the trachea and the larynx, and pass it onto the deep cervical nodes.

### Retropharyngeal Nodes

The retropharyngeal nodes lie in front of the prevertebral fascia and behind the buccopharyngeal fascia covering the posterior wall of the pharynx. They extend laterally in front of the lateral mass of the atlas and along the lateral border of the longus capitis. They drain the pharynx, the auditory tube, the soft palate, the posterior part of the hard palate, and the nose. Their efferents pass to the upper lateral group of deep cervical nodes.

### Waldeyer's Ring

The ring comprises lingual, palatine, tubal and nasopharyngeal tonsils.

## MAIN LYMPH TRUNKS AT THE ROOT OF THE NECK

1. The ***thoracic duct*** is the largest lymph trunk of the body. It begins in the abdomen from the upper end of the cisterna chyli enters the thorax through aortic opening, traverses the thorax, and ends on the left side of the root of the neck by opening into the angle of junction between the left internal jugular vein and the left subclavian vein. Before its termination, it forms an arch at the level of the transverse process of vertebra C7 rising 3 to 4 cm above the clavicle. Apart from its tributaries in the abdomen and thorax, the thoracic duct receives (in the neck):
   a. The left jugular trunk
   b. The left subclavian trunk
   c. The left bronchomediastinal trunk.

   It drains most of the body, except for the right upper limb, the right halves of the head, the neck and the thorax and the superior surface of the liver.

2. **The right *jugular trunk*** drains half of the head and neck.
3. The **right *subclavian trunk*** drains the upper limb.
4. The ***bronchomediastinal trunk*** drains the lung, half of the mediastinum and parts of the anterior walls of the thorax and abdomen.
5. On the right side, the subclavian, jugular and bronchomediastinal trunks unite to form the ***right lymph trunk*** which ends in a manner similar to the thoracic duct.

## CLINICAL ANATOMY

- The deep cervical lymph nodes lie on the internal jugular vein. These nodes often become adherent to the vein in malignancy or in tuberculosis. Therefore, during operation on such patients, the vein is also resected. These are examined from behind with the neck slightly flexed.
- Superficial cervical, supraclavicular and lymph nodes of anterior triangle can easily be palpated (Fig. 8.36).
- Chronic infection of the palatine tonsil causes enlargement of jugulodigastric lymph nodes which adhere to the internal jugular vein.
- Painful enlargement of the submandibular lymph nodes is common because infections in tongue, mouth and cheek are quite common. These nodes may be affected by tubercular bacteria.
- The spinal root of accessory nerve may get entangled in the enlarged lymph nodes situated in the posterior triangle of neck. While taking biopsy of the lymph node, one must be careful not to injure the accessory nerve lest trapezius gets damaged.
- The left supraclavicular nodes are called Virchow's lymph nodes. Cancer from stomach and testis may metastasize into these lymph nodes, which may become palpable.
- **Common causes of lymph node enlargement**
  a. *Local causes:* Acute infection, chronic infection, malignancy of any part of the body.
  b. *General causes:* Tuberculosis, secondary syphilis, Hodgkin's disease, lymphatic leukaemia.

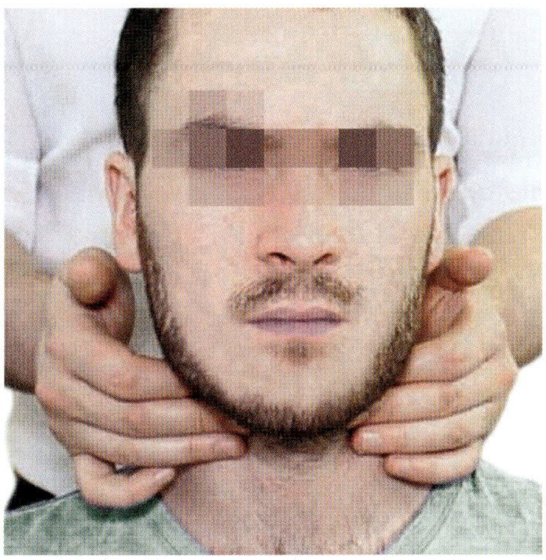

**Fig. 8.36:** Palpation of the lymph nodes of neck

## DISSECTION

Identify the lymph nodes in the submental, the submandibular, the parotid, the mastoid and the occipital regions including the deep cervical nodes. Dissect the main lymph trunk present at the root of the neck.

## STYLOID APPARATUS

- The styloid process with its attached structures is called the styloid apparatus.
- The *styloid process* is a long, slender and pointed bony process projecting downwards, forwards and slightly medially from the temporal bone. Its proximal part is enclosed by tympanic plate (tympanohyal). Its distal part gives attachment to muscles and ligaments (stylohyoid). It descends between the external and internal carotid arteries to reach the side of the pharynx. It is interposed between the parotid gland laterally and the internal jugular vein medially.

### Attachments of Styloid Process

The structures attached to the process are three muscles and two ligaments:

1. ***Styloglossus** muscle* arises from the anterior surface of the styloid process and is inserted into the side of the tongue.
2. ***Stylopharyngeus** muscle* arises from the medial surface of the base of the styloid process and is inserted on the posterior border of the lamina of the thyroid cartilage.
3. ***Stylohyoid*** extends between posterior surface of styloid process and hyoid bone. It splits at its lower end to enclose the intermediate tendon of digastric muscle.
4. ***Stylomandibular ligament*** is attached laterally to styloid process above and angle of mandible below.
5. ***Stylohyoid ligament*** extends from the tip of the styloid process to the lesser cornua of the hyoid bone.

### Features

1. The apparatus is of diverse origin (Fig. 8.37).
   a. Embryologically, styloid process comprises two parts: (i) Tympanohyal is proximal part and is ensheathed by tympanic plate, and (ii) stylohyal is the distal part
   b. The styloid process, the stylohyoid ligament and stylohyoid muscle are derived from the second branchial arch; the stylopharyngeus from the third arch; the styloglossus from occipital myotomes; and the stylomandibular ligament from a part of the deep fascia of neck.
2. The *five attachments resemble the reins of a chariot.* Two of these reins (ligaments) are nonadjustable, whereas the other three (muscles) are adjustable and are controlled each by a separate cranial nerve—seventh, ninth and twelfth nerves.
3. External carotid artery crosses tip of styloid process superficially and pierces stylomandibular ligament.
4. Facial nerve crosses the base of styloid process laterally after it emerges from stylomastoid foramen.

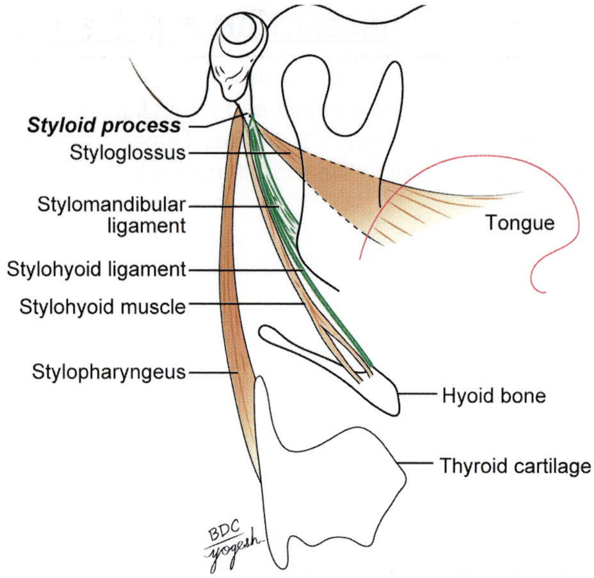


**Fig. 8.37:** The styloid apparatus

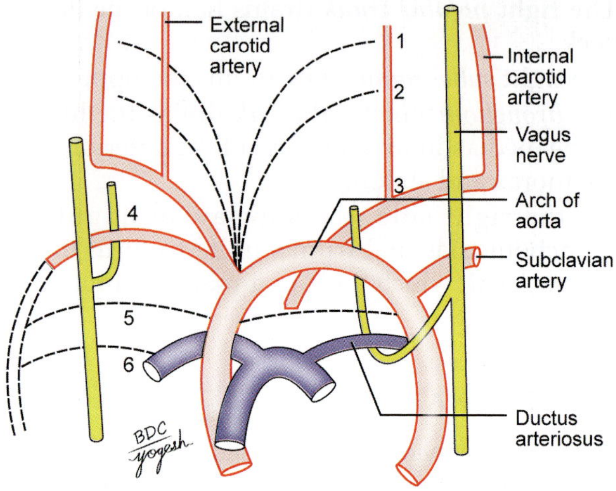


**Fig. 8.38:** Relation to recurrent laryngeal nerve

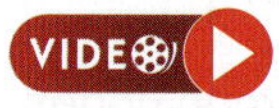


**Video 3.8 Thyroid Gland**

## DEVELOPMENT OF THE ARTERIES

| | |
|---|---|
| Brachiocephalic artery | Right aortic sac |
| Right subclavian artery | Proximal part from the right 4th aortic arch artery and remaining part from right 7th cervical intersegmental artery |
| Left subclavian artery | Only left 7th cervical intersegmental artery |
| Common carotid artery | Third aortic arch proximal to external carotid bud |
| Internal carotid artery | Third aortic arch, distal to the external carotid bud and original dorsal aorta cranial to the attachment of third aortic arch |
| External carotid artery | Develop as sprout from the third aortic arch |
| Pulmonary trunk | Part of truncus arteriosus |
| Arch of aorta | Left aortic sac<br>• Left 4th aortic arch<br>• Left dorsal aorta |

***Relation to recurrent laryngeal nerve:*** Recurrent laryngeal is given off from vagi in relation to distal part of 6th arch artery. Since this distal part forms ligamentum arteriosum on left side only, the recurrent laryngeal nerve hooks around this ligamentum in thorax to reach tracheo-oesophageal groove (Fig. 8.38).

On the right side, there is no ligamentum arteriosum, the recurrent laryngeal nerve slips upwards in the neck and hooks around the right subclavian artery to reach the tracheo-oesophageal groove.

### *Facts to Remember*

- Thyroid gland is the largest endocrine and the most vascular gland of the body.
- The most common ectopic site of thyroid gland is within tongue. The most common site of thyroglossal cyst is subhyoid.
- Parathyroid glands lie along the anastomotic channel between posterior branch of superior thyroid artery and ascending branch of inferior thyroid artery.
- Internal carotid artery comprises 4 parts: Cervical, petrous, cavernous and cerebral.
- Scalenus anterior can press upon the subclavian artery and brachial plexus, causing nervous and vascular changes in upper limb.
- Phrenic nerve (C4) supplies motor fibres to musculature of diaphragm. It carries sensory fibres from peritoneum underlying diaphragm, mediastinal pleura and pericardium.
- Styloid apparatus comprises styloglossus (XII), stylohyoid (VII), stylopharyngeus muscles (IX); and stylohyoid and stylomandibular ligaments.

### BDC's Anatomy *e*-book

1. Follicular cells and activity of thyroid gland
2. Thyroglossal cyst and fistula
3. Blood–thymic barrier
4. Further reading
5. Viva voce questions

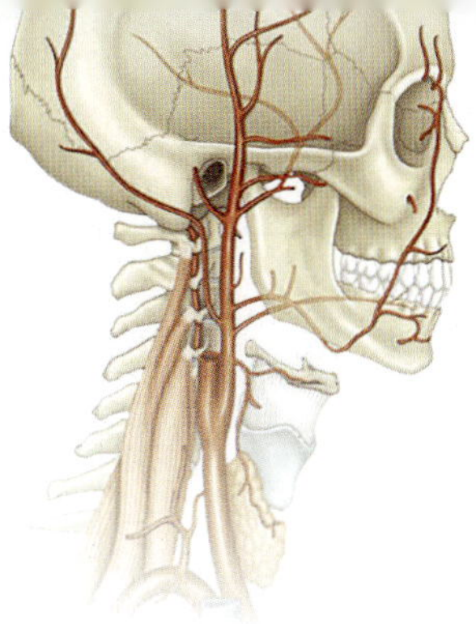

Chapter 9

# Prevertebral and Paravertebral Regions

The prevertebral region of the neck extends from the base of skull, from the C1 to T2 vertebrae. The paravertebral region of the neck lies on either side of the prevertebral region and extends from the transverse process of C1 vertebra to the first rib (Fig. 9.1).

***Prevertebral region:*** It contains:

1. Prevertebral (anterior vertebral) muscles: Rectus capitis anterior, rectus capitis lateralis, longus colli (cervicis) and longus capitis
2. 1st and 2nd parts of vertebral arteries
3. Joints of the neck.

***Paravertebral region:*** It contains:

1. Three scalene muscles
2. Cervical plexus and its branches
3. Phrenic nerve
4. Cervical pleura.

## PREVERTEBRAL MUSCLES (ANTERIOR VERTEBRAL MUSCLES)

There are four prevertebral or anterior vertebral muscles (Figs 9.2 to 9.4, Plate 9.1):

1. Rectus capitis anterior
2. Rectus capitis lateralis
3. Longus colli (cervicis)
4. Longus capitis.

### Features

- All these are covered by thick prevertebral fascia.
- They are weak flexors of the head and neck.
- They are supplied by ventral primary rami of cervical spinal nerves.

The origin, insertion, nerve supply and actions of these muscles are described in Table 9.1.

#### DISSECTION

Remove the scalenus anterior muscle. Identify deeply placed anterior and posterior intertransverse muscles. Cut through the anterior intertransverse muscles to expose the second part of vertebral artery. First part was seen as the branch arising from the first part of the subclavian artery. Its third part was seen in the suboccipital triangle. The fourth part lies in the cranial cavity.

## VERTEBRAL ARTERY

The vertebral artery arises from the posterosuperior aspect of the 1st part of the subclavian artery near its commencement (Fig. 9.5, Flowchart 9.1).

### Course

It passes upward to enter the foramina transversarium of the 6th cervical vertebra and traverses upward in foramina transversarium of upper 6 cervical vertebrae.

After emerging from the foramina transversarium of the 1st cervical vertebrae, this artery winds backward around the lateral mass of atlas. Further, the artery enters the cranial cavity through the foramen magnum.

In the cranial cavity, at the lower border of pons, it joins with the similar artery of the opposite side to form *basilar artery*.

### Parts of Vertebral Artery

Based on the location, the vertebral artery is divided into four parts as follows:

1. *First (cervical part)* extends from the 1st part of subclavian artery to the foramen transversarium of C6 vertebra. The 1st part of vertebral artery is present in the *scalenovertebral triangle*.
2. *Second (vertebral part)* lies within the foramen transversaria of C6 to C1 vertebrae.
3. *Third (suboccipital part)* extends from foramen transversarium of C1 vertebra to the foramen magnum of skull. The loop of third part of vertebral artery dampens down the arterial pulsation within the cranial cavity. It lies within the suboccipital triangle.
4. *Fourth (intracranial part)* extends from foramen magnum to the lower border of the pons.

**Plate 9.1:** Prevertebral muscles

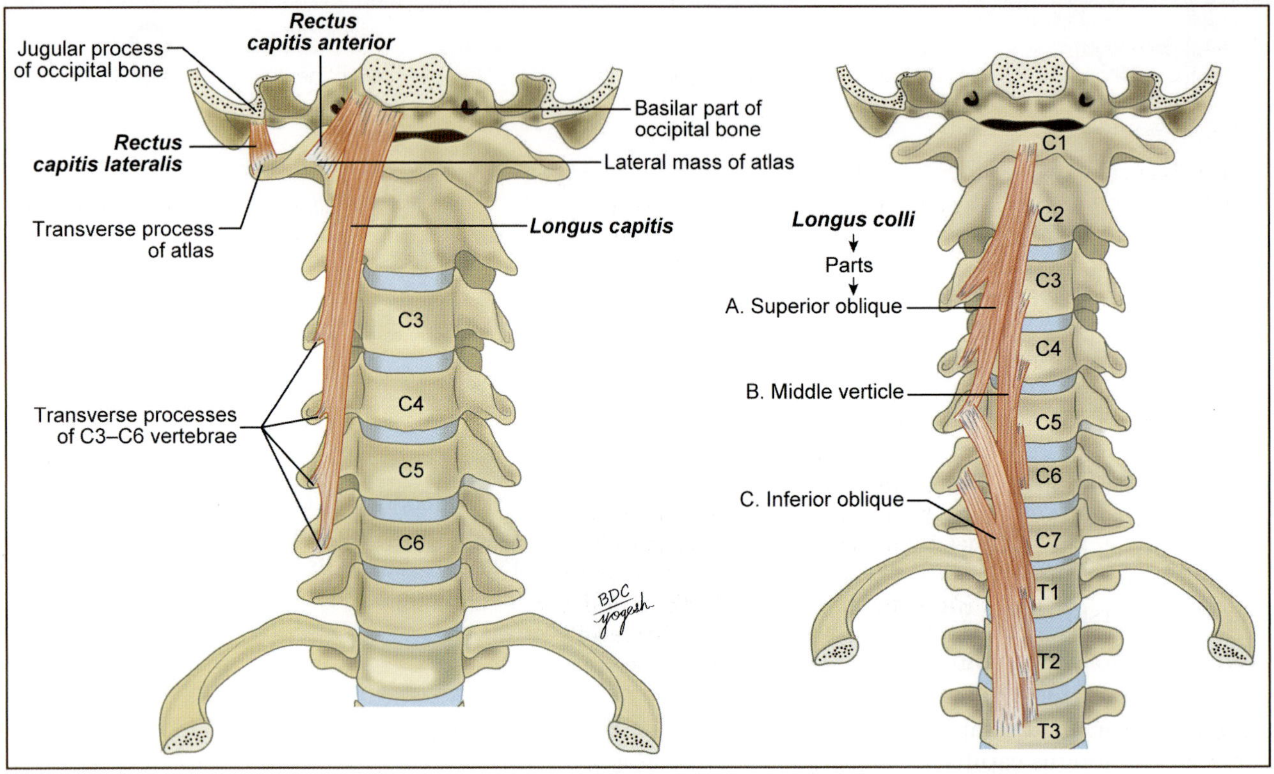


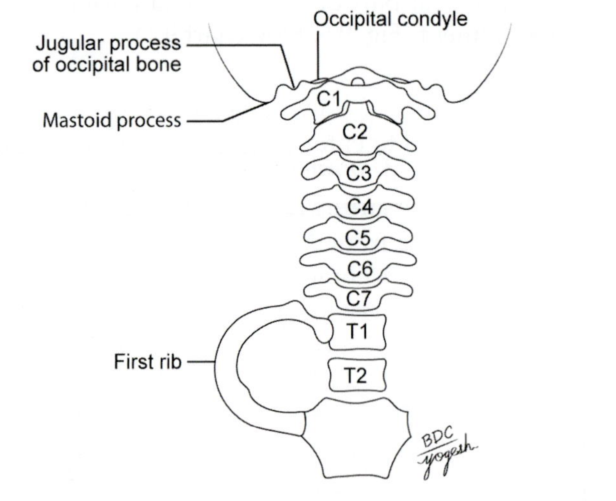


**Fig. 9.1:** Bony framework of the pre- and paravertebral regions and the root of the neck

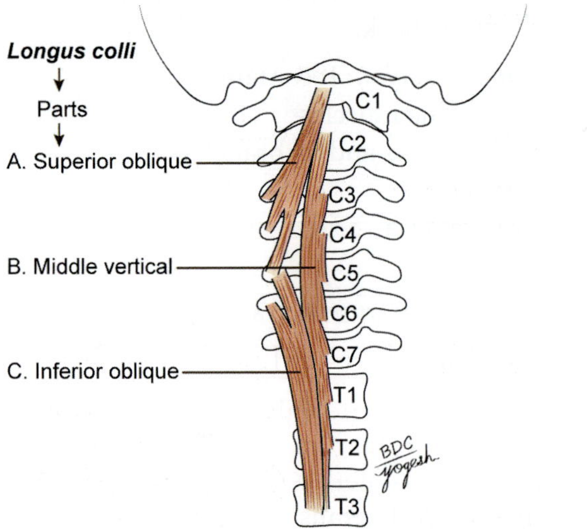


**Fig. 9.3:** Longus colli muscle

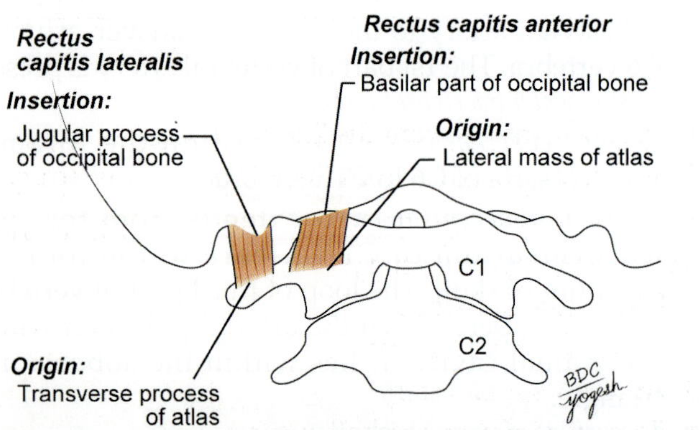


**Fig. 9.2:** Rectus capitis anterior and rectus capitis lateralis muscles

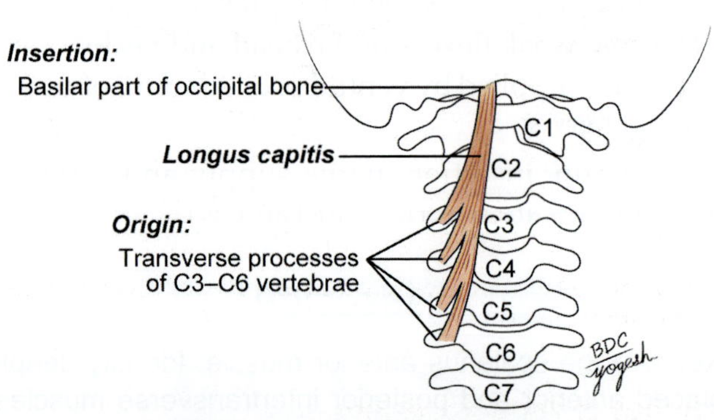


**Fig. 9.4:** Longus capitis muscle

**TABLE 9.1: The origin, insertion, nerve supply and actions of prevertebral muscles**

| *Muscle* | *Origin* | *Insertion* | *Nerve supply* | *Actions* |
|---|---|---|---|---|
| **Rectus capitis anterior** This is a very short and flat muscle. It lies deep to the longus capitis | Anterior surface of lateral mass of ***atlas*** | Basilar part of the occipital bone | Ventral ramus of nerve C1 | Flexes the head |
| **Rectus capitis lateralis** This is a short, flat muscle | Upper surface of transverse process of ***atlas*** | Inferior surface of jugular process of the occipital bone | Ventral rami of nerves C1, C2 | Flexes the head laterally |
| **Longus colli (cervicis)** This muscle extends from the atlas to the C3 vertebra. It has upper and lower oblique parts and a middle vertical part | a. ***Upper oblique part*** is from the anterior tubercles of the transverse processes of C3, C4, C5 vertebrae<br>b. ***Lower oblique part*** is from bodies of upper 2–3 thoracic vertebrae<br>c. ***Middle vertical part*** is from bodies of upper 3 thoracic and lower 3 cervical vertebrae | a. ***Upper oblique part*** is into the anterior tubercle of the atlas<br>b. ***Lower oblique part*** is into the anterior tubercles of the transverse processes of 5th and 6th cervical vertebrae<br>c. ***Middle vertical part*** is into bodies of 2, 3, 4 vertebrae cervical vertebrae | Ventral rami of nerves C3–C8 | a. Flexes the neck<br>b. Oblique parts flex the neck laterally<br>c. Lower oblique part rotates the neck to the opposite side |
| **Longus capitis** It overlaps the longus colli. It is thick above and narrow below | Anterior tubercles of transverse processes of cervical 3–6 vertebrae | Inferior surface of basilar part of occipital bone | Ventral rami of nerves C1–C3 | Flexes the head |

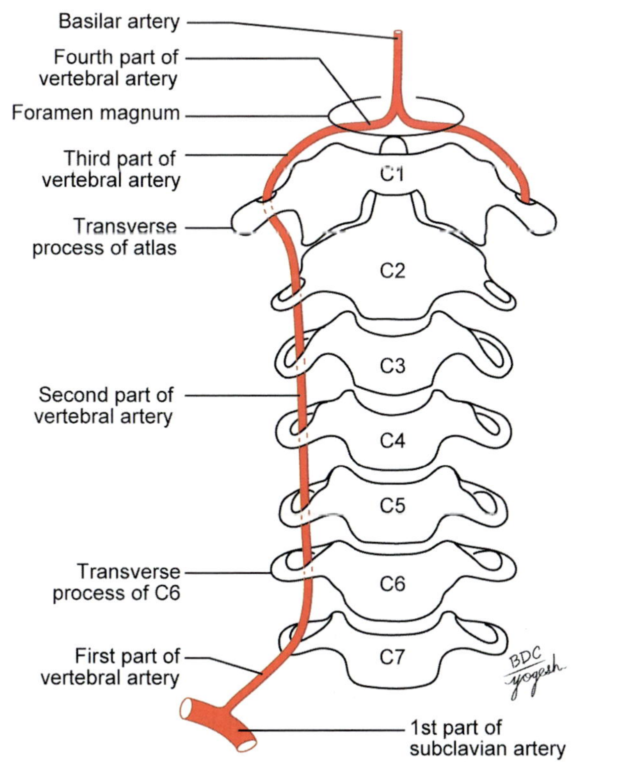


**Fig. 9.5:** Scheme showing parts of the vertebral artery, as seen from the front

## Branches of Vertebral Artery

*First part* has no branches.

**Flowchart 9.1:** Vertebral artery

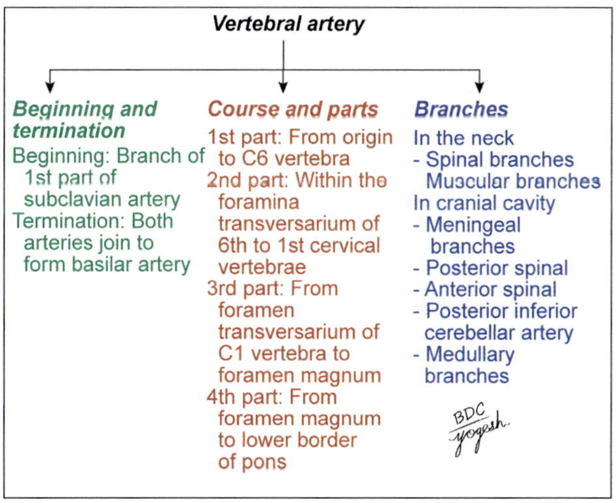


***In the neck:***

1. Spinal branches from the 2nd part of the artery
2. Muscular branches from the 3rd part of the artery.

***In the cranial cavity:*** They arise from the 4th (cranial) part of the vertebral artery.

1. Meningeal branches
2. Posterior spinal artery
3. Anterior spinal artery
4. Posterior inferior cerebellar artery
5. Medullary branches.

### Development of Vertebral Artery (Fig. 9.6)

1. *First part*: Extends from subclavian artery to foramen transversarium of sixth cervical vertebra – develops from dorsal division of seventh cervical intersegmental artery.
2. *Second part*: Extends through foramina transversarium from sixth to first cervical vertebrae – develops from postcostal anastomosis.
3. *Third part*: Extends from foramina transversarium and rests on posterior arch of the atlas – develops from spinal branch of first cervical intersegmental artery.
4. *Fourth part*: Intracranial part – develops from preneural division of spinal branch of basilar artery.

## TRACHEA

The trachea (Latin rough air vessel) is a non-collapsible, wide tube, forming the beginning of the lower respiratory passages. It is kept patent because of the presence of C-shaped cartilaginous 'rings' in its wall. The cartilages are deficient posteriorly, this part of the wall being made up of muscle (trachealis) and fibrous tissue. The soft posterior wall allows expansion of the oesophagus during passage of food.

### Dimensions

The *trachea* is about 10 to 15 cm long. Its upper half lies in the neck and its lower half in the superior mediastinum. The external diameter measures 2 cm in the male and 1.5 cm in the female. The lumen is smaller in the living than in cadavers. It is about 3 mm at 1 year of age, and corresponds to the age in years during childhood, with a maximum of 12 mm at puberty.

Trachea divides into right and left principal bronchi at the level of lower border of T6 vertebra (42nd *Grey's Anatomy*) (Previous concept: Trachea bifurcates at the lower border of T4 vertebra.)

### Cervical Part of Trachea

1. The trachea begins at the lower border of the cricoid cartilage opposite the lower border of vertebra C6. It runs downwards and slightly backward in front of the oesophagus, follows the curvature of the spine, and enters the thorax in the median plane
2. In the neck, the trachea is comparatively superficial and has the following relations.

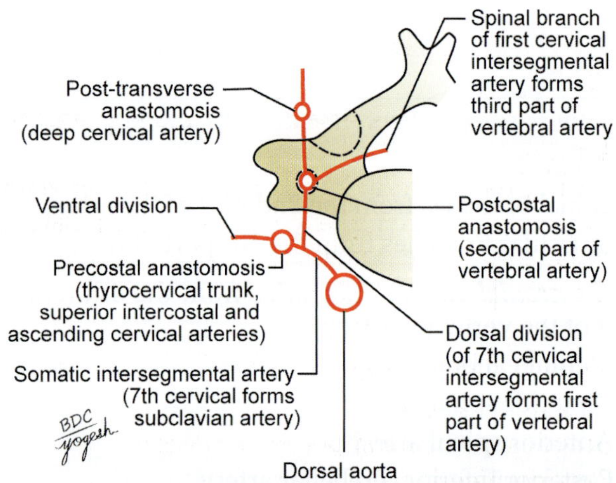


**Fig. 9.6:** Development of vertebral artery

### Anterior

1. Isthmus of the thyroid gland covering the second and third tracheal rings (*see* Fig. 8.2)
2. Inferior thyroid veins below the isthmus (*see* Fig. 8.9)
3. Pretracheal fascia enclosing the thyroid and the inferior thyroid veins
4. Sternohyoid and sternothyroid muscles (*see* Fig. 8.5)
5. Investing layer of the deep cervical fascia and the suprasternal space
6. The skin and superficial fascia
7. In children, the left brachiocephalic vein extends into the neck and then lies in front of the trachea.

### Posterior

1. Oesophagus
2. Longus colli
3. Recurrent laryngeal nerve in the tracheo-oesophageal groove.

### On Each Side

1. The corresponding lobe of the thyroid gland.
2. The common carotid artery within the carotid sheath.

### Vessels and Nerves

*Arterial supply*: Inferior thyroid arteries.

*Venous drainage*: Left brachiocephalic vein.

*Lymphatic drainage*: Peritracheal and paratracheal lymph nodes.

*Nerve supply*: Trachea is supplied by autonomic nerves as follows:

A. *Parasympathetic nerves*: They come from vagus and recurrent laryngeal nerves. These are sensory and secretomotor to mucous membrane and motor to trachealis muscle
B. *Sympathetic nerves*: They come from middle cervical ganglion along the inferior thyroid artery. These are vasomotor.

### CLINICAL ANATOMY

- The trachea may be compressed by pathological enlargements of the thyroid, the thymus, lymph nodes and the aortic arch. This causes dyspnoea, irritative cough and often a husky voice.
- ***Tracheostomy*** is an emergency operation done in cases of laryngeal obstruction (foreign body, diphtheria, carcinoma, etc.). It is commonly done in the retrothyroid region after retracting the isthmus of the thyroid gland.

## OESOPHAGUS

The oesophagus is a muscular food passage lying between the trachea and the vertebral column.

The oesophagus is a downward continuation of the pharynx and begins at the lower border of the cricoid cartilage, opposite the lower border of the body of vertebra C6. It passes downwards behind the trachea, traverses the superior and posterior mediastina of the thorax and ends by opening into the cardiac end of the stomach in the abdomen. It is about 25 cm long.

It has three parts:

1. Cervical
2. Thoracic
3. Abdominal.

### Cervical Part

The cervical part of the oesophagus is related:

1. *Anteriorly*, to the trachea and to the right and left recurrent laryngeal nerves.
2. *Posteriorly*, to the longus colli muscle and the vertebral column.
3. *On each side*, to the corresponding (*see* Fig. 8.5) lobe of the thyroid gland; and on the left side, to the thoracic duct.

The cervical part of the oesophagus is supplied by the inferior thyroid arteries. Its veins drain into the left brachiocephalic vein. Its lymphatics pass to the deep cervical lymph nodes. The oesophagus is narrowest at its junction with the pharynx, the junction being the narrowest part of the gastrointestinal tract, except for the vermiform appendix.

For thoracic part of oesophagus study, *see* Chapter 20, *BD Chaurasia's Human Anatomy, Volume 1.*

### CLINICAL ANATOMY

Oesophagus has four natural constrictions (Fig. 9.7).

1. *First constriction*: At pharyngoesophageal junction, 15 cm (6 inches) from incisor teeth. It is produced by cricopharyngeus part of inferior constrictor muscle of pharynx.
2. *Second constriction*: At the crossing of arch of the aorta, 23 cm (9 inches) from incisor teeth.
3. *Third constriction*: At the crossing of the left principal bronchus, 28 cm (11 inches) from incisor teeth.
4. *Fourth constriction*: At the passage through the diaphragm, 40 cm (15 inches) from incisor teeth.

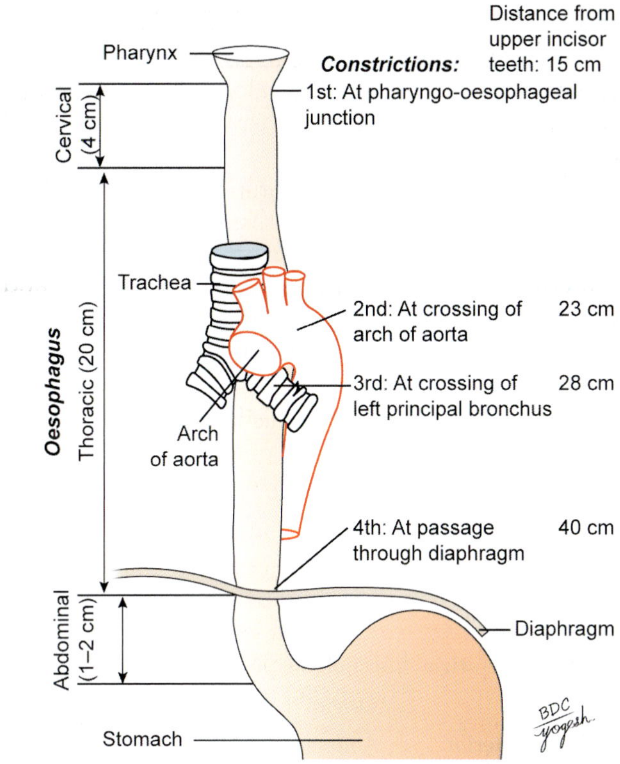


**Fig. 9.7:** Natural constrictions of the oesophagus

## PARAVERTEBRAL REGION

### SCALENE MUSCLES

There are usually three scalene muscles (Plate 9.2):

1. Scalenus anterior
2. Scalenus medius
3. Scalenus posterior.

### Features

1. The scalenus medius is the largest and the scalenus posterior is the smallest of three
2. These muscles extend from the transverse processes of cervical vertebrae to the first two ribs
3. They can, therefore, either elevate these ribs or bend the cervical part of the vertebral column laterally.

*Note*: Sometimes a fourth, rudimentary scalene muscle, the ***scalenus minimus*** is present. It arises from the anterior border of the transverse process of vertebra C7 and is inserted into the inner border of the 1st rib behind the groove for the subclavian artery and into the dome of the cervical pleura. The *suprapleural membrane* is regarded as the expansion of this muscle. Contraction of the scalenus minimus pulls the dome of the cervical pleura.

The origin, insertion, nerve supply and actions of these muscles are described in Table 9.2.

### Relations of Scalene Anterior Muscles (Fig. 9.8)

The scalenus anterior is a *key* muscle of the lower part of the neck because of its intimate relations to many important structures in this region. It is a useful surgical landmark.

#### *Anterior relations*

1. Prevertebral fascia
2. Phrenic nerve
3. Two arteries – transverse cervical and suprascapular arteries
4. Two veins – anterior jugular and subclavian veins
5. Two muscles – inferior belly of omohyoid and clavicular head of sternocleidomastoid
6. Clavicle.

#### *Posterior relations*

1. Roots of brachial plexus
2. Subclavian artery
3. Scalenus medius and posterior muscles
4. Cervical pleura
5. Suprapleural membrane.

Plate 9.2: Scalene muscles

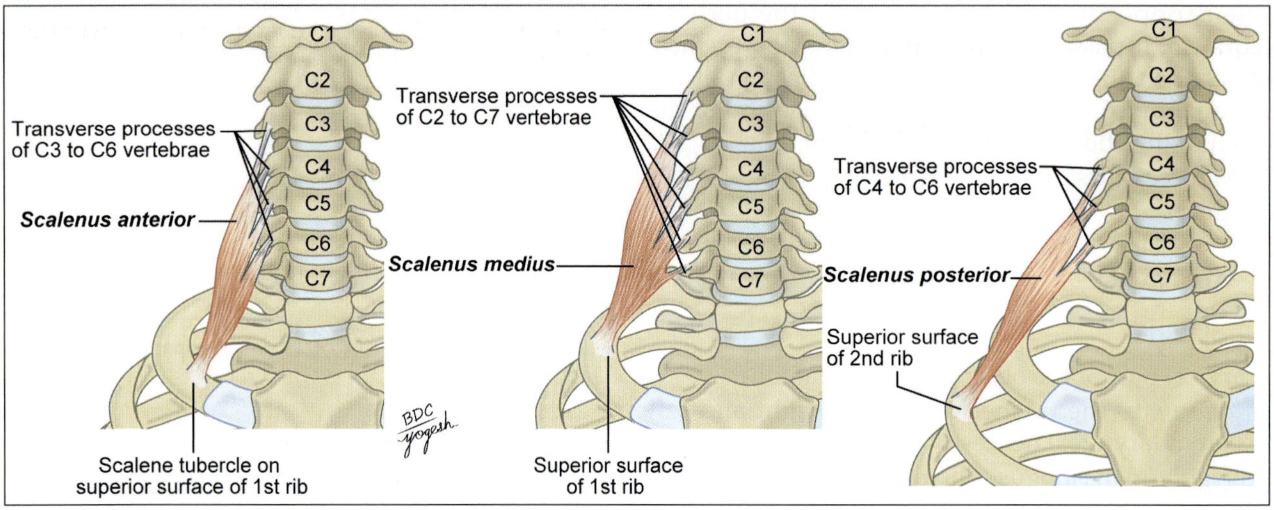


**TABLE 9.2: The origin, insertion, nerve supply and actions of scalene muscles**

| *Muscle* | *Origin* | *Insertion* | *Nerve supply* | *Actions* |
|---|---|---|---|---|
| 1. **Scalenus anterior** | Anterior tubercles of transverse processes of **C3 to C6** vertebrae | Scalene tubercle and adjoining ridge on the superior surface of the ***1st rib*** (between subclavian artery and vein) | Ventral rami of nerves C4–C6 | a. Anterolateral flexion of cervical spine<br>b. Rotates cervical spine to opposite side<br>c. Elevates the 1st rib during inspiration<br>d. Stabilises the neck along with other muscles |
| 2. **Scalenus medius** | a. Posterior tubercles of transverse processes of **C2 to C7** vertebrae<br>b. Transverse process of axis and sometimes also of the atlas vertebra | Superior surface of the ***1st rib*** behind the groove for the subclavian artery | Ventral rami of nerves C3–C8 | a. Lateral flexion of the cervical spine<br>b. Elevation of 1st rib<br>c. Stabilises neck along with other muscles |
| 3. **Scalenus posterior** | Posterior tubercles of transverse processes of **C4 to C6** vertebrae | Outer surface of the ***2nd rib*** behind the tubercle for the serratus anterior | Ventral rami of nerves C6–C8 | a. Lateral flexion of cervical spine<br>b. Elevation of the 2nd rib<br>c. Stabilises neck along with other muscles |

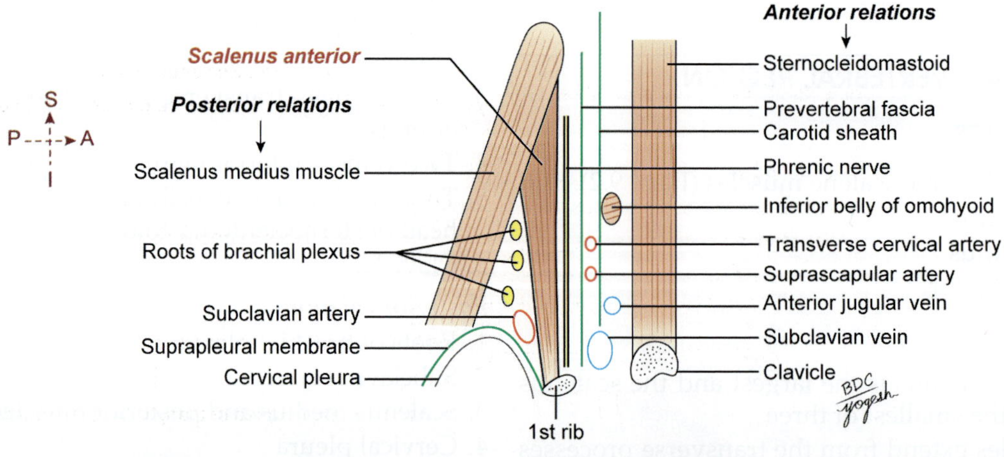


Fig. 9.8: Lateral view of the scalene muscles with a few related structures

***Relation of medial border***

1. Forms the lateral boundary of scalenovertebral triangle
2. Vertebral artery and contents of scalenovertebral triangle.

***Relations of lateral border:*** Trunks of brachial plexus emerge deep to the lateral border.

## SCALENE TRIANGLE

It is also called *subclavian triangle*. It is a narrow triangular gap bounded as follows (Fig. 9.9):

*Inferiorly (base)*: 1st rib
*Medially*: Scalenus anterior
*Laterally*: Scalenus medius
*Contact*: It gives passage to:

1. Subclavian artery
2. Trunks of brachial plexus

*Note*: ***Scalene syndrome*** occurs due to compression of the lower trunk of brachial plexus and the subclavian artery in the scalene triangle. It may occur due to the cervical rib or spasm of scalene muscle. Due to compression of subclavian artery, there will be ischaemic pain and absence of radial pulse. The compression of lower trunk (C8, T1) produces tingling sensation and numbness or sensory loss along the medial border of forearm and hand, and the paralysis and muscle wasting of intrinsic muscles of hand.

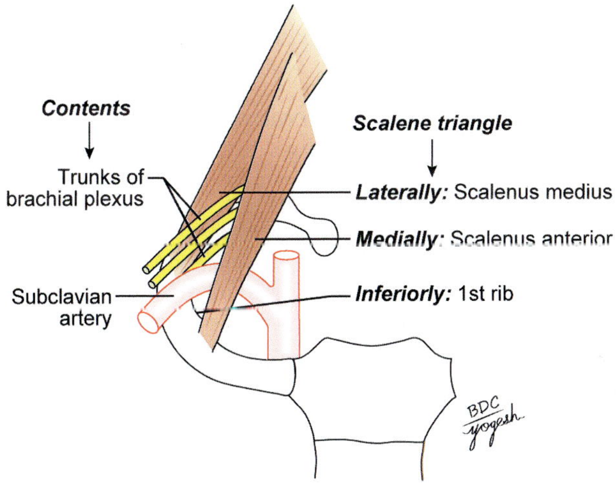


**Fig. 9.9:** Scalene triangle

## SCALENOVERTEBRAL TRIANGLE

It is also called *triangle of the vertebral artery*. It is a bilaterally placed triangular space at the root of the neck (Fig. 9.10, Flowchart 9.2).

### Boundaries

*Medial:* Lower oblique part of longus colli
*Lateral:* Scalenus anterior
*Apex:* Transverse process of C6 vertebra
*Base:* 1st part of subclavian artery
*Floor (posterior wall):*

1. Transverse process of C7 vertebra
2. Ventral ramus of C8 spinal nerve
3. Neck of 1st rib
4. Cupola of cervical pleura

*Roof:* Carotid sheath.

### Contents

1. 1st part of vertebral artery and accompanying vein
2. Thyrocervical trunk
3. Inferior thyroid artery
4. Sympathetic chain with stellate ganglion
5. Thoracic duct on the left
6. Ansa subclavia

*Note*: *Ansa subclavia* is an anterior root of nerve fibres connecting the middle and inferior cervical sympathetic ganglia. It loops around the 1st part of subclavian artery.

**Flowchart 9.2:** Scalenovertebral triangle

***Scalenovertebral triangle***
Triangle of vertebral artery

***Boundaries***
Medial: Lower oblique part of longus colli
Lateral: Scalenus anterior
Apex: Transverse process of C6 vertebra
Base: 1st part of subclavian artery
Floor: Transverse process of C7 vertebra, ventral ramus of C8 spinal nerve, neck of 1st rib, cupola of cervical pleura
Roof: Carotid sheath

***Contents***
1st part of vertebral artery
Thyrocervical trunk
Inferior thyroid artery
Sympathetic chain with stellate ganglion
Thoracic duct on the left
Ansa subclavia

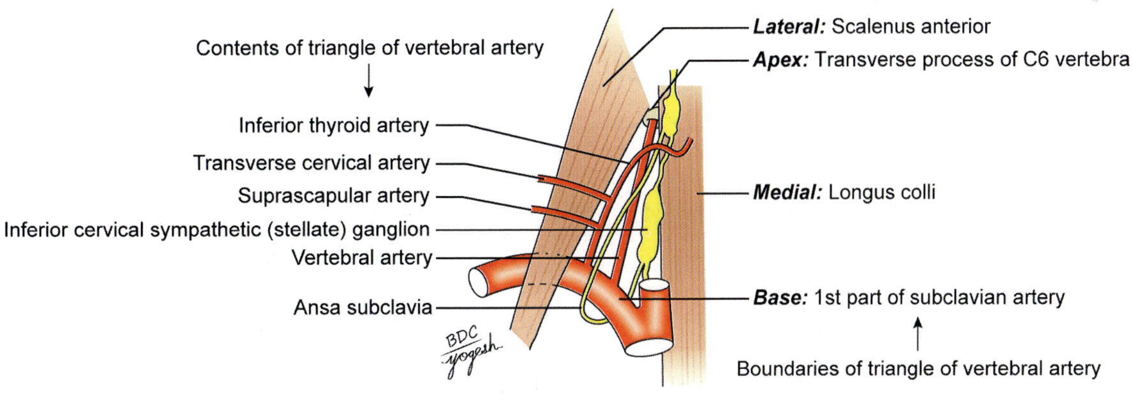


**Fig. 9.10:** Triangle of vertebral artery (right anterior view, Note: Thoracic duct is a content of the left triangle of vertebral artery)

## DISSECTION

Clean and define the cervical parts of the trachea and oesophagus.

Scalenus anterior has been seen in relation to subclavian artery. Scalenus medius is one of the muscles forming floor of posterior triangle of neck.

Scalenus posterior lies deep to the medius.

## CERVICAL PLEXUS

### Formation

The cervical plexus is formed by the ventral rami of C1 to C4 spinal nerves (Fig. 9.11). The rami emerge between the anterior and posterior tubercles of the cervical transverse processes, grooving the costotransverse bars. The four roots are connected with one another to form three loops.

### Position and Relations of the Plexus

The plexus is related:

1. *Posteriorly*, to the muscles which arise from the posterior tubercles of the transverse processes, i.e. the levator scapulae and the scalenus medius
2. *Anteriorly*, to the prevertebral fascia, the internal jugular vein and the sternocleidomastoid.

### Branches

#### Superficial (Cutaneous) Branches

1. Lesser occipital (C2)
2. Great auricular (C2, C3)
3. Transverse (anterior) cutaneous nerve of the neck (C2, C3)
4. Supraclavicular (C3, C4).

These are described in Chapter 3.

### Deep Branches

#### Communicating Branches

1. Grey rami pass from the superior cervical ganglion to the roots of C1–C4 nerves
2. A branch from C1 joins the hypoglossal nerve and carries fibres for supply of the thyrohyoid and geniohyoid muscles (directly) and the superior belly of the omohyoid through the descendens hypoglossi
3. A branch each from C2, C3 to the sternocleidomastoid and branches from C3 and C4 to the trapezius communicate with the accessory nerve.

#### Muscular Branches

Muscles supplied solely by cervical plexus:

1. Rectus capitis anterior from C1
2. Rectus capitis lateralis from C1, C2
3. Longus capitis from C1 to C3
4. Lower root of ansa cervicalis (descendens cervicalis) from C2, C3 (to sternohyoid, sternothyroid and inferior belly of omohyoid).

Muscles supplied by cervical plexus along with the brachial plexus or the spinal accessory nerve are:

1. Sternocleidomastoid from C2 to C3 along with accessory nerve
2. Trapezius from C3 to C4 along with accessory nerve
3. Levator scapulae from C3 to C5 (dorsal scapular nerve)
4. The diaphragm from phrenic nerve from C3 to C5
5. Longus colli from C3 to C8
6. Scalenus medius from C3 to C8
7. Scalenus anterior from C4 to C6
8. Scalenus posterior from C6 to C8.

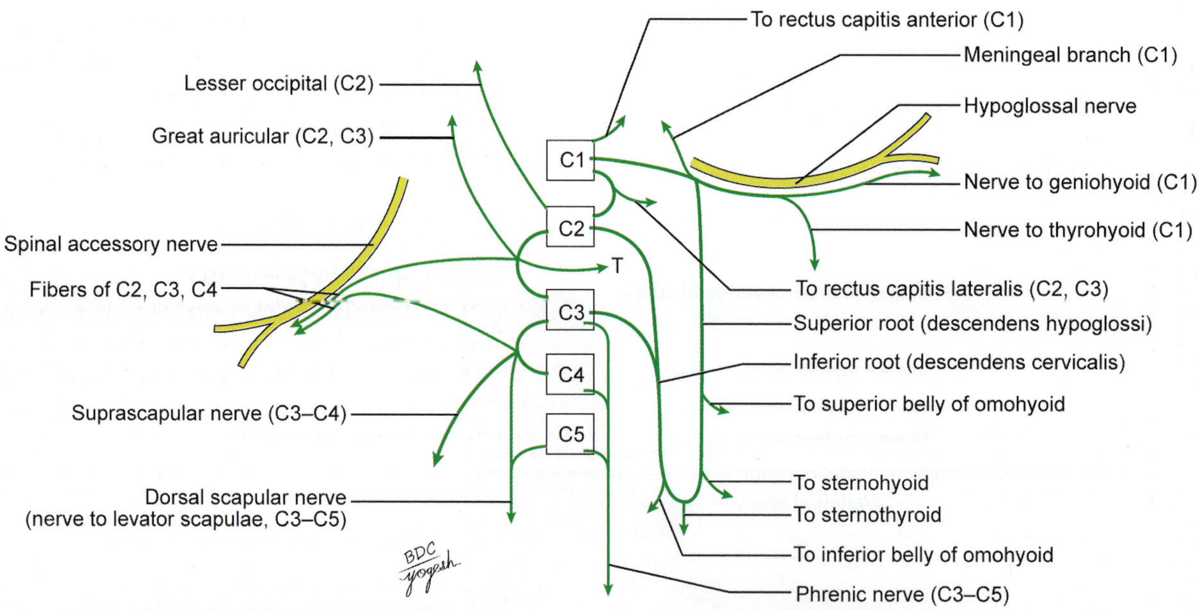


**Fig. 9.11:** Cervical plexus and its branches (T: transverse cutaneous nerve of neck [C2, C3], *Note*: Grey rami communicantes and branches for longus capitis, longus coli, scalene muscles are not shown to maintain the clarity)

## PHRENIC NERVE

This is a ***mixed*** nerve carrying motor fibres to the diaphragm and sensory fibres from the diaphragm, pleura, pericardium and part of the peritoneum (Fig. 9.12, Flowchart 9.3).

### Origin

Phrenic nerve arises chiefly from the fourth cervical nerve but receives contributions from third and fifth cervical nerves. The contribution from C5 may come directly from the root or indirectly through the nerve to the subclavius. In the latter case, the contribution is known as the *accessory phrenic nerve*.

### Course and Relations in the Neck

1. The nerve is formed at the lateral border of the scalenus anterior, opposite the middle of the sternocleidomastoid, at the level of the upper border of the thyroid cartilage.
2. It runs vertically downwards on the anterior surface of the scalenus anterior. Since the muscle is oblique, the nerve appears to cross it obliquely from lateral to medial border. In this part of its course, the nerve is related anteriorly to the prevertebral fascia, the inferior belly of the omohyoid, the transverse cervical artery, the suprascapular artery, the internal jugular vein, the sternocleidomastoid and the thoracic duct on left side (Fig. 9.12).
3. After leaving the anterior surface of scalenus anterior, the nerve runs downwards on the cervical pleura behind the commencement of the brachiocephalic vein. Here, it crosses the internal thoracic artery (either anteriorly or posteriorly) from lateral to medial side, and enters the thorax behind the first costal cartilage. On the left side, the nerve leaves (crosses) the medial margin of the scalenus anterior at a higher level and crosses in front of the first part of the subclavian artery.

### Branches

1. It supplies diaphragm from its under surface through four sets of branches on each side — anteromedial, anterolateral, posteromedial and posterolateral.
2. *Right phrenic nerve* — right half of the diaphragm, part of right crus.
3. *Left phrenic nerve* — left half of the diaphragm, left crus and part of right crus
4. Also supplies pleura and peritoneum.

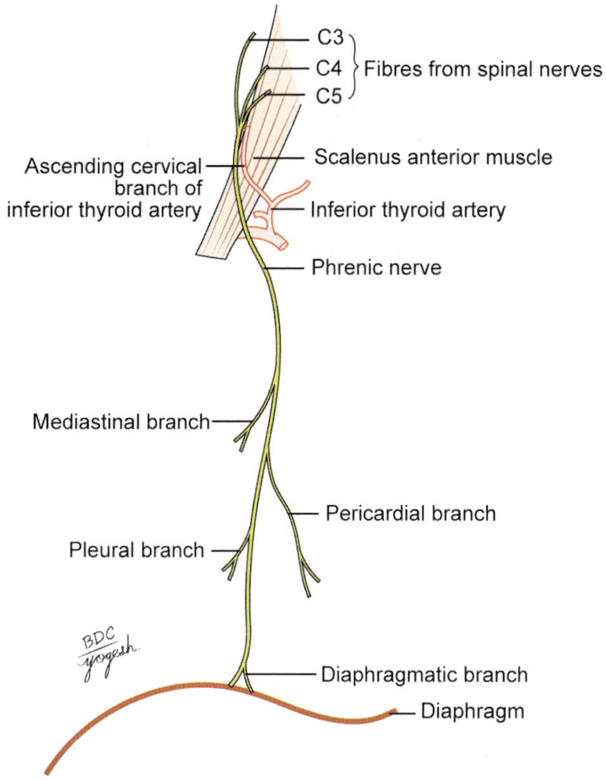


**Fig. 9.12:** Formation, course and distribution of phrenic nerve

**Flowchart 9.3:** Phrenic nerve

***Phrenic nerve***
Root value: C3, C4, C5

| ***Formation*** | ***Course and relations*** | ***Branches*** |
|---|---|---|
| Branch of ventral primary rami of C3 to C5 | In neck: Runs on anterior surface of scalenus anterior<br>In thorax: It runs just medial to mediastinal pleura<br>Right nerve passes through diaphragmatic opening of IVC<br>Left nerve pierces left cupola of diaphragm | 1. Diaphragm<br>2. Pleura<br>3. Peritoneum |

***Clinical integration:*** Surgical identification (association with ascending cervical branch of inferior thyroid artery), avulsion of phrenic nerve, accessory phrenic nerve (C5), referred pain of diaphragm

### CLINICAL ANATOMY

- ***Surgical identification:*** In the neck, phrenic nerve is accompanied by ascending cervical branch of inferior thyroid artery. It may help for the identification of the phrenic nerve.
- ***Avulsion of phrenic nerve (old surgical method):*** Crushing or avulsion of phrenic nerve was done to paralyze half part of the diaphragm. It was useful in the treatment of severe lung disease.
- ***Accessory phrenic nerve (root value C5):*** It is the branch of nerve to subclavius (C5). It may descend in front of subclavian vein and then join phrenic nerve in the thorax (Fig. 9.13). Accessory phrenic nerve, if present, may damage the subclavian vein during avulsion of phrenic nerve → severe bleeding.
- ***Referred pain of diaphragm:*** Pain from the diaphragm get referred from phrenic nerve (C3–C5) to the shoulder region through supraclavicular nerves (C3–C4).

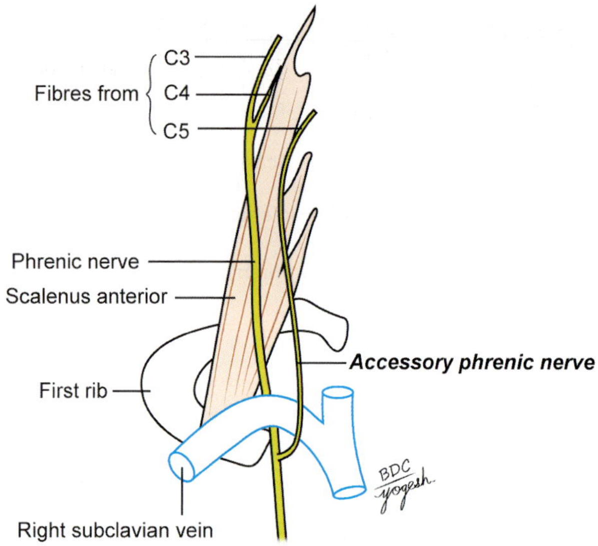


Fig. 9.13: Accessory phrenic nerve

## JOINTS OF THE NECK

The joints of the neck include (Flowchart 9.4, Table 9.3):

1. Craniovertebral joints
   A. Atlanto-occipital joints
   B. Atlanto-axial joints
2. Joints between lower cervical vertebrae (typical cervical joints).

### Typical Cervical Joints between the Lower Six Cervical Vertebrae (Figs 9.14a to e)

The bodies of cervical vertebra are united by intervertebral disc. On each side of the disc are small synovial joints called joints of Luschka or uncovertebral joints. The adjacent vertebrae are connected by several ligaments; which are as follows:

1. *Anterior longitudinal ligament* passes from the anterior surface of the body of one vertebra to another. Its upper end reaches the basilar part of the occipital bone (Fig. 9.14c).
2. *Posterior longitudinal ligament* is present on the posterior surface of the vertebral bodies within the vertebral canal. Its upper end reaches the body of the axis vertebra beyond which it continues as the *membrana tectoria*.
3. *Intertransverse ligaments* connect adjacent transverse processes.
4. *Interspinous ligaments* connect adjacent spines.
5. *Supraspinous ligaments* connect the tips of the spines of vertebrae from the seventh cervical to the sacrum. In the cervical region, they are replaced by the ligamentum nuchae.
6. ***Ligamentum nuchae*** is triangular in shape. Its apex lies at the seventh cervical spine and its base at the external occipital crest. Its anterior border is attached to cervical spines, while the posterior border is free and provides attachment to the investing layer of deep cervical fascia. The ligament gives origin to the splenius, rhomboids and trapezius muscles (Fig. 9.14e).

**Flowchart 9.4:** Joints of neck and their types

***Joints of neck and their types***

***Craniovertebral joints***
Atlanto-occipital joints
- Ellipsoid synovial
Median atlantoaxial joint
- Pivot synovial
Lateral atlantoaxial joints
- Plane synovial

***Typical cervical joints***
Between vertebral bodies
- Secondary cartilagenous
Joints of Luschka
- Plane synovial
Between articular processes
- Plane synovial
Between laminae, spines and transverse processes
- Syndesmosis (fibrous)

**TABLE 9.3: Joints of neck and classification**

| *Joint* | *Classification* |
|---|---|
| 1. Craniovertebral joints | |
| A. Atlanto-occipital joints | Ellipsoidal variety of synovial joint |
| B. Atlantoaxial joints | |
| i. Median atlantoaxial joints | Pivot variety of synovial joint |
| ii. Lateral atlantoaxial joints | Plane synovial joints |
| 2. Typical cervical joints | |
| A. Joints between vertebral bodies | Secondary cartilaginous joints |
| B. Joints of Luschka (between the lateral margins of vertebral bodies) | Plane synovial joints |
| C. Joints between vertebral arches | |
| i. Joints between articular processes (zygapophyseal joints/facet joints) | Plane synovial joints |
| ii. Intervertebral syndesmosis (joints between adjacent laminae, spines and transverse processes) | Syndesmosis type of fibrous joints |

### Joint between Vertebral Arches

The joint between superior and inferior articular processes of adjacent vertebrae is plane joint of synovial variety. The articular processes slope inferiorly to allow rotation of neck. These are also called zygapophyseal/ facet joints.

The laminae of adjacent vertebrae are united by ligamentum flava, made up of elastic fibres. It ends at C2 level (Fig. 9.14a).

### Joints between Atlas, Axis and Occipital Bone

1. The atlanto-occipital and the atlantoaxial joints are designed to permit free movements of the head on the neck (vertebral column).
2. The axis vertebra and the occipital bone are connected by very strong ligaments. Between these two bones, the atlas is held like a washer. The axis of movement

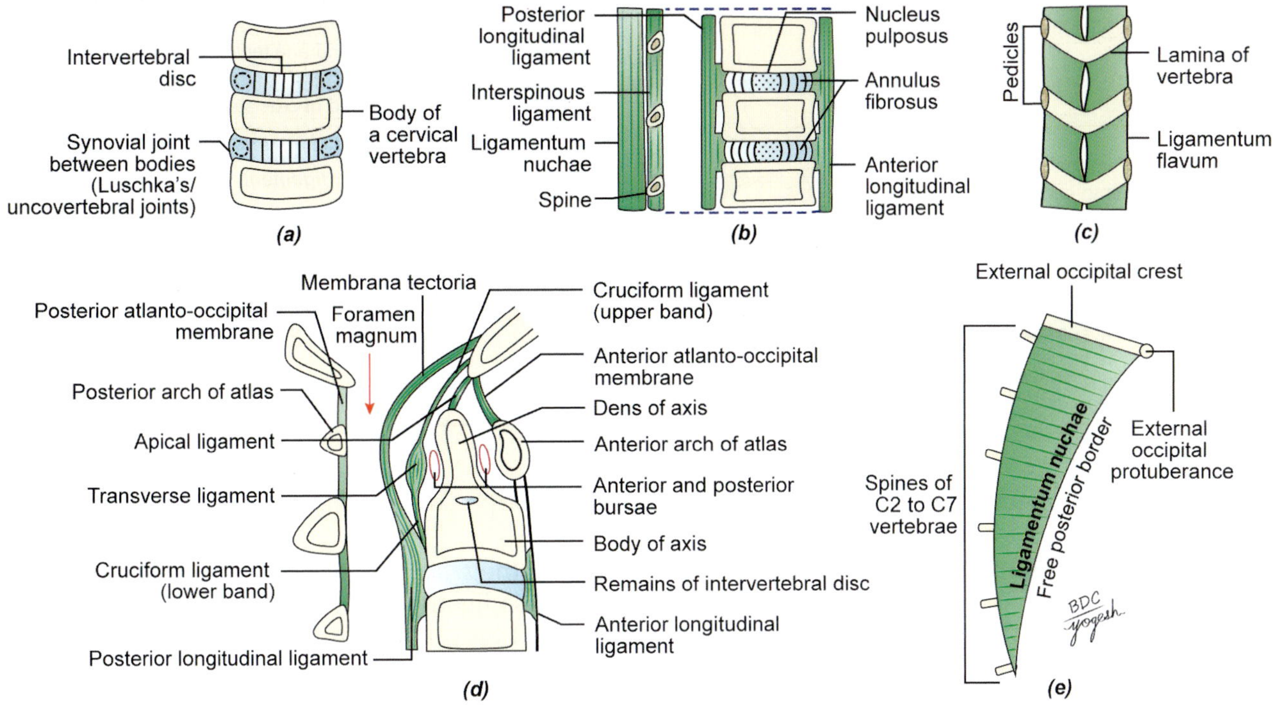


**Figs 9.14a to e:** (a) Joints between vertebral bodies as seen from front, (b) side view showing the ligaments, (c) anterior view of the ligamentum flava, (d) median section through the foramen magnum and upper two cervical vertebrae showing the ligaments in this region, and (e) ligamentum nuchae

between the atlas and skull is transverse, permitting flexion and extension (nodding), whereas the axis of movement between the axis and the atlas is vertical, permitting rotation of the head.

*Competency:*

**AN43.1** Describe and demonstrate the movements with muscles producing the movements of atlanto-occipital joint and atlantoaxial joint.

## Atlanto-occipital Joints

### Types and Articular Surfaces

These are synovial joints of the ellipsoid variety (Fig. 9.15).

***Above:*** The convex occipital condyles.

***Below:*** The superior articular facets of the atlas vertebra. These are concave. The articular surfaces are elongated and are directed forwards and medially.

### Ligaments

1. ***Fibrous capsule*** *(capsular ligament)* surrounds the joint. It is thick posterolaterally and thin anteromedially.
2. ***Anterior atlanto-occipital membrane*** extends from the anterior margin of the foramen magnum above to the upper border of the anterior arch of the atlas below. Laterally, it is continuous with the anterior part of the capsular ligament, and anteriorly, it is strengthened by the cord-like anterior longitudinal ligament.
3. ***Posterior atlanto-occipital membrane*** extends from the posterior margin of the foramen magnum above, to the upper border of the posterior arch of the atlas below. Inferolaterally, it has a free margin that arches over the vertebral artery and the first cervical nerve. Laterally, it is continuous with the posterior part of the capsular ligament.

### Arterial and Nerve Supply

The joint is supplied by the vertebral artery and the first cervical nerve.

### Movements

Since these are ellipsoid joints, they permit movements around two axes (Figs 9.16a to c). Flexion and extension (nodding) occur around a transverse axis. Slight lateral flexion is permitted around an anteroposterior axis.

1. *Flexion* is brought about by the longus capitis and the rectus capitis anterior.
2. *Extension* is done by the rectus capitis posterior major and minor, the obliquus capitis superior, the semispinalis capitis, the splenius capitis and the upper part of the trapezius.
3. *Lateral bending* is produced by the rectus capitis lateralis, the semispinalis capitis, the splenius capitis, the sternocleidomastoid and the trapezius.

## Atlantoaxial Joints

### Types and Articular Surfaces

These joints comprise (Fig. 9.15, Flowchart 9.5):

1. A pair of lateral atlantoaxial joints between the inferior facets of the atlas and the superior facets of the axis. These are plane joints.
2. A median atlantoaxial joint between the dens (odontoid process) and the anterior arch and between

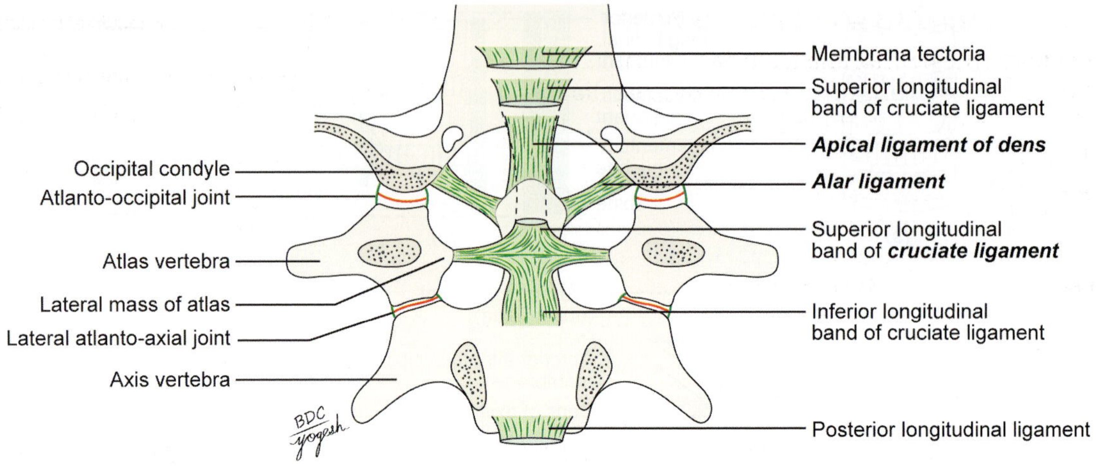


**Fig. 9.15:** Ligaments connecting the axis with occipital bone (coronal section passing through occipital condyles, posterior view)

**Flowchart 9.5:** Atlanto-occipital joint

***Atlanto-occipital joint***
Ellipsoid synovial joint

- ***Articular surfaces***
  - Superior: Occipital condyles
  - Inferior: Facets of atlas
- ***Ligaments***
  - Fibrous capsule
  - Anterior atlanto-occipital membrane
  - Posterior atlanto-occipital membrane
- ***Supply***
  - Vertebral artery
  - C1 nerve
- ***Movements***
  - Flexion
    - Longus capitis
    - RCA
  - Extension
    - RCP major
    - RCP minor
    - Splenius capitis
    - Semispinalis capitis

(RCA: Rectus capitis anterior, RCP major: Rectus capitis posterior major, RCP minor: Rectus capitis posterior minor)

dens and transverse ligament of the atlas. It is a pivot joint. The joint has two separate synovial cavities—anterior and posterior.

### *Ligaments*

The lateral atlantoaxial joints are supported by:

a. Capsular ligament all around.
b. Lateral part of the anterior longitudinal ligament.
c. Ligamentum flavum.
d. Accessory atlantoaxial ligament presents between posterior surface of body of axis and lateral masses of atlas vertebra.

The median atlantoaxial joint is strengthened by the following:

a. The anterior smaller part of the joint between the anterior arch of the atlas and the dens is surrounded by a loose capsular ligament.
b. The posterior larger part of the joint between the dens and transverse ligament (often called a bursa) is often continuous with one of the atlanto-occipital joints. Its main support is the transverse ligament which forms a part of the cruciform ligament of the atlas.

The *transverse ligament* is attached on each side to the medial surface of the lateral mass of the atlas. In the median plane, its fibres are prolonged upwards to the basiocciput and downwards to the body of the axis, thus forming the *cruciform ligament of the atlas vertebra*. The transverse ligament embraces the narrow neck of the dens, and prevents its dislocation.

### *Movements* (Figs 9.16a to c)

Movements at all three joints are rotatory and take place around a vertical axis. The dens forms a pivot around which the atlas rotates (carrying the skull with it). The movement is limited by the alar ligaments.

The rotatory movements are brought about by the obliquus capitis inferior, the rectus capitis posterior major and the splenius capitis of one side, acting with the sternocleidomastoid of the opposite side.

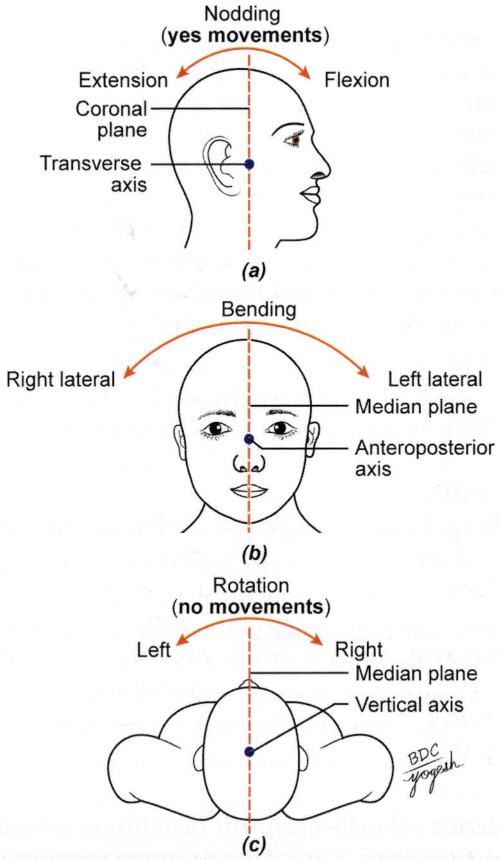


**Figs 9.16a to c:** Various movements of the neck

### Ligaments Connecting Axis with Occipital Bone

These ligaments are the membrana tectoria, the cruciate ligament, the apical ligament of the dens and the alar ligaments. They support both the atlanto-occipital and atlantoaxial joints.

1. ***Membrana tectoria*** is an upward continuation of the posterior longitudinal ligament. It lies posterior to the transverse ligament. It is attached inferiorly to the posterior surface of the body of the axis and superiorly to the basiocciput (within the foramen magnum).
2. ***Cruciate ligament*** (*see* transverse ligament).
3. The *apical ligament of the dens* extends from the apex of the dens to the basiocciput inferior to the attachment of the cruciate ligament. It is the continuation of the notochord.
4. ***Alar ligament***, one on each side, extends from the upper part of the lateral surface of the dens to the medial surface of the occipital condyles. These are strong ligaments that limit the rotation and flexion of the head. They are relaxed during extension.

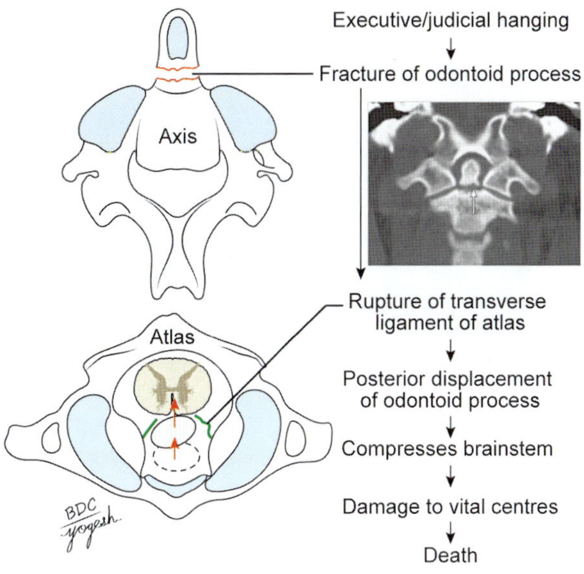


**Fig. 9.17:** Fracture of the dens during hanging

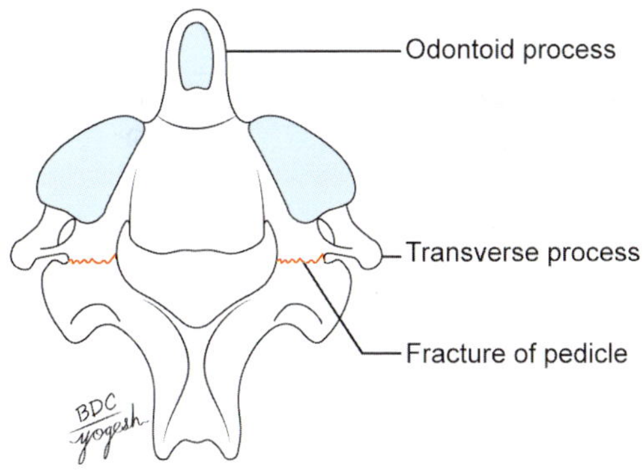


**Fig. 9.18:** Hangman's fracture

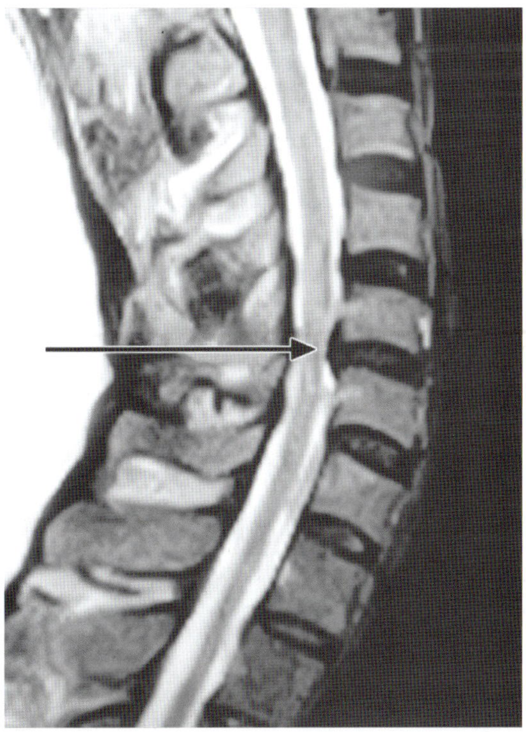

**Fig. 9.19:** Posterior intervertebral disc prolapse

## CLINICAL ANATOMY

- Death in execution by ***hanging*** is due to dislocation of the dens following rupture of the transverse ligament of the dens, which then crushes the spinal cord and medulla. However, hanging can also cause fracture through the axis, or separation of the axis from the third cervical vertebra (Fig. 9.17).
- ***Hangman's fracture*** is the fracture of pedicles of axis vertebra (Fig. 9.18). It may occur in automobile accidents or fall from height.
- ***Cervical spondylosis:*** Injury or degenerative changes of old age may rupture the thin lateral parts of the annulus fibrosus (of the intervertebral disc) resulting in prolapse of the nucleus pulposus. This is known as disc prolapse or spondylosis and may be lateral or median. Although, it is commonest in the lumbar region, it may occur in the lower cervical region. This causes shooting pain along the distribution of the cervical nerve pressed. A direct posterior prolapse may compress the spinal cord (Fig. 9.19).
- Cervical vertebrae may be fractured, or dislocated by a fall on the head with acute flexion of the neck. In the cervical region, the vertebrae can dislocate without any fracture of the articular processes due to their horizontal position.
- Pithing of frog takes place when the cruciate ligament of median atlantoaxial joint ruptures, crushing the vital centres in medulla oblongata, resulting in immediate death. This occurs in judicial hanging as well.
- The degenerative changes or spondylitis may occur in the cervical spine, leading to narrowed intervertebral foramen, causing pressure on the spinal nerves (Fig. 9.20).

***Competency:***
**AN29.5** Describe and demonstrate attachments of: Scalenus anterior and scalenus medius

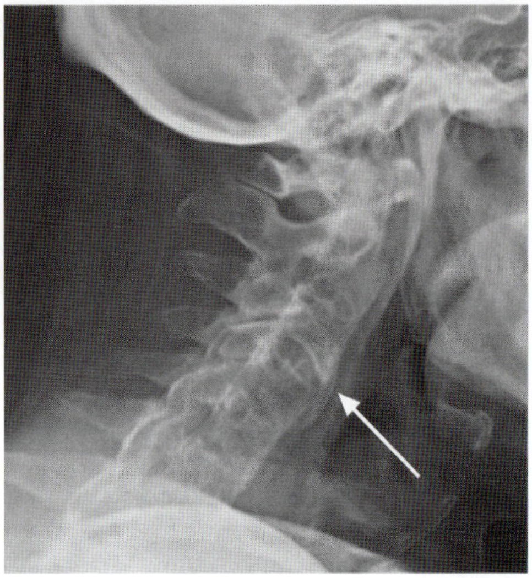

Fig. 9.20: Spondylitis

### Facts to Remember

- Vertebral artery comprises four parts:
  a. First part in neck
  b. Second part in forearm transversaria of C6 to C1 vertebrae
  c. Third part on the posterior arch of atlas
  d. Fourth part through foramen magnum in the cranial cavity.
- Apical ligament is a remnant of notochord
- Median atlantoaxial joint is a pivot type of joint, permitting movement of 'No'
- Atlanto-occipital joint is an ellipsoid joint permitting movement of 'Yes'
- Transverse ligament of atlas is part of the cruciate ligament. It keeps the dens of axis in position.

### BDC's Anatomy *e*-book

1. Relations of vertebral artery
2. Cervical pleura
3. Further reading
4. Viva voce questions

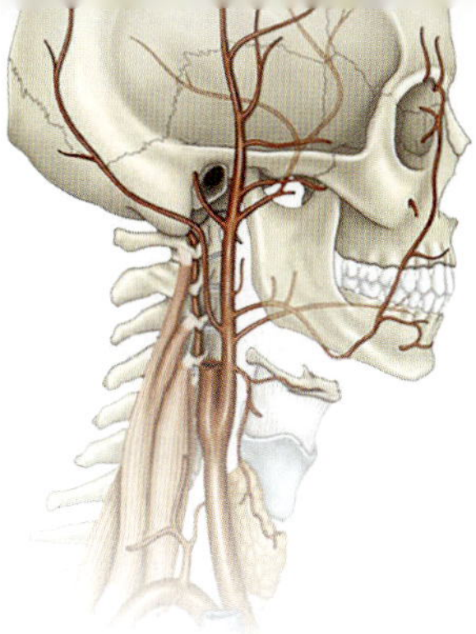

Chapter

10

# Back of the Neck

The back of the neck extends from external occipital protuberance and superior nuchal line above and spine of C7 vertebra and horizontal line passing through the acromion processes of both scapulae below. Important structures of back of neck are as follows:

1. Ligamentum nuchae
2. Extensor muscles of neck
3. Suboccipital triangle
4. Arterial anastomosis around the semispinalis capitis
5. 3rd part of vertebral artery.

## SURFACE LANDMARKS

1. *External occipital protuberance*: It is a bony prominence felt at the upper end of nuchal furrow. It demarcates the junction of head and neck (Fig. 10.1).
2. *Nuchal furrow*: It is a vertical groove in the midline on the back of neck.
3. *Superior nuchal lines*: These are upward arched bony lines extending laterally from the external occipital protuberance.
4. *Spine of 7th cervical vertebra*: It is a round, bony projection at the lower end of nuchal furrow (Fig. 10.1).

   *Note*: Spine of other cervical vertebrae are covered by ligamentum nuchae, hence they cannot be felt.
5. *Acromion process*: It can be felt as a bony edge at the summit of the shoulder (*akros* = highest and *omos* = shoulder in Greek) (Fig. 10.1).

## LAYERS OF BACK OF THE NECK

The layers of back of the neck are as follows:

1. Skin
2. Superficial fascia
3. Deep fascia
4. Muscle

## SKIN OF BACK OF THE NECK

The skin of the nape or back of the neck, and of the back of the scalp is supplied by medial branches of the dorsal rami of C2 the *greater occipital nerve;* C3 the *third occipital nerve*. Each posterior primary ramus divides into a medial branch and a lateral branch, both of which supply the intrinsic muscles of the back.

The medial branch in this region supplies the skin as well. The *dorsal ramus of C1* does not divide into medial and lateral branches, and is distributed only to the muscles bounding the suboccipital triangle.

## SUPERFICIAL FASCIA

The superficial fascia of the back is thick and tough. It contains cutaneous nerves and vessels. The cutaneous nerves include greater occipital, third occipital, and cutaneous branches of C4 and C5 nerves. The superficial fascia also contains occipital artery and minute branch from the second part of vertebral artery.

## DEEP FASCIA

The deep fascia of back is having two components:

1. *Investing layer of deep cervical fascia* which encloses the trapezius posteriorly.
2. Ligamentum nuchae.

### Ligamentum Nuchae

The *ligamentum nuchae* is a triangular fibrous sheet that separates muscles of the two sides of the neck.

Ligamentum nuchae comprises:

- Superior border—attached to external occipital crest.
- Anterior border—attached to posterior tubercles of atlas and spines of C2–C7 vertebrae.
- Free posterior border lies between external occipital protuberance and spine of C7.

*Note:* Ligamentum nuchae is not a ligament of neck as it does not connect the adjacent bone and it does not have structure of typical ligament [*Reference* 42nd edn. *Gray's Anatomy*]. *Previous concept:* Ligamentum nuchae is a fibroelastic sheet. *Recent concept:* The ligamentum nuchae has two parts:

Dorsal median raphe and median fascial septum.

***Median fascial septum*** lies deep to the dorsal raphe. It extends from the dorsal raphe to the vertebral column, up to the tips of spines of cervical vertebrae. Superiorly, it is attached to the external occipital crest and posterior tubercle of atlas. Median fascial septum does not give rise to any muscle.

## DISSECTION

Extend the incision from external occipital protuberance (i), to the spine of the seventh cervical vertebra (Fig. 10.1). Give a horizontal incision from spine of 7th cervical vertebra or vertebra prominens (iv), till the acromion process (v). This will expose the upper part and apex of posterior triangle of neck. Look for the occipital artery at its apex.

Extend the incision from vertebra prominens to spine of lumbar 5 vertebra. Reflect the skin laterally along an oblique line from spine of T12 (ii), till the deltoid tuberosity.

Close to the median plane in the superficial fascia are seen the greater occipital nerve and occipital artery.

Cut through trapezius muscle vertically at a distance of 2 cm from the median plane. Reflect it laterally and identify the accessory nerve, superficial branch of transverse cervical artery and ventral rami of 3rd and 4th cervical nerves.

Latissimus dorsi has already been exposed by the students dissecting the upper limb. Otherwise extend the incision from T12 spine till L5 spine. Reflect the skin till lateral side of the trunk and define the margins of broad thin latissimus dorsi. This muscle and trapezius form the first layer of muscles.

The 2nd layer comprises splenius muscle, levator scapulae, rhomboid major, rhomboid minor, serratus posterior superior and serratus posterior inferior muscles. The splenius is the highest of these muscles.

Levator scapulae forms part of the muscular floor of the posterior triangle. It is positioned between scalenus medius below and splenius capitis above. Follow its nerve and blood supply from dorsal scapular nerve and deep branch of transverse cervical artery, respectively.

Spinal root of accessory nerve and fibres from C3 and C4 to trapezius muscle lie on the levator scapulae.

Rhomboid minor and major lie on same plane as levator scapulae. Both are supplied by dorsal scapular nerve (C5).

Deep to the two rhomboid muscles is thin aponeurotic serratus posterior superior muscle from spines of C7 and T1–T2 vertebrae to be inserted into 2nd–5th ribs. Serratus posterior inferior muscle arises from T11 to T12 spines and thoracolumbar fascia and is inserted into 9th–12th ribs.

The 3rd layer is composed of erector spinae or sacrospinalis with its three subdivisions and semispinalis with its three divisions.

Erector spinae arises from the dorsal surface of sacrum and ascends up the lumbar region. There it divides into three subdivisions, the medial one is spinalis—inserted into the spines, the intermediate one is longissimus—inserted into the transverse processes, and the lateral one is iliocostalis—inserted into the ribs. Each of these divisions is made of short parts, fresh slips arising from the area where the lower slips are inserted.

Deep to erector spinae is the semispinalis again made up of three parts: Semispinalis thoracis, semispinalis cervicis, and semispinalis capitis.

Both these muscles are innervated by the dorsal rami of cervical, thoracic, lumbar and sacral nerves.

Muscles of 4th layer are the multifidus, rotatores, interspinales, intertransversarii and suboccipital muscles.

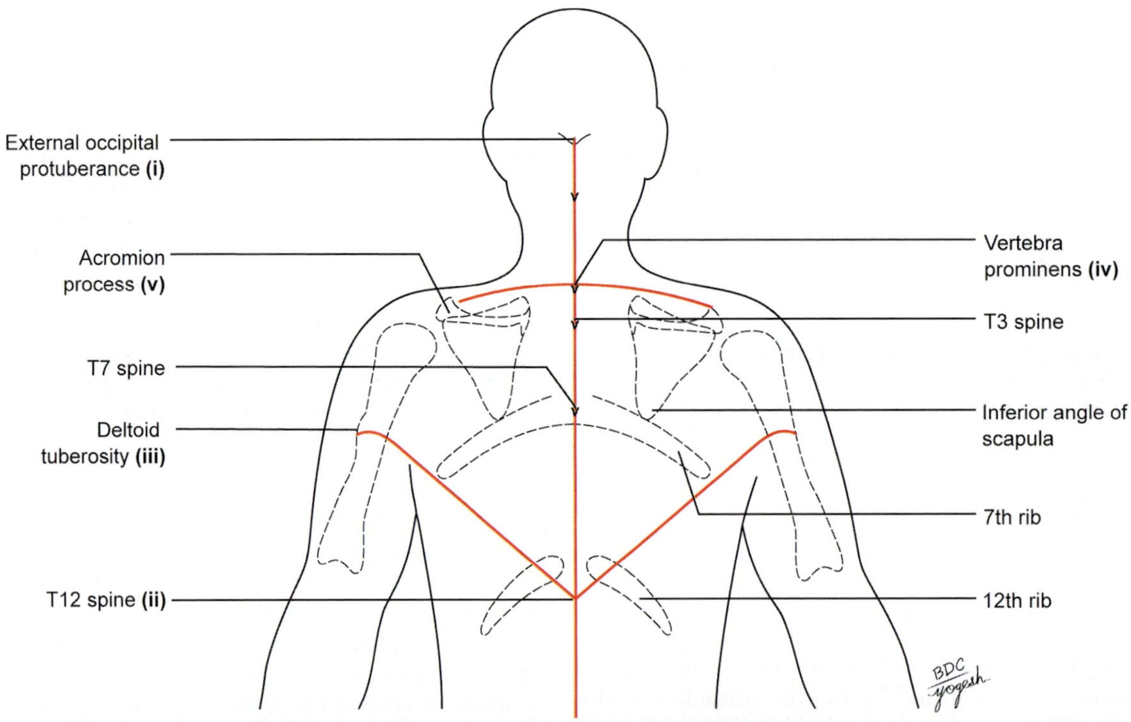


**Fig. 10.1:** Lines of dissection of back

**Competency:**

AN42.3 Describe the position, direction of fibres, relations, nerve supply, actions of semispinalis capitis and splenius capitis.

## MUSCLES OF THE BACK

The muscles of the back are grouped into the following layers (Flowchart 10.1):

A. ***Immigrant muscles*** (extrinsic or superficial most layers): They are the muscles that connect axial skeleton with the upper limb. They consist of the following (Table 10.1, Plate 10.1):
   1. *First layer*: Trapezius and latissimus dorsi.
   2. *Second layer*: Levator scapulae, rhomboid minor, rhomboid major.
   3. *Third layer*: Serratus posterior superior, serratus posterior inferior (not described here).

B. ***Intrinsic or deep muscles:*** The muscles of these layers are true muscles of the back and are supplied by dorsal rami of spinal nerves. These muscles are arranged in four layers as follows:
   1. *First layer (external layer)*: Splenius capitis, splenius cervicis.
   2. *Second layer (intermediate layer)*: It is group of erector spinae (sacrospinalis) muscles that includes iliocostalis, longissimus, and spinalis.
   3. *Third layer (deep layer)*: Semispinalis, multifidus, rotatores.

**TABLE 10.1: Origin and insertion of muscles connecting the upper limb to the vertebral column – Immigrant axioappendicular muscles of back (extrinsic muscles of back)**

| *Muscle* | *Origin* | *Insertion* | *Nerve supply* | *Actions* |
|---|---|---|---|---|
| **Trapezius**<br>The right and left muscles together form a trapezium that covers the upper half of the back. Upper fibres descend, lower fibres ascend and middle fibres pass horizontally | • Medial 1/3rd of superior nuchal line<br>• External occipital protuberance<br>• Ligamentum nuchae<br>• C7 spine<br>• T1–T12 spines<br>• Corresponding supraspinous ligaments | • *Upper fibres* into the posterior border of lateral one-third of clavicle and adjacent superior and inferior surfaces<br>• *Middle fibres* into the medial margin of the acromion process and upper lip of the crest of spine of the scapula<br>• *Lower fibres* on the smooth triangular area at the medial end of the spine, with a bursa intervening | • Spinal part of accessory nerve (XI)<br>• Branches from C3, C4 | *Upper fibres*: Along with levator scapulae – elevation of scapula (shrugging of shoulder)<br>*Middle fibres*: Along with rhomboid major and minor – retraction of scapula<br>*Lower fibres*: Along with serratus anterior – rotates the scapula in overhead abduction of arm |
| **Latissimus dorsi**<br>It covers a large area of the lower back, and is overlapped by the trapezius | • Posterior 1/3rd of the outer lip of iliac crest<br>• Posterior layer of lumbar fascia; thus attaching the muscle to the lumbar and sacral spines<br>• Spines of T7–T12, lower four ribs<br>• Inferior angle of the scapula | The muscle winds round the lower border of the teres major, and forms the posterior fold of the axilla<br>The tendon is twisted upside down and is inserted into floor of the intertubercular sulcus | Thoracodorsal nerve (C6–C8) (nerve to latissimus dorsi) | • Adduction, extension, and medial rotation of the shoulder as in swimming, rowing, climbing, pulling, folding the arm behind the back, and scratching the opposite scapula<br>• Violent expiratory effort like coughing, sneezing, etc.<br>• Climbing muscle |
| **Levator scapulae** | • Transverse processes of C1, C2<br>• Posterior tubercles of the transverse processes of C3, C4 | Superior angle and upper part of medial border (up to triangular area) of the scapula | • A branch from dorsal scapular nerve (C5)<br>• Branches from C3, C4 | • Elevation of scapula<br>• Steadies the scapula during movements of the arm |
| **Rhomboid minor** | • Lower part of ligamentum nuchae<br>• Spines C7 and T1 | Base of the triangular area at the root of the spine of the scapula | Dorsal scapular nerve (C5) | Retraction of scapula |
| **Rhomboid major** | • Spines of T2–T5<br>• Supraspinous ligaments | Medial border of scapula below the root of the spine | Dorsal scapular nerve (C5) | Retraction of scapula |
| **Serratus posterior superior** | Ligamentum nuchae, spines of T1–T3 vertebrae | Upper borders of 2nd–5th ribs | 2nd–5th intercostal nerves | Elevates 2nd–5th ribs |
| **Serratus posterior inferior** | Spines of T11–L2 vertebrae | Lower borders of 9th–12th ribs | 9th–12th intercostal nerves | Depress the lower ribs |

**Plate 10.1:** Immigrant axioappendicular muscles of back

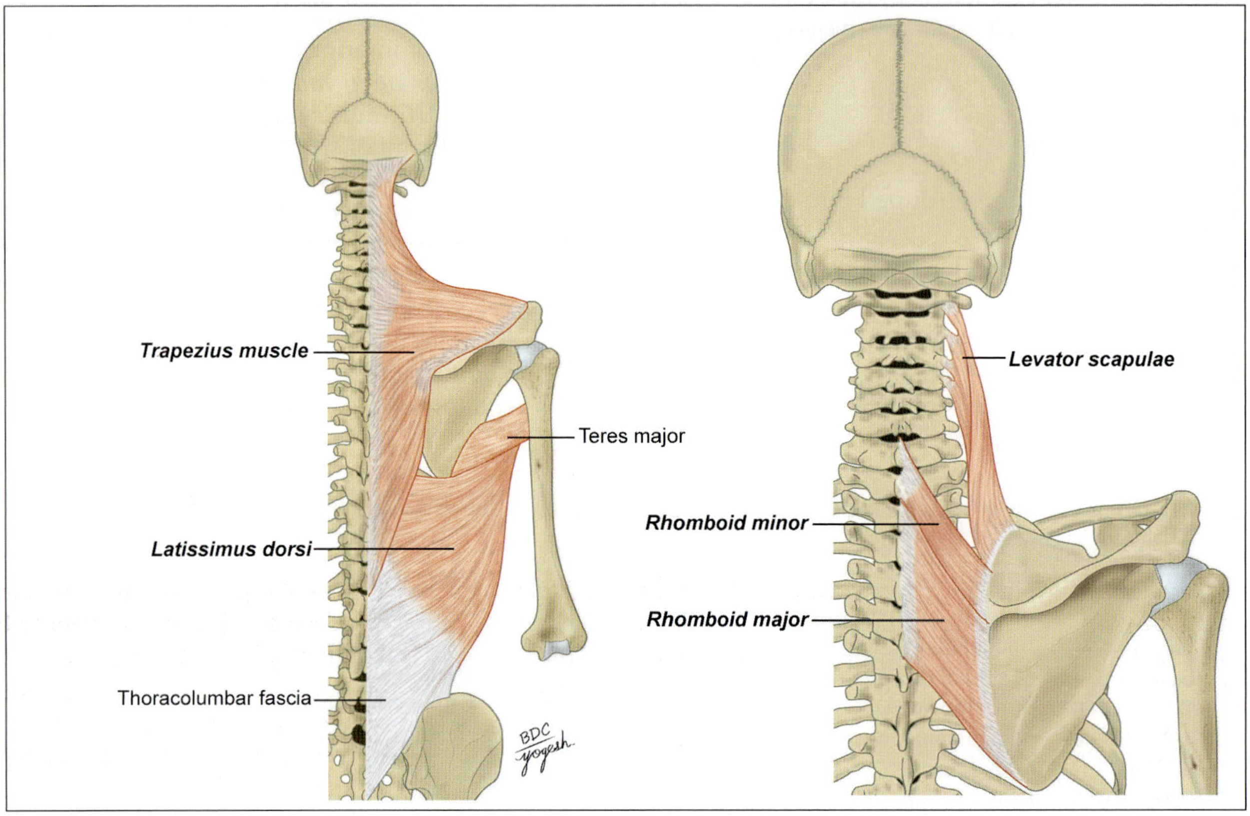


**Flowchart 10.1:** Muscles of back

**Muscles of back**

| Immigrant muscles of back | Layer 1 | Layer 2 | Layer 3 | Layer 4 |
|---|---|---|---|---|
| Trapezius<br>Latissimus dorsi<br>Levator scapulae<br>Rhomboid minor<br>Rhomboid major<br>Serratus posterior superior<br>Serratus posterior inferior | **Splenius muscles**<br>Splenius capitis<br>Splenius cervicis | Erector spinae group<br>A. Iliocostalis:<br>- Iliocostalis cervicis<br>- Iliocostalis thoracis<br>- Iliocostalis lumborum<br>B. Longissimus:<br>- Longissimus capitis<br>- Longissimus cervicis<br>- Longissimus thoracis<br>C. Spinalis:<br>- Spinalis capitis<br>- Spinalis cervicis<br>- Spinalis thoracis | Spinotransverse group<br>A. Semispinalis:<br>- Semispinalis capitis<br>- Semispinalis cervicis<br>- Semispinalis thoracis<br>B. Multifidus<br>C. Rotatores:<br>- Rotatores capitis<br>- Rotatores cervicis<br>- Rotatores thoracis | A. Levator costarum<br>B. Interspinales:<br>- Interspinales cervicis<br>- Interspinales thoracis<br>- Interspinales lumborum<br>C. Intertransversarii:<br>- Intertransversarii colli<br>- Intertransversarii lumborum<br>D. Suboccipital muscles:<br>- RCP major<br>- RCP minor<br>- Obliquus capitis superior<br>- Obliquus capitis inferior |

(RCP major: Rectus capitis posterior major, RCP minor: Rectus capitis posterior minor)

4. *Fourth layer (deepest layer)*: Levator costarum, interspinales, intertransversarii, suboccipital muscles.

## Intrinsic or Deep Muscles of Back

### Muscles of First Layer

**Splenius muscles** (Plate 10.2)

- They are two in number: ***Splenius cervicis*** and ***splenius capitis***.
- These cover the deeper muscles like a bandage.
- *Origin:* From lower half of ligamentum nuchae and spines of upper 6 thoracic vertebrae. These curve in a half spiral fashion and separate into splenius cervicis and splenius capitis.
- *Splenius cervicis* gets inserted into the posterior tubercles of transverse processes of C1–C4 vertebrae. Splenius capitis forms the floor of the posterior triangle and gets inserted into the mastoid process beneath the sternocleidomastoid muscle.
- It is supplied by dorsal rami of C1–C6 nerves.

### Muscles of Second Layer

It is group of erector spinae (sacrospinalis) muscles that includes iliocostalis, longissimus, and spinalis.

*Erector spinae* is supplied by posterior rami of the spinal nerves. It extends from the sacrum to the skull.

*Origin:* Mainly from the back of sacrum between median and lateral sacral crests, from the dorsal segment of iliac

**Plate 10.2:** Splenius capitis and splenius cervicis

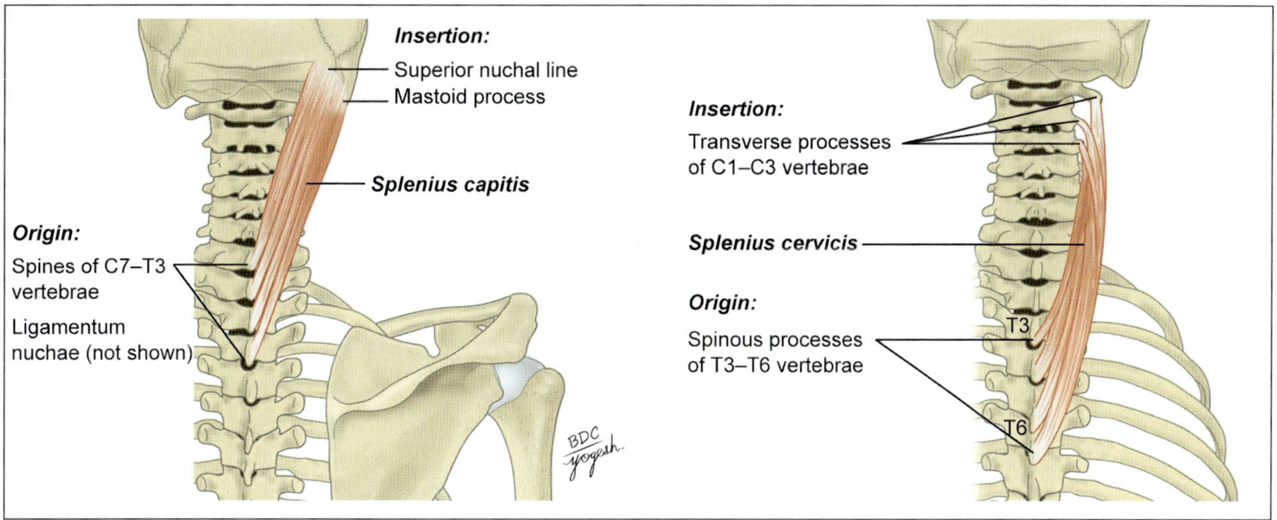


crest and related ligaments. Soon it splits into three columns: Iliocostalis, longissimus, and spinalis (Plate 10.3).

1. ***Iliocostalis*** is the lateral column and comprises Plate 10.3:
   a. Iliocostalis lumborum
   b. Iliocostalis thoracis
   c. Iliocostalis cervicis.

   These are short slips and are inserted into angles of the ribs and posterior tubercles of cervical transverse process. Origin of the higher slips is medial to the insertion of the lower slips.
2. ***Longissimus*** is the middle column and is composed of (Plate 10.3):
   a. Longissimus thoracis—inserted into transverse processes of thoracic vertebrae.
   b. Longissimus cervicis—inserted into transverse process of C2–C6 vertebrae.
   c. Longissimus capitis—inserted into mastoid process.
3. ***Spinalis*** is the medial column, extending between lumbar and cervical spines. Its parts are (Plate 10.3):
   a. Spinalis lumborum
   b. Spinalis thoracis
   c. Spinalis cervicis.

### Muscles of Third Layer (Plate 10.4)

This layer consists of (Plate 10.4):

1. ***Semispinalis*** extends between transverse processes and spines of the vertebrae. It has three parts:
   a. Semispinalis thoracis
   b. Semispinalis cervicis
   c. Semispinalis capitis.

   It only lies in the upper half of vertebral column. Semispinalis capitis is its biggest component. It arises from transverse processes of C3–T4 vertebrae, passes up next to the median plane, and gets inserted into the medial area between superior and inferior nuchal lines of the occipital bone.
2. ***Multifidus*** is one of the oblique deep muscles. It arises from mammillary process of lumbar vertebrae to be inserted into 2–3 higher spinous processes.
3. ***Rotatores*** are the deepest group. These pass from root of transverse process to the root of the spinous process. These are well developed in thoracic region. It has two components:
   a. Rotatores longi
   b. Rotatores brevis.

### Muscles of Fourth Layer (Plate 10.5)

1. ***Levatores costarum*** consists of 12 small triangular muscles that connect the thoracic vertebrae with the adjacent ribs. Located along either side of the posterior aspect of the thoracic vertebra they descend adjacent to the spine, spanning the thoracic region from C7 to T12 levels.
2. ***Interspinales*** muscles are short, paired muscles that belong to the deepest layer of the intrinsic muscles of the back. They extend between adjacent spinous processes of the vertebral column. It has three components:
   a. Interspinales cervicis
   b. Interspinales thoracis
   c. Interspinales lumborum.
3. ***Intertransversarii*** are small muscles of the back found between contiguous transverse processes of the cervical, lumbar, and some thoracic, vertebrae. It has two components:
   a. Intertransversarii colli
   b. Intertransversarii lumborum.
4. ***Suboccipital muscles*** are located inferior to the external occipital protuberance and the inferior nuchal line. These includes four pairs of small muscles:
   a. Rectus capitis posterior major
   b. Rectus capitis posterior minor
   c. Obliquus capitis inferior
   d. Obliquus capitis superior

**Plate 10.3:** Iliocostalis, longissimus and spinalis muscles

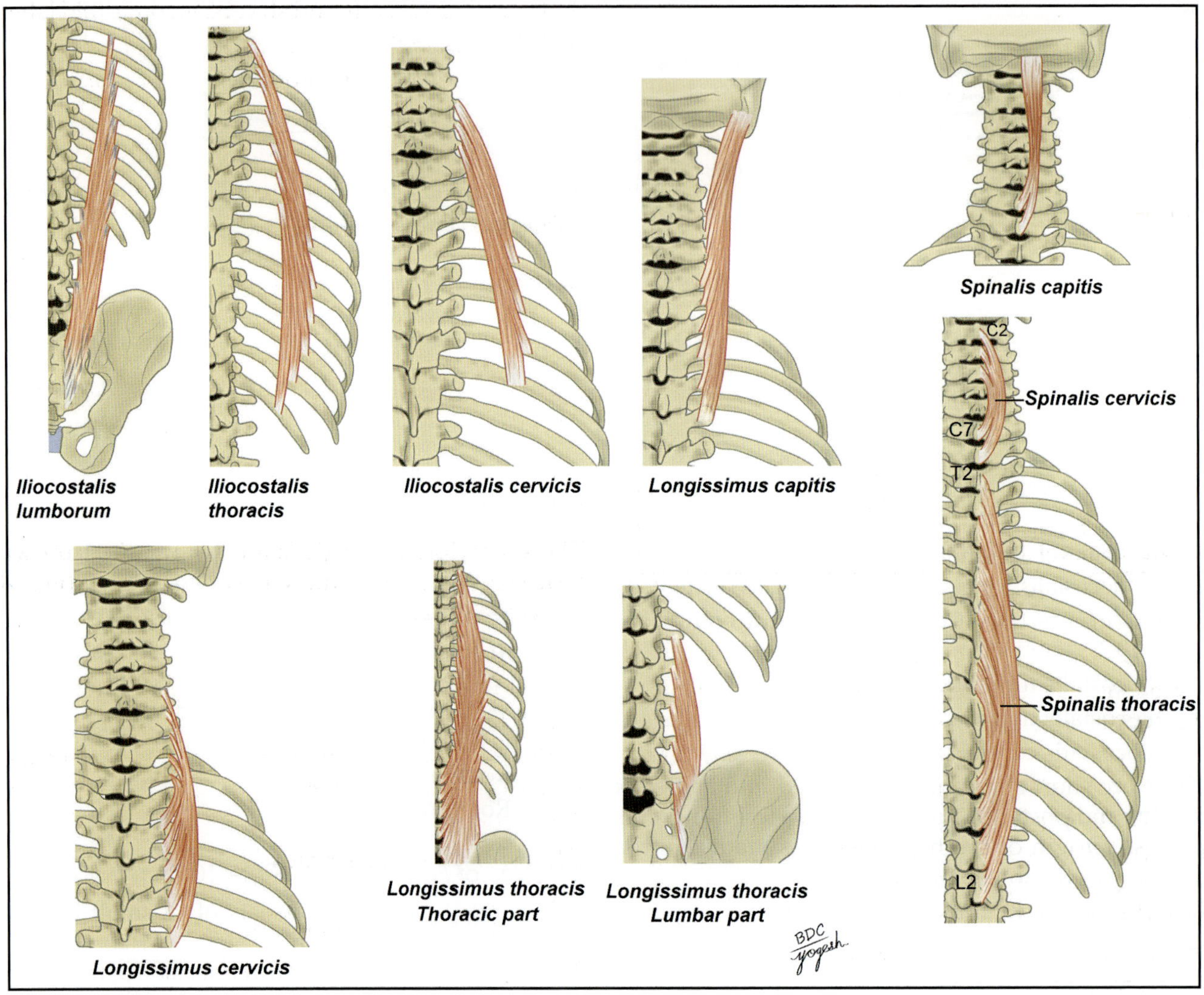


**Plate 10.4:** Semispinalis, multifidus and rotatores muscles

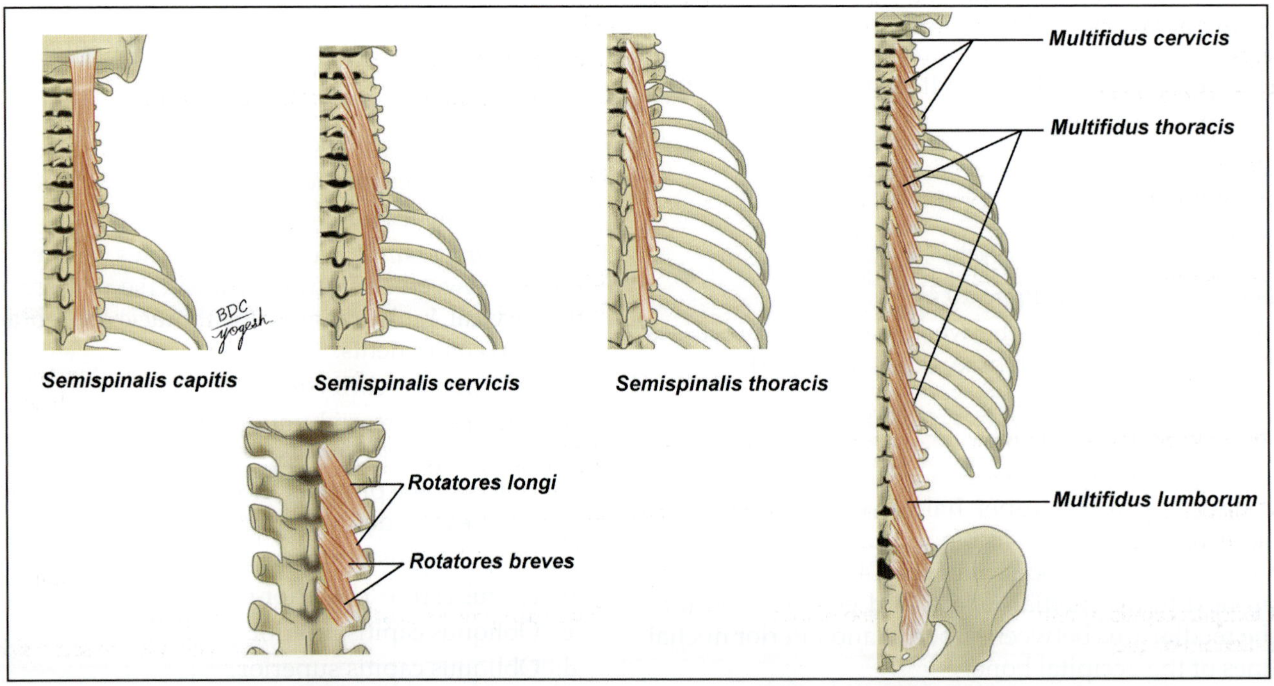

**Plate 10.5:** Levator costarum, interspinales and intertransversarii

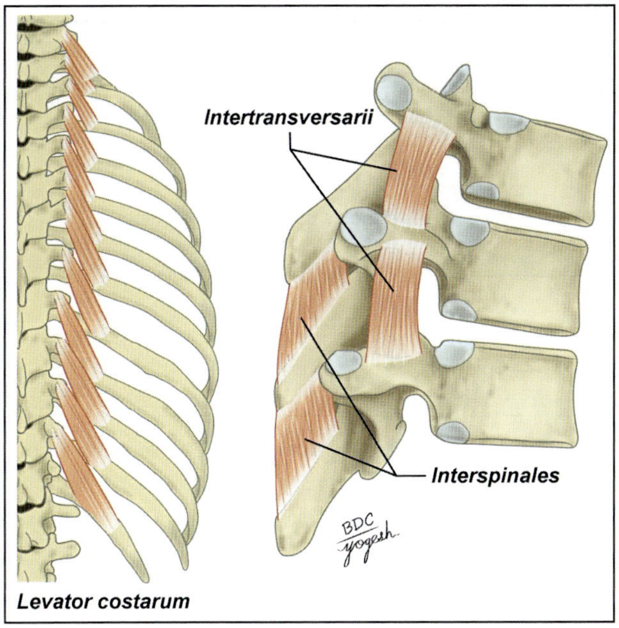


## SUBOCCIPITAL REGION

The suboccipital region is located deep in the upper part of the neck (Table 10.2, Plate 10.6).

### Boundaries

*Above:* Inferior nuchal line

*Below:* Spine and laminae of axis vertebra

*Laterally:* Mastoid process and transverse processes of atlas and axis vertebrae.

In this region, the following structures are present:
1. Suboccipital muscles
2. Suboccipital triangle and its contents.

### Exposure of Suboccipital Triangle

To expose the suboccipital triangle, the following structure or layers need to be reflected:
1. Skin
2. Superficial fascia
3. Cutaneous nerves and vessels: Greater and 3rd occipital nerves, occipital artery
4. Trapezius medially and sternocleidomastoid laterally
5. Splenius capitis
6. Semispinalis capitis and longissimus capitis.

### Suboccipital Muscles

The origin, insertion, nerve supply and actions of suboccipital muscles are described in Table 10.2.

The suboccipital triangle is a muscular space situated deep in the suboccipital region.

*Competency:*
AN42.2 Describe and demonstrate the boundaries and contents of suboccipital triangle.

## SUBOCCIPITAL TRIANGLE

The suboccipital triangle is a triangular intermuscular space located deep in the suboccipital region (Fig. 10.2, Flowchart 10.2).

### Boundaries

*Superomedially*

*Rectus capitis posterior major* muscle supplemented by the *rectus capitis posterior minor*.

*Superolaterally*

*Obliquus capitis superior* muscle.

*Inferiorly*

*Obliquus capitis inferior* muscle.

*Roof*
1. *Medially:* Dense fibrous tissue covered by the semispinalis capitis.
2. *Laterally:* Longissimus capitis and occasionally the splenius capitis.

*Floor*
1. Posterior arch of atlas.
2. Posterior atlanto-occipital membrane.

**TABLE 10.2: Origin, insertion, nerve supply and actions of suboccipital muscles**
(*Note*: All the suboccipital muscles are supplied by dorsal ramus of C1 nerve, i.e. suboccipital nerve)

| *Muscle* | *Origin* | *Insertion* | *Actions* |
|---|---|---|---|
| 1. **Rectus capitis posterior major** | Spine of axis | Lateral part of the area below the inferior nuchal line | 1. Mainly postural<br>2. Acting alone, it turns the chin to the same side<br>3. Acting together, the two muscles extend the head |
| 2. **Rectus capitis posterior minor** | Posterior tubercle of atlas | Medial part of the area below the inferior nuchal line | 1. Mainly postural<br>2. Extends the head |
| 3. **Obliquus capitis superior** (superior oblique) | Transverse process of atlas | Lateral area between the nuchal lines | 1. Mainly postural<br>2. Extends the head<br>3. Flexes the head laterally |
| 4. **Obliquus capitis inferior** (inferior oblique) | Spine of axis | Transverse process of atlas | 1. Mainly postural<br>2. Turns chin to the same side |

**Plate 10.6:** Suboccipital muscles (posterior view)

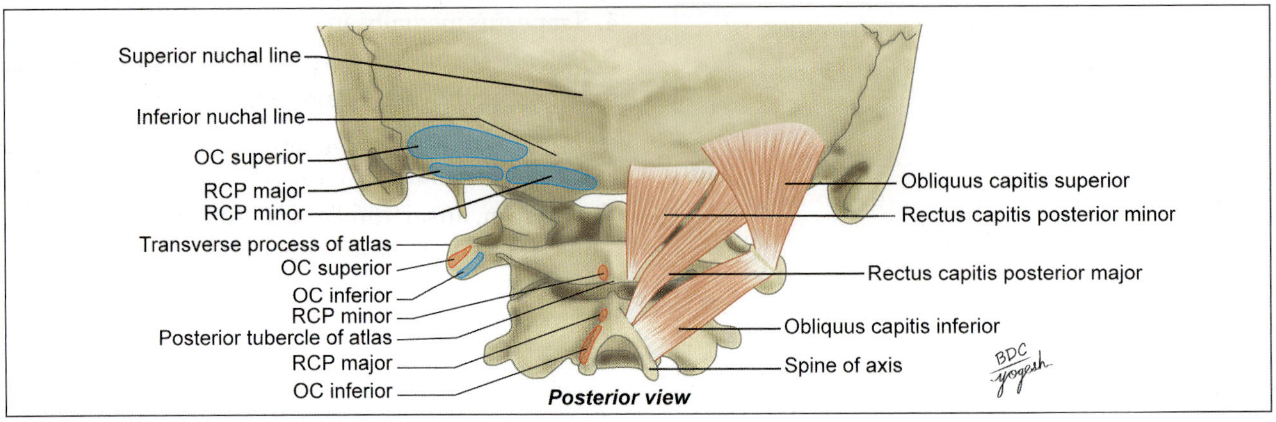


(OC inferior: Obliquus capitis inferior, OC superior: Obliquus capitis superior, RCP major: Rectus capitis posterior major, RCP minor: Rectus capitis posterior minor)

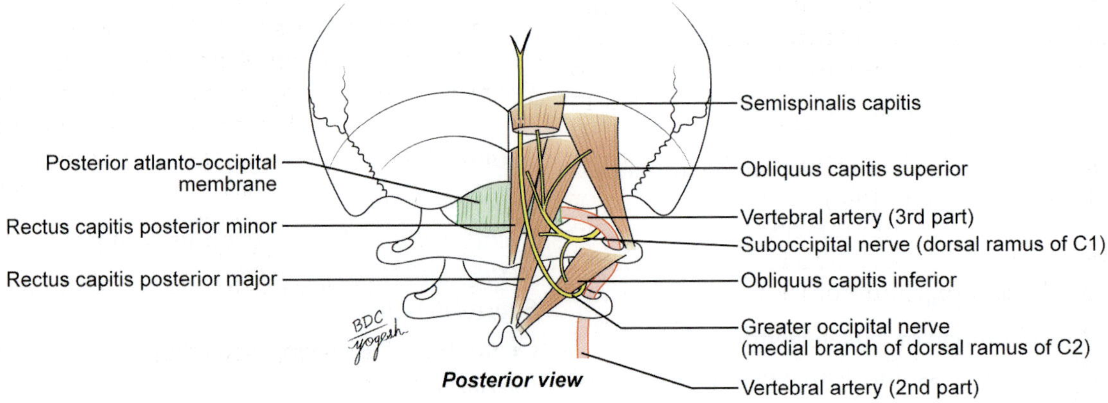


**Fig. 10.2:** Suboccipital triangle: Boundaries, floor and contents

**Flowchart 10.2:** Suboccipital triangle

***Suboccipital triangle***
Triangular intermuscular space

| ***Boundaries*** | ***Roof*** | ***Floor*** | ***Content*** |
|---|---|---|---|
| Superomedial: RCP major, RCP minor<br>Superolateral: Obliquus capitis superior<br>Inferior: Obliquus capitis inferior | Dense fibrous tissue<br>Semispinalis capitis<br>Longissimus capitis | Posterior arch of atlas<br>Posterior atlanto-occipital membrane | Suboccipital plexus of veins<br>Suboccipital nerve<br>Third part of vertebral artery<br>Greater occipital nerve |

*Note*:

***Vertebral artery:*** It is the first and largest branch of the first part of the subclavian artery. Its only the third part appears in the suboccipital triangle (Fig. 10.3). This part appears at the foramen transversarium of the atlas, grooves the atlas, and leaves the triangle by passing deep to the lateral edge of the posterior atlanto-occipital membrane. The artery is separated from the posterior arch of the atlas by the first cervical nerve and its dorsal and ventral rami (For details, *see* Chapter 9).

***Suboccipital plexus of veins*** lies in and around the suboccipital triangle, and drains the muscular, occipital veins, the internal vertebral venous plexus, and the condylar emissary vein. It itself drains into the deep cervical and vertebral plexus of veins.

***Greater occipital nerve*** is the larger medial branch of the dorsal ramus of the second cervical nerve. It is the *thickest cutaneous nerve* in the body. It crosses the suboccipital triangle and pierces the semispinalis capitis and trapezius muscles to ramify on the back of the head reaching up to the vertex. It supplies the semispinalis capitis in addition to the scalp (Fig. 10.2).

***Third occipital nerve*** is the slender medial branch of the dorsal ramus of the third cervical nerve. After piercing the semispinalis capitis and the trapezius, it ascends medial to the greater occipital nerve. It supplies the skin to the back of the neck up to the external occipital protuberance.

***Deep cervical artery*** is a branch of the costocervical trunk of the subclavian artery. It passes into the back of the neck just above the neck of the 1st rib. It ascends deep to the *semispinalis capitis* and anastomoses with the descending branch of the occipital artery.

## Contents

1. Suboccipital plexus of veins
2. Suboccipital nerve (dorsal ramus of C1 nerve)
3. Third part of vertebral artery
4. Greater occipital nerve (medial branch of dorsal ramus of C2).

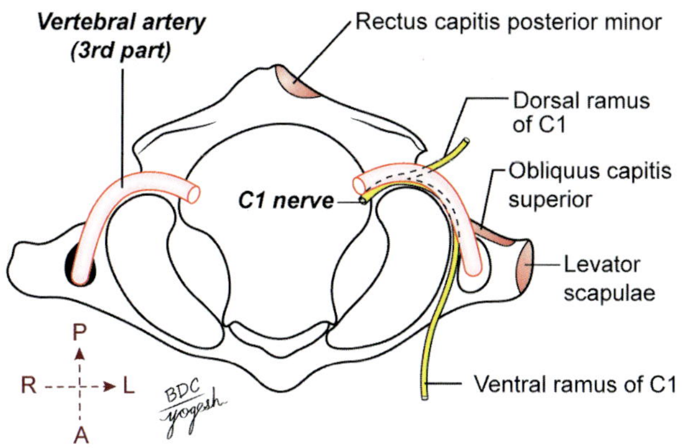


**Fig. 10.3:** Relationship of the vertebral artery to the atlas vertebra and to the first cervical nerve, as seen from above

## OCCIPITAL ARTERY

It arises from the external carotid artery, opposite the origin of the facial artery. It runs backwards and upwards deep to the lower border of the posterior belly of the digastric, crossing the carotid sheath, and the accessory and hypoglossal nerves. Next it runs deep to the mastoid process and to the muscles attached to it—the sternocleidomastoid, digastric, splenius capitis and longissimus capitis. The artery then crosses the rectus capitis lateralis, the obliquus capitis superior and the semispinalis capitis muscles at the apex of the posterior triangle. Finally, it pierces the trapezius 2.5 cm from the midline and comes to lie along the greater occipital nerve. In the superficial fascia of the scalp, it has a tortuous course.

Its branches in this region are:

a. Mastoid
b. Meningeal
c. Muscular: 2 branches to sternocleidomastoid muscle.

## SUBOCCIPITAL NERVE

The suboccipital nerve is the *dorsal ramus of C1 nerve*. It emerges backward between the vertebral artery and the posterior arch of atlas (Fig. 10.4). It ends by giving 5 muscular branches to the following muscles:

1. Rectus capitis posterior major
2. Rectus capitis posterior minor
3. Obliquus capitis superior
4. Obliquus capitis inferior
5. Semispinalis capitis

The branch to oblique capitis inferior gives a communicating branch to the greater occipital nerve.

*Note*: Suboccipital nerve does not give any subcutaneous branch. Ventral primary ramus of C1 nerve joins the ventral ramus of C2 nerve and takes part in the formation of cervical plexus.

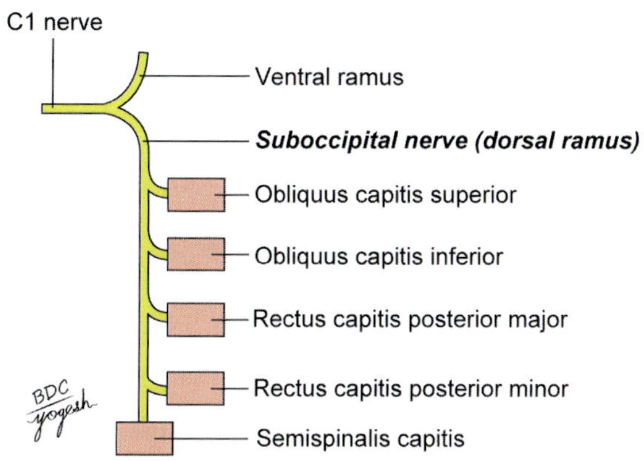


**Fig. 10.4:** Suboccipital nerve (dorsal ramus)

## CLINICAL ANATOMY

- ***Neck rigidity***, seen in cases with meningitis, is due to spasm of the extensor muscles. This is caused by irritation of the nerve roots during their passage through the subarachnoid space which is infected. Passive flexion of neck and straight leg raising test cause pain as the nerves are stretched (Figs 10.5 and 10.6).
- ***Cisternal puncture*** is done when lumbar puncture fails. The patient either sits up or lies down in the left lateral position. A needle is introduced in the midline above the spine of axis in forward and upward direction parallel to an imaginary line extending from external acoustic meatus to nasion. It passes through the posterior atlanto-occipital membrane between the posterior arch of atlas and the posterior margin of foramen magnum. The needle enters the cerebellomedullary cistern and small amount of CSF is withdrawn.
- Neurosurgeons approach the posterior cranial fossa through this region.

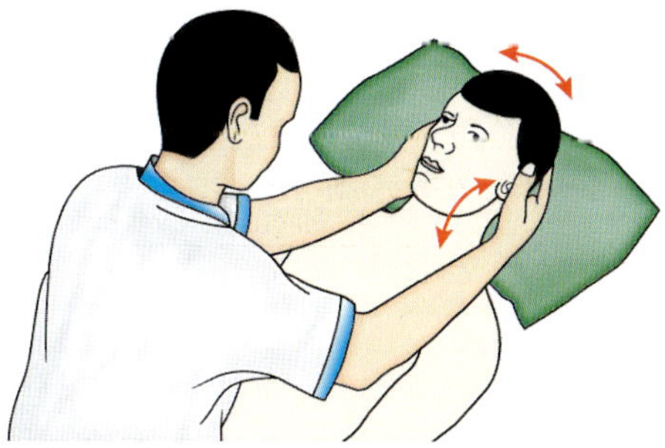

**Fig. 10.5:** Passive flexion of neck

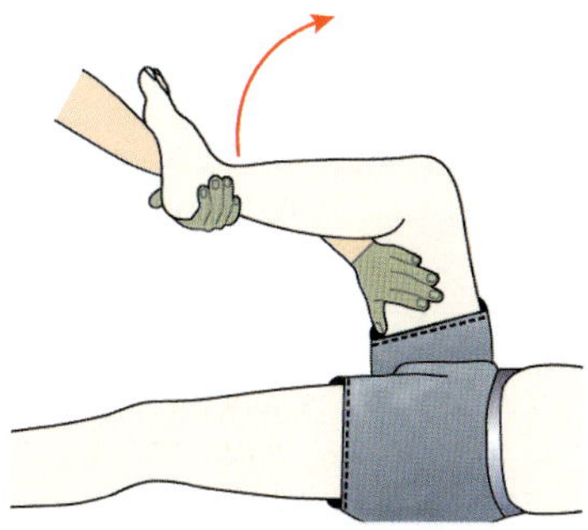

**Fig. 10.6:** Straight leg raising test causes pain in meningitis

## DISSECTION

It is deep triangle in the area between the occiput and the spine of 2nd cervical (the axis) vertebra. The deepest muscles are the muscles of suboccipital triangle.

Cut the attachments of trapezius from superior nuchal line and reflect it towards the spine of scapula. Cut the splenius capitis from its attachment on the mastoid process and reflect it downwards. Clean the superficial fascia over the semispinalis capitis medially and longissimus capitis laterally. Reflect longissimus capitis downwards from the mastoid process.

Cut through semispinalis capitis and turn it towards lateral side. Define the boundaries and contents of the suboccipital triangle.

VIDEO

**Video 3.10** Muscles of the Back

### *Facts to Remember*

- Artery lying on posterior arch of atlas is the third part of vertebral artery.
- Greater occipital nerve is the thickest cutaneous nerve of the body.
- The spinal process of C7 vertebra can be palpated at the root of the neck on the back.
- Suboccipital nerve does not give any subcutaneous branch.

### BDC's Anatomy *e*-book

1. Intrinsic muscles of the back – first or external layer
2. Intrinsic muscles of the back – second or intermediate layer
3. Intrinsic muscles of the back – third or deep layer
4. Intrinsic muscles of neck – fourth or deepest layer
5. Further reading
6. Viva voce questions

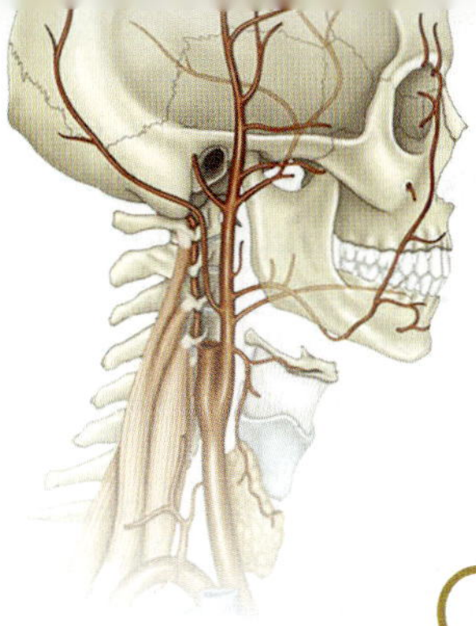

Chapter

# 11

# Contents of Vertebral Canal

## VERTEBRAL CANAL

When the vertebrae are put in a sequence, their vertebral foramina lie one below the other forming a continuous canal which is called the *vertebral canal*. This canal contains the three meninges with their spaces and the spinal cord including the cauda equina. The intervertebral foramina are a pair of foramina between the pedicles of the adjacent vertebrae. Each foramen contains dorsal and ventral roots, trunk and dorsal and ventral primary rami of the spinal nerve, and spinal vessels.

***Competency:***
**AN42.1** Describe the contents of the vertebral canal.

### CONTENTS

The vertebral canal contains the following structures from without inwards (Fig. 11.1).

1. Epidural or extradural space
2. Thick dura mater or pachymeninx
3. Subdural capillary space
4. Delicate arachnoid mater
5. Wide subarachnoid space containing cerebrospinal fluid (CSF)
6. Firm pia mater. The arachnoid and pia together form the leptomeninges.
7. Spinal cord or spinal medulla and the cauda equina.

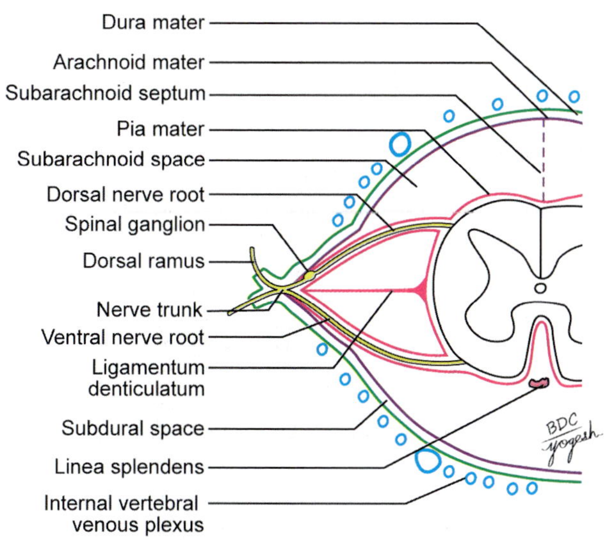


**Fig. 11.1:** Schematic transverse section showing the spinal meninges

*Note*: The spinal cord is considered along with the brain in Chapter 5, *BD Chaurasia's Human Anatomy, Volume 4*. The other contents are described below.

**DISSECTION**

Clean the spines and laminae of the entire vertebral column by removing all the muscles attached to them. Trace the dorsal rami of spinal nerves towards the intervertebral foramina. Saw through the spines and laminae of the vertebrae carefully and detach them so that the spinal medulla/spinal cord encased in the meninges becomes visible.

Clean the external surface of dura mater enveloping the spinal cord by removing fat and epidural plexus of veins. Carefully cut through a small part of the dura mater by a fine median incision. Extend this incision above and below. See the delicate arachnoid mater. Incise it. Push the spinal cord to one side and try to identify the ligamentum denticulatum. Define the attachments of the dorsal and ventral nerve roots on the surface of spinal cord and their union to form the trunk of the spinal nerve. Cut the trunk of all spinal nerves on both the sides. Gently pull the spinal cord with cauda equina out from the vertebral canal.

### Epidural Space

Epidural space lies between the spinal dura mater, and the periosteum with ligaments lining the vertebral canal.

It contains:

a. Loose areolar tissue
b. Semiliquid fat
c. Spinal arteries on their way to supply the deeper contents
d. Internal vertebral venous plexus.

The *spinal arteries* arise from different sources at different levels; they enter the vertebral canal through the intervertebral foramina, and supply the spinal cord, the spinal nerve roots, the meninges, the periosteum and ligaments.

Venous blood from the spinal cord drains into the epidural or internal vertebral plexus.

### Spinal Dura Mater

Spinal dura mater is a thick, tough fibrous membrane which forms a loose sheath around the spinal cord (Fig. 11.2). It is continuous with the meningeal layer of the cerebral dura mater. The spinal dura extends from the foramen magnum to the lower border of the second sacral vertebra; whereas the spinal cord ends at the lower border of first lumbar vertebra. The dura gives tubular prolongations to the dorsal and ventral nerve roots and to the spinal nerves as they pass through the intervertebral foramina.

### Subdural Space

Subdural space is a capillary or potential space between the dura and the arachnoid, containing a thin film of serous fluid. This space permits movements of the dura over the arachnoid. The space is continued for a short distance onto the spinal nerves and is in free communication with the lymph spaces of the nerves.

### Arachnoid Mater

Arachnoid mater is a thin, delicate and transparent membrane that loosely invests the entire central nervous system (Fig. 11.2). Inferiorly, it extends, like the dura up to the lower border of the second sacral vertebra. It is adherent to the dura only where some structures pierce the membrane and where the ligamentum denticulata are attached to the dura mater.

### Subarachnoid Space

Subarachnoid space is a wide space between the pia and the arachnoid, filled with ***cerebrospinal fluid*** (**CSF**). It surrounds the brain and spinal cord like a water cushion. The spinal subarachnoid space is wider than the space around the brain. It is widest below the lower end of the spinal cord where it encloses the cauda equina.

*Note:* **Lumbar puncture** is usually done in the lower widest part of the space, between 3rd and 4th lumbar vertebrae (Fig.11.3)

### Spinal Pia Mater (Figs 11.1 and 11.2)

1. Spinal pia mater is thicker, firmer, and less vascular than the cerebral pia, but both are made up of two layers:
   a. Outer ***epi-pia*** containing larger vessels.
   b. Inner ***pia-glia*** *or pia-intima* which is in contact with nervous tissue.

   Between the two layers, there are many small blood vessels and also cleft-like spaces which communicate with the subarachnoid space. The pia mater closely invests the spinal cord, and is continued below the spinal cord as the ***filum terminale***.
2. Posteriorly, the pia is adherent to the posterior median septum of the spinal cord, and is also connected to the arachnoid by a fenestrated ***subarachnoid septum***.
3. Anteriorly, the pia is folded into the anterior median fissure of the spinal cord. It thickens at the mouth of the fissure to form a median, longitudinal glistening band, called the ***linea splendens*** (Fig. 11.1).
4. On each side between the ventral and dorsal nerve roots, the pia forms a narrow vertical ridge, called the ***ligamentum denticulatum*** ***(Fig. 11.2)***. This is so-called because it gives off a series of triangular tooth-like processes which project from its lateral free border. Each ligament has 21 processes; the first at the level of the foramen magnum, and the last between twelfth thoracic and first lumbar spinal nerves. Each process passes through the arachnoid to the dura between two *adjacent spinal nerves*. The processes suspend the spinal cord in the middle of the subarachnoid space.
5. The ***filum terminale*** is a delicate, thread-like structure about 20 cm long. It extends from the apex of the conus medullaris to the dorsum of the first piece of the coccyx. It is composed chiefly of pia mater, although a few nerve fibres rudiments of 2nd and 3rd coccygeal nerves are found adherent to the upper part of its outer surface. The central canal of the spinal cord extends into it for about 5 mm.
6. The filum terminale is subdivided into a part lying within the dural sheath called the ***filum terminale internum***; and a part lying outside the dural sheath, below the level of the second sacral vertebra called the ***filum terminale externum***. The filum terminale internum is 15 cm long, and the externum is 5 cm long.
7. ***Pial sheaths*** surround the nerve roots crossing the subarachnoid space, and the vessels entering the substance of the spinal cord.

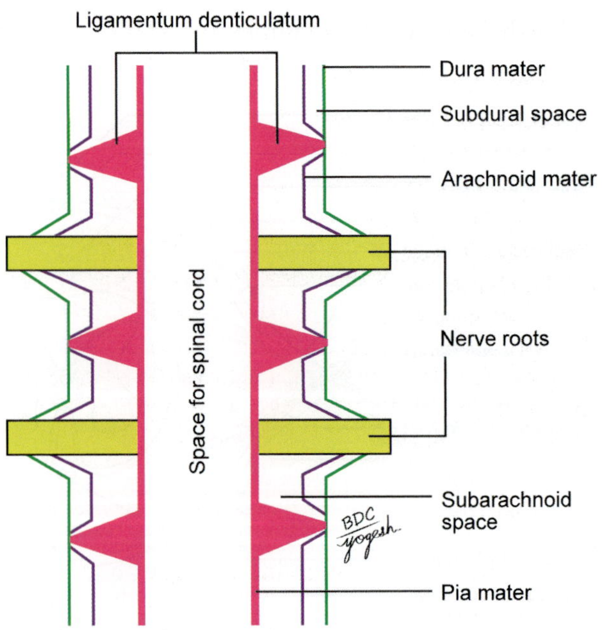


**Fig. 11.2:** Ligamentum denticulatum and its relationship to the dura mater and to the arachnoid mater

Head and Neck 11

## CLINICAL ANATOMY

- ***Leptomeningitis:*** Inflammation due to infection of leptomeninges, i.e. pia mater and arachnoid mater is known as ***meningitis***. This is commonly tubercular or pyogenic. It is characterized by fever, marked headache, neck rigidity, often accompanied by delirium and convulsions, and a changed biochemistry of CSF. CSF pressure is raised, its proteins and cell contents are increased, and sugars and chloride are selectively diminished.
- ***Lumbar puncture in adult:*** Patient is lying on side with maximally flexed spine. A line is taken between highest points of iliac spine at L4 level. Skin locally anaesthetized, and lumbar puncture needle with trocar inserted carefully between L3 and L4 spines. Needle courses through skin, fat, supraspinous and interspinous ligaments, ligamentum flava, epidural space, dura, arachnoid, subarachnoid space to release CSF (Fig. 11.3).
- ***Lumbar puncture in infant/children:*** During 2nd month of life, spinal cord usually reaches L3 level. Lumbar puncture needle is introduced in flexed spine between L4 and L5.
- ***Cisternal puncture:*** This procedure is rather difficult and dangerous. Cerebellomedullary cistern is approached through posterior atlanto-occipital membrane.
- ***Lumbar epidural:*** The epidural space is the space between vertebral canal and dura mater. The epidural space is deeper in the midline. The procedure is same as lumbar puncture, the needle should reach only in the epidural space and not deep to it in the dura mater. Epidural space is utilized for giving anaesthesia or analgesia (Fig. 11.4).
- ***Caudal epidural:*** The needle is passed through sacral hiatus, which lies equidistant from the right and left posterior superior iliac spines. The needle passes through posterior sacrococcygeal ligament and enters the sacral canal. Then the hub of needle is lowered so that it passes along sacral canal. This space lies below S2 (Fig. 11.3).

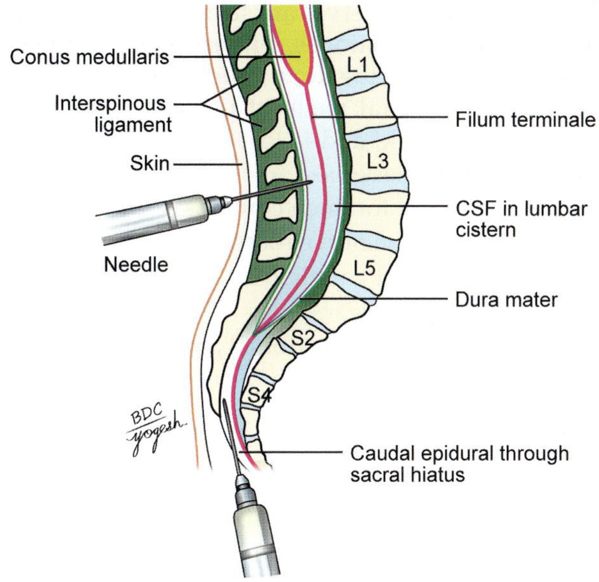


**Fig. 11.3:** Lumbar puncture in an adult

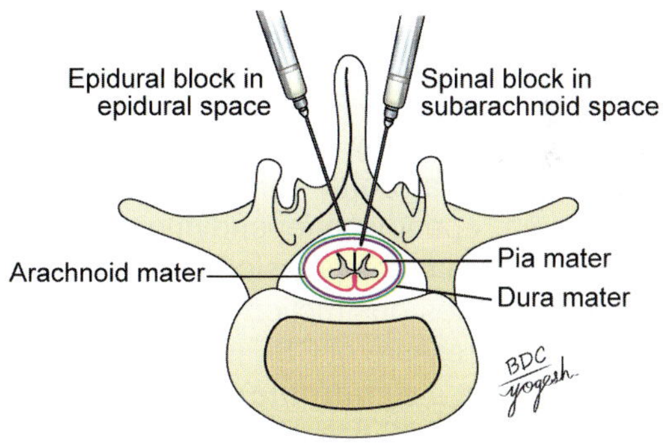


**Fig. 11.4:** Lumbar epidural anaesthesia and spinal block

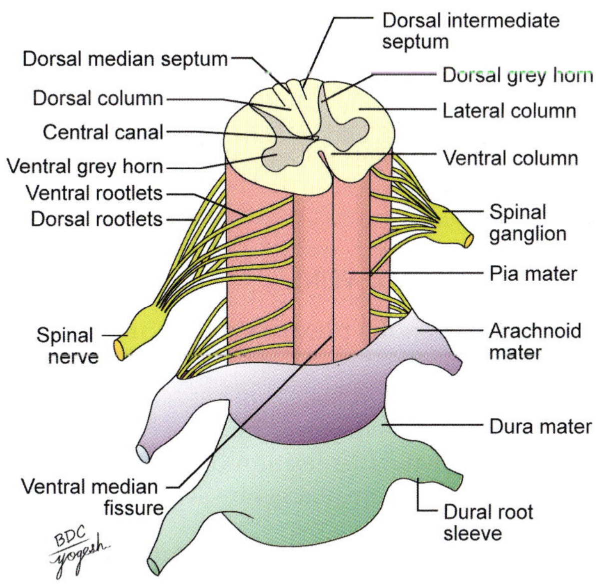


**Fig. 11.5:** Formation of spinal nerve

## SPINAL NERVES

The spinal cord gives rise to 31 pairs of *spinal nerves:* Eight cervical, twelve thoracic, five lumbar, five sacral, and one coccygeal. Each nerve is attached to the cord by two roots—ventral motor and dorsal sensory. Each dorsal nerve root bears a ganglion. The ***ventral and dorsal nerve roots*** unite in the intervertebral foramen to form the ***nerve trunk*** which soon divides into ***ventral and dorsal rami*** (Fig. 11.5).

The uppermost nerve roots pass horizontally from the spinal cord to reach the intervertebral foramina. Lower down they have to pass with increasing obliquity, as the spinal cord is much shorter than the vertebral column. Below the termination of the spinal cord at the level of 1st lumbar vertebra, the obliquity becomes more marked.

Below the lower end of the spinal cord, the roots form a bundle known as the ***cauda equina*** because of its resemblance to the tail of a horse.

The roots of spinal nerves are surrounded by sheaths derived from the meninges. The ***pial and arachnoid sheaths*** extend up to the dura mater. The ***dural sheath*** encloses the terminal parts of the roots, continues over the nerve trunk, and is lost by merging with the epineurium of the nerve.

An intervertebral foramen contains:

a. The ends of the nerve roots
b. The dorsal root ganglion
c. The nerve trunk
d. The beginning of the dorsal and ventral rami
e. A spinal artery
f. An intervertebral vein.

## CLINICAL ANATOMY

- ***Compression of the spinal cord*** by a tumour gives rise to paraplegia or quadriplegia, depending on the level of compression.
- Compression of roots of spinal nerves may be caused by prolapse of an intervertebral disc, by osteophytes (formed in osteoarthritis), by a cervical rib, or by an extramedullary tumour. Such compression results in shooting pain along the distribution of the nerve.
- ***Spinal tumours*** may arise from dura mater—meningioma, glial cells—glioma, nerve roots—neurofibroma, ependyma–ependymoma, and other tissues. Apart from compression of the spinal cord, the tumour causes obstruction of the subarachnoid space so that pressure of CSF is low below the level of lesion (***Froin's syndrome***). There is yellowish discolouration of CSF below the level of obstruction. CSF reveals high level of protein but the cell content is normal. ***Queckenstedt's test*** does not show a sudden rise and a sudden fall of CSF pressure by coughing or by brief pressure over the jugular veins. Spinal block can be confirmed either by myelography, CT scan or MRI scan.
- Compression of the cauda equina gives rise to flaccid paraplegia, saddle anaesthesia and sphincter disturbances. This is called the ***cauda equina syndrome***.

## VERTEBRAL SYSTEM OF VEINS

The vertebral venous plexus assumes importance in cases of (Fig. 11.6):

1. Carcinoma of the prostate causing secondaries in the vertebral column and the skull.
2. Chronic empyema (collection of pus in the pleural cavity) causing brain abscess by septic emboli.

### Anatomy of the Vertebral Venous Plexus/Batson Venous Plexus

The vertebral venous system is made up of a valveless, complicated network of veins with a longitudinal pattern. It runs parallel to and anastomoses with the superior and inferior venae cavae. This network has three intercommunicating subdivisions.

1. ***Epidural plexus:*** Lies in the vertebral canal outside the dura mater. The plexus consists of a postcentral and a prelaminar portion. Each portion is drained by two vessels. The plexus drains the structures in the vertebral canal, and is itself drained at regular intervals by segmental veins—vertebral, posterior intercostal, lumbar and lateral sacral.
2. ***Plexus within the vertebral bodies:*** It drains backwards into the epidural plexus, and anterolaterally into the external vertebral plexus.
3. ***External vertebral venous plexus:*** It consists of anterior vessels lying in front of the vertebral bodies, and the posterior vessels on the back of the vertebral arches and on adjacent muscles. It is drained by segmental veins.

The suboccipital plexus of veins is a part of the external plexus. It lies in the suboccipital triangle. It receives the occipital veins of the scalp is connected with the transverse sinus by emissary veins and drains into the subclavian veins.

### Communications and Implications

Valveless vertebral system of veins communicates:

1. Above with the intracranial venous sinuses.
2. Below with the pelvic veins, the portal vein, and the caval system of veins.

The veins are *valveless* and the blood can flow in them in either direction. An increase in intrathoracic or intra-abdominal pressure, brought about by coughing and straining, may cause blood to flow in the plexus away from the heart, either upwards or downwards. Such periodic changes in venous pressure are clinically important because they make possible the spread of tumours or infections. For example, cells from pelvic, abdominal, thoracic and breast tumours may enter the venous system, and may ultimately lodge in the vertebrae, the spinal cord, the skull, or the brain.

The common primary sites of tumours causing secondaries in vertebrae are the breast and the prostate.

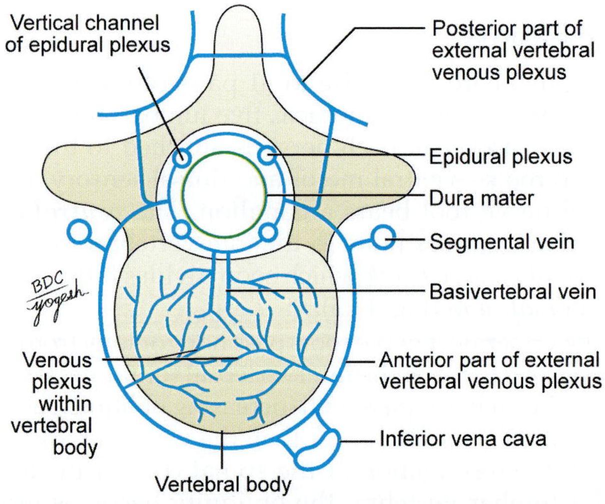


**Fig. 11.6:** The vertebral system of veins

### Facts to Remember

- Spinal cord in adult ends at lower border of lumbar one vertebra.
- Spinal dura mater and arachnoid mater extend till second sacral vertebra.
- Spinal pia mater comprises an outer epi-pia and an inner pia-intima.
- Ligamenta denticulata of pia mater are two vertical ridges with 21 tooth-like processes which suspend the spinal cord in the subarachnoid space.
- The lowest or 21st process lies between T12 and L1 spinal nerves.
- Through the vertebral venous plexus, secondaries of prostate or breast can reach up to the cranial cavity.

### BDC's Anatomy e-book

1. Viva voce questions
2. Nomenclature of spinal nerves

Chapter

# 12

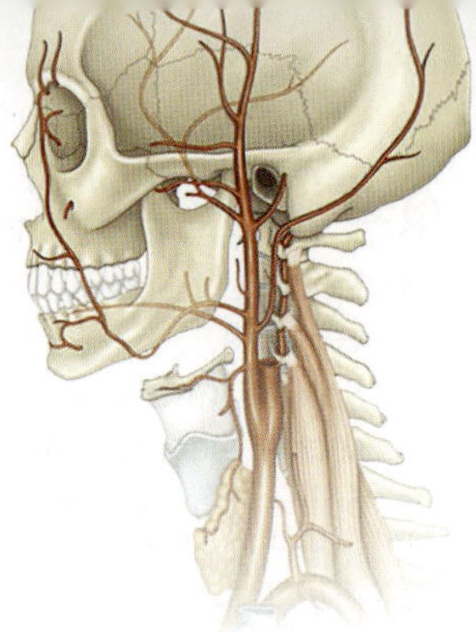

# Cranial Cavity

Cranial cavity contains the brain, meninges, venous sinuses, all cranial nerves, four petrosal nerves, parts of internal carotid artery and a part of the vertebral artery besides the special senses. The anterior branch of middle meningeal artery lies at the pterion and is prone to rupture resulting in extradural haemorrhage.

The convex upper wall of the cranial cavity is called the ***vault***. It is uniform and smooth.

The ***base of the cranial cavity*** is uneven and presents three cranial fossae (anterior, middle and posterior) lodging the uneven base of the brain.

## CONTENTS OF CRANIAL CAVITY

The cranial cavity contains:

1. Brain
2. Meninges
   - Outer dura mater
   - Middle arachnoid mater
   - Inner pia mater
3. Hypophysis cerebri
4. Intracranial parts of cranial nerves
5. Dural venous sinuses including cavernous sinus
6. *Arteries*: Internal carotid arteries, 4th part of vertebral arteries, circle of Willis, and middle meningeal arteries.

### DISSECTION

Detach the epicranial aponeurosis, if not already done, laterally till the inferior temporal line. In the region of the temple, detach the temporalis muscle with its overlying fascia and reflect these downwards over the pinna.

***Removal of skull cap or calvaria***

Draw a horizontal line across the skull 1 cm above the orbital margins and 1 cm above the inion. Saw through the skull. Be careful in the temporal region as skull is rather thin there. Separate the inner table of skull from the fused endosteum and dura mater.

***Removal of the brain***

To remove the brain and its enveloping meninges, the structures leaving or entering the brain through various foramina of the skull have to be carefully detached/incised. Start from the anterior aspect by detaching falx cerebri from the crista galli.

Put 2–3 blocks under the shoulders so that head falls backwards. This will expose the olfactory bulb, which may be lifted from the underlying anterior cranial fossa. Identify optic nerve, internal carotid artery, infundibulum passing towards hypophysis cerebri. Divide all three structures. Cut through the oculomotor and trochlear nerves in relation to free margin of tentorium cerebelli. Divide the attachment of tentorium from the petrous temporal bone.

Identify and divide trigeminal, abducent, facial, and vestibulocochlear nerves. Then cut glossopharyngeal, vagus, accessory and hypoglossal nerves. All these nerves have to be cut first on one side and then on the other side. Lastly identify the two vertebral arteries entering the skull through foramen magnum on each side of the spinal medulla. With a sharp knife, cut through these structures. Thus, the whole brain with the meninges can be gently removed from the skull. Preserve it in 5% formaldehyde.

Cut through the dura mater on the ventral aspect of brain till the inferolateral borders along the superciliary margin. Pull upwards the fold of dura mater present between the adjacent medial surfaces of cerebral hemispheres. This will be possible till the occipital lobe of brain. Pull backwards a similar but much smaller fold between two lobes of cerebellum, i.e. falx cerebelli.

Separating the cerebrum from the cerebellum is a double fold of dura mater called tentorium cerebelli. Pull it out in a horizontal plane by giving incision along the petrous temporal bone.

Learn about the folds of dura mater, i.e. falx cerebri, tentorium cerebelli, falx cerebelli, diaphragma sellae including trigeminal cave from the specimen with the help of base of skull. Make a paper model of these dural folds for recapitulation.

*Competency:*
**AN30.3** Describe and identify dural folds and dural venous sinuses.

## CEREBRAL DURA MATER

The dura mater is the outermost, thickest and toughest membrane covering the brain (*dura* = hard) (*mater* = mother) (Figs 12.1a to c).

### LAYERS OF DURA MATER

There are **two layers** of dura:

1. Outer or ***endosteal layer*** which serves as an internal periosteum or endosteum or endocranium for the skull bones.
2. Inner or ***meningeal layer*** which surrounds the brain. The meningeal layer is continuous with the spinal dura mater.

The two layers are fused to each other at all places, except where the cranial venous sinuses are enclosed between them.

#### Endosteal Layer or Endocranium

1. The endocranium is continuous:
   a. With the periosteum lining the outside of the skull or pericranium through the sutures and foramina.
   b. With the periosteal lining of the orbit through the superior orbital fissure.
2. It provides ***sheaths*** for the cranial nerves, the sheaths fuse with the epineurium outside the skull.
3. Its outer surface is adherent to the inner surface of the cranial bones by a number of fine fibrous and vascular processes. The adhesion is most marked at the sutures, on the base of the skull and around the foramen magnum.

*Note*: Over the optic nerve, the dura forms a sheath which becomes continuous with the sclera.

#### Meningeal Layer

At places, the meningeal layer of dura mater is folded on itself to form partitions which divide the cranial cavity into compartments which lodge different parts of the brain. The folds are (Fig. 12.1b):

1. Falx cerebri
2. Tentorium cerebelli
3. Falx cerebelli
4. Diaphragma sellae.

#### Blood Supply

The outer layer is richly vascular. The inner meningeal layer is more fibrous and requires little blood supply.

1. The vault or supratentorial space is supplied by the middle meningeal artery.
2. The anterior cranial fossa and the dural lining is supplied by meningeal branches of the anterior ethmoidal, posterior ethmoidal and ophthalmic arteries.
3. The middle cranial fossa is supplied by the middle meningeal, accessory meningeal, and internal carotid arteries; and by meningeal branches of the ascending pharyngeal artery.
4. The posterior cranial fossa is supplied by meningeal branches of the vertebral, occipital and ascending pharyngeal arteries.

#### Nerve Supply

1. The dura of the *vault* has only a few sensory nerves which are derived mostly from the ophthalmic division of the trigeminal nerve.

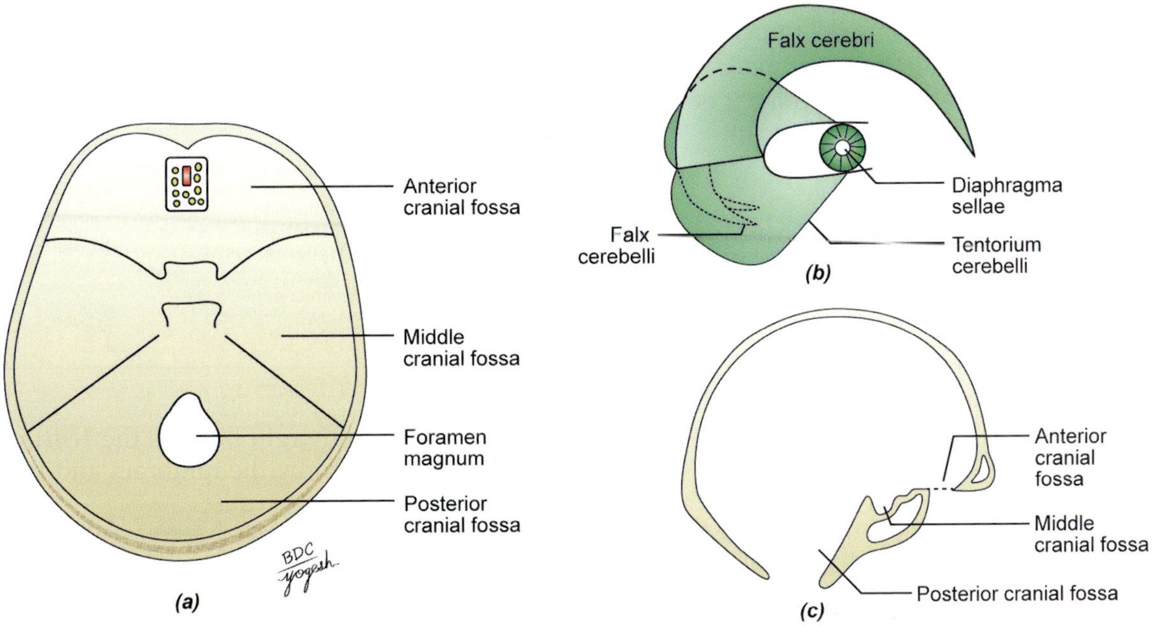


**Figs 12.1a to c:** The cranial cavity: (a) Three cranial fossae, (b) folds of meningeal layer of dura mater, and (c) sagittal section

2. The dura of the floor has a rich nerve supply and is quite sensitive to pain (Figs 12.1a and 12.1c).
   a. *Anterior cranial fossa* is supplied mostly by the anterior ethmoidal nerve and partly by the maxillary nerve.
   b. *Middle cranial fossa* is supplied by the maxillary nerve in its anterior half, and by branches of the mandibular nerve and from the trigeminal ganglion in its posterior half.
   c. *Posterior cranial fossa* is supplied chiefly by recurrent branches from first, second and third cervical spinal nerves and partly by meningeal branches of the ninth and tenth cranial nerves.

## FOLDS OF DURA MATER

### Falx Cerebri

The falx cerebri is a large sickle-shaped fold of dura mater occupying the median longitudinal fissure between the two cerebral hemispheres (Figs 12.2a to c, Flowchart 12.1).

#### Parts

***Ends:*** It has two ends:

1. *Anterior end* is narrow, and is attached to the crista galli.
2. *Posterior end* is broad, and is attached along the median plane to the upper surface of the tentorium cerebelli.

***Margins:*** The falx cerebri has two margins:

1. *Upper margin* is convex and is attached to the lips of the sagittal sulcus.
2. *Lower margin* is concave and free.

***Surfaces:*** The falx cerebri has *right* and *left surfaces* each of which is related to the medial surface of the corresponding cerebral hemisphere.

#### Related Venous Sinuses

Three important venous sinuses are present in relation to this fold.

1. *Superior sagittal sinus* lies along the upper margin.
2. *Inferior sagittal* sinus along the lower margin.
3. *Straight sinus* along the line of attachment of the falx to the tentorium cerebelli (Figs 12.2a to c).

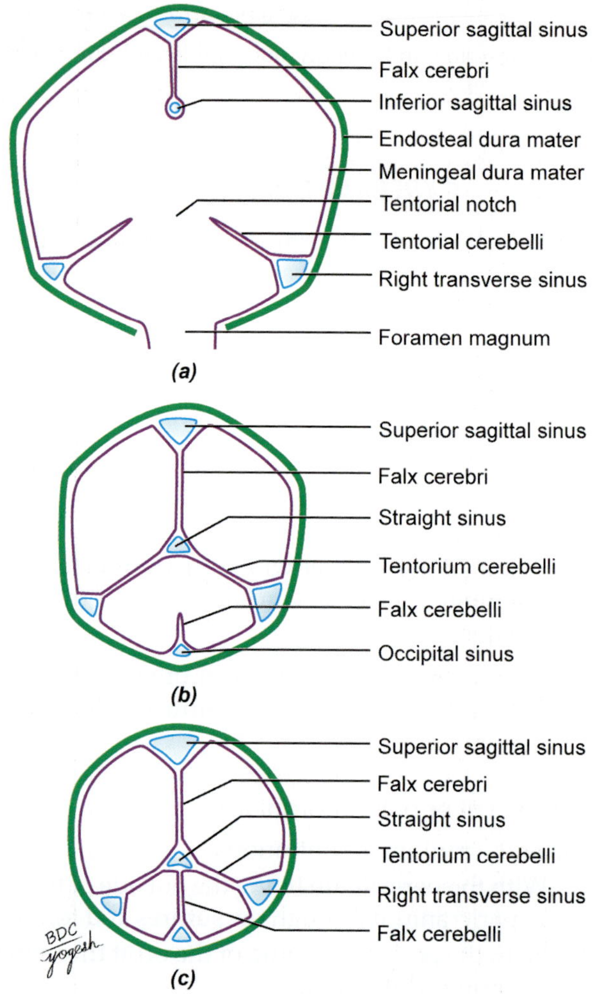


**Figs 12.2a to c:** Coronal sections through the posterior cranial fossa showing folds of dura mater and the venous sinuses enclosed in them: (a) Section through the tentorial notch (anterior part of the fossa), (b) section through the middle part of the fossa, and (c) section through the posterior most part

**Flowchart 12.1:** Falx cerebri

***Falx cerebri***

| *Definition* | *Parts* | *Related sinuses* |
|---|---|---|
| Large sickle-shaped<br>Fold of dura mater<br>Lies in median longitudinal fissure of brain | Anterior end: Attached to crista galli<br>Posterior end: Attached to tentorium cerebelli<br>Upper margin: Attached to sagittal sulcus<br>Lower margin: Concave, free | Superior sagittal sinus<br>Inferior sagittal sinus<br>Straight sinus |

BDC yogesh

### Tentorium Cerebelli

The tentorium cerebelli is a tent-shaped fold of dura mater, forming the roof of the posterior cranial fossa (Figs 12.3 and 12.4, Flowchart 12.2). It separates the cerebellum from the occipital lobes of the cerebrum, and broadly divides the cranial cavity into supratentorial and infratentorial compartments. The infratentorial compartment is the posterior cranial fossa containing the hindbrain and the lower part of the midbrain.

#### Parts

***Margins:*** The tentorium cerebelli has a free margin and an attached margin.

1. *Anterior free margin* is U-shaped and free. The ends of the 'U' are attached anteriorly to the anterior clinoid processes. This margin bounds the ***tentorial notch*** which is occupied by the midbrain and the anterior part of the superior vermis.
2. *Outer or attached margin* is convex. Posterolaterally, it is attached to the lips of the transverse sulci on the occipital bone, and on the posteroinferior angle of the parietal bone. Anterolaterally, it is attached to the superior border of the petrous temporal bone and to

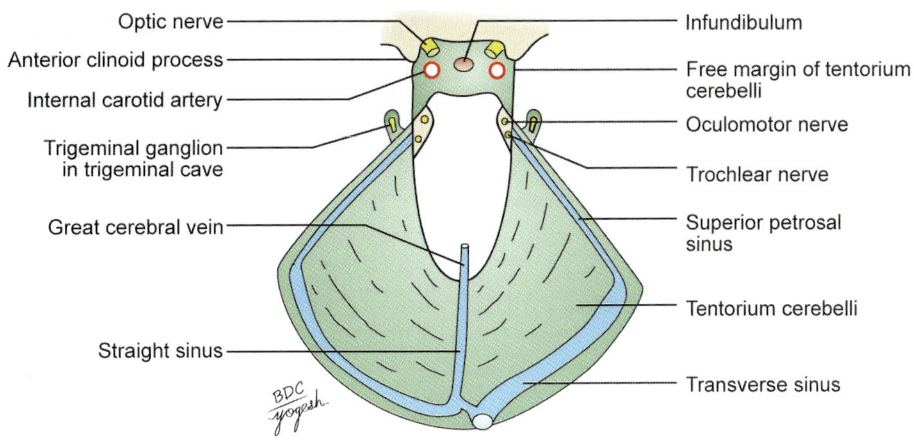


**Fig. 12.3:** Tentorium cerebelli and diaphragma sellae seen from above

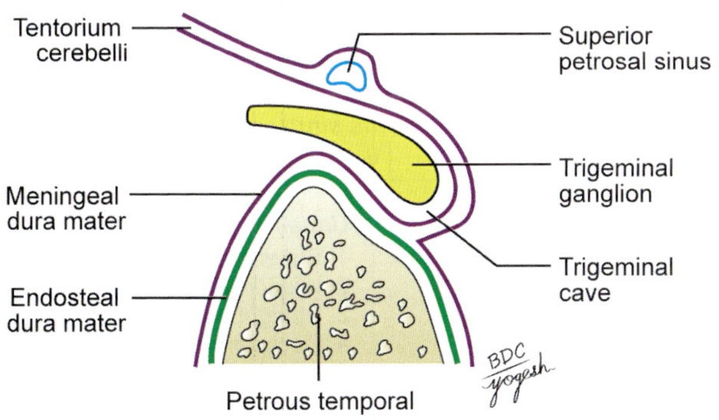


**Fig. 12.4:** Parasagittal section through the petrous temporal bone and meninges to show the formation of the trigeminal cave

**Flowchart 12.2:** Tentorium cerebelli

***Tentorium cerebelli***

***Definition***
- Tent-shaped fold of dura mater
- Forms roof of posterior cranial fossa
- Separates cerebellum from occipital lobe

***Parts***
- Free margin
  - U-shaped
  - Encloses tentorial notch
- Attached margin
  - Convex fixed
  - Extends along posterior clinoid process, superior border of temporal bone and transverse sulcus
- Upper surface:
  - Gives attachment to falx cerebri
- Lower surface
  - Gives attachment to falx cerebelli

***Related sinuses***
- Transverse sinus
- Superior petrosal sinus
- Straight sinus

BDC yogesh

the posterior clinoid processes. Along the attached margin, there are the transverse and superior petrosal venous sinuses.

***Surfaces:*** The tentorium cerebelli has two surfaces—superior and inferior.

1. *Superior surface* is convex and slopes to either side from the median plane. The falx cerebri is attached to this surface in the midline; the straight sinus lies along the line of this attachment. The superior surface is related to the occipital lobes of the cerebrum.
2. *Inferior surface* is concave and fits the convex superior surface of the cerebellum. The falx cerebelli is attached to its posterior part (Fig. 12.2c).

*Note*:

The ***trigeminal* or *Meckel's cave*** is a recess of dura mater present in relation to the attached margin of the tentorium. It is formed by evagination of the inferior layer of the tentorium over the trigeminal impression on the petrous temporal bone. It contains the trigeminal ganglion (Fig. 12.4).

The free and attached margins of the tentorium cerebelli cross each other near the apex of the petrous temporal bone. Anterior to the point of crossing, there is a triangular area which forms the posterior part of the roof of cavernous sinus, and is pierced by the 3rd and 4th cranial nerves.

## Falx Cerebelli

The falx cerebelli is a small sickle-shaped fold of dura mater projecting forwards into the posterior cerebellar notch (Fig. 12.2c).

### Parts

1. *Base* of the sickle is attached to the posterior part of the inferior surface of the tentorium cerebelli in the median plane.
2. *Apex* of the sickle is frequently divided into two parts which are lost on the sides of the foramen magnum.
3. *Posterior margin* is convex and is attached to the internal occipital crest. It encloses the occipital sinus.
4. *Anterior margin* is concave and free.

## Diaphragma Sellae

The diaphragma sellae is a small circular, horizontal fold of dura mater forming the roof of the hypophyseal fossa (Figs 12.5a and b). The diaphragma has a ***central aperture*** through which the stalk of the hypophysis cerebri passes.

### Attachments

1. *Anteriorly* – to the tuberculum sellae
2. *Posteriorly* – to the dorsum sellae.
3. *On each side* – continuous with the dura mater of the middle cranial fossa.

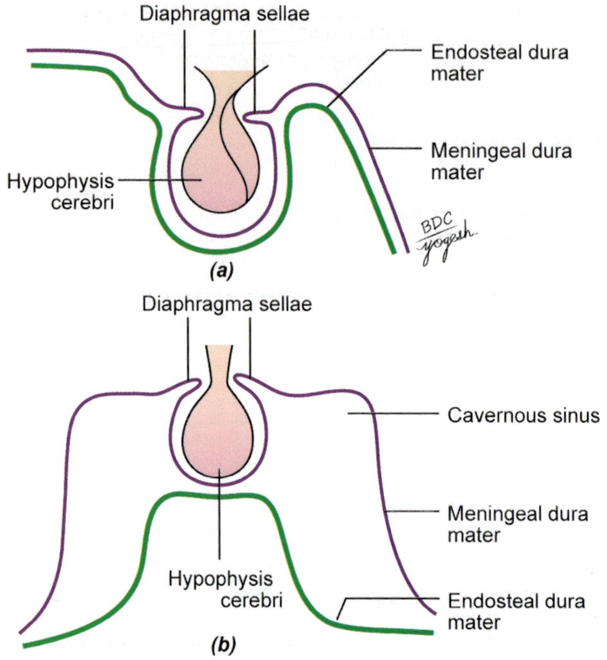


**Figs 12.5a and b:** Diaphragma sellae as seen in: (a) Sagittal section and (b) coronal section

*Competency:*
**AN30.4** Describe clinical importance of dural venous sinuses.

## CLINICAL ANATOMY

***Pain-sensitive intracranial structures:*** They are:

a. The large cranial venous sinuses and their tributaries from the surface of the brain
b. Dural arteries
c. The dural floor of the anterior and posterior cranial fossae
d. Arteries at the base of the brain.

***Headache:*** It may be caused by:

a. Dilatation of intracranial arteries
b. Dilatation of extracranial arteries
c. Traction or distension of intracranial pain sensitive structures
d. Infection and inflammation of intracranial and extra-cranial structures supplied by the sensory, cranial and cervical nerves.

***Extradural and subdural haemorrhages:*** Their differences are listed in Table 12.1.

**TABLE 12.1: Differences between extradural and subdural haemorrhages**

| *Feature* | *Extradural (epidural) haemorrhage* | *Subdural haemorrhage* |
|---|---|---|
| Location | Between the skull and endosteal layer of dura mater | Between the dura mater and arachnoid mater |
| Involved vessels | Arteries (middle meningeal artery) | Veins |
| Symptoms | Rapid onset of symptoms (sudden onset of paralysis) | Gradual increasing symptoms |
| Blood in CSF | Absent | Present |
| CT scan appearance of hematoma | Biconvex lens | Crescent-shaped |

## VENOUS SINUSES OF DURA MATER

***Definition:*** The dural venous sinuses are the venous spaces or channels present in the dura mater. These are lined by *endothelium*.

### Features of Dural Venous (Flowchart 12.3)

1. The dural venous sinuses are formed by two ways:
   a. By separation of two layers of dura mater
   b. By folding of meningeal layer on itself.

**Flowchart 12.3:** Dural venous sinuses

***Dural venous sinuses***
Venous channels in dura mater

***Paired***
1. Cavernous
2. Superior petrosal
3. Inferior petrosal
4. Transverse
5. Sigmoid
6. Sphenoparietal
7. Petrosquamous

***Unpaired***
1. Superior sagittal
2. Inferior sagittal
3. Straight
4. Occipital
5. Anterior intercavernous
6. Posterior intercavernous
7. Basilar plexus of veins

2. Lined by endothelium only
3. Muscle coat is absent in their walls
4. Devoid of valves in their lumen
5. Receive blood and CSF both
6. Communicates with veins outside the skull through emissary veins. It helps to maintain the constant blood pressure in the sinuses.

### Classification of Dural Venous Sinuses

There are 23 venous sinuses, of which 8 are paired and 7 are unpaired.

*Paired venous sinuses*

There is one sinus each on right and left side.

1. Cavernous sinus
2. Superior petrosal sinus
3. Inferior petrosal sinus
4. Transverse sinus
5. Sigmoid sinus
6. Sphenoparietal sinus
7. Petrosquamous sinus
8. Middle meningeal sinus/veins

*Unpaired venous sinuses*

These are median in position.

1. Superior sagittal sinus
2. Inferior sagittal sinus
3. Straight sinus
4. Occipital sinus
5. Anterior intercavernous sinus
6. Posterior intercavernous sinus
7. Basilar plexus of veins

## CAVERNOUS SINUS

Cavernous sinus is a large dural venous sinus that lies between the two layers of the dura mater (Figs 12.6a and b, Flowchart 12.4).

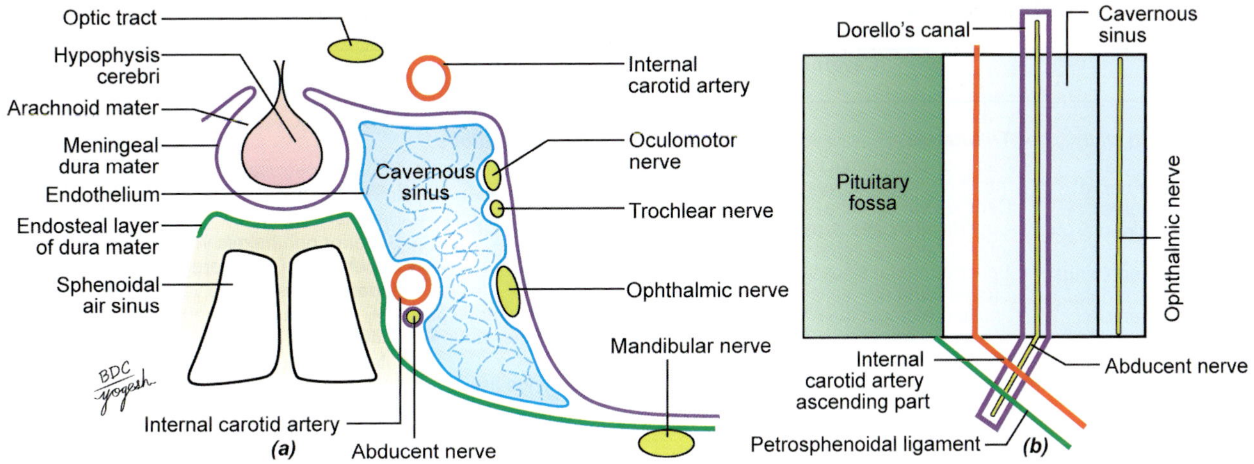


**Figs 12.6a and b:** (a) Coronal section through the middle cranial fossa showing the relations of the cavernous sinus and (b) Dorellos's canal (*Courtesy*: Prof. SN Kazi)

**Flowchart 12.4:** Cavernous sinuses: Location, parts, extent and relations

**Cavernous sinus**

- ***Definition***
  - Dural venous sinus
  - Lies in two layers of dura
  - Size: 2 x 1 cm
- ***Location***
  - In middle cranial fossa
  - On either side of body of sphenoid
- ***Parts***
  - Roof and lateral wall: Formed by meningeal layer of dura mater
  - Floor and medial wall: Formed by endosteal layer of dura mater
- ***Extent***
  - Anteriorly: Up to superior orbital fissure
  - Posteriorly: Up to apex of petrous temporal bone
- ***Relations***
  - Superior: Optic chiasma, optic tract, olfactory tract, ICA, anterior perforated sub.
  - Inferior: Foramen lacerum, junction of body and greater wing of sphenoid
  - Medial: Pituitary gland, sphenoidal air sinus
  - Laterally: Temporal lobe with uncus
  - Anteriorly: Superior orbital fissure
  - Posteriorly: Petrous part of temporal bone

***Size:*** It is about 2 cm long, and 1 cm wide.

***Location:*** Each cavernous sinus lies in the middle cranial fossa, on either side of the body of sphenoid bone.

## Parts (Structure)

The cavernous sinus lies between two layers of dura mater. Each cavernous sinus has a roof, floor, and two walls (medial and lateral).

1. Roof and lateral wall is formed by the meningeal layer of dura mater.
2. Floor and medial wall is formed by the endosteal layer of dura mater.

*Note*: The interior of the cavernous sinus is divided into a number of spaces or caverns by trabeculae. The trabeculae are much less conspicuous in the living than in the dead.

## Extent

Each sinus extends.

*Anteriorly*: Up to the medial end of superior orbital fissure.

*Posteriorly*: Up to the apex petrous part of temporal bone.

## Relations

*Superior:* Optic tract, optic chiasma, olfactory tract, internal carotid artery and anterior perforated substance.

*Inferior:* Foramen lacerum and the junction of the body and greater wing of the sphenoid bone.

*Medial:* Hypophysis cerebri and sphenoidal air sinus.

*Lateral:* Temporal lobe with uncus.

*Anterior:* Superior orbital fissure and the apex of the orbit.

*Posterior:* Apex of the petrous temporal and the crus cerebri of the midbrain.

## Structures within the Lateral Wall of the Sinus (from above downwards) (Flowchart 12.5)

1. Oculomotor nerve
2. Trochlear nerve
3. Ophthalmic nerve

*Note:*

1. *Oculomotor nerve*: In the anterior part of the sinus, it divides into superior and inferior divisions which leave the sinus by passing through the superior orbital fissure.
2. *Trochlear nerve:* In the anterior part of the sinus, it crosses superficial to the oculomotor nerve, and enters the orbit through the superior orbital fissure.
3. *Ophthalmic nerve:* In the anterior part of the sinus, it divides into the lacrimal, frontal and nasociliary nerves.
4. *Maxillary nerve:* It does not pass through cavernous sinus or its lateral wall. It courses beneath the dura mater of middle cranial fossa. It passes below the level of cavernous sinus by piercing cavum trigeminale (refer to Gray's Anatomy, 42nd edition).

The structures in the lateral wall and on the medial aspect of the sinus are separated from blood by the endothelial lining.

**Flowchart 12.5:** Cavernous sinus: Structures in wall, tributaries and communications

***Cavernous sinus***

***Structures in wall***

Within lateral wall:
- Oculomotor nerve
- Trochlear nerve
- Ophthalmic nerve

Passing through sinus:
- ICA
- Abducent nerve

***Tributaries***

- Superior ophthalmic vein
- Inferior ophthalmic vein
- Central vein of retina
- Superficial middle cerebral vein
- Inferior cerebral veins
- Sphenoparietal sinus
- Frontal trunk of middle meningeal vein

***Communications***

- Transverse sinus ⟷ Superior petrosal sinus
- Internal jugular vein ⟷ Inferior petrosal sinus
- Pterygoid venous plexus ⟷ Emissary veins
- Facial vein ⟷ Superior ophthalmic vein, emissary veins
- Superior sagittal sinus ⟷ Superficial middle cerebral vein, superior anastomotic vein
- Internal vertebral venous plexus ⟷ Basilar venous plexus
- Opposite cavernous sinus ⟷ Anterior and posterior intercavernous sinuses

***Clinical integration:*** Cavernous sinus thrombosis, carotid-cavernous sinus fistula

### Structures Passing through the Medial Aspect of the Sinus

1. *Internal carotid artery* with the venous and sympathetic plexus around it.
2. *Abducent nerve.*

*Note*: The abducent nerve enters the cavernous sinus by passing inferior to the petrosphenoidal ligament within a dural tunnel (***Dorello's canal***) (Fig. 12.6b) just posterior to the short ascending portion of the cavernous carotid artery, and then runs on the inferolateral side of the horizontal portion of the cavernous carotid artery, just medial to the ophthalmic nerve at the lateral wall of the sinus, known as the ***infratrochlear or Parkinson's triangle.*** It gives access to the horizontal portion of the cavernous carotid artery and the abducent nerve (Fig. 12.7).

### Tributaries or Incoming Channels (Figs 12.8 and 12.9)

#### *From the orbit*

1. Superior ophthalmic vein.
2. Branch of the inferior ophthalmic vein or sometimes the vein itself.
3. Central vein of the retina may drain either into the superior ophthalmic vein or into the cavernous sinus.

#### *From the brain*

1. Superficial middle cerebral vein.
2. Inferior cerebral veins from the temporal lobe.

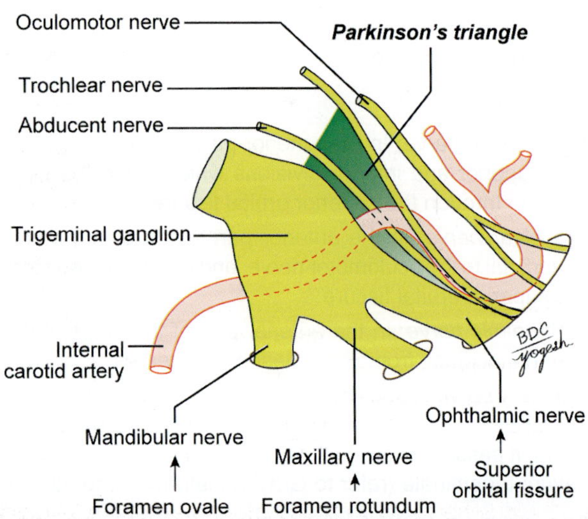


**Fig. 12.7:** Infratrochlear or Parkinson's triangle

#### *From the meninges*

1. Sphenoparietal sinus.
2. Frontal trunk of the middle meningeal vein.
3. From the face—facial vein → deep facial vein → pterygoid plexus → emissary vein → cavernous sinus.

### Draining Channels or Communications

The cavernous sinus drains (Figs 12.10 and 12.11):

1. Into the transverse sinus through the superior petrosal sinus.
2. Into the internal jugular vein through the inferior petrosal sinus and through a plexus around the internal carotid artery.
3. Into the pterygoid plexus of veins through the emissary veins passing through the foramen ovale, the foramen lacerum and the emissary sphenoidal foramen.
4. Into the facial vein through the superior ophthalmic vein.
5. The right and left cavernous sinuses communicate with each other through the anterior and posterior intercavernous sinuses and the basilar plexus of veins.

All these communications are valveless, and blood can flow through them in either direction.

### Factors Helping Expulsion of Blood from the Sinus

1. Expansile pulsations of the internal carotid artery within the sinus
2. Gravity
3. Position of the head

## CLINICAL ANATOMY

- ***Thrombosis of the cavernous sinus*** may be caused by sepsis in the dangerous area of the face, in nasal cavities, and paranasal air sinuses. This gives rise to the following symptoms:
  - **a. *Nervous symptoms:***
    - Severe pain in the eye and forehead in the area of distribution of ophthalmic nerve.
    - Involvement of the third, fourth and sixth cranial nerves resulting in paralysis of the muscles supplied.

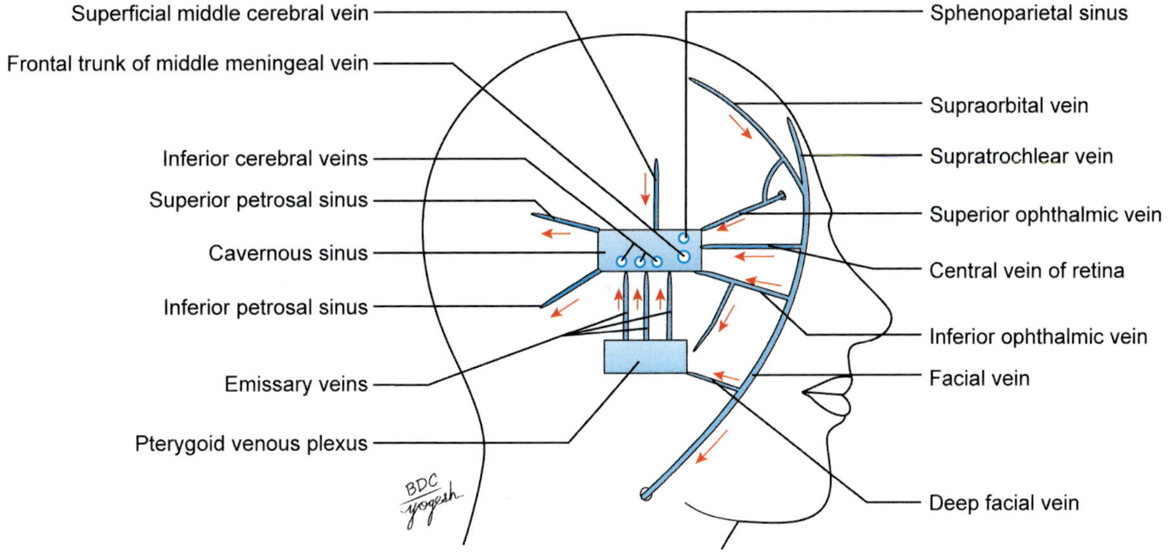


**Fig. 12.8:** Side view of the tributaries and communications of the cavernous sinus. Arrows show the direction of blood flow

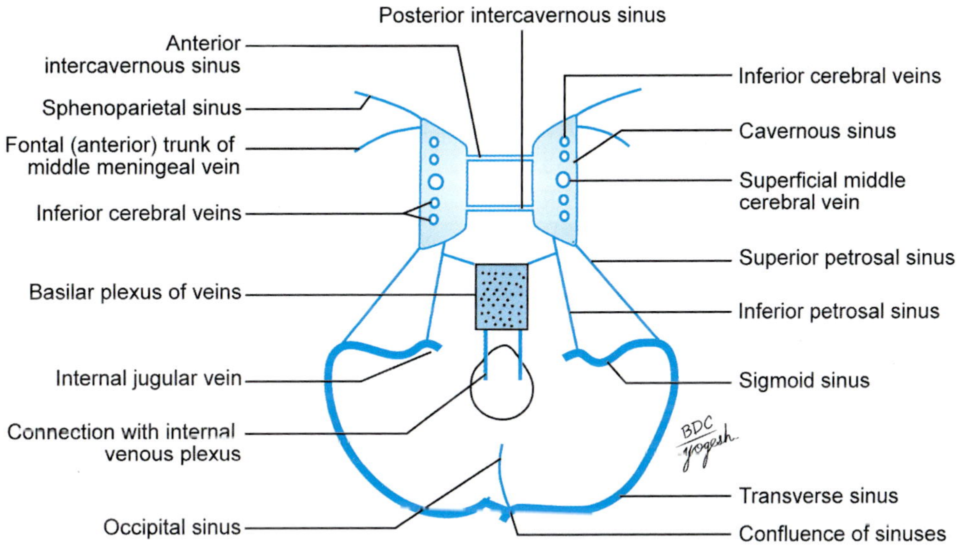


**Fig. 12.9:** Superior view of the tributaries and communications of the cavernous sinus. Arrows show the direction of blood flow

b. ***Venous symptoms:*** Marked oedema of eyelids, cornea and root of the nose, with exophthalmos due to congestion of the orbital veins.

- A communication between the cavernous sinus and the internal carotid artery may be produced by head injury. When this happens the eyeball protrudes and pulsates with each heartbeat. It is called the ***pulsating exophthalmos***.

## DISSECTION

Define the cavernous sinuses situated on each side of the body of the sphenoid bone. Cut through it between the anterior and posterior ends and locate its contents. Define its connections with the other venous sinuses and veins.

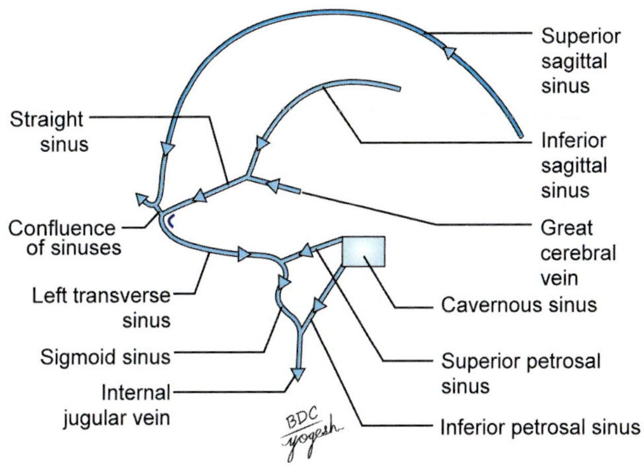


**Fig. 12.10:** Scheme to show the lateral view of the intracranial venous sinuses. Arrowheads show the direction of blood flow

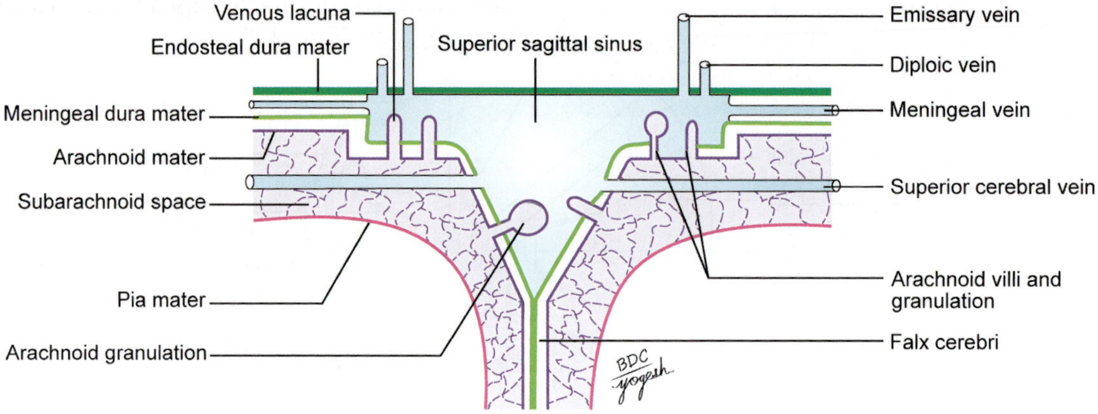


**Fig. 12.11:** Coronal section through superior sagittal sinus showing arrangement of the meninges, the arachnoid villi and granulations, and the various (emissary, diploic, meningeal and cerebral) veins in its relation

## OTHER SINUSES

### Superior Sagittal Sinus

The superior sagittal sinus occupies the upper convex, attached margin of the falx cerebri (Figs 12.10 and 12.11).

It begins anteriorly at the crista galli by the union of tiny meningeal veins. Here it communicates with the veins of the frontal sinus, and occasionally with the veins of the nose, through the foramen caecum. As the sinus runs upwards and backwards, it becomes progressively larger in size. It is triangular on cross-section. It ends near the internal occipital protuberance by turning to one side, usually the right, and becomes continuous with the right transverse sinus (Fig. 12.10). It generally communicates with the opposite sinus. The junction of all these sinuses is called the ***confluence of sinuses***.

The *interior* of the sinus shows:

1. Openings of the superior cerebral veins.
2. Openings of venous lacunae, usually three on each side.
3. Arachnoid villi and granulations projecting into the lacunae as well as into the sinus (Fig. 12.11).
4. Numerous fibrous bands crossing the inferior angle of the sinus.

*Tributaries:*

1. Superior cerebral veins which never open into the venous lacunae (Fig. 12.11).
2. Parietal emissary veins (Table 12.2).
3. Venous lacunae, usually three on each side which first, receive the diploic and meningeal veins, and then open into the sinus.
4. Occasionally, a vein from the nose opens into the sinus when the foramen caecum is patent.

### Inferior Sagittal Sinus

The inferior sagittal sinus, a small channel, lies in the posterior two-thirds of the lower, concave free margin of the falx cerebri. It ends by joining the great cerebral vein to form the straight sinus (Fig. 12.10).

**TABLE 12.2: Emissary veins: Valveless and communicate intracranial with extracranial veins**

| *Sinus* | *Connection* | *Veins* |
|---|---|---|
| Superior sagittal sinus | Parietal emissary vein<br>Foramen caecum<br>Middle meningeal vein | Veins of scalp, nasal veins<br>Pterygoid veins |
| Transverse sinus | Petrosquamous | External jugular |
| Sigmoid sinus | Mastoid vein<br>Hypoglossal vein<br>Posterior condylar vein | Posterior auricular<br>IJV<br>Suboccipital vein |
| Cavernous sinus | Emissary veins<br>Veins around ICA<br>Ophthalmic vein<br>Inferior petrosal | Pterygoid veins<br>IJV<br>Facial vein<br>IJV |

ICA: Internal carotid artery; IJV: Internal jugular vein

### Straight Sinus

The straight sinus lies in the median plane within the junction of falx cerebri and the tentorium cerebelli. It is formed anteriorly by the union of the inferior sagittal sinus with the great cerebral vein, and ends at the internal occipital protuberance by continuing as the transverse sinus usually left (Fig. 12.10).

### Transverse Sinuses

The transverse sinuses are large sinuses. The right sinus usually larger than the left, is situated in the posterior part of the attached margin of the tentorium cerebelli. The right transverse sinus is usually a continuation of the superior sagittal sinus, and the left sinus a continuation of the straight sinus. Each sinus extends from the internal occipital protuberance to the posteroinferior angle of the parietal bone at the base of mastoid process where it bends downwards and becomes the sigmoid sinus.

*Tributaries:*

1. Superior petrosal sinus
2. Inferior cerebral veins
3. Inferior cerebellar veins
4. Diploic (posterior temporal) vein
5. Inferior anastomotic vein.

### Sigmoid Sinuses

Each sinus, right or left, is the direct continuation of the transverse sinus (Fig. 12.9). It is S-shaped, hence the name. It extends from the posteroinferior angle of the parietal bone to the posterior part of the jugular foramen where it becomes the superior bulb of the internal jugular vein. It grooves the mastoid part of the temporal bone, where *it is separated anteriorly from the mastoid antrum and mastoid air cells by only a thin plate of bone.*

*Tributaries*:

1. Mastoid and condylar emissary veins
2. Cerebellar veins
3. Internal auditory vein.

### Occipital Sinus

The occipital sinus is small, and lies in the attached margin of the falx cerebelli. It begins near the foramen magnum and ends in the confluence of sinuses (Fig. 12.9).

### Sphenoparietal Sinuses

The sphenoparietal sinuses, right and left, lie along the posterior free margin of the lesser wing of the sphenoid bone, and drain into the anterior part of the cavernous sinus. Each sinus may receive the frontal trunk of the middle meningeal vein (Fig. 12.10).

### Superior Petrosal Sinuses

The superior petrosal sinuses lie in the anterior part of the attached margin of the tentorium cerebelli along the upper border of the petrous temporal bone. It drains the cavernous sinus into the transverse sinus (Fig. 12.9).

### Inferior Petrosal Sinuses

The inferior petrosal sinuses, right and left, lie in the corresponding petro-occipital fissure, and drain the cavernous sinus into the superior bulb of the internal jugular vein.

### Basilar Plexus of Veins

The basilar plexus of veins lies over the clivus of the skull. It connects the two inferior petrosal sinuses and communicates with the internal vertebral venous plexus.

### Middle Meningeal Veins

The middle meningeal veins form two main trunks, one frontal or anterior and one parietal or posterior, which accompany the two branches of the middle meningeal artery.

1. The ***frontal trunk*** may end either in the pterygoid plexus through the foramen ovale, or in the sphenoparietal or cavernous sinus.
2. The ***parietal trunk*** usually ends in the pterygoid plexus through the foramen spinosum. The meningeal veins are nearer to the bone than the arteries, and are, therefore, more liable to injury in fractures of the skull.

### Intercavernous Sinuses

The anterior and posterior intercavernous sinuses connect the cavernous sinuses. They pass through the diaphragma sellae, one in front and the other behind the infundibulum (Fig. 12.9).

## CLINICAL ANATOMY

- ***Thrombosis of the superior sagittal sinus*** may be caused by spread of infection from the nose, scalp and diploe. This gives rise to:
  - A considerable rise in intracranial tension due to defective absorption of CSF.
  - Delirium and sometimes convulsions due to congestion of the superior cerebral veins.
  - Paraplegia of the upper motor neuron type due to bilateral involvement of the paracentral lobules of cerebrum where the lower limbs and perineum are represented.
- Spread of infection or thrombosis from the sigmoid and transverse sinuses to the superior sagittal sinus may cause impaired CSF drainage into the latter and may, therefore, lead to the development of hydrocephalus. Such a hydrocephalus associated with sinus thrombosis following ear infection is known as ***otitic hydrocephalus***.
- ***Thrombosis of the sigmoid sinus*** is always secondary to infection in the middle ear/otitis media, or in the mastoid process called mastoiditis.
- During operations on the mastoid process, one should be careful about the sigmoid sinus, so that it is not exposed.

## HYPOPHYSIS CEREBRI (PITUITARY GLAND)

The hypophysis cerebri is a small endocrine gland situated in relation to the base of the brain. It is often called the ***master of the endocrine orchestra*** because it produces a number of hormones which control the secretions of many other endocrine glands of the body (Figs 12.12a and b).

### Location

The gland lies in the hypophyseal fossa or ***sella turcica*** or pituitary fossa. The fossa is roofed by the diaphragma sellae. The stalk of the hypophysis cerebri pierces the diaphragma sellae and is attached above to the floor of the third ventricle.

### Measurements

The gland is oval in shape, and measures 8 mm anteroposteriorly and 12 mm transversely. It weighs about 500 mg.

### Relations

#### Superior

1. Diaphragma sellae
2. Optic chiasma
3. Tubercinerium
4. Infundibular recess of the third ventricle

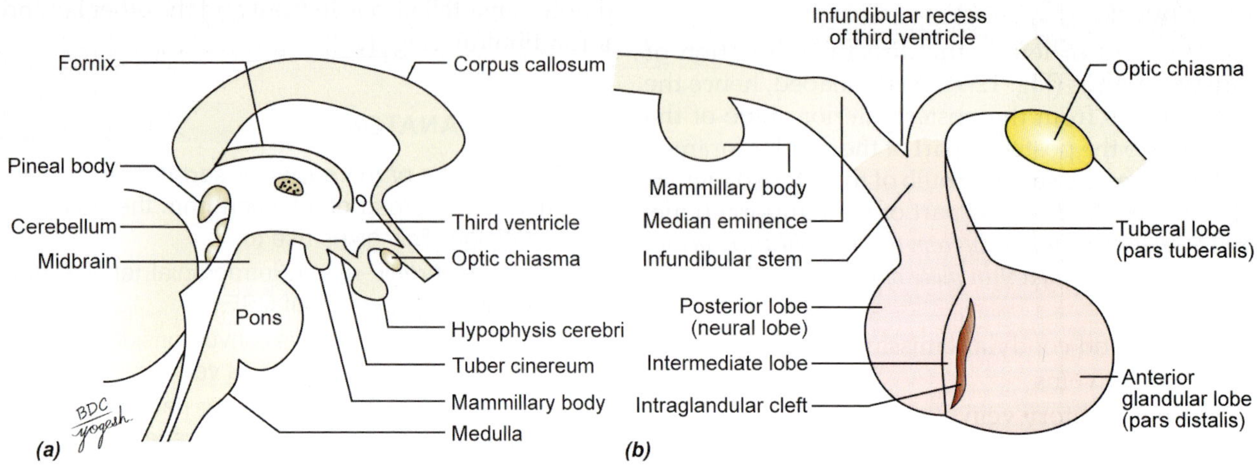


**Figs 12.12a and b:** (a) Sagittal section of diencephalon and the brainstem showing structures at the base of brain including hypophysis cerebri, (b) parts of the hypophysis cerebri as seen in a sagittal section

### Inferior

1. Irregular venous channels between the two layers of dura mater lining the floor of the hypophyseal fossa.
2. Hypophyseal fossa.
3. Sphenoidal air sinuses

### Lateral

Cavernous sinus with its contents.

> ***Competency:***
> **AN43.4** Describe the development and developmental basis of congenital anomalies of face, palate, tongue, branchial apparatus, pituitary gland, thyroid gland and eye. Development of pituitary gland is given here. Development of other organs is given with their respective chapters.

## Subdivisions/Parts and Development

The gland has two main parts: *Adenohypophysis* and *neurohypophysis* which differ from each other embryologically, morphologically and functionally (Figs 12.12a and b, Plate 12.1).

The adenohypophysis develops as an upward growth called the ***Rathke's pouch*** from the ectodermal roof of the stomodeum. The neurohypophysis develops as a downward growth from the floor of the diencephalon, and is connected to the hypothalamus by neural pathways.

The subdivisions of each part are given below:

### Adenohypophysis

1. ***Anterior lobe*** **or** ***pars anterior, pars distalis, or pars glandularis:*** This is the largest part of the gland (Fig. 12.11).
2. ***Intermediate lobe*** **or** ***pars intermedia:*** This is in the form of a thin strip which is separated from the anterior lobe by an intraglandular cleft, a remnant of the lumen of Rathke's pouch.
3. ***Tuberal lobe*** **or** ***pars tuberalis:*** It is an upward extension of the anterior lobe that surrounds and forms part of the infundibulum.

### Neurohypophysis

1. ***Posterior lobe*** **or** ***neural lobe, pars posterior:*** It is smaller than the anterior lobe and lies in the posterior concavity of the larger anterior lobe.
2. ***Infundibular stem,*** which contains the neural connections of the posterior lobe with the hypothalamus.
3. ***Median eminence*** of the tuber cinerium which is continuous with the infundibular stem.

## Arterial Supply

The hypophysis cerebri is supplied by the following branches of the internal carotid artery (Fig. 12.13).

1. One superior hypophyseal artery on each side.
2. One inferior hypophyseal artery on each side.

## Venous Drainage

Short veins emerge on the surface of the gland and drain into neighbouring dural venous sinuses. The hormones pass out of the gland through the venous blood, and are carried to their target cells.

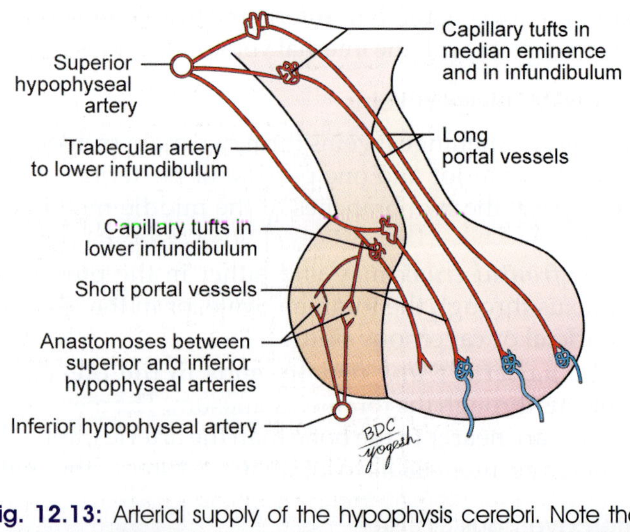


**Fig. 12.13:** Arterial supply of the hypophysis cerebri. Note that the neurohypophysis is supplied by the superior and inferior hypophyseal arteries, and the adenohypophysis, exclusively by the portal vessels

Head and Neck 12

**Plate 12.1:** Histology of hypophysis cerebri

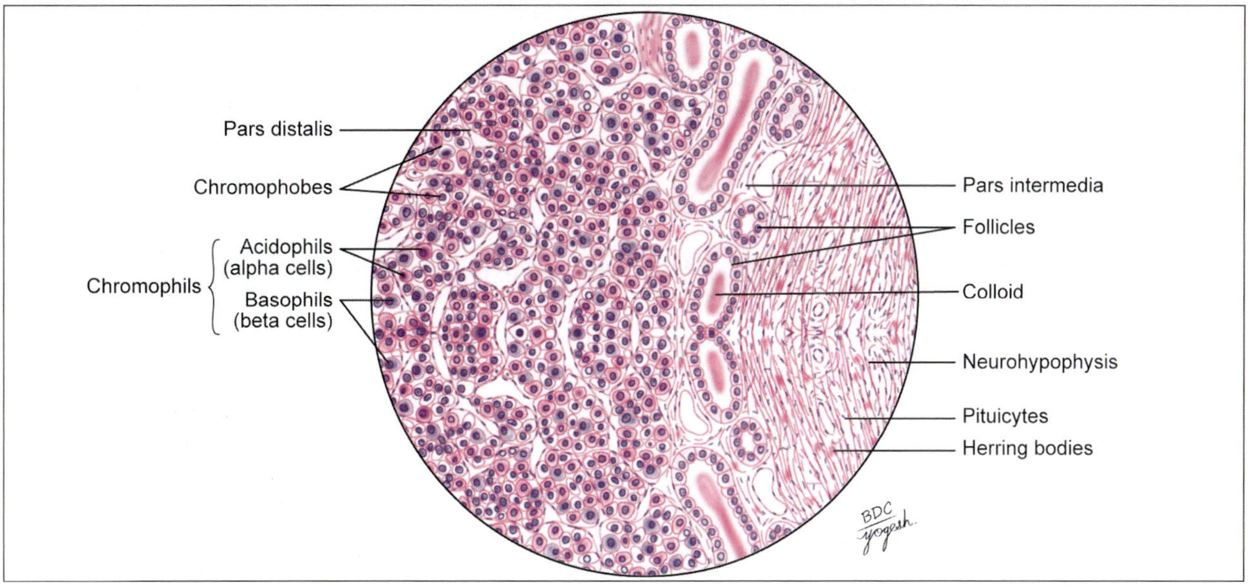


***Competency:***

**AN43.2** Identify, describe and draw the microanatomy of pituitary gland, thyroid, parathyroid gland, tongue, salivary glands, tonsil, epiglottis, cornea, retina. Histology of other organs is given with their respective chapters.

## Histology of Pituitary Gland

Pituitary gland consists of (Plate 12.1)

- Adenohypophysis that have pars distalis, pars intermedia, and pars tuberalis
- Neurohypophysis

***Adenohypophysis*** shows clumps or cords of cells separated by fenestrated capillaries. These cells consist of:

*Acidophils*: Having pink granules

- Somatotrophs (50%) secrete growth hormone
- Lactotropes (15–20%) secrete prolactin

*Basophils*: Having dark blue granules

- Corticotropes (15–20%) secrete ACTH
- Gonadotropes (10%) secrete LH and FSH
- Thyrotropes (5%) secrete TSH

***Pars intermedia*** consists of a series of colloid-filled cysts/vesicles that secrete MSH.

***Neurohypophysis*** consists of nonmyelinated axons and ***pituicytes***. Bodies of these neurons lie in supraoptic and paraventricular nuclei of hypothalamus. Neurohypophysis secretes vasopressin/ADH and oxytocin.

## Hypothalamo-hypophyseal Portal System

1. Each ***superior hypophyseal artery*** supplies:
   a. Ventral part of the hypothalamus
   b. Upper part of the infundibulum
   c. Lower part of the infundibulum through a separate long descending branch, called the trabecular artery.
2. Each ***inferior hypophyseal artery*** divides into medial and lateral branches which join one another to form an arterial ring around the posterior lobe. Branches from this ring supply the posterior lobe and also anastomose with branches from the superior hypophyseal artery.
3. The anterior lobe or pars distalis is supplied exclusively by ***portal vessels*** arising from capillary tufts formed by the superior hypophyseal arteries. The long portal vessels drain the median eminence and the upper infundibulum, and the short portal vessels drain the lower infundibulum.
4. The hypothalamohypophyseal tract begins in the preoptic and paraventricular nuclei of the hypothalamus. Its short fibres terminate in relation to capillary tufts of portal vessels, providing the possibility for a neural control of the secretory activity of the anterior lobe. The long fibres of the neurosecretory tract pass to the posterior lobe and terminate near vascular sinusoids.

   The hormones related to the posterior lobe are:
   a. *Vasopressin*, antidiuretic hormone (ADH) which acts on kidney tubules.
   b. *Oxytocin*, which promotes contraction of the uterine and mammary smooth muscle.

These hormones are actually secreted by the hypothalamus, from where these are transported through the hypothalamohypophyseal tract to the posterior lobe of the gland.

***Competency:***

**AN30.5** Explain effect of pituitary tumours on visual pathway.

## CLINICAL ANATOMY

***Pituitary tumours*** give rise to two main categories of symptoms:

A. *General symptoms* due to pressure over surrounding structures:
   a. Sella turcica is enlarged in size.

b. Pressure over the central part of optic chiasma causes bitemporal hemianopia and tubular vision (Figs 12.14a and b).
c. Pressure over the hypothalamus may cause one of the hypothalamic syndromes like obesity of ***Frolich's syndrome*** in cases with Rathke's pouch tumours.
d. A large tumour may press upon the third ventricle, causing a rise in intracranial pressure.

B. *Specific symptoms* depending on the cell type of the tumour.
a. Acidophil or eosinophil adenoma causes acromegaly in adults and gigantism in younger patients.
b. Basophil adenoma causes Cushing's syndrome.
c. Chromophobe adenoma causes effects of hypopituitarism.
d. Posterior lobe damage causes diabetes insipidus, although the lesion in these cases usually lies in the hypothalamus.

## DISSECTION

Identify diaphragma sellae over the hypophyseal fossa. Incise it radially and locate the hypophysis cerebri lodged in its fossa. Take it out and examine it in detail with the hand lens.

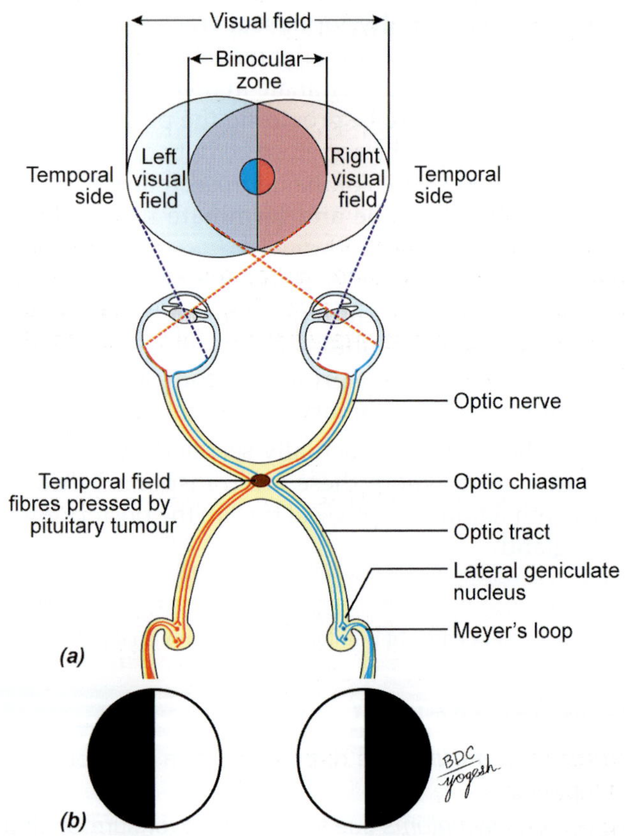


**Figs 12.14a and b:** Bitemporal hemianopia due to pressure of pituitary tumour on the central part of optic chiasma

## TRIGEMINAL GANGLION

This is the *sensory ganglion* (***Gasserian ganglion***) of the 5th cranial nerve (Fig. 12.15). It is homologous with the dorsal nerve root ganglia of spinal nerves. All such ganglia are made up of pseudounipolar nerve cells, with a 'T'-shaped arrangement of their process; one process arises from the cell body which then divides into a central and a peripheral process.

The ganglion is crescentic or semilunar in shape, with its convexity directed anterolaterally.

### Situation and Meningeal Relations

The ganglion lies on the *trigeminal impression,* on the anterior surface of the petrous temporal bone near its apex. It occupies a special space of dura mater, called the *trigeminal or **Meckel's cave**.* There are two layers of dura below the ganglion. The cave is lined by pia-arachnoid, so that the ganglion along with the motor root of the trigeminal nerve is surrounded by CSF. The ganglion lies at a depth of about 5 cm from the preauricular point.

### Relations (Fig. 12.15)

*Medially*
1. Internal carotid artery
2. Posterior part of cavernous sinus

*Laterally:* Middle meningeal artery

*Superiorly:* Parahippocampal gyrus

*Inferiorly*
1. Motor root of trigeminal nerve
2. Greater petrosal nerve
3. Apex of the petrous temporal bone
4. The foramen lacerum.

### Associated Root and Branches

The central processes of the ganglion cells form the large ***sensory root*** of the trigeminal nerve which is attached to pons at its junction with the middle cerebellar peduncle.

The peripheral processes of the ganglion cells form three divisions of the trigeminal nerve, namely the

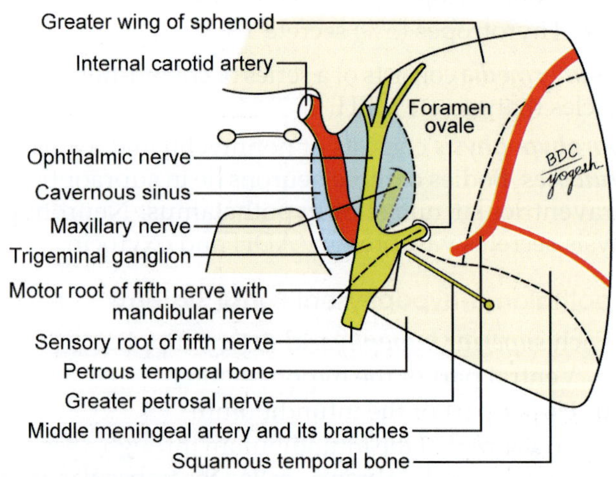


**Fig. 12.15:** Superior view of the middle cranial fossa showing some of its contents

Ophthalmic V1 (*see* Chapter 13), maxillary V2 (*see* Chapter 15) and mandibular V3 (*see* Chapter 6).

The small ***motor root*** of the trigeminal nerve is attached to the pons superomedial to the sensory root. It passes under the ganglion from its medial to the lateral side, and joins the mandibular nerve at the foramen ovale.

#### Blood Supply

The ganglion is supplied by twigs from:
1. Internal carotid
2. Middle meningeal
3. Accessory meningeal arteries
4. By the meningeal branch of the ascending pharyngeal artery.

### CLINICAL ANATOMY

- Intractable facial pain due to trigeminal neuralgia or carcinomatosis may be abolished by injecting alcohol into the ganglion. Sometimes cutting of the sensory root is necessary (Fig. 12.16).
- Congenital cutaneous naevi on the face (port wine stains) map out accurately the areas supplied by one or more divisions of the V cranial nerve.

### DISSECTION

Identify trigeminal ganglion situated on the anterior surface of petrous temporal bone near its apex. Define the three branches emerging from its convex anterior surface.

## MIDDLE MENINGEAL ARTERY

It is the largest branch of 1st part of maxillary artery.

***Course:*** It ascends upward in the infratemporal fossa, deep to lateral pterygoid muscle. Here, it is encircled by two roots of auriculotemporal nerve. It enters the middle cranial fossa through foramen spinosum.

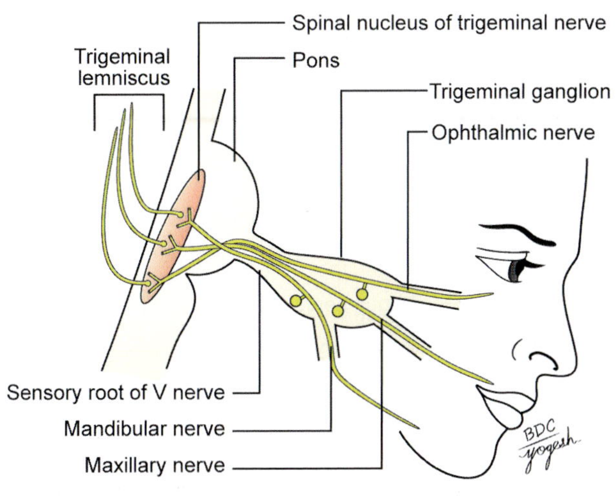


**Fig. 12.16:** Pathways of fibres from the skin of face

In the middle cranial fossa, the artery runs forward and laterally in extradural course and terminates by dividing into two terminal branches:
1. Anterior or frontal
2. Posterior or parietal

#### *Branches*

1. Frontal or anterior branch: It crosses pterion and supplies meninges.
2. Parietal or posterior branch: It also supplies meninges.
3. Ganglion branch to trigeminal ganglion.
4. Petrosal branch to hiatus for the greater petrosal nerve.
5. Superior tympanic branch to tensor tympani muscle
6. Temporal branches to temporal fossa.

### CLINICAL ANATOMY

- The middle meningeal artery is of great surgical importance because it can be torn in head injuries resulting in ***extradural haemorrhage****. The frontal* or *anterior branch* is commonly involved. The haematoma presses on the motor area, giving rise to hemiplegia of the opposite side. The anterior division can be approached surgically by making a hole in the skull over the pterion, 4 cm above the midpoint of the zygomatic arch.
- Rarely, the parietal or posterior branch is implicated, causing contralateral deafness. In this case, the hole is made at a point 4 cm above and 4 cm behind the external acoustic meatus.

### DISSECTION

Dissect the middle meningeal artery which enters the skull through foramen spinosum. It is an important artery for the supply of endocranium, inner table of skull and diploe. Examine the other structures seen in cranial fossae after removal of brain. These are the cranial nerves, internal carotid artery, petrosal nerves and fourth part of vertebral artery.

***Competency:***
**AN30.1** Describe the cranial fossae and identify related structures.

## OTHER STRUCTURES SEEN IN CRANIAL FOSSAE AFTER REMOVAL OF BRAIN

#### Various Structures

The structures seen after removal of the brain are:
- 12 cranial nerves
- Four petrosal nerves
- Cavernous part of internal carotid artery
- 4th part of the vertebral artery.

## DISSECTION

Following structures are seen in the anterior cranial fossa: Crista galli, cribriform plate of ethmoid, orbital part of frontal bone, and lesser wing of sphenoid.

*Following structures are seen in the middle cranial fossa:* Middle meningeal vessels, diaphragma sellae pierced by infundibulum, oculomotor nerves, internal carotid arteries, optic nerve, posterior cerebral artery, and great cerebral vein.

*Following structures are seen in the posterior cranial fossa:* Facial, vestibulocochlear, glossopharyngeal, vagus, accessory, hypoglossal nerves, vertebral arteries, and spinal root of accessory nerve.

## Cranial Nerves (Plate 12.2, Fig. 12.17)

1. *First* or ***olfactory nerve*** is seen in the form of 15 to 20 filaments on each side that pierce the cribriform plate of the ethmoid bone.
2. *Second* or ***optic nerve*** passes through the optic canal with the ophthalmic artery (Fig. 12.17).
3. *Third* or ***oculomotor*** and *fourth* or ***trochlear nerves*** pierce the posterior part of the roof of the cavernous sinus formed by crossing of the free and attached margins of the tentorium cerebelli; next they run in the lateral wall of the cavernous sinus. They enter the orbit through the superior orbital fissure.
4. *Fifth* or ***trigeminal nerve*** has a large sensory root and a small motor root. The roots cross the apex of the petrous temporal bone beneath the superior petrosal sinus, to enter the middle cranial fossa.
5. *Sixth* or ***abducent nerve*** pierces the lower part of the posterior wall of the cavernous sinus near the apex of the petrous temporal bone. It runs forwards by the side of the dorsum sellae beneath the petrosphenoidal ligament to reach the centre of the cavernous sinus.
6. *Seventh* or ***facial*** and *eighth* or *statoacoustic* or ***vestibulocochlear nerves*** pass through the internal acoustic meatus with the labyrinthine vessels.
7. *Ninth* or ***glossopharyngeal***, *tenth* or ***vagus*** and *eleventh* or ***accessory nerves*** pierce the dura mater at the jugular foramen and pass out through it. The *glossopharyngeal* nerve is enclosed in a separate sheath of dura mater, while vagus and accessory nerves are enclosed in one sheath. The spinal part of the accessory nerve first enters the posterior cranial fossa through the foramen magnum, and then passes out through the jugular foramen along with cranial part.
8. The two parts of the *twelfth* or ***hypoglossal nerve*** pierce the dura mater separately opposite the hypoglossal canal and then pass out through it.

## Petrosal Nerves

### Greater Petrosal Nerve

It carries gustatory and parasympathetic fibres. It arises from the geniculate ganglion of the facial nerve, and enters the middle cranial fossa through the hiatus for the greater petrosal nerve on the anterior surface of the petrous temporal bone. It proceeds towards the foramen lacerum, where it joins the deep petrosal nerve which carries sympathetic fibres to form the nerve of the pterygoid canal (*see* Table A.2).

The nerve of the pterygoid canal passes through the pterygoid canal to reach the pterygopalatine ganglion. The parasympathetic fibres relay in this ganglion. Postganglionic parasympathetic fibres arising in the ganglion ultimately supply the lacrimal gland and the mucosal glands of the nose, palate and pharynx. The

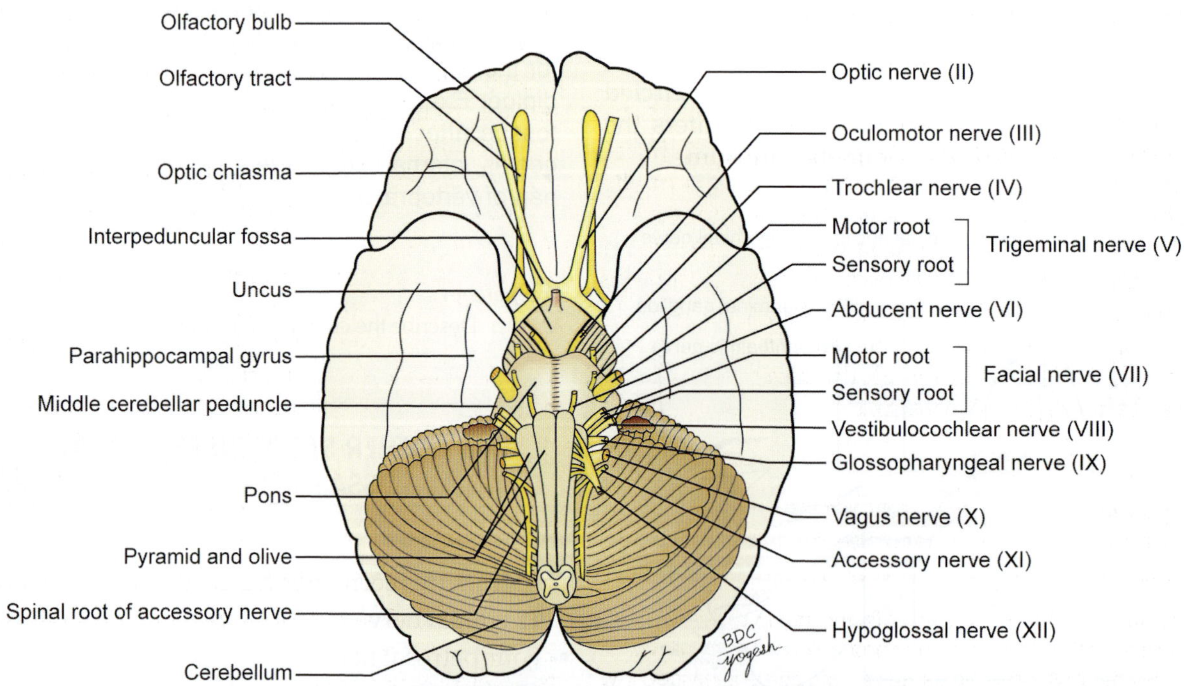


**Fig. 12.17:** Highlights of the cranial nerves

**Plate 12.2:** Identification of cranial nerve in cranial fossae

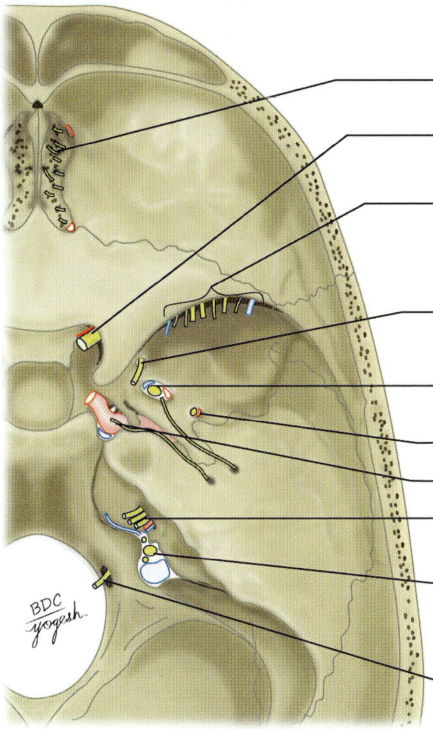


gustatory or taste fibres do not relay in the ganglion and are distributed to the palate.

### Deep Petrosal Nerve

It is sympathetic in nature. It is a branch of the sympathetic plexus around the internal carotid artery. It contains postganglionic fibres from the superior cervical sympathetic ganglion. The nerve joins the greater petrosal nerve to form the nerve of the pterygoid canal. The sympathetic fibres are distributed through the branches of the pterygopalatine ganglion.

### Lesser Petrosal Nerve

It is parasympathetic in nature. It is a branch of the tympanic plexus, deriving its preganglionic parasympathetic fibres from the tympanic branch of the glossopharyngeal nerve. It emerges through the hiatus for the lesser petrosal nerve, situated just lateral to the hiatus for the greater petrosal nerve, passes out of the skull through the foramen ovale, and ends in the otic ganglion. Postganglionic fibres arising in the ganglion supply the parotid gland through the auriculotemporal nerve (*see* Table A.2 in Appendix).

### External Petrosal Nerve

It is sympathetic in nature. It is an inconstant branch from the sympathetic plexus around the middle meningeal artery to the geniculate ganglion of the facial nerve.

*Note: Internal carotid artery* begins in the neck as one of the terminal branches of the common carotid artery at the level of the upper border of the thyroid cartilage. Its course is divided into the four parts: Cervical, petrous, cavernous and cerebral (*see* Chapter 8 for details).

*Fourth part of the vertebral artery* enters the posterior cranial fossa through the foramen magnum after piercing the dura mater near the skull. It has been studied in Chapter 9.

VIDEO

**Video 3.12 Cranial Cavity:** Introduction, Dura mater, venous sinuses, cavernous sinus.

### *Facts to Remember*

- Meningeal layer of dura mater forms falx cerebri and falx cerebelli in sagittal plane and tentorium cerebelli and diaphragma sellae in horizontal plane.
- Only spinal ganglia present in the cranial cavity is the trigeminal ganglion.
- Only mixed branch of trigeminal is the mandibular branch. The other two are purely sensory.
- Anterior branch of middle meningeal artery lies on the inner aspect of *pterion* and is liable to injury, leading to extradural haemorrhage.
- Trigeminal ganglion lies in Meckel's cave – formed by meningeal layer of dura mater.
- Rathke's pouch give rise to adenohypophysis.
- Herring bodies are located in neurohypophysis and they are the nerve terminals of hypothalamo-hypophyseal tracts containing vasopressin and antidiuretic hormones.

### BDC's Anatomy *e*-book

1. Molecular regulation of development of pituitary gland
2. Trigeminal nerve
3. Further reading
4. Viva voce questions

Chapter

# 13

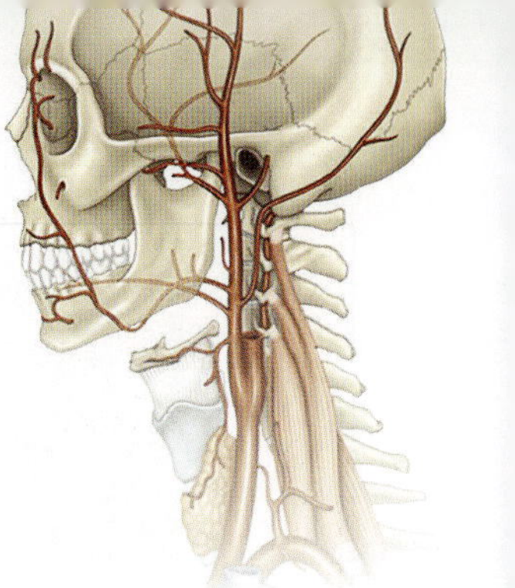

# Contents of the Orbit

## BONY ORBITS

These are pyramidal bony cavities, situated one on each side of the root of the nose. They provide sockets for rotatory movements of the eyeballs. They also protect the eyeballs (Figs 13.1 and 13.2, Plate 13.1).

The long or ***orbital axis*** of the orbit passes backwards and medially. The medial walls of the two orbits are parallel and the lateral walls are set at right angles to each other (Fig. 13.1). The axis passing through centres of anterior and posterior poles of the eyeball is known as ***visual axis***. It makes an angle of 20–25° with the orbital axis.

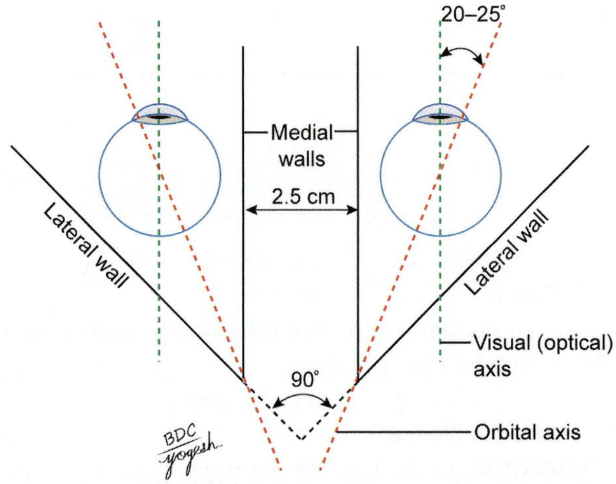


**Fig. 13.1:** Visual and orbital axes

### BOUNDARIES OF BONY ORBIT

Each orbit resembles a four-sided pyramid. Thus, it has (Plate 13.1, Fig. 13.2):

1. *Apex* – situated at the posterior end of orbit at the medial end of superior orbital fissure.
2. *Base* – seen as the orbital opening on the face.
3. *Four walls*: Roof, floor, lateral and medial walls.

#### Roof

It is concave from side-to-side. It is formed:

1. Mainly by the orbital plate of the frontal bone.
2. It is completed posteriorly by the lesser wing of the sphenoid.

##### Features

1. ***Lacrimal fossa***, placed anterolaterally, lodges the lacrimal gland.
2. ***Optic canal*** lies posteriorly, at the junction of the roof and medial wall.
3. ***Trochlear fossa*** lies anteromedially. It provides attachment to the fibrous pulley or trochlea for the tendon of the *superior oblique muscle.*

#### Lateral Wall

This is the thickest and strongest of all the walls of the orbit. It is formed:

1. By the anterior surface of the greater wing of the sphenoid bone, posteriorly.
2. By the orbital surface of the frontal process of the zygomatic bone, anteriorly.

##### Features

1. ***Superior orbital fissure*** occupies the posterior part of the junction between the roof and lateral wall.
2. ***Foramen for the zygomatic nerve*** is seen in the zygomatic bone.
3. ***Whitnall's* or *zygomatic tubercle*** is a palpable elevation on the zygomatic bone just within the orbital margin. It provides attachment to the lateral check ligament of eyeball.

#### Floor

It slopes upwards and medially to join the medial wall. It is formed:

1. Mainly by the orbital surface of the maxilla.
2. By the lower part of the orbital surface of the zygomatic bone, anterolaterally.
3. Orbital process of the palatine bone, at the posterior angle.

##### Features

1. ***Inferior orbital fissure*** occupies the posterior part of the junction between the lateral wall and floor. Through this fissure, the orbit communicates with

**Plate 13.1:** Bony orbit

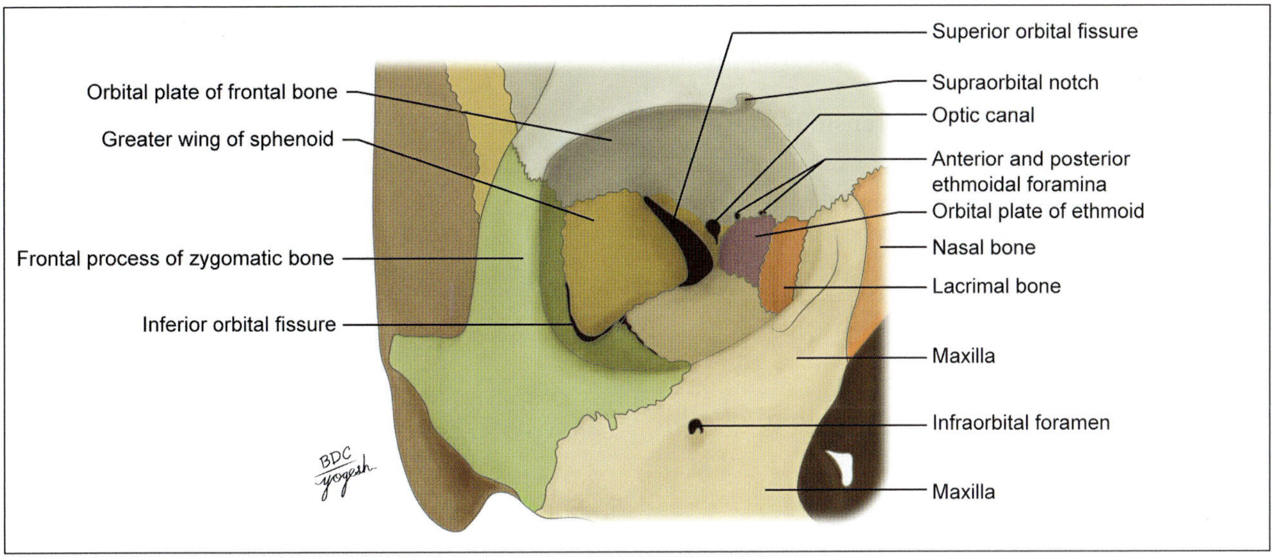


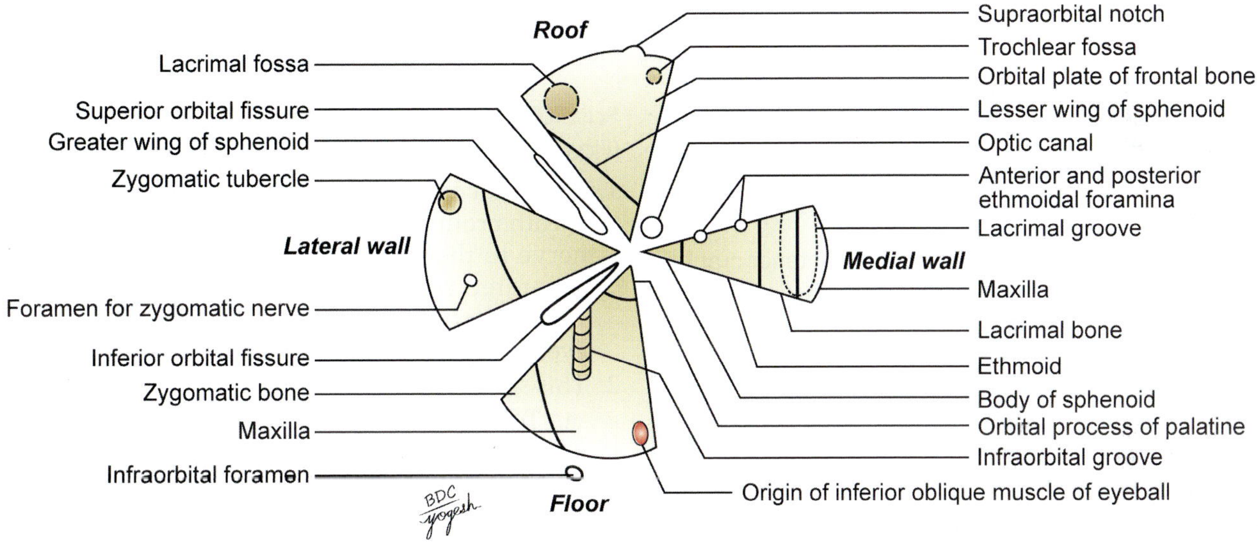


**Fig. 13.2:** Features of bony orbit. The four walls of the pyramidal cavity have been separated to show their details

the infratemporal fossa anteriorly and with the pterygopalatine fossa posteriorly.

2. ***Infraorbital groove*** runs forwards in relation to the floor.
3. A small depression on anteromedial part of the floor gives origin to *inferior oblique muscle.*

## Medial Wall

It is very thin. From before backwards, it is formed by:

1. Frontal process of the maxilla
2. Lacrimal bone
3. Orbital plate of the ethmoid
4. Body of the sphenoid bone.

### Features

1. The ***lacrimal groove*** lies anteriorly on the medial wall. It is bounded anteriorly by the anterior lacrimal crest of the frontal process of the maxilla, and posteriorly by posterior lacrimal crest of the lacrimal bone. The floor of the groove is formed by the maxilla in front and by the lacrimal bone behind. The groove lodges the lacrimal sac which lies deep to the lacrimal fascia bridging the lacrimal groove. The groove leads inferiorly, through the nasolacrimal duct, to the inferior meatus of the nose.
2. ***Anterior and posterior ethmoidal foramina*** lie on the frontoethmoidal suture, at the junction of the roof and medial wall.

## Foramina in Relation to the Orbit

1. *Inferior orbital fissure* transmits:
   a. *Zygomatic nerve,*
   b. *Orbital branches of the pterygopalatine ganglion,*
   c. *Infraorbital nerve and vessels,* and the communication between the inferior ophthalmic vein and the pterygoid plexus of veins.

2. *Infraorbital groove and canal* transmit the corresponding nerve and vessels.
3. *Zygomatic foramen* transmits the zygomatic nerve.
4. *Anterior ethmoidal foramen* transmits the corresponding nerve and vessels.
5. *Posterior ethmoidal foramen* only transmits vessels of same name.

*Note*: The structures passing through the optic canal and through the superior orbital fissure have been described in cranial fossae.

## CONTENTS OF ORBITS

### Contents

1. *Eyeball:* Eyeball occupies anterior one-third of orbit (For details, *see* Chapter 19).
2. *Fascia:* Orbital and bulbar.
3. *Muscles:* Extraocular and intraocular.
4. *Vessels:* Ophthalmic artery, superior and inferior ophthalmic veins, and lymphatics.
5. *Nerves:* Optic, oculomotor, trochlear and abducent; branches of ophthalmic and maxillary nerves, and sympathetic nerves.
6. *Lacrimal gland* (For details, *see* Chapter 2).
7. *Orbital fat.*

### DISSECTION

Strip the endosteum from the floor of the anterior cranial fossa. Gently break the orbital plate of frontal bone forming the roof of the orbit and remove it in pieces so that orbital periosteum is clearly visible. Medially, the ethmoidal vessels and nerves should be preserved. Posteriorly, identify the optic canal and superior orbital fissure and structures traversing these. Define the orbital fascia and fascial sheath of eyeball.

Divide the orbital periosteum along the middle of the orbit anteroposteriorly. Cut through it horizontally close to anterior margin of orbit.

### Orbital Fascia or Periorbita

It forms the *periosteum* of the bony orbit (Fig. 13.3).

#### Features

1. Due to the loose connection to bone, it can be easily stripped. Posteriorly, it is continuous with the dura mater and with the sheath of the optic nerve. Anteriorly, it is continuous with the periosteum lining the bones around the orbital margin.
2. There is a gap in the periorbita over the inferior orbital fissure. This gap is bridged by connective tissue with some smooth muscle fibres in it. These fibres constitute the ***orbitalis muscle***.
3. At the upper and lower margins of the orbit, the orbital fascia sends off flap-like continuations into the eyelids. These extensions form the ***orbital septum***.
4. A process of the fascia holds the fibrous ***pulley*** of the tendon of the superior oblique muscle in place.

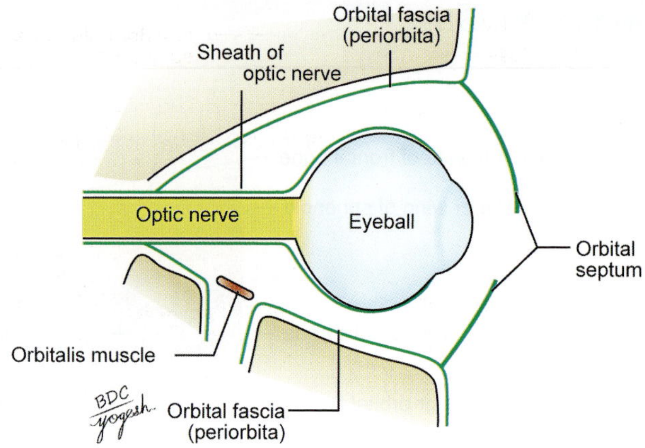


**Fig. 13.3:** Orbital fascia and fascial sheath of the eyeball as seen in a parasagittal section

5. Another process forms the ***lacrimal fascia*** which bridges the lacrimal groove.

*Note*: ***Orbitalis muscle*** is a smooth muscle that bridges the inferior orbital fissure. It is considered a rudimentary muscle. It is fused with the orbital fascia. It receives sympathetic innervation, and its function is not known.

### Fascial Sheath of Eyeball or Bulbar Fascia

(Figs 13.4 and 13.5)

1. ***Tenon's capsule*** forms a thin, loose membranous sheath around the eyeball, extending from the optic nerve to the sclerocorneal junction or limbus. It is separated from the sclera by the episcleral space which is traversed by delicate fibrous bands. The eyeball can freely move within this sheath.
2. This *sheath* is pierced by:
   a. Tendons of the various extraocular muscles.
   b. Ciliary vessels and nerves around the entrance of the optic nerve.
3. This sheath gives off a number of expansions.
   a. *Tubular sheath* covers each orbital muscle.

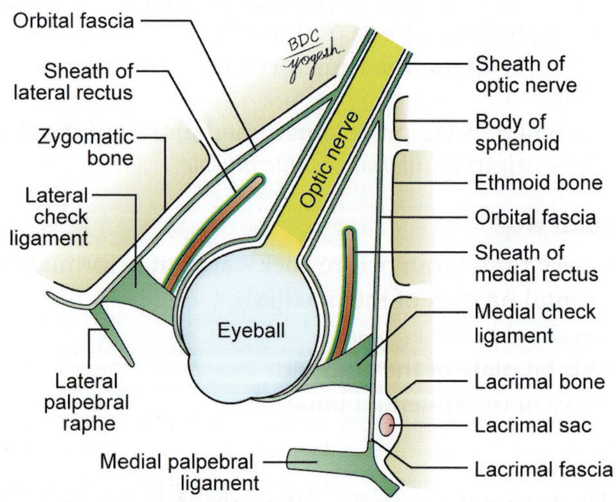


**Fig. 13.4:** Orbital fascia and fascial sheath of the eyeball as seen in the transverse section

Head and Neck 13

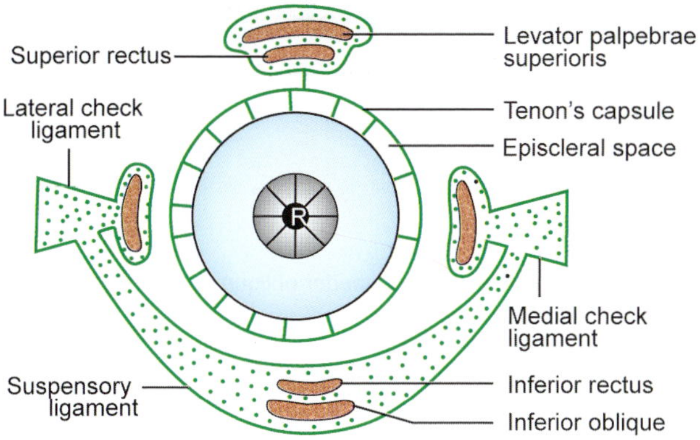


**Fig. 13.5:** Fascial sheath of the eyeball as seen in coronal section

b. ***Medial check ligament*** is a strong triangular expansion from the sheath of the medial rectus muscle; it is attached to the lacrimal bone.

c. ***Lateral check ligament*** is a strong triangular expansion from the sheath of the lateral rectus muscle; it is attached to the zygomatic bone (Fig. 13.4).

4. ***Suspensory ligament of Lockwood:*** The lower part of Tenon's capsule is thickened, and is named the *suspensory ligament of the eye* or the *suspensory ligament of Lockwood* (Fig. 13.5). It is expanded in the centre and narrow at its extremities, and is slung like a hammock below the eyeball. It is formed by union of the margins of the sheaths of the inferior rectus and the inferior oblique muscles with the medial and lateral check ligaments.

**DISSECTION**

Identify and preserve the trochlear nerve entering the superior oblique muscle in the superomedial angle of the orbit. Find the frontal nerve lying in the midline on the levator palpebrae superioris. It divides into two terminal divisions in the anterior part of orbit.

Beneath the levator palpebrae superioris is the superior rectus muscle. The upper division of oculomotor nerve lies between these two muscles. Along the lateral wall of the orbit, look for lacrimal nerve and artery to reach the superolateral corner of the orbit.

Follow the tendon of superior oblique muscle passing superolaterally beneath the superior rectus to be inserted into sclera behind the equator. After identification, divide frontal nerve, levator palpebrae superioris and superior rectus in the middle of the orbit and reflect them apart. Identify the optic nerve and other structures crossing it. These are nasociliary nerve, ophthalmic artery and superior ophthalmic vein. With the optic nerve find two long ciliary nerves and 12–20 short ciliary nerves. Remove the orbital fat and look carefully in the posterior part of the interval between the optic nerve and lateral rectus muscle along the lateral wall of the orbit and identify the pinhead-sized ciliary ganglion. Trace the roots connecting it to the nasociliary nerve and nerve to inferior oblique muscle.

Lastly, identify the abducent nerve closely adherent to the medial surface of lateral rectus muscle. Incise the inferior fornix of conjunctiva and palpebral fascia. Elevate the eyeball and remove the fat and fascia to identify the origin of inferior oblique muscle from the floor of the orbit anteriorly.

Identify the levator palpebrae superioris and superior rectus above the eyeball, superior oblique superomedially, medial rectus medially, lateral rectus laterally, and inferior rectus inferiorly.

The voluntary muscles are miniature ribbon muscles, having short tendons of origin and long tendons of insertion.

*Competency:*

**AN31.1** Describe and identify extraocular muscles of eyeball, along with a note on its attachment, action and clinical anatomy.

## EXTRAOCULAR MUSCLES

The extraocular muscles of the eyeball are classified into two groups: Involuntary and voluntary (Plate 13.2, Flowchart 13.1).

### Involuntary Muscles

1. ***Superior tarsal muscle*** is the deeper portion of the levator palpebrae superioris. It is inserted on the upper margin of the superior tarsus. It elevates the upper eyelid.
2. ***Inferior tarsal muscle*** extends from the fascial sheath of the inferior rectus and inferior oblique to the lower margin of the inferior tarsus. It possibly depresses the lower eyelid.
3. ***Orbitalis*** bridges the inferior orbital fissure. Its action is uncertain.

### *Nerve Supply*

Involuntary muscles of the eye are supplied by postganglionic sympathetic fibres from superior cervical ganglion.

### Voluntary Extraocular Muscles

1. Four recti:
   a. Superior rectus
   b. Inferior rectus
   c. Medial rectus
   d. Lateral rectus
2. Two obliques:
   a. Superior oblique
   b. Inferior oblique
3. Levator palpebrae superioris.

### *Recti Muscles*

#### *Origin*

1. All recti arise from a *common annular tendon* or ***tendinous ring* of Zinn**. The ring is attached to the middle part of superior orbital fissure and around optic canal (Fig. 13.6).

**Plate 13.2:** Extraocular muscles (right lateral view, parasagittal section, lateral wall of orbit is removed to visualize its interior)

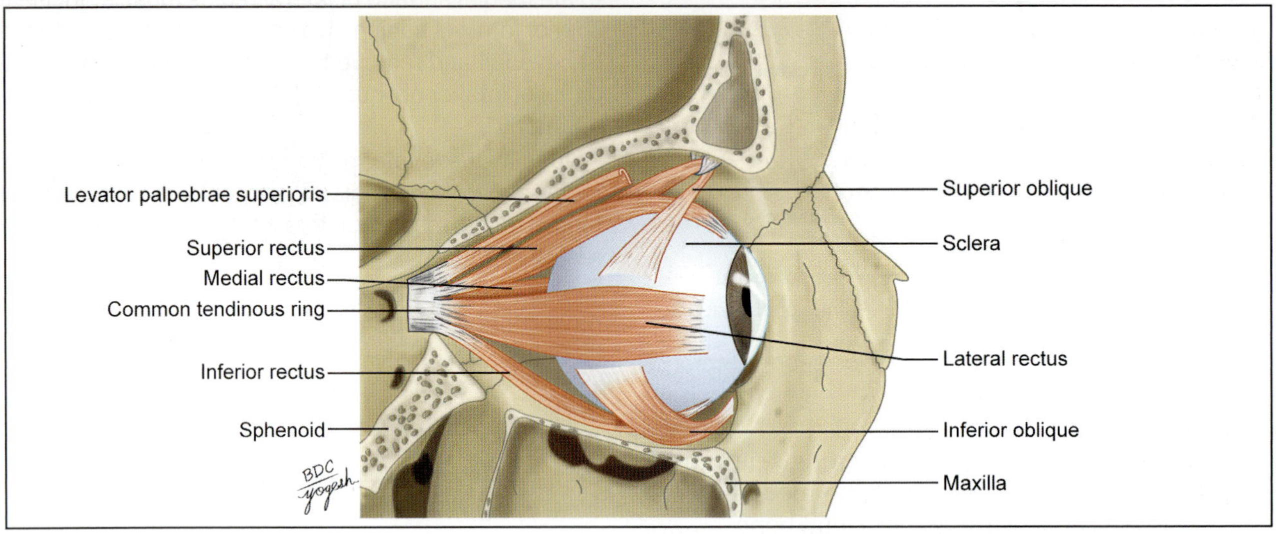


**Flowchart 13.1:** Extraocular voluntary muscles

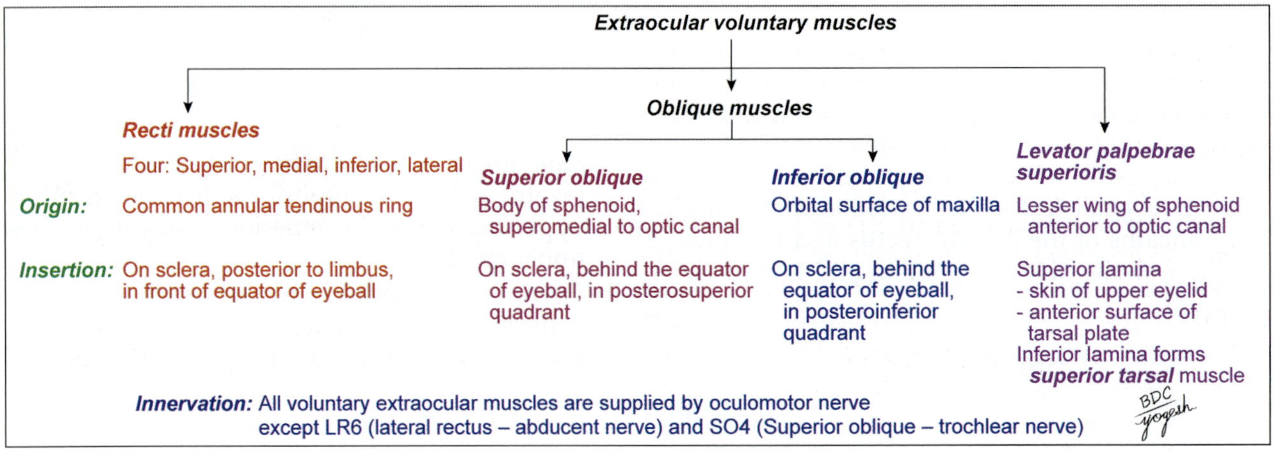


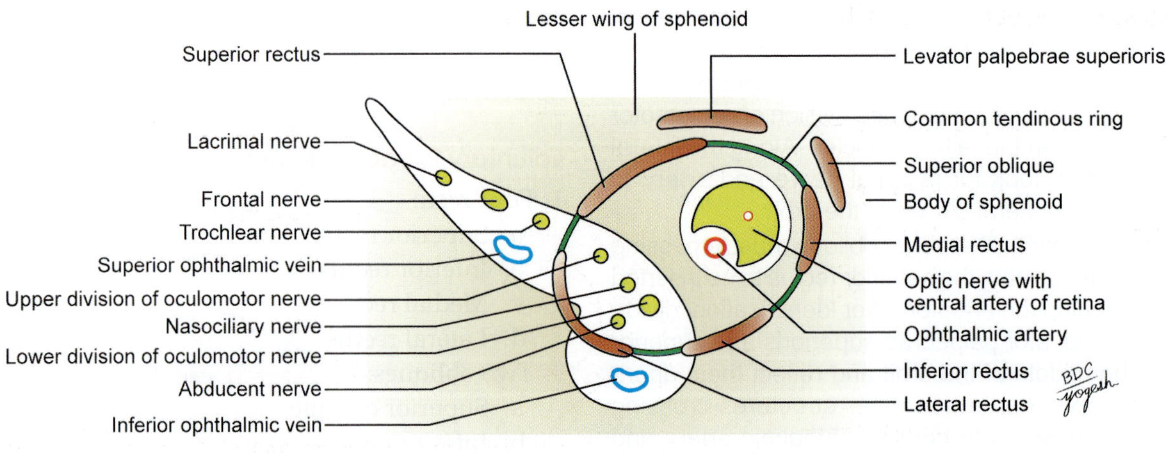


**Fig. 13.6:** Apical part of the orbit showing the origin of the extraocular muscles, the common tendinous ring and the structures passing through superior orbital fissure (seen from front)

2. The lateral rectus has an additional small tendinous head which arises from the orbital surface of the greater wing of the sphenoid bone lateral to the tendinous ring. Through the gap between the two heads abducent nerve passes.

***Insertion:*** The recti are inserted into the sclera, a little posterior to the limbus (corneoscleral junction). The average distances of the insertions from the cornea are: Superior 7.7 mm; inferior 6.5 mm, medial 5.5 mm; lateral 6.9 mm (Fig. 13.7).

### Oblique Muscles

#### Origin

1. The superior oblique arises from the undersurface of lesser wing of the sphenoid, superomedial to the optic canal (Fig. 13.6).
2. The inferior oblique arises from the orbital surface of the maxilla, lateral to the lacrimal groove. The muscle is situated near the anterior margin of the orbit.

#### Insertion (Fig. 13.8)

1. The tendon of the superior oblique passes through a fibrocartilaginous pulley attached to the trochlear fossa of the frontal bone. The tendon then passes laterally, downwards and backward below the superior rectus. It is inserted into the sclera behind the equator of the eyeball in posterolateral quadrant.
2. The inferior oblique is fleshy throughout. It passes laterally, upwards and backwards below the inferior rectus and then deep to the lateral rectus. The inferior oblique is inserted close to the superior oblique a little below and posterior to the latter.

### Levator Palpebrae Superioris

***Origin:*** The levator palpebrae superioris arises from the orbital surface of the lesser wing of the sphenoid bone, anterosuperior to the optic canal and to the origin of the superior rectus (Plate 13.2, Fig. 13.6).

***Insertion:*** The flat tendon of the levator splits into a superior or voluntary and an inferior or involuntary lamellae. Superior lamella of the levator is inserted into the anterior surface of the superior tarsus, and into the skin of the upper eyelid. The inferior lamella (smooth part) is inserted into the upper margin of the superior tarsus and into superior conjunctival fornix.

### Nerve Supply

1. The superior oblique is supplied by the IV cranial or trochlear nerve (SO4) (Fig. 13.9).

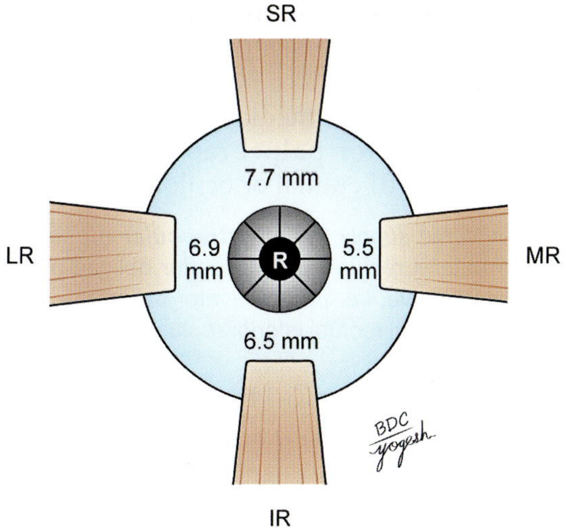


**Fig. 13.7:** Insertion of recti muscles

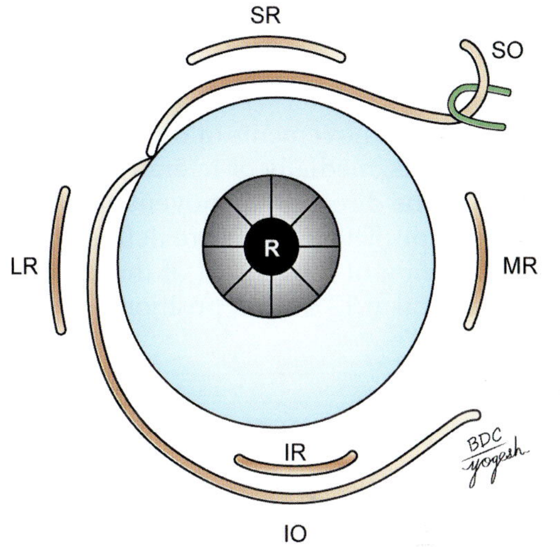


**Fig. 13.8:** Scheme to show the insertion of the oblique muscles of the eyeball

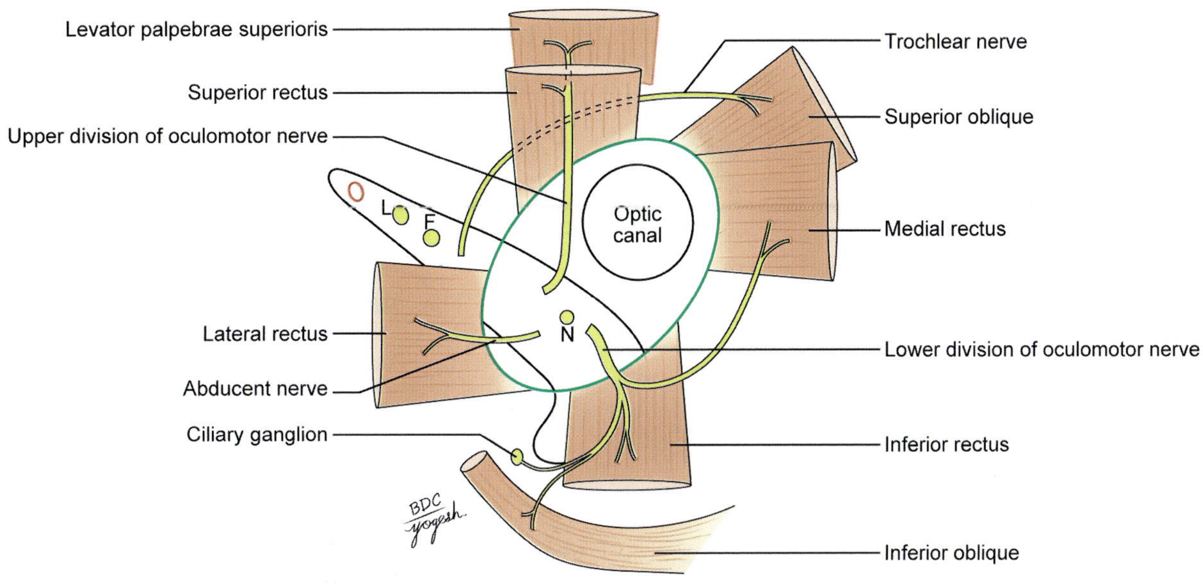


**Fig. 13.9:** Scheme showing the nerve supply of the extraocular muscles

2. The lateral rectus is supplied by the VI cranial or abducent nerve (LR6).
3. The remaining four and a half extraocular muscles; superior, inferior and medial recti; inferior oblique; and part of levator palpebrae superioris are all supplied by the III cranial or oculomotor nerve.

[*Mnemonics: Nerve supply of the* ***extraocular muscles: "LR6 SO4 rest 3"*** Lateral rectus by **VI**; **S**uperior **o**blique by **IV**; **Rest** are by **III** cranial nerve, i.e. part of levator palpebrae superioris, superior rectus, medial rectus, inferior rectus and inferior oblique]

### *Actions* (Figs 13.10 and 13.11)

1. ***Movements of the eyeball***
   a. *Around a transverse axis:*
      - Upward rotation or elevation (33°)
      - Downwards rotation or depression (33°)
   
   b. *Around a vertical axis:*
      - Medial rotation or adduction (50°)
      - Lateral rotation or abduction (50°)
   
   c. *Around an anteroposterior axis:*
      - Intorsion
      - Extorsion
   
   The rotatory movements of the eyeball upwards, downwards, medially or laterally, are defined in terms of the direction of movement of the centre of the pupil. The torsions are defined in terms of the direction of movement of the upper margin of the pupil at 12 o'clock position.

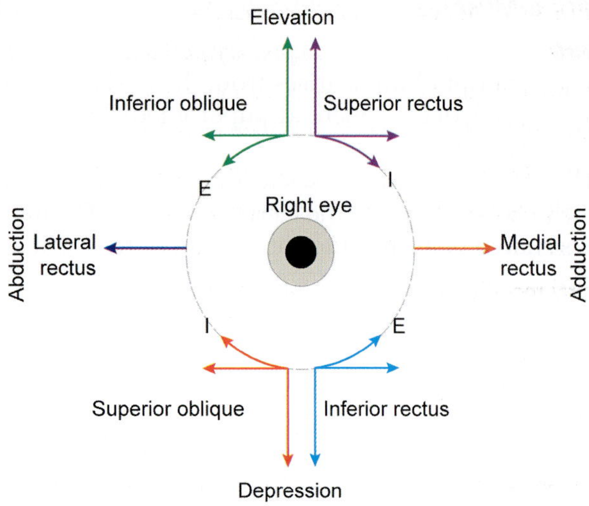


**Fig. 13.10:** Actions of extraocular muscles (I: Intorsion, E: Extorsion)

2. ***Actions of individual muscles*** are shown in Table 13.1.
3. ***Single*** **or** ***pure movements*** are produced by combined actions of muscles. Similar actions get added together, while opposing actions cancel each other enabling pure movements (Table 13.2).
4. ***Combined movements of the eyes:*** The movements given above can take place in various combinations. Normally, movements of the two eyes are harmoniously coordinated. Such coordinated movements of both eyes are called ***conjugate ocular movements***.

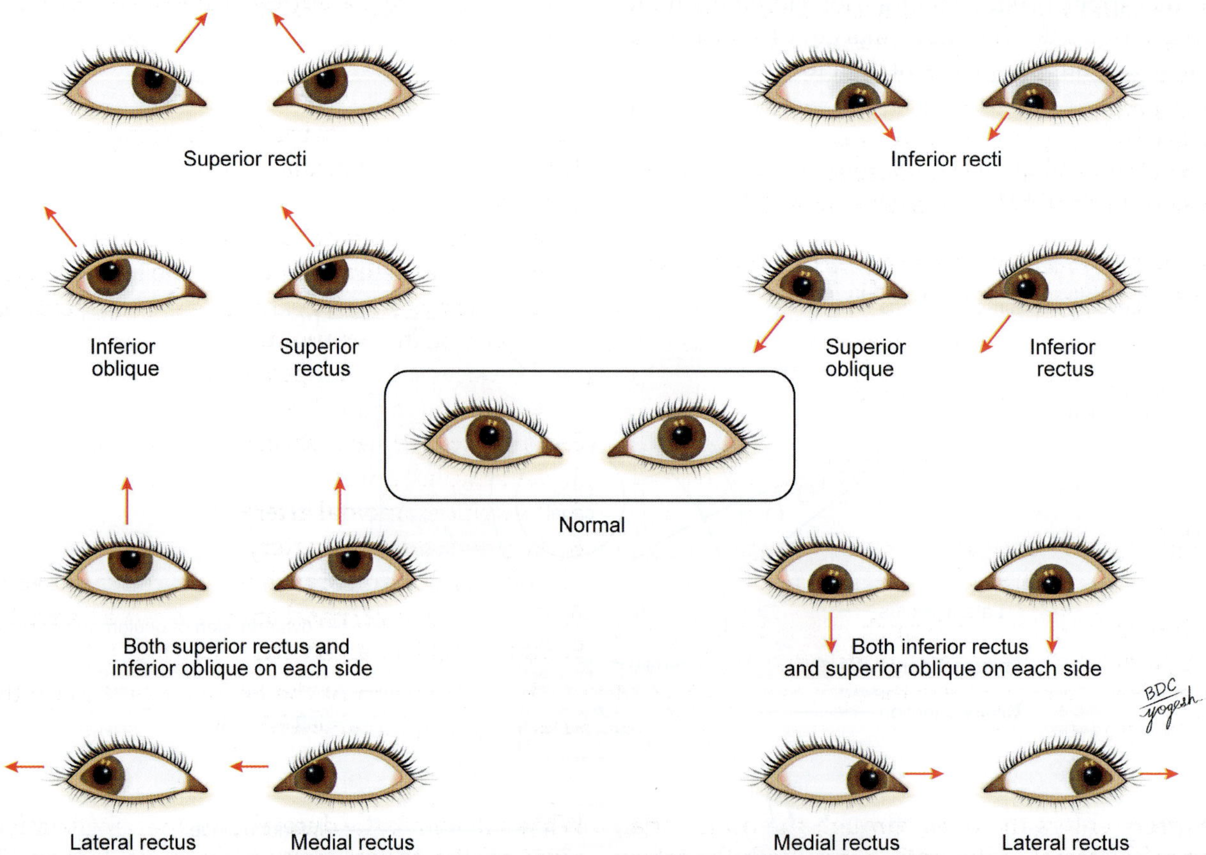


**Fig. 13.11:** Muscles for conjugate movements of the eyes

**TABLE 13.1: Actions of individual muscles**

| *Muscle* | *In primary position* |
|---|---|
| Superior oblique (SO) | Depression, abduction, intorsion |
| Inferior oblique (IO) | Elevation, abduction, extorsion |
| Inferior rectus (IR) | Depression, adduction, extorsion |
| Superior rectus (SR) | Elevation, adduction, intorsion |
| Medial rectus (MR) | Only adduction |
| Lateral rectus (LR) | Only abduction |

**TABLE 13.2: Single *or* pure movements of the eyeball**

| *Movement of eyeball* | *Muscles* |
|---|---|
| Upward rotation or elevation | Superior rectus, inferior oblique |
| Downward rotation or depression | Inferior rectus, superior oblique |
| Medial rotation or adduction | Medial rectus, superior rectus, inferior rectus |
| Lateral rotation or abduction | Lateral rectus, superior oblique, inferior oblique |
| Intorsion | Superior oblique, superior rectus |
| Extorsion | Inferior oblique, inferior rectus |

## CLINICAL ANATOMY

- Weakness or paralysis of a muscle causes ***squint*** or ***strabismus***, which may be concomitant or paralytic. Concomitant squint is congenital; there is no limitation of movement, and no diplopia (Fig. 13.12).
- In ***paralytic squint***, movements are limited, diplopia and vertigo are present, head is turned in the direction of the function of paralysed muscle, and there is a false orientation of the field of vision.
- ***Nystagmus*** is characterized by involuntary, rhythmical oscillatory movements of the eyes. This is due to incoordination of the ocular muscles. It may be either vestibular or cerebellar, or even congenital.

*Note*: Terms medial squint or internal strabismus and lateral squint or external strabismus are currently not in use.

*Competency:*

**AN31.2** Describe and demonstrate vessels in the orbit.

## VESSELS OF THE ORBIT

### OPHTHALMIC ARTERY

#### Origin

The ophthalmic artery is a branch of the cerebral part of the internal carotid artery, given off medial to the anterior clinoid process close to the optic canal (Figs 13.13 and 13.14, Flowchart 13.2).

#### Course and Relations

1. The artery enters the orbit through the optic canal, lying inferolateral to the optic nerve. Both the artery and nerve lie in a common dural sheath.

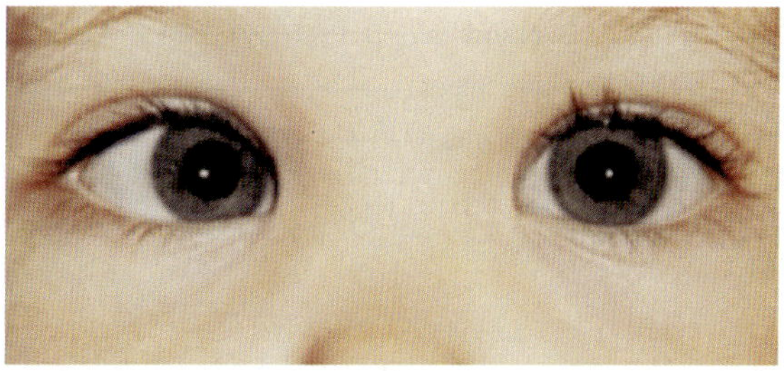

**Fig. 13.12:** Medial squint of the right eye

**Flowchart 13.2:** Ophthalmic artery

***Ophthalmic artery***
Main artery of eyeball

- ***Beginning***: Branch of internal carotid artery; Enters orbit through optic canal
- ***Termination***: Supratrochlear; Dorsal nasal branch
- ***Branches***: Central artery of retina; Lacrimal artery; Posterior ciliary artery: Long, short; Supraorbital artery; Posterior ethmoidal artery; Anterior ethmoidal artery; Medial palpebral branches; Dorsal (external) nasal artery; Supratrochlear artery

2. In the orbit, the artery pierces the dura mater, ascends over the lateral side of the optic nerve, and crosses above the nerve from lateral to medial side along with the nasociliary nerve. It then runs forwards along the medial wall of the orbit between the superior oblique and the medial rectus muscles and parallel to the nasociliary nerve.
3. It terminates near the medial angle of the eye by dividing into the supratrochlear and dorsal nasal branches.

#### Branches

The ophthalmic artery has the following branches:

1. Central artery of retina
2. Lacrimal artery
   a. Glandular branches to lacrimal gland
   b. Two palpebral branches – one for each eyelid
   c. Two zygomatic branches – zygomaticofacial and zygomaticotemporal
   d. Recurrent meningeal branches
   e. Muscular branches.
3. Posterior (long and short) ciliary arteries
4. Supraorbital artery
5. Posterior ethmoidal artery
6. Anterior ethmoidal artery
7. Medial palpebral branches – one for each eyelid
8. Dorsal (external) nasal artery (terminal branch)
9. Supratrochlear artery (terminal branch).

The distribution of the branches of the ophthalmic artery is given in Table 13.3.

#### *Central Artery of Retina*

While still within the dural sheath, the ophthalmic artery gives off the *central artery of the retina*. Figure 13.10 is the first and most important branch of the ophthalmic

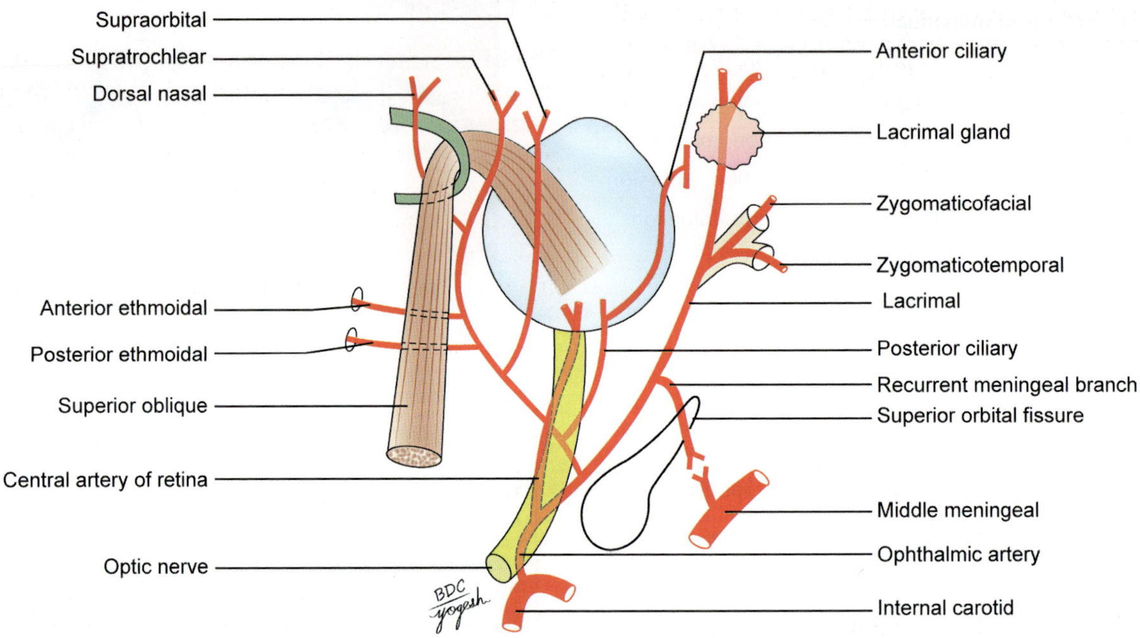


**Fig. 13.13:** Arteries of the eyeball

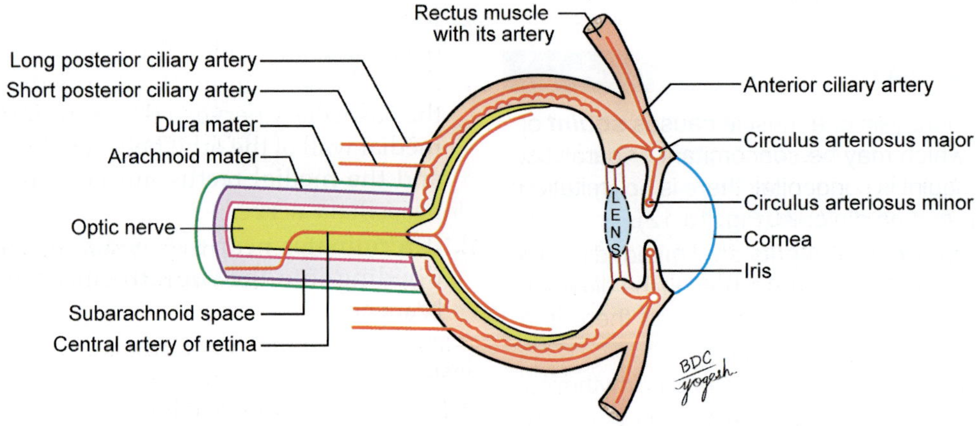


**Fig. 13.14:** Branches of ophthalmic artery

**TABLE 13.3: Branches of the ophthalmic artery**

| ***Branches*** | ***Course and distribution*** |
|---|---|
| **Central artery of retina** | Supply the retina |
| **Lacrimal artery** | |
| Glandular branches | Lacrimal gland |
| Two palpebral branches | One for each eyelid |
| Two zygomatic branches | Enter canals in the zygomatic bone. One branch appears on the face through the zygomaticofacial foramen. The other appears on the temporal surface of the bone through the zygomaticotemporal foramen |
| Recurrent meningeal branches | Runs backwards to enter the middle cranial fossa through the superior orbital fissure |
| Muscular branches | Muscles of the orbit |
| **Branches arising from the main trunk** | |
| Posterior (long and short) ciliary arteries | Supply chiefly the choroid and iris |
| Supraorbital and supratrochlear branches | Supply the skin of the forehead |
| Anterior and posterior ethmoidal branches | Enter foramina in the medial wall of the orbit to supply the ethmoidal air sinuses. They then enter the anterior cranial fossa. The terminal branches of the anterior ethmoidal artery enter the nose and supply part of it. |
| Medial palpebral branches | Supply the eyelids |
| Dorsal nasal branch | Supplies the upper part of the nose |

artery. It first lies below the optic nerve. It pierces the dural sheath of the nerve and runs forwards for a short distance between these two. It then enters the substance of the nerve and runs forwards in its centre to reach the optic disc (Fig. 13.9). Here it divides into branches that supply the retina (*see* Fig. 19.6).

### CLINICAL ANATOMY

- The anterior ciliary arteries arise from the muscular branches of ophthalmic artery. The muscular arteries are important in this respect.
- The central artery of the retina is an ***end artery***. It does not have effective anastomoses with other arteries. Occlusion of the artery results in ***blindness***. The intraocular part of the artery can be seen, in the living, through an ***ophthalmoscope*** (*see* Fig. 19.12).

### DISSECTION

Trace the ophthalmic artery after it was seen to cross over the optic nerve along with nasociliary nerve and superior ophthalmic vein. Identify its branches especially the central artery of the retina which is an 'end artery'.

## OPHTHALMIC VEINS

***Superior ophthalmic vein:*** It accompanies the ophthalmic artery. It lies above the optic nerve. It receives tributaries corresponding to the branches of the artery, passes through the superior orbital fissure, and drains into the cavernous sinus. It communicates anteriorly with the supraorbital and angular veins.

***Inferior ophthalmic vein:*** It runs below the optic nerve. It receives tributaries from the lacrimal sac, the lower orbital muscles, and the eyelids, and ends either by joining the superior ophthalmic vein or drains directly into the cavernous sinus. It communicates with the pterygoid plexus of veins by small veins passing through the inferior orbital fissure.

### Lymphatics of the Orbit

The lymphatics drain into the preauricular parotid lymph nodes.

***Competency:***
**AN31.2** Describe and demonstrate nerves of the orbit.

## NERVES OF THE ORBIT

These are:

1. Optic (II)
2. Ciliary ganglion
3. Oculomotor (III) and trochlear (IV)
4. Abducent (VI)
5. Branches of ophthalmic (V1) and maxillary divisions (V2) of the trigeminal nerve
6. Sympathetic nerves.

## OPTIC NERVE

The optic nerve is the nerve of sight. It is made up of the axons of cells in the ganglionic layer of the retina. It emerges from the eyeball 3 or 4 mm nasal to its posterior pole. It runs backwards and medially and passes through the optic canal to enter the middle cranial fossa where it joins the optic chiasma.

The nerve is about 4 cm long, out of which 25 mm are intraorbital, 5 mm intracanalicular, and 10 mm intracranial. The entire nerve is enclosed in three meningeal sheaths. The subarachnoid space extends around the nerve up to the eyeball.

### Relations in the Orbit

1. At the apex of the orbit, the nerve is closely surrounded by the recti muscles. The ciliary ganglion lies between the optic nerve and the lateral rectus.
2. The central artery and vein of the retina pierce the optic nerve inferomedially about 1.25 cm behind the eyeball.
3. The optic nerve is crossed superiorly by the ophthalmic artery, the nasociliary nerve and the superior ophthalmic vein.
4. The optic nerve is crossed inferiorly by the nerve to the medial rectus.
5. Near the eyeball, the nerve is surrounded by fat containing the ciliary vessels and nerves.

### Structure

1. There are about 1.2 million myelinated fibres in each optic nerve, out of which about 53% cross in the optic chiasma.
2. The optic nerve is not a nerve in the strict sense as there is no neurolemmal sheath. It is actually a tract. It cannot regenerate, if it is cut. Developmentally, the optic nerve and the retina are a direct prolongation of the brain.

*Note*: Optic nerve has no neurilemmal sheath, and has no power of regeneration. It is a tract and not a nerve.

### CLINICAL ANATOMY

- The anastomoses between tributaries of facial vein and ophthalmic veins may result in spread of infection from the orbital and nasal regions to the cavernous sinus leading to its thrombosis.
- ***Optic neuritis*** is characterized by pain in and behind the eye on ocular movements and on pressure. The ***papilloedema*** is less but loss of vision is more. When the optic disc is normal as seen by an ophthalmoscope the same condition is called retrobulbar neuritis. The common causes are demyelinating diseases of the central nervous system, any septic focus in the teeth or paranasal sinuses, meningitis, encephalitis, syphilis, and even vitamin B deficiency.
- Optic atrophy may be caused by a variety of diseases. It may be primary or secondary.

## CILIARY GANGLION

The ciliary ganglion is a peripheral parasympathetic ganglion (Fig. 13.15, Flowchart 13.3).

*Size:* It is about 1–2 mm in diameter (about the size of pin's head).

### *Neuronal relationship*

*Topographic relation:* It is connected with the nasociliary nerve.

*Functional relation:* It is functionally related to the oculomotor nerve.

### *Location*

It is situated near the apex of the orbit between the optic nerve and the origin of the lateral rectus muscle. It hangs from the nasociliary nerve. The ganglion lies medial to the ophthalmic artery.

Roots (connections and distribution) (Fig. 13.16)

The ciliary ganglion has three roots:

1. *Parasympathetic* or *secretomotor root*: It consists of pre- and post-ganglionic fibres.
   a. *Preganglionic fibres* begin from the Edinger-Westphal nucleus located in the midbrain at the level of superior colliculus. These fibres pass through the oculomotor nerve and then they branch to the inferior oblique. These fibres relay in the *ciliary ganglion*.
   b. *Postganglionic fibres* from the cells of ciliary ganglion join the *short ciliary nerve* and supply the two intraocular muscles – *sphincter pupillae and ciliary muscles*.
2. *Sympathetic root*: The lateral horn cells of T1 segment of spinal cord give rise to preganglionic sympathetic fibres. They traverse to T1 nerve, sympathetic chain, and relay in superior cervical sympathetic ganglion. Postganglionic fibres pass along the plexus around the internal carotid and then ophthalmic artery. These fibres pass through the ciliary ganglion without relay and join the short ciliary nerves. They supply blood vessels of the eyeball and *dilator pupillae* muscle.
3. *Sensory root*: These are the fibres of *nasociliary nerve*. They pass through the ganglion without relay. They carry general sensation from the eyeball.

**Flowchart 13.3:** Ciliary ganglion

***Ciliary ganglion***
Size: 1–2 mm

- ***Neurological connection***
  - Topographic: Nasociliary nerve
  - Functional: Oculomotor nerve
- ***Location***
  - At the apex of orbit
  - Hangs from nasociliary nerve
- ***Surfaces***
  - ***Parasympathetic***: Edinger-Westphal nucleus in midbrain → III cranial nerve → inferior division → nerve to inferior oblique → relay in ciliary ganglion → short ciliary nerves → sphincter pupillae, ciliary muscles
  - ***Sympathetic***: Lateral horn cells of T1 → superior cervical ganglion → relay → plexus around ICA → plexus around ophthalmic artery → ciliary ganglion → short ciliary nerves → dilator pupillae
  - ***Sensory***: Fibres of nasociliary nerve

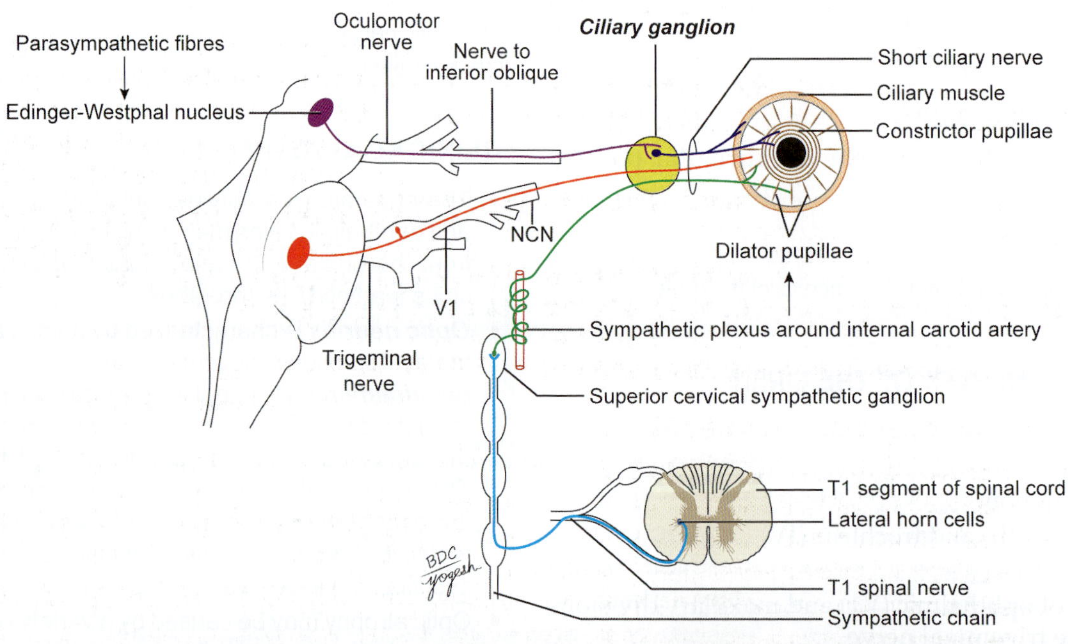


**Fig. 13.15:** Ciliary ganglion (V1: Ophthalmic nerve, NCN: Nasociliary nerve)

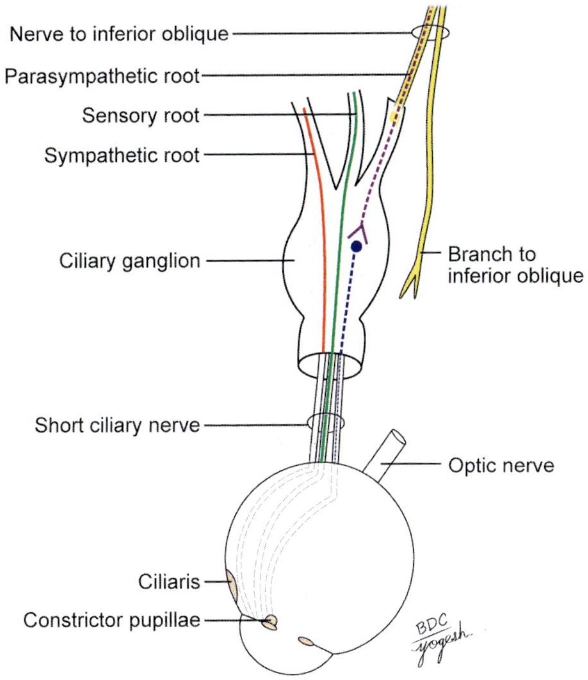


**Fig. 13.16:** Roots and branches of ciliary ganglion

### *Functions/branches*

The ciliary ganglion gives off 8–10 short ciliary nerves which divides into 15–20 branches. These small branches pierce the sclera around the entrance of the optic nerve. These fibres from ciliary ganglion perform the following functions:

1. Parasympathetic fibres – motor to sphincter pupillae and ciliary muscle.
2. Sympathetic fibres – vasomotor to vessels and motor to dilator pupillae muscle.
3. Sensory fibres carry general sensation from the eyeball.

***Ciliary nerve block:*** It produces dilatation of pupil before cataract surgery.

## OCULOMOTOR NERVE

Course of oculomotor (III) nerve is shown by Flowchart 13.4.

## TROCHLEAR NERVE

Course of trochlear (IV) nerve is shown by Flowchart 13.5 and Fig. 13.17.

## ABDUCENT NERVE

Course of abducent (VI) nerve is depicted by Flowchart 13.6, Figs 13.18 and 13.9 (details can be read from Chapter 6, *BD Chaurasia's Human Anatomy, Volume 4*).

## BRANCHES OF OPHTHALMIC DIVISION OF TRIGEMINAL NERVE

The ophthalmic (V1) is the smallest branch of trigeminal nerve (others are maxillary and mandibular nerves) (Flowchart 13.7).

**Flowchart 13.4:** Oculomotor nerve—III nerve

***Nucleus at level of superior colliculus***
↓
Lies between midbrain and pons
↓
Passes through lateral wall of cavernous sinus
↓
Superior orbital fissure:
- Small upper branch
- Large lower branch

↓
In orbit

**Small upper branch supplies:**
- Half of levator palpebrae superioris
- Superior rectus

**Large lower branch supplies:**
- Medial rectus
- Inferior rectus
- Inferior oblique

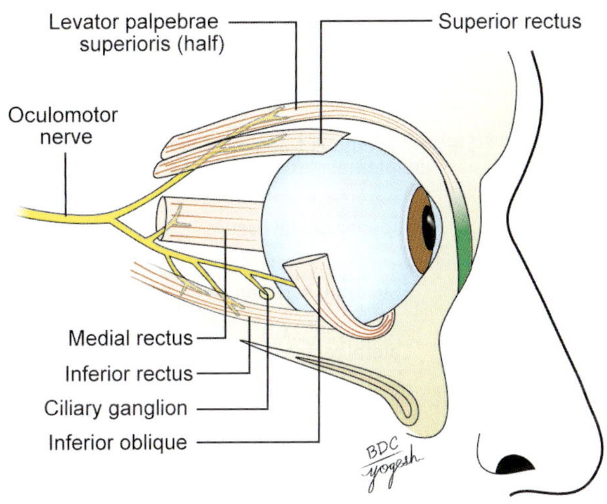


**Fig. 13.17:** Distribution of oculomotor nerve

**Flowchart 13.5:** Trochlear—IV nerve

***Nucleus at level of inferior colliculus***
↓
Courses around midbrain
↓
Lateral wall of cavernous sinus
↓
Superior orbital fissure
↓
In orbit
↓
Supplies superior oblique muscle

The ophthalmic nerve is purely sensory nerve. It arises from the anterolateral aspect of trigeminal ganglion in the middle cranial fossa. Then the nerve enters the lateral wall of the cavernous sinus and runs forward below the trochlear nerve and above the maxillary nerve. In the lateral wall of cavernous sinus, the ophthalmic nerve divides into three terminal branches: Lacrimal, frontal, and nasociliary (*mnemonic*: LFN). All the branches enter the orbit through the superior orbital fissure.

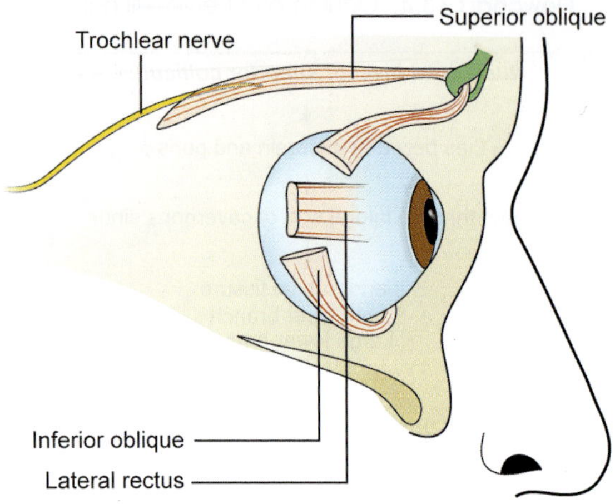


**Fig. 13.18:** Course of trochlear nerve

**Flowchart 13.6:** Abducent nerve—VI nerve

***Nucleus at level of lower pons (abducent nerve)***
↓
Dorello's canal
↓
Lies in cavernous sinus in relation to internal carotid artery
↓
Superior orbital fissure
↓
In orbit, supplies
↓
Lateral rectus muscle

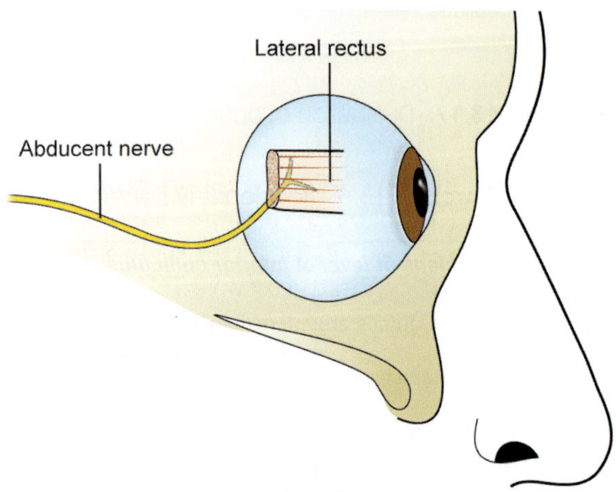


**Fig. 13.19:** Distribution of abducent nerve

## Branches

Following are the branches of ophthalmic division of trigeminal nerve (Figs 13.20a and b).

1. Frontal nerve:
   a. Supratrochlear
   b. Supraorbital.
2. Nasociliary nerve:
   a. Branch to ciliary ganglion
   b. 2–3 long ciliary nerves

**Flowchart 13.7:** Ophthalmic nerve (V1)

***Ophthalmic nerve (V1)***

***Origin, course***
- The smallest branch of V nerve
- Arises from trigeminal ganglion
- Traverses through lateral wall of cavernous sinus

***Branches***
All branches enter orbit through superior orbital fissure

- ***Frontal***: Supratrochlear; Supraorbital
- ***Nasociliary***: Branch to ciliary ganglion; 2–3 long ciliary nerves; Posterior ethmoidal; Intratrochlear; Anterior ethmoidal
- ***Lacrimal***: Branch to upper eyelid; Secretomotor fibres to the lacrimal gland

   c. Posterior ethmoidal
   d. Intratrochlear
   e. Anterior ethmoidal.
3. Lacrimal:
   a. Branch to upper eyelid
   b. Secretomotor fibres to the lacrimal gland.

## Lacrimal Nerve

This is the smallest of the three terminal branches of ophthalmic nerve (Fig. 13.15a). It enters the orbit through lateral part of superior orbital fissure and runs forwards along the upper border of lateral rectus muscle, in company with lacrimal artery. Anteriorly, it receives communication from zygomaticotemporal nerve, passes deep to the lacrimal gland, and ends in the lateral part of the upper eyelid.

The lacrimal nerve supplies the lacrimal gland, the conjunctiva and the upper eyelid. Its own fibres to the gland are sensory. The secretomotor fibres to the gland come from the greater petrosal nerve through its communication with the zygomaticotemporal nerve.

## Frontal Nerve

This is the largest of the three terminal branches of the ophthalmic nerve. It begins in the lateral wall of the anterior part of the cavernous sinus. It enters the orbit through the lateral part of the superior orbital fissure, and runs forwards on the superior surface of the levator palpebrae superioris. At the middle of the orbit, it divides into a small supratrochlear branch and a large supraorbital branch.

1. The ***supratrochlear nerve*** emerges from the orbit above the trochlea about one finger breadth from the median plane. It supplies the conjunctiva, the upper eyelid, and a small area of the skin of the forehead above the root of the nose.
2. The ***supraorbital nerve*** emerges from the orbit through the supraorbital notch or foramen about two fingers breadth from the median plane. It divides into medial and lateral branches which runs upwards over the forehead and scalp. It supplies the conjunctiva, the central part of the upper eyelid, the *frontal air sinus* and the skin of the forehead and scalp up to the vertex, or even up to the lambdoid suture.

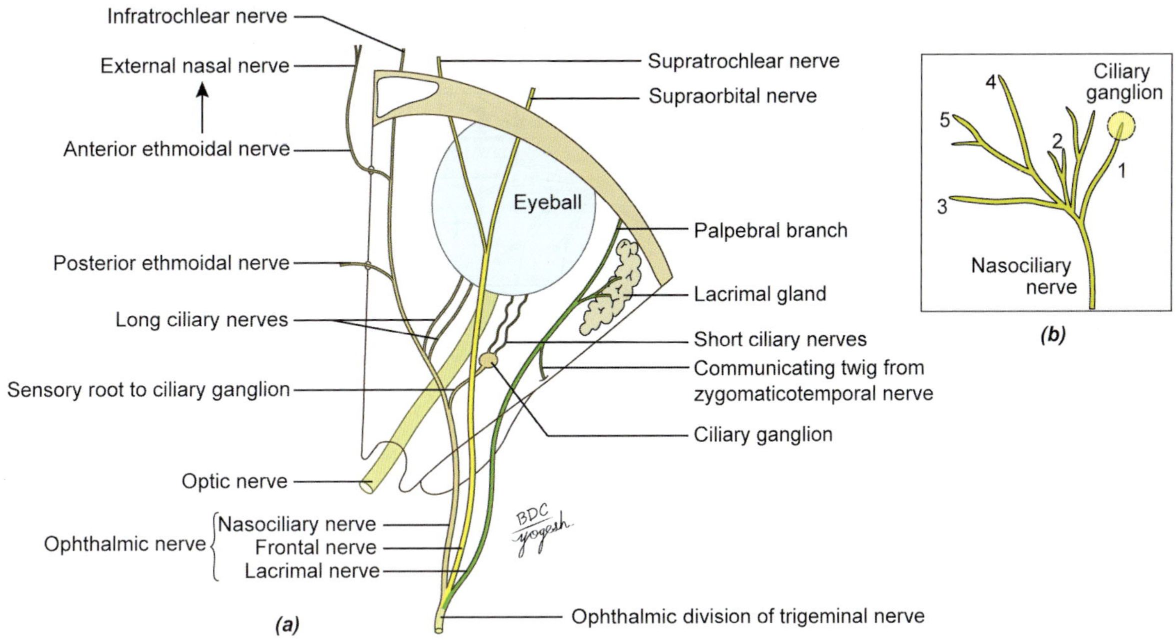


**Figs 13.20a and b:** (a) Branches of right ophthalmic nerve including III, IV, VI cranial nerves and the extraocular muscles and (b) branches of nasociliary: (1) Branch to ciliary ganglion; (2) Long ciliary; (3) Posterior ethmoidal; (4) Infratrochlear; (5) Anterior ethmoidal

### Nasociliary Nerve

This is one of the terminal branches of the ophthalmic division of the trigeminal nerve. It begins in the lateral wall of the anterior part of the cavernous sinus. It enters the orbit through the middle part of the superior orbital fissure between the two divisions of the oculomotor nerve. It crosses above the optic nerve from lateral to medial side along with ophthalmic artery and runs along the medial wall of the orbit between the superior oblique and the medial rectus. It ends at the anterior ethmoidal foramen by dividing into the infratrochlear and anterior ethmoidal nerves. Its branches are as follows:

1. A *communicating branch to the ciliary ganglion* forms the sensory root of the ganglion. It is often mixed with the sympathetic root.
2. Two or three ***long ciliary nerves*** run on the medial side of the optic nerve, pierce the sclera, and supply sensory nerves to the cornea, the iris and the ciliary body. They also carry sympathetic nerves to the dilator pupillae.
3. The ***posterior ethmoidal nerve*** passes through the posterior ethmoidal foramen and supplies the ethmoidal and sphenoidal air sinuses.
4. The ***infratrochlear nerve*** is the smaller terminal branch of the nasociliary nerve given off at the anterior ethmoidal foramen. It emerges from the orbit below the trochlea for the tendon of the superior oblique and appears on the face above the medial angle of the eye. It supplies the conjunctiva, the lacrimal sac and caruncle, the medial ends of the eyelids and the upper half of the external nose.
5. The ***anterior ethmoidal nerve*** is the larger terminal branch of the nasociliary nerve. It leaves the orbit by passing through the anterior ethmoidal foramen. It appears, for a very short distance, in the anterior cranial fossa, above the cribriform plate of the ethmoid bone. It then descends into the nose through a slit at the side of the anterior part of the crista galli. In the nasal cavity, it lies deep to the nasal bone. It gives off two ***internal nasal branches***—medial and lateral to the mucosa of the nose. Finally, it emerges at the lower border of the nasal bone as the ***external nasal nerve*** which supplies the skin of the lower half of the nose.

## SOME BRANCHES OF MAXILLARY DIVISION OF THE TRIGEMINAL NERVE

### Infraorbital Nerve (Fig. 13.21)

It is the continuation of the maxillary nerve. It enters the orbit through the *inferior orbital fissure*. It then runs forwards on the floor of the orbit or the roof of the maxillary sinus, at first in the *infraorbital groove* and then in the *infraorbital canal* remaining outside the periosteum of the orbit. It emerges on the face through the *infraorbital foramen* and terminates by dividing into palpebral, nasal and labial branches. The nerve is accompanied by the infraorbital branch of the third part of the maxillary artery and the accompanying vein.

### Branches

1. ***Middle superior alveolar nerve*** arises in the infraorbital groove, runs in the lateral wall of the maxillary sinus, and supplies the upper premolar teeth.
2. ***Anterior superior alveolar nerve*** arises in the infraorbital canal, and runs in a sinuous canal having a complicated course in the anterior wall of the maxillary sinus. It supplies the upper incisor and canine teeth, the maxillary sinus, and the anteroinferior part of the nasal cavity where it communicates with branches of anterior ethmoidal and anterior palatine nerves.

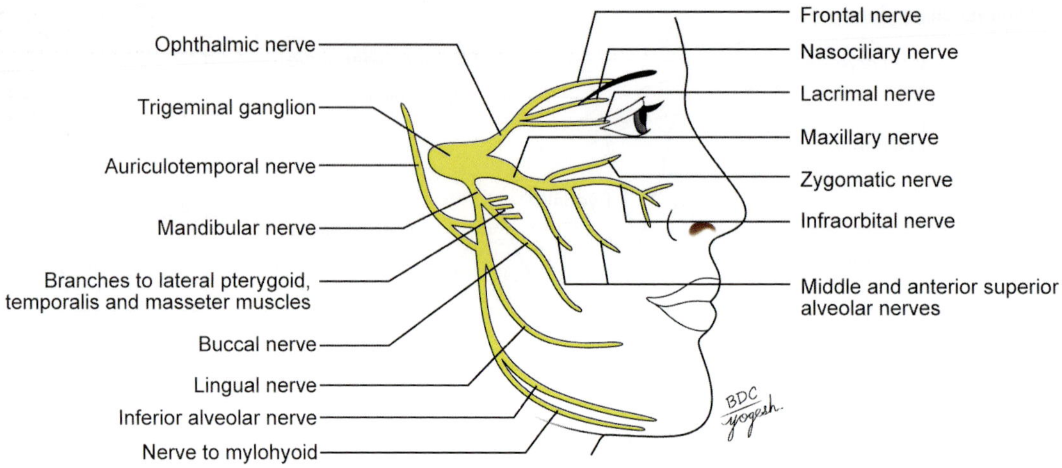


**Fig. 13.21:** Some branches of ophthalmic, maxillary and mandibular branches of trigeminal nerve

3. *Terminal branches*—***palpebral, nasal and labial***—supply a large area of skin on the face. They also supply the mucous membrane of the upper lip and cheek.

### Zygomatic Nerve

It is a branch of the maxillary nerve, given off in the pterygopalatine fossa. It enters the orbit through the lateral end of the inferior orbital fissure, and runs along the lateral wall, outside the periosteum, to enter the zygomatic bone. Just before or after entering the bone, it divides into its two terminal branches, the *zygomaticofacial* and *zygomaticotemporal nerves* which supply the skin of the face and of the anterior part of the temple. The communicating branch to the lacrimal nerve, which contains secretomotor fibres to the lacrimal gland, arises from the zygomaticotemporal nerve, and runs in the lateral wall of the orbit. Detailed description is given in *see* Chapter 15.

## SYMPATHETIC NERVES OF THE ORBIT

Sympathetic nerves arise from the internal carotid plexus and enter the orbit through the following sources.

1. The dilator pupillae of the iris is supplied by sympathetic nerves that pass through the ophthalmic nerve, the nasociliary nerve, and its long ciliary branches.
2. Other sympathetic nerves enter the orbit as follows:
   a. A plexus surrounds the ophthalmic artery.
   b. A direct branch from the internal carotid plexus passes through the superior orbital fissure and joins the ciliary ganglion.
   c. Other filaments pass along the oculomotor, trochlear, abducent, and ophthalmic nerves. All these sympathetic nerves are vasomotor in function.

VIDEO

Video 3.13 **Orbit**

### *Facts to Remember*

- Levator palpebrae superioris is partly supplied by III nerve and partly by sympathetic fibres.
- Central artery of retina is an end artery.
- Nerve supply of extraocular muscles is LR6, SO4, rest (levator palpebrae superioris, SR, MR, IR and IO) by III.
- Edinger-Westphal is the nucleus for the supply of ciliaris muscles and constrictor pupillae muscles. The fibres supply these muscles after relaying in the ciliary ganglion.
- Elevation and depression of the cornea occur around a transverse axis.
- Adduction and abduction of the cornea take place around a vertical axis.
- Intorsion and extorsion occur around an anteroposterior axis.

### BDC's Anatomy *e*-book

1. Actions of individual muscles according to their axes
2. Actions of individual muscles according to the position of eye
3. Single or pure movements of the eyeball
4. Further reading
5. Viva voce questions

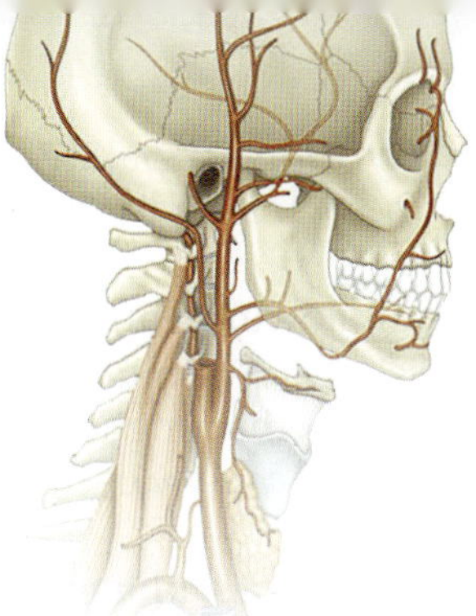

Chapter

14

# Mouth and Pharynx

## ORAL CAVITY

Oral cavity is used for ingestion of food and fluids. It is continued posteriorly into the oropharynx, the middle part of the muscular pharynx. In its upper part, opens the posterior part of the nasal cavity and the inlet of larynx opens into its lower part. Roof of oral cavity is formed by the hard and the soft palates. Tongue is the biggest occupant of the oral cavity, described in Chapter 17. The cavity also contains 32 teeth in an adult.

### Divisions

The oral or mouth cavity is divided into:

1. An outer, smaller portion – vestibule
2. An inner larger part – oral cavity proper.

***Competency:***

**AN36.1** Describe and demonstrate the structures of the vestibule of the mouth and oral cavity proper.

### VESTIBULE

1. The vestibule of the mouth is a narrow space *bounded* externally by the lips and cheeks, and internally by the teeth and gums (Figs 14.1a and b).
2. It *communicates*:
   a. With the exterior through the oral fissure.
   b. With the mouth open, it communicates freely with the oral cavity proper. Even when the teeth are occluded a small communication remains behind the third molar tooth.
3. The ***parotid duct*** opens on the inner surface of the cheek opposite the crown of the upper second molar tooth. Numerous ***labial and buccal glands*** (mucous) situated in the submucosa of the lips and cheeks open into the vestibule. Four or five ***molar glands*** (mucous), situated on the buccopharyngeal fascia, also open into the vestibule.
4. Except for the teeth, the entire vestibule is lined by mucous membrane. The mucous membrane forms median folds that pass from the lips to the gums, and are called the ***frenula of the lips***.

### CLINICAL ANATOMY

- The ***papilla of the parotid duct*** in the vestibule of the mouth provides access to the parotid duct for the injection of the radio-opaque dye to locate calculi in the duct system or the gland.
- ***Koplik's spots*** are seen as white pinpoint spots around the opening of the parotid duct in measles. These are diagnostic of the disease.

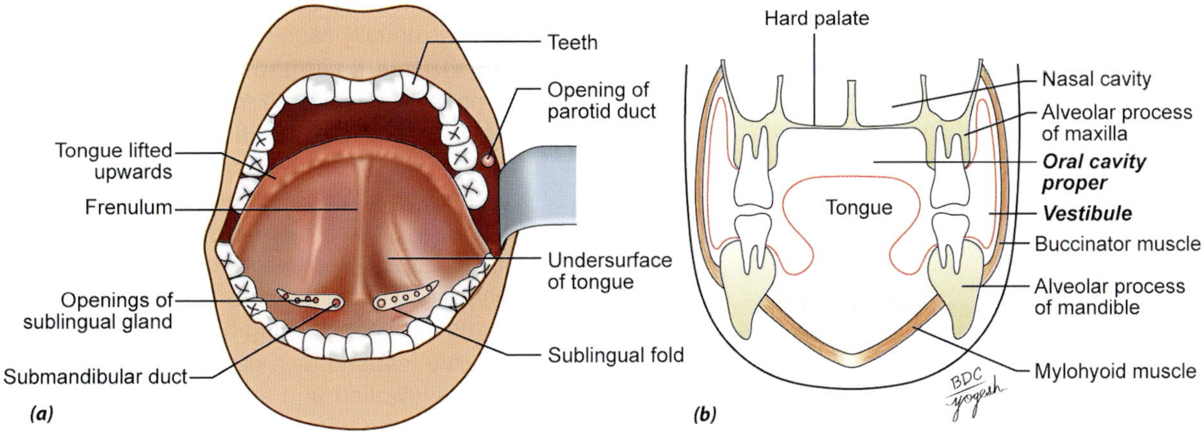


**Figs 14.1a and b:** (a) Interior of the mouth cavity and (b) subdivisions of the oral cavity in coronal section

## LIPS

1. The lips are fleshy folds lined externally by skin and internally by mucous membrane. The ***mucocutaneous junction*** lines the 'edge' of the lip, part of the mucosal surface is also normally seen.
2. ***Layers:*** Each lip is *composed* of:
   a. Skin
   b. Superficial fascia
   c. The orbicularis oris muscle
   d. The submucosa, containing mucous labial glands and blood vessels
   e. Mucous membrane.
3. The lips bound the ***oral fissure***. They meet laterally at the angles of the mouth. The inner surface of each lip is supported by a ***frenulum*** which ties it to the gum. Philtrum is a median vertical groove on the outer surface of the upper lip.
4. *Lymphatics* of the central part of the lower lip drain to the submental nodes; the lymphatics from the rest of the lower lip pass to the submandibular nodes.

*Note*: ***Vermilion*** or ***red margin*** is a mucocutaneous junction. The free margin of the lip shows vermilion. Large number of the blood vessels that are present beneath the epithelium gives red colour to the lip.

## CHEEKS (BUCCAE)

1. The cheeks are fleshy flaps, forming a large part of each side of the face. They are continuous in front with the lips, and the junction is indicated by the *nasolabial sulcus* (*furrow*) which extends from the side of the nose to the angle of the mouth.
2. ***Layers:*** Each cheek is *composed of:*
   a. Skin
   b. Superficial fascia containing some facial muscles, the parotid duct, mucous molar glands, vessels and nerves.
   c. The buccinator covered by buccopharyngeal fascia and pierced by the parotid duct.
   d. Submucosa, with mucous buccal glands.
   e. Mucous membrane.
3. The *buccal pad of fat* is best developed in infants. It lies on the buccinator partly deep to the masseter and partly in front of it.
4. The *lymphatics* of the cheek drain chiefly into the submandibular and preauricular nodes, and partly also to the buccal and mandibular nodes.

## ORAL CAVITY PROPER

1. Boundaries:
   *Anterolaterally* – Teeth, the gums and the alveolar arches of the jaws.
   *Roof* – Formed by the hard palate and the soft palate.
   *Floor* – Occupied by the tongue posteriorly, and presents the sublingual region anteriorly, below the tip of the tongue.
   *Posteriorly* – The cavity communicates with the pharynx through the ***oropharyngeal isthmus*** (*isthmus of fauces*) which is bounded superiorly by the soft palate, inferiorly by the tongue, and on each side by the palatoglossal arches.
2. The ***sublingual region*** presents the following features:
   a. In the median plane, there is a fold of mucosa passing from the inferior aspect of the tongue to the floor of the mouth. This is the *frenulum* of the tongue.
   b. On each side of the frenulum, there is a ***sublingual papilla***. On the summit of this papilla, there is the opening of submandibular duct.
   c. Running laterally and backwards from the sublingual papilla, there is the ***sublingual fold*** which overlies the sublingual gland. A few sublingual ducts open on the edge of this fold.
3. *Lymphatics* from the anterior part of the floor of the mouth pass to the submental nodes. Those from the hard palate and soft palate pass to the retropharyngeal and upper deep cervical nodes. The gums and the rest of the floor drain into the submandibular nodes.

### Gums (Gingivae)

1. The gums are the soft tissues which envelop the alveolar processes of the upper and lower jaws and surround the necks of the teeth. These are composed of dense fibrous tissue covered by stratified squamous epithelium.
2. Each gum has two parts:
   a. The free part surrounds the neck of the tooth like a collar.
   b. The *attached part* is firmly fixed to the alveolar arch of the jaw. The fibrous tissue of the gum is continuous with the periosteum lining the alveoli (periodontal membrane).
3. Nerve supply of gums is shown in Table 14.1.
4. *Lymphatics* of the upper gums pass to the submandibular nodes. The anterior part of the lower gums drains into the submental nodes, whereas the posterior part drains into the submandibular nodes.

### CLINICAL ANATOMY

- ***Ludwig's angina*** is the cellulitis of the floor of the mouth. The tongue is forced upwards leading to swelling both below the chin and within the mouth. The disease is usually caused due to a caries molar tooth.
- ***Gingivitis*** is an inflammation of the gums. Its commonest cause is an improper oral hygiene. If it remains untreated, it usually results in tooth loss. It can be identified as swollen red gums, tenderness of gum, pus, or ulceration of gums.
- ***Pyorrhea*** or ***periodontitis*** is an inflammatory condition affecting tissue surrounding the teeth. It has a clinical presentation of pus discharge at the margins of gums and foul-smelling breath.
- In ***scurvy*** (caused by a deficiency of vitamin C), the gums are swollen and spongy, and bleed on touch. In gingivitis, the edges of the gums are red and bleed easily.

**TABLE 14.1: Nerve supply of gums**

| *Upper gums* | *Nerve supply* |
|---|---|
| Labial side | Posterior, middle and anterior superior alveolar nerves (V2) |
| Lingual side | Anterior palatine and nasopalatine nerves (from pterygopalatine ganglion) |
| ***Lower gums*** | |
| Labial side | Buccal branch of mandibular and incisive branch of mental nerve (V3) |
| Lingual side | Lingual nerve (V3) |

## TEETH

The teeth form part of the masticatory apparatus and are fixed to the jaws. In man, the teeth are replaced only once *(diphyodont)* in contrast with nonmammalian vertebrates where teeth are constantly replaced throughout life *(polyphyodont)*. The teeth of the first set (dentition) are known as *milk*, or *deciduous teeth*, and the second set, as *permanent teeth*.

### Number of Teeth (Figs 14.2a and b)

The ***deciduous teeth*** are 20 in number. In each half of each jaw, there are two incisors, one canine, and two molars.

The ***permanent teeth*** are 32 in number, and consist of two incisors (Latin *to cut*), one canine (Latin *dog*), two premolars (Latin *millstone*), and three molars in each half of each jaw.

### Parts of a Tooth

Each tooth has three parts:

1. *Crown*, projecting above or below the gum.
2. *Root*, embedded in the jaw beneath the gum.
3. *Neck*, between the crown and root and surrounded by the gum (Fig. 14.3).

### Structure

Structurally, each tooth is composed of (Fig. 14.3):

1. Pulp in the centre
2. Dentine surrounding the pulp.
3. Enamel covering the projecting part of dentine, or crown.
4. Cementum surrounding the embedded part of the dentine.
5. Periodontal membrane.

The ***pulp*** is loose fibrous tissue containing vessels, nerves and lymphatics, all of which enter the pulp cavity through the apical foramen. The pulp is covered by a layer of tall columnar cells, known as *odontoblasts* which are capable of replacing dentine any time in life.

The ***dentine*** is a calcified material containing spiral tubules radiating from the pulp cavity. Each tubule is occupied by a protoplasmic process from one of the odontoblasts. The calcium and organic matter are in the same proportion as in bone.

The ***enamel*** is the hardest substance in the body. It is made up of crystalline prisms lying roughly at right angles to the surface of the tooth.

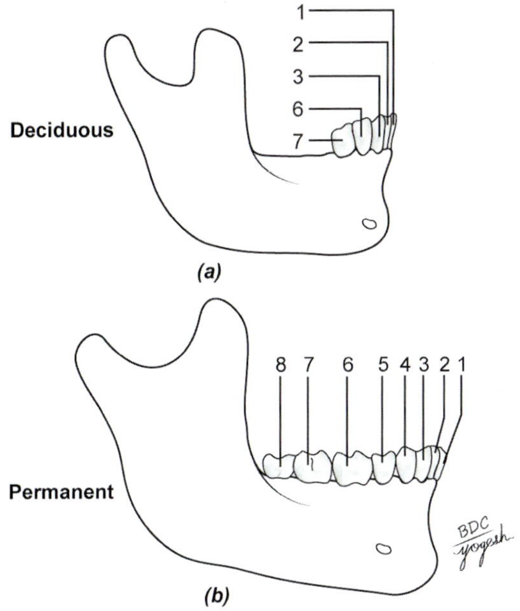


**Figs 14.2a and b:** Deciduous and permanent teeth: (1) Central incisor; (2) Lateral incisor; (3) Canine; (4) 1st premolar; (5) 2nd premolar; (6) 1st molar; (7) 2nd molar; (8) 3rd molar

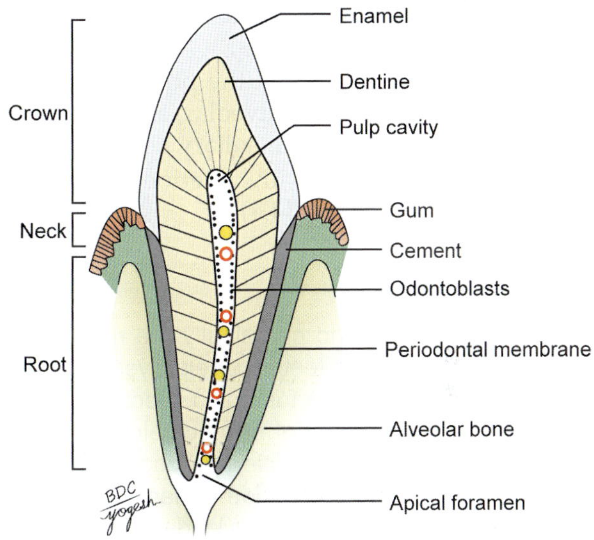


**Fig. 14.3:** Parts of a tooth

The ***cementum*** resembles bone in structure, but like enamel and dentine, there is neither any blood supply nor any nerve supply. Over the neck, the cementum commonly overlaps the cervical end of enamel; or, less commonly, it may just meet the enamel. Rarely, it stops short of the enamel (10%) leaving the cervical dentine covered only by gum.

The ***periodontal membrane*** *(ligament)* holds the root in its socket. This membrane acts as a periosteum to both the cementum as well as the bony socket.

### Form and Function (Crowns and Roots)

1. The shape of a tooth is adapted to its function. The *incisors are cutting teeth,* with chisel-like crowns. The upper and lower incisors overlap each other like the blades of a pair of scissors. *The canines are holding and*

tearing teeth, with conical and rugged crowns. These are better developed in carnivores. Each *premolar* has two cusps and is, therefore, also called a *bicuspid* tooth. The *molars are grinding teeth,* with square crowns, bearing four or five cusps on their crowns.

2. The incisors, canines and premolars have single roots, with the exception of the first upper premolar which has a bifid root. The upper molars have three roots, of which two are lateral and one is medial. The lower molars have only two roots—an anterior and a posterior.

## Eruption of Teeth

The *deciduous teeth* begin to erupt at about the 6th month, and all get erupted by the end of the 2nd year or soon after. The teeth of the lower jaw erupt slightly earlier than those of the upper jaw. The approximate ages of eruption of deciduous and permanent teeth are given in Table 14.2.

## Blood Supply of Teeth

Both upper and lower are supplied by branches of maxillary artery.

## Nerve Supply of Teeth

The pulp and periodontal membrane have the same nerve supply which is as follows:

1. *Upper teeth* are supplied by the posterior superior alveolar, middle superior alveolar, and the anterior superior alveolar nerves (maxillary nerve).
2. *Lower teeth* are supplied by the inferior alveolar nerve (mandibular nerve) (Fig. 14.4).

## CLINICAL ANATOMY

- Being the hardest and chemically the most stable tissues in the body, the teeth are selectively preserved after death and may be fossilized. Because of this, the teeth are very helpful in medicolegal practice for identification of otherwise unrecognizable dead bodies. The teeth also provide by far the best data to study evolutionary changes and the relationship between ontogeny and phylogeny.
- Decalcification of enamel and dentine with consequent softening and gradual destruction of the tooth is known as ***dental caries***. A caries tooth is tender on mastication.
- Infection of apex of root (apical abscess) occurs only when the pulp is dead. The condition can be recognized in a good radiograph.
- Irregular dentition is common in rickets and the upper permanent incisors may be notched, the notching corresponds to a small segment of a large circle. Even in congenital syphilis, the same teeth are notched, but the notching corresponds to a large segment of a small circle (*Hutchinson's teeth*).
- The third molar teeth, also called ***wisdom teeth***, usually erupt between 18 and 20 years. These may not erupt normally due to less space and may get ***impacted*** causing enormous pain.

**TABLE 14.2: Usual time of eruption of teeth and time of shedding of deciduous teeth**

| *Tooth* | *Eruption time* |
|---|---|
| **Deciduous** (Fig. 14.2a) | |
| Central incisor | 6–9 months |
| Lateral incisor | 8–10 months |
| First molar | 12–20 months |
| Canine | 16–20 months |
| Second molar | 20–39 months |
| **Permanent** (Fig. 14.2b) | |
| First molar | 6–7 years |
| Central incisor | 7–8 years |
| Lateral incisor | 8–9 years |
| First premolar | 10–11 years |
| Second premolar | 11–12 years |
| Canine | 12–13 years |
| Second molar | 12–14 years |
| Third molar | 18–25 years |

*Note*: The teeth of the lower jaw erupt slightly earlier than those of the upper jaw.

- Time of eruption of the teeth helps in assessing the age of the person.
- The upper canine teeth are called as the 'eye teeth' as these have long roots which reach up to the medial angle of the eye. Infection of these roots may spread in the facial vein and even lead to thrombosis of the cavernous sinus.
- The upper teeth need separate injections of the anaesthetic on both the buccal and palatal surfaces of the maxillary process just distal to the tooth. The thin layer of bone permits rapid diffusion of the drug up to the tooth.

## Types of Teeth

The humans have *heterodont teeth*, i.e. the teeth are of different types. According to the structure, the teeth are classified as incisors, canines, premolars, and molars (Figs 14.5a and b).

### Incisors

These are chisel-like teeth (incisor = to cut in Latin) used to cut the food. There are total eight incisors, four in upper jaw and four are in lower jaw. There are two incisors in each quadrant (out of 4 quadrants) and they are named as follows:

1. Maxillary central incisor
2. Maxillary lateral incisor
3. Mandibular central incisor
4. Mandibular lateral incisor.

In children, incisors erupt as deciduous teeth that later get replaced by permanent teeth. The mandibular central incisor erupts first followed by maxillary central incisors, mandibular lateral incisors, and finally maxillary lateral incisors. Each incisor has five surfaces: Labial, lingual, mesial (medial), distal (lateral), and biting or incisal surfaces. Maxillary incisors are present in premaxillary

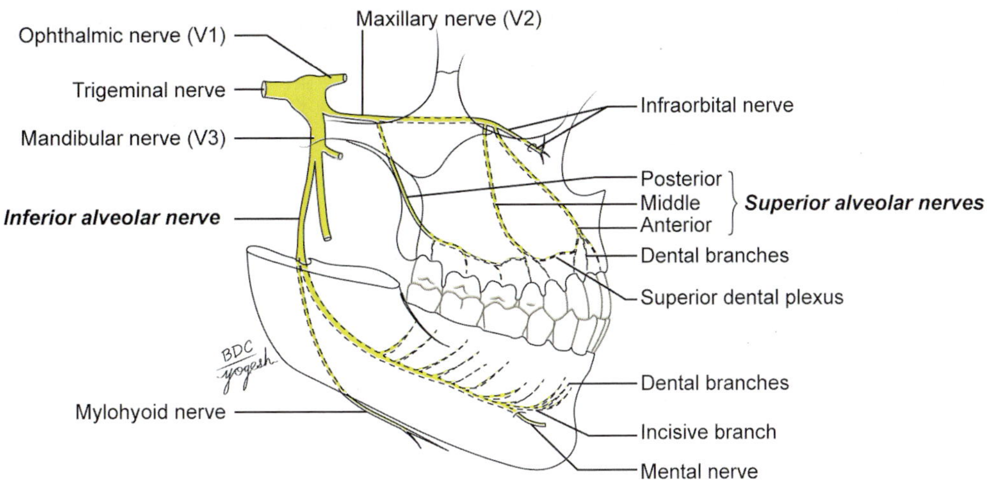


**Fig. 14.4:** Nerve supply of teeth

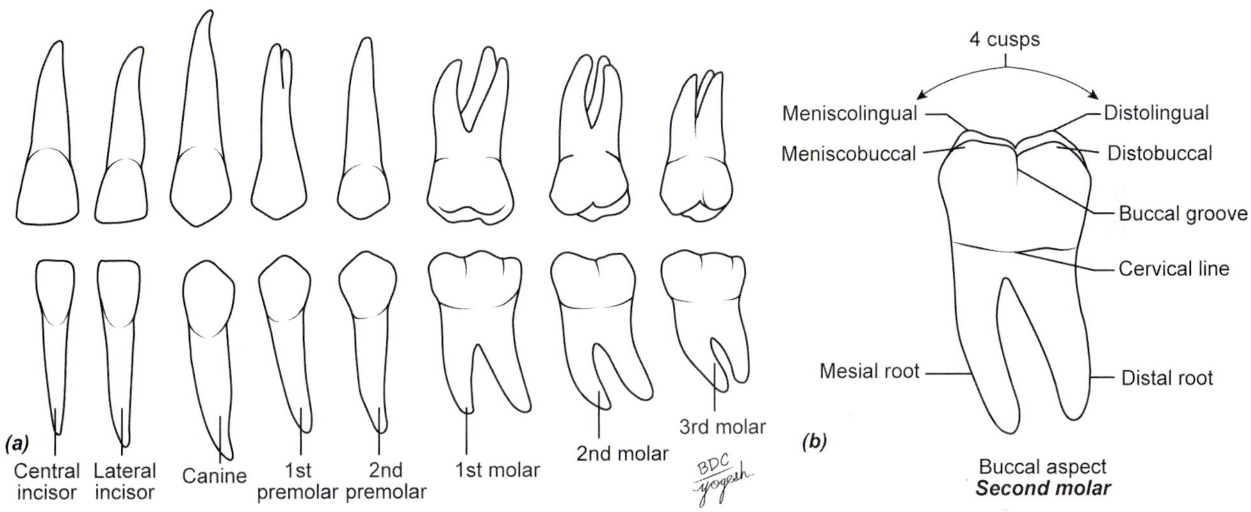


**Figs 14.5a and b:** (a) Types of the permanent tooth (upper and lower teeth of the right side) and (b) buccal aspect of second molar tooth

portion of the maxilla. The lower edge of incisors partially covers the labial surface of mandibular incisor. Incisors have a single root and a sharp incisal edge. The incisors are useful for biting, cutting off pieces of food.

### Canines

These are pointed teeth. There are total four canines, one in each quadrant and they are named as maxillary canines and mandibular canines. They lie behind and adjacent to the lateral incisors. They have single, pointed cusp and a single root. They have the longest root. They are prominent in carnivorous animal, hence called *canines*. They are the last deciduous teeth to erupt. They are used to tear the food.

### Premolars *(Bicuspids)*

They are located behind the canine and in front of molars. There are eight premolars, two in each quadrant. They are named as first premolar (close to midline) and second premolar (farthest from the midline). Each premolar has at least two cusps (hence called *bicuspids*). The first premolar has two roots, and second premolar has single root. There are no premolars in the primary dentition. They are designated to crush the food.

### Molars

They are located behind the canine in deciduous dentition and behind the premolars in permanent dentition. There are twelve molars (grinders in Latin), three on each quadrant. They are named as first, second, and third molars. The molars have 4–5 cups (four cups in upper molars and five cups in lower molars). Mandibular molars have two roots, whereas maxillary molars have three roots. Third molar tooth is known as *wisdom tooth*. It is mostly seen as impacted. They are designated for grinding the food.

## STAGES OF DEVELOPMENT OF DECIDUOUS TEETH

1. *Stages of dental lamina*: During the 6th week of development, epithelium (ectoderm) in the region of developing alveolar process (U-shaped zone) thickens to form dental lamina (Fig. 14.6).

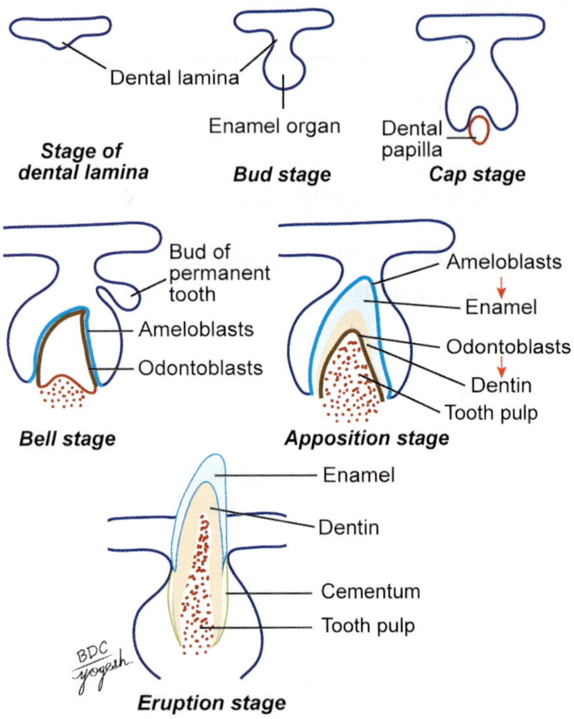


**Fig. 14.6:** Development of tooth

2. *Bud stage*: In each alveolar process, the dental lamina thickens at ten places and forms tooth buds (enamel organ) that grow towards underlying mesoderm.
3. *Cap stage*: Mass of mesenchyme (mostly neural crest cells) occupies the core of enamel organ and makes enamel organ cap-shaped. In the 8th week, enamel organs appear. This mass of the mesenchyme forms the dental papilla. In 10th week, enamel organs become cap-shaped.
4. *Bell stage*: Cells of the enamel organ facing dental papilla become columnar and form ameloblasts.

   Cells of the dental papilla facing ameloblasts, later form an epithelium-like layer called odontoblasts. Enamel organ soon forms:
   - outer cell layer as outer dental epithelium,
   - inner cell layer as inner dental epithelium (ameloblasts), and
   - central core loose mesenchymal cells as stellate reticulum or enamel reticulum.

   Growing dental cap forms a bell-shaped structure over underlying dental papilla; hence, called bell stage.
5. *Apposition stage*: Ameloblasts lay down enamel on the outer surface of basement membrane separating ameloblasts and odontoblasts, whereas odontoblast lays down dentin on deeper surface of basement membrane. The ameloblasts move towards outer dental epithelium through satellite reticulum. Finally, outer epithelium, reticulum and ameloblasts disappear, leaving behind dental cuticle of Nasmyth (a thin layer) over enamel. On the formation of dentin, regressing odontoblast leaves behind their cytoplasmic processes (called odontoblastic processes or Tomes processes) that remain trapped in dentin.

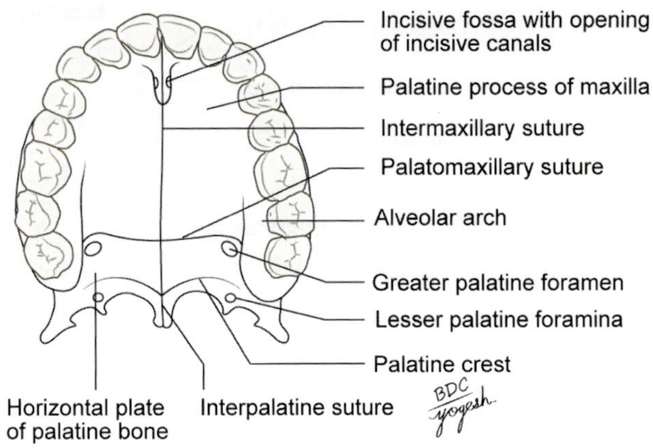


**Fig. 14.7:** Hard palate

   Continuous deposition of dentin reduces pulp cavity to a narrow pulp canal. Blood vessels and nerves reach tooth through the pulp canal. Mesenchymal cells covering the root of the tooth modify to form cementoblasts. The cementoblasts lay down a layer of dense bone called cementum. Cementum is produced just before the birth. Mesenchymal cells covering cementum form periodontal ligament that connects root of the tooth with jaw bone. After birth, before eruption of tooth, periodontal ligament appears.
6. *Eruption stage*: Growth of the root produces eruption of tooth. Eruption age of various teeth is listed in Table 14.2.

***Formation of permanent teeth:*** These develop from the dental buds arising from the dental lamina and lie on the medial side of each developing milk tooth.

## HARD PALATE

It is a partition between the nasal and oral cavities. Its anterior 2/3rd are formed by the palatine processes of the maxillae; and its posterior 1/3rd by the horizontal plates of the palatine bones (Plate 14.1 and Fig. 14.7).

### *Features*

1. *Anterolateral margins* of the palate are continuous with the alveolar arches and gums.
2. *Posterior margin* gives attachment to the soft palate.
3. *Superior surface* forms the floor of the nose.
4. *Inferior surface* forms the roof of the oral cavity.

### Vessels and Nerves

***Arteries:*** Greater palatine branch of maxillary artery.

***Veins:*** Drain into the pterygoid plexus of veins.

***Nerves:*** Greater palatine and nasopalatine branches of the pterygopalatine ganglion suspended by the maxillary nerve.

***Lymphatics:*** The lymphatics drain mostly to the upper deep cervical nodes and partly to the retropharyngeal nodes.

Plate 14.1: Hard palate (inferior view)

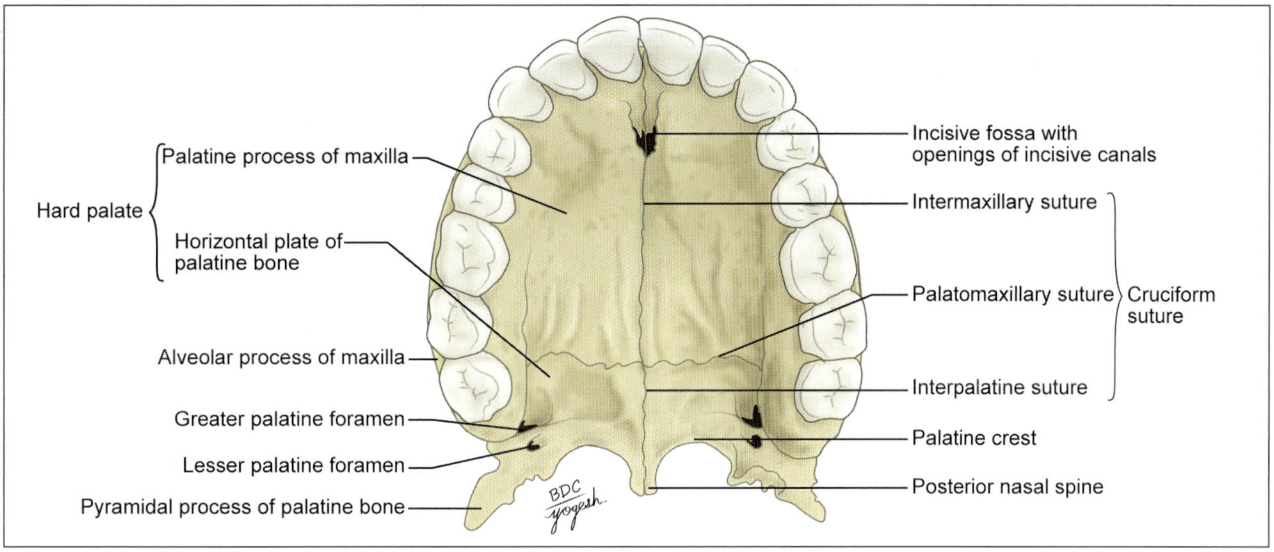


**DISSECTION**

Cut through the centre of the frontal bone, internasal suture, intermaxillary sutures, chin, hyoid bone, thyroid, cricoid and tracheal cartilages; carry the incision through the septum of nose, nasopharynx, tongue, and both the palates.

Cut through the centre of the remaining occipital bone and cervical vertebrae. This will complete the *sagittal section of head and neck.*

***Hard palate:*** Strip the mucoperiosteum of hard palate.

***Soft palate:*** Remove the mucous membrane of the soft palate in order to identify its muscles. Also remove the mucous membrane over palatoglossal and palatopharyngeal arches and salpingopharyngeal fold to visualise the subjacent muscles.

*Competency:*

AN36.2 Describe the: (1) morphology, relations, blood supply and applied anatomy of palatine tonsil, (2) composition of soft palate.

## SOFT PALATE

It is a movable, muscular fold, suspended from the posterior border of the hard palate.

It separates the nasopharynx from the oropharynx, the crossroads between the food and air passages (Fig. 14.8 and Flowchart 14.1).

### External Features

The soft palate has two surfaces—anterior and posterior:

1. ***Anterior (oral) surface*** is concave and is marked by a median raphe.
2. ***Posterior surface*** is convex, and is continuous superiorly with the floor of the nasal cavity.

The soft palate has two borders—superior and inferior:

1. ***Superior border*** is attached to the posterior border of the hard palate, blending on each side with the pharynx.

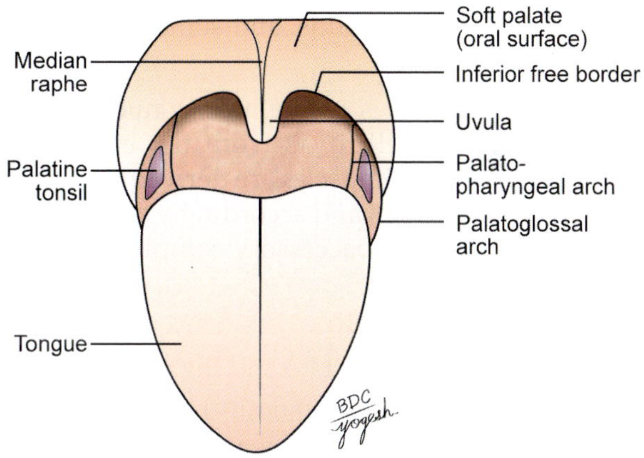


Fig. 14.8: Soft palate with palatine tonsils

2. ***Inferior border*** is free and bounds the pharyngeal isthmus. From its middle, there hangs a conical projection, called the ***uvula.*** From each side of the base of the uvula (Latin *small grape*), two curved folds of mucous membrane extend laterally and downwards as follows:
   a. The anterior fold is called the ***palatoglossal arch*** or anterior pillar of fauces. It contains the palatoglossus muscle and reaches the side of the tongue at the junction of its oral and pharyngeal parts. This fold forms the lateral boundary of the oropharyngeal isthmus or isthmus of fauces.
   b. The posterior fold is called the ***palatopharyngeal arch*** or posterior pillar of fauces. It contains the palatopharyngeus muscle. It forms the posterior boundary of the tonsillar fossa, and merges inferiorly with the lateral wall of the pharynx.

### Structure

The soft palate is a fold of mucous membrane containing the following parts:

- The palatine aponeurosis which is the flattened tendon of the tensor veli palatini forms the fibrous basis of the

**Flowchart 14.1:** Soft palate

**Soft palate**
Movable mucomuscular flap

***External features***
Two surfaces
- Anterior (oral): Median raphe
- Posterior
Two borders: Superior, inferior (free)
Two mucosal arches
- Palatoglossal, palatopharyngeal

***Structure***
Mucosa
Posterior surface:
Pseudostratified ciliated columnar epithelium
Anterior surface:
Nonkeratinized stratified squamous epithelium
Submucosa
Palatine aponeurosis
Muscles

***Muscles***
Tensor veli palatini
Levator veli palatini
Palatoglossus
Palatopharyngeus
Musculus uvulae

***Nerve supply***
Motor: All muscles by cranial root of accessory nerve except tensor veli palatini (by mandibular nerve)
General sensation: Glossopharyngeal, lesser palatine nerves
Taste sensation
- Lesser palatine nerve
Secretomotor: Pterygopalatine ganglion

palate. Near the median plane, the aponeurosis splits to enclose the musculus uvulae.

- The levator veli palatini and the palatopharyngeus lie on the superior surface of the palatine aponeurosis.
- The palatoglossus lies on the inferior or anterior surface of the palatine aponeurosis.
- Numerous mucous glands, and some taste buds are present.

Soft palate comprises epithelium, connective tissue and muscles. Epithelium is from the ectoderm of maxillary process. The muscles are derived from 1st, 4th and 6th branchial arches and accordingly are innervated by mandibular and vagoaccessory complex.

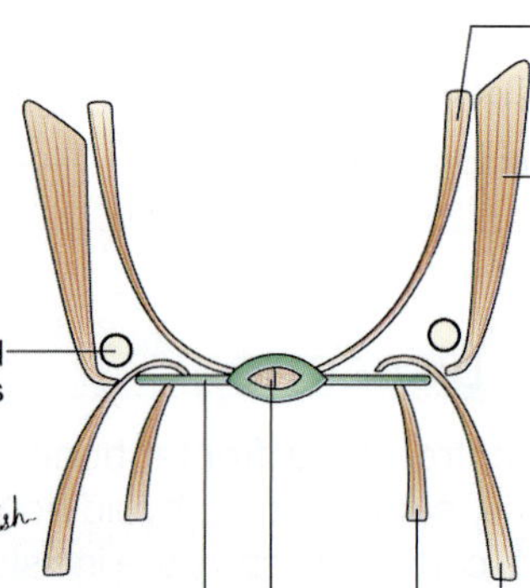


**Fig. 14.9:** Muscles of soft palate

## Muscles of the Soft Palate

They are as follows (Plate 14.2 and Fig. 14.9):

1. Tensor palati (tensor veli palatini)
2. Levator palati (levator veli palatini)
3. Musculus uvulae
4. Palatoglossus
5. Palatopharyngeus.

The origin, insertion and actions of these muscles are given in Table 14.3.

## Blood Supply

### Arteries

1. Greater palatine branch of maxillary artery.
2. Ascending palatine branch of facial artery.
3. Palatine branch of ascending pharyngeal artery.

### Veins

They pass to the pterygoid and tonsillar plexuses of veins.

### Lymphatics

Drain into the upper deep cervical and retropharyngeal lymph nodes.

## Nerve Supply

1. ***Motor nerves***. All muscles of the soft palate except the tensor veli palatini are supplied by the pharyngeal plexus. The fibres of this plexus are derived from the cranial part of the accessory nerve through the vagus. The tensor veli palatini is supplied by the mandibular nerve.
2. **General *sensory nerves*** are derived from:
   a. The middle and posterior lesser palatine nerves, which are branches of the maxillary nerve through the pterygopalatine ganglion.
   b. The glossopharyngeal nerve.
3. ***Special sensory*** or *gustatory nerves,* carrying *taste sensations* from the oral surface, are contained in the lesser palatine nerves. The fibres travel through the greater petrosal nerve to the geniculate ganglion of the facial nerve and from there to the nucleus of the tractus solitarius.
4. ***Secretomotor nerves*** are also contained in the lesser palatine nerves. They are derived from the superior salivatory nucleus and travel through the greater petrosal nerve.

## Passavant's Ridge

Some of the upper fibres of the palatopharyngeus pass circularly deep to the mucous membrane of the pharynx, to form a sphincter internal to the superior constrictor. These fibres constitute Passavant's muscle which on contraction raises a ridge called the Passavant's ridge on the posterior wall of the nasopharynx. When the soft palate is elevated it comes in contact with this ridge, the two together closing the pharyngeal isthmus between the nasopharynx and the oropharynx (Fig. 14.10).

**Plate 14.2:** Muscles of the soft palate

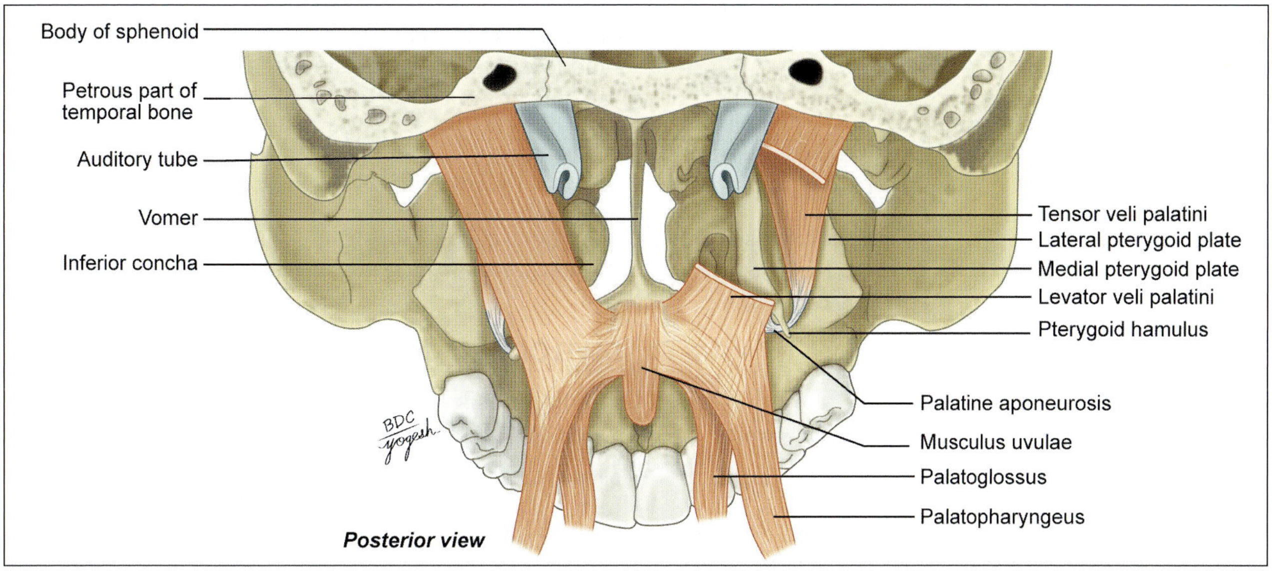


**TABLE 14.3: Origin, insertion and actions of muscles of the soft palate** (Plate 14.2 and Fig. 14.9)

| *Muscle* | *Origin* | *Insertion* | *Actions* |
|---|---|---|---|
| 1. **Tensor veli palatini**<br>This is a thin, triangular muscle | a. Lateral side of auditory tube<br>b. Adjoining part of the base of the skull (greater wing and scaphoid fossa of sphenoid bone) | Muscle descends, converges to form a delicate tendon which winds round the pterygoid hamulus, passes through the origin of the buccinator, and flattens out to form the palatine aponeurosis. Aponeurosis is attached to:<br>a. Posterior border of hard palate<br>b. Inferior surface of palate behind the palatine crest | a. Tightens the soft palate, chiefly the anterior part<br>b. Opens the auditory tube to equalize air pressure between the middle ear and the nasopharynx |
| 2. **Levator veli palatini**<br>This is a cylindrical muscle that lies deep to the tensor veli palatini | a. Inferior aspect of auditory tube<br>b. Adjoining part of inferior surface of petrous temporal bone | Muscle enters the pharynx by tube passing over the upper concave margin of the superior constrictor, runs downwards and medially and spreads out in the soft palate. It is inserted into the upper surface of the palatine aponeurosis | a. Elevates soft palate and closes the pharyngeal isthmus<br>b. Opens the auditory tube like the tensor veli palatini |
| 3. **Musculus uvulae**<br>This is a longitudinal strip placed on each side of the median plane, within the palatine aponeurosis | a. Posterior nasal spine<br>b. Palatine aponeurosis | Mucous membrane of uvula | Pulls up the uvula |
| 4. **Palatoglossus** | Oral surface of palatine aponeurosis | Descends in the palatoglossal arch, to the side of the tongue at the junction of its oral and pharyngeal parts | Pulls up the root of the tongue, approximates the palatoglossal arches, and thus closes the oropharyngeal isthmus |
| 5. **Palatopharyngeus**<br>It consists of two fasciculi that are separated by the levator veli palatini (also *see* Passavant's ridge) | a. Anterior fasciculus from posterior border of hard palate<br>b. Posterior fasciculus from the palatine aponeurosis | Descends in the palatopharyngeal arch and spreads out to form the greater part of longitudinal muscle coat of pharynx. It is inserted into:<br>a. Posterior border of the lamina of the thyroid cartilage<br>b. Wall of the pharynx and its median raphe | Pulls up the wall of the pharynx and shortens it during swallowing |

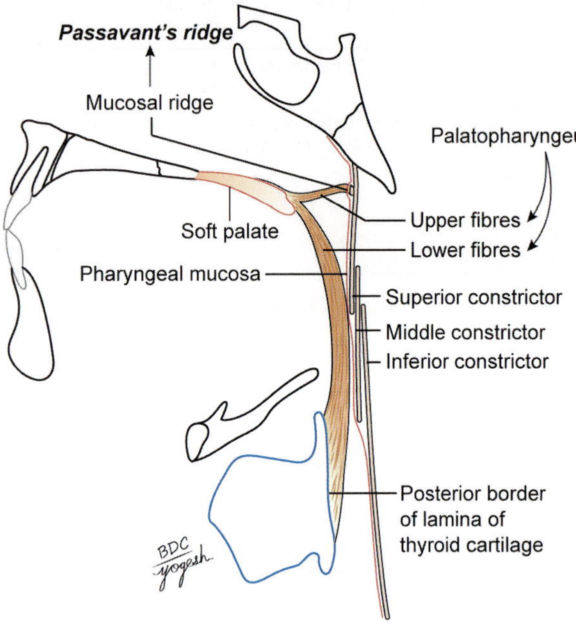


Fig. 14.10: Passavant's ridge

### Movements and Functions of the Soft Palate

1. Soft palate separates the oropharynx from nasopharynx during swallowing to prevent the entry of food into nose.
2. Separates oral cavity from oropharynx to facilitate chewing and breathing simultaneously.
3. Voice modulation.
4. Protection of nasal mucosa by diverting airflow through the mouth during sneezing.
5. Prevent entry of mucous into nose during coughing.

## CLINICAL ANATOMY

- ***Paralysis of the soft palate*** in lesions of the vagus nerve produces:
  1. Nasal regurgitation of liquids
  2. Nasal twang in voice
  3. Flattening of the palatal arch
  4. Deviation of uvula to normal side (Fig. 14.11).
- Choking by food/fluid causes laryngeal obstruction and asphyxia. Heimlich manoeuver can remove the obstruction.

**Heimlich Manoeuvre**

Stand behind the patient. Pass your arm under his arm. Put hand in his epigastrium; one hand made into a fist and other hand over fist. Give 3–4 abdominal thrusts directed upwards and backwards. This helps in squeezing residual air from lungs in trachea, and larynx, dislodges the foreign body and relieves laryngeal obstruction.

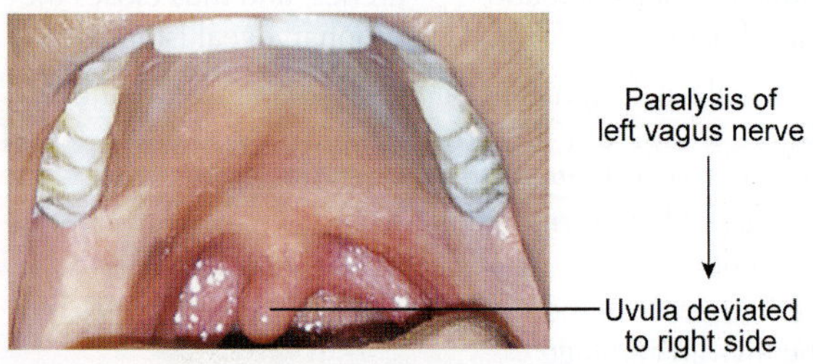


Fig. 14.11: Uvula deviated to right side in paralysis of left vagus nerve

*Competency:*

**AN43.4** Describe the development and developmental basis of congenital anomalies of face, palate, tongue, branchial apparatus, pituitary gland, thyroid gland and eye (Palate is described here. For the rest of organs, please see respective chapters.)

## DEVELOPMENT OF PALATE

Palatogenesis takes place between 5th week and 12th week of IUL (Fig. 14.12 and Flowchart 14.2).

*Primary palate:* In sixth week, the intermaxillary segment forms a shelf-like projection (that later bears upper four incisor teeth), called primary palate or median palatine process. Later, primary palate forms premaxillary part of the maxilla.

*Secondary palate:* In sixth week, two mesenchymal projections extend from the inner aspects of maxillary processes. These projections are called secondary palate or lateral palatine processes. During 7th–8th weeks, the lateral palatine processes elongate and fuse:

1. With each other in the midline
2. With nasal septum
3. With posterior part of the primary palate.

*Formation of definitive palate:* The primary palate fuses with secondary palate to form definitive palate. Incisive foramen divides primary and secondary palates.

- Anterior three-fourths of the definitive palate ossifies and forms hard palate.
- Posterior one-fourth of the definitive palate remains unossified and forms soft palate with uvula.

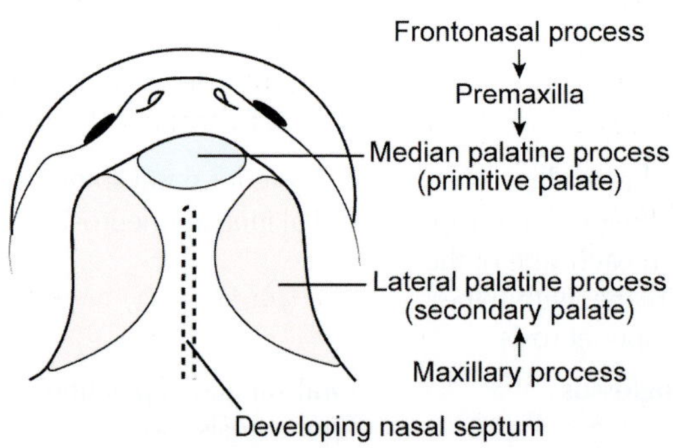


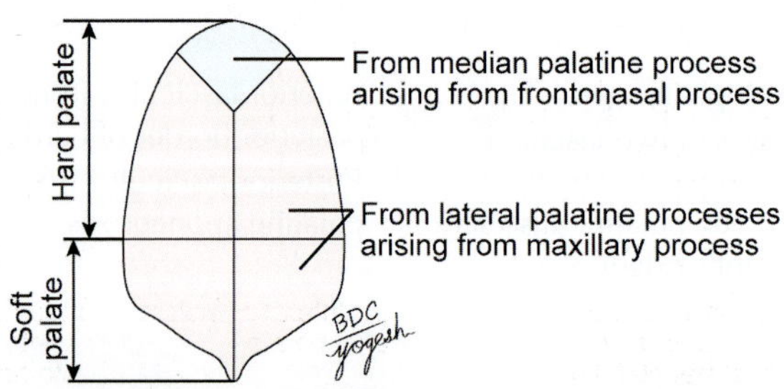


Fig. 14.12: Development of the palate

**Flowchart 14.2:** Development of the palate

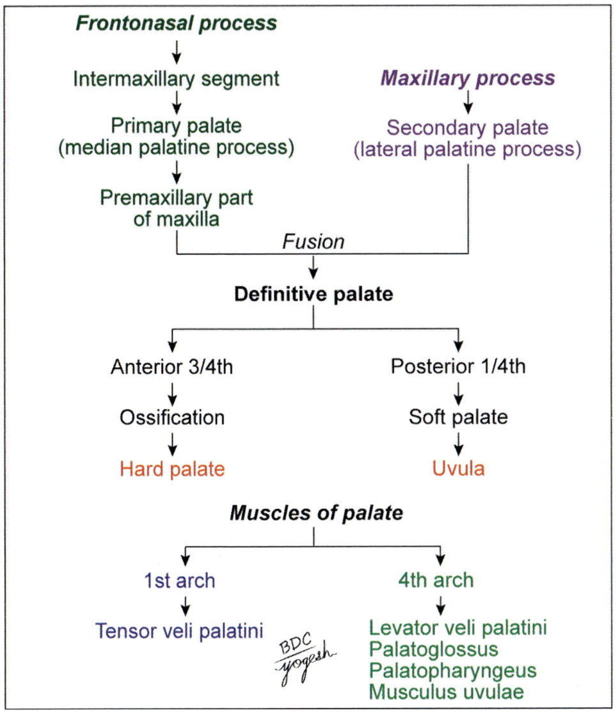


**Flowchart 14.3:** Cleft palate

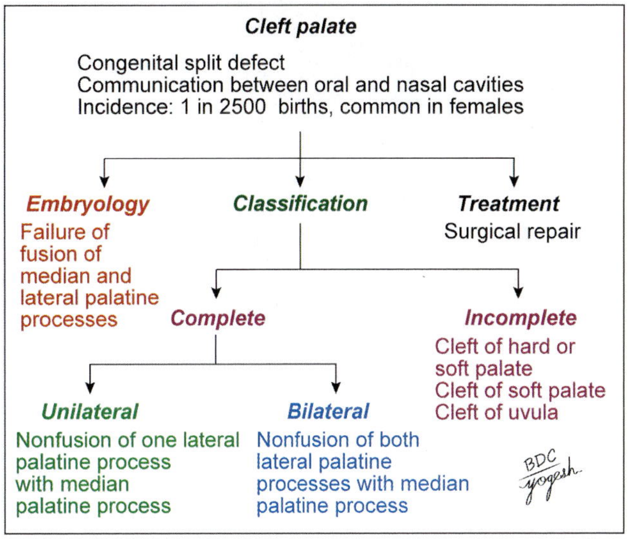


- Small persistent nasopalatine canal in the median plane of premaxilla forms the incisive fossa. In the incisive fossa, right and left incisive canals open.

*Muscles of palate:* Mesoderm of branchial arches invades soft palate to form muscles as follows:

- Tensor veli palatini – from 1st arch
- Levator veli palatini, palatoglossus, palatopharyngeus, musculus uvulae – from 4th arch.

## CLINICAL ANATOMY

### Cleft palate

- Cleft palate is a congenital split defect of palate that causes communication between oral and nasal cavities (Figs 14.13 and 14.14, Flowchart 14.3). Patient with cleft palate usually has eating, speech, and dental problems. The commonest cause is multifactorial inheritance.
- *Incidence*
  - 1 in 2500 births.
  - Cleft palate is more common in females (67%).
  - Incidence of cleft palate is not related to the maternal age.
  - If a couple has a child with cleft palate, there are 2% chances that another baby will have cleft palate.
  - Unilateral cleft of upper lip is the commonest congenital anomaly of face.
- *Embryological basis*
  - Nonfusion of median and lateral palatine processes, and the nasal septum results in cleft palate.
- Classification: Cleft palate may be complete or incomplete (partial) (Flowchart 14.3).
  1. Complete cleft palate may be unilateral or bilateral.
     - *Unilateral complete cleft palate*: It results due to nonfusion of one lateral palatine process of the maxilla with the median palatine process of premaxilla and also the nonfusion of the two lateral palatine processes. It is always associated with harelip on the same side of the defect.
     - *Bilateral complete cleft palate*: It results due to nonfusion of both the lateral palatine process of maxilla and the median palatine process of premaxilla.
  2. Incomplete cleft palate may be cleft of hard and soft palate or only the cleft of soft palate or uvula.

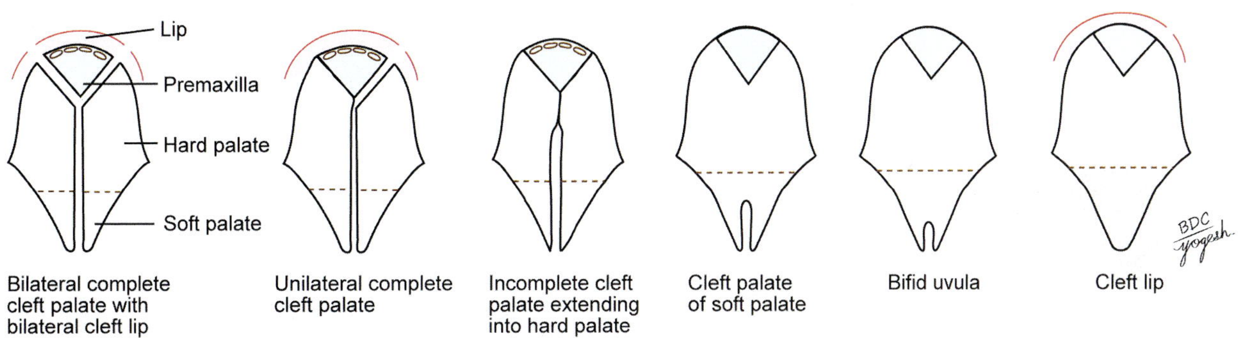


**Fig. 14.13:** Types of congenital cleft palate

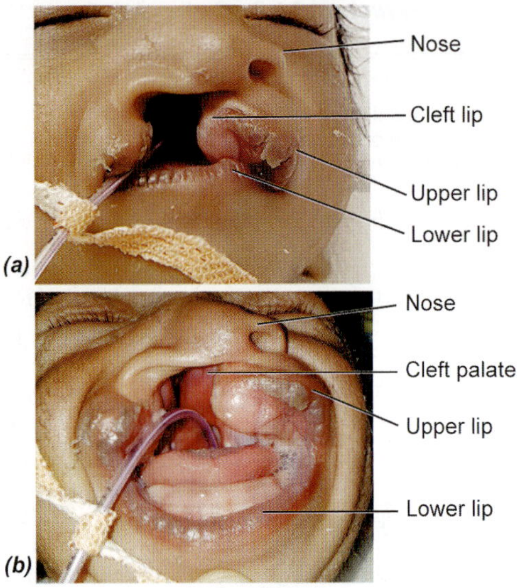


**Figs 14.14a and b:** A 5-day-old baby with unilateral cleft lip and cleft palate (on the right side)

***Competency:***

**AN36.3** Describe and demonstrate the muscles, nerve supply, blood supply and lymphatic drainage of the pharynx.

## PHARYNX

The pharynx (Latin *throat*) is a wide muscular tube, situated behind the nose, the mouth and the larynx. Clinically, it is a part of the upper respiratory passages where infections are common. The upper part of the pharynx transmits only air, the lower part (below the inlet of the larynx), only food, but the middle part is a common passage for both air and food. The nasopharynx part of pharynx is connected to the middle ear via the pharyngotympanic tube (Figs 14.15 to 14.18).

### Dimensions of Pharynx

*Length:* About 12–14 cm.

*Width:*

1. Upper part is the widest (3.5 cm) and non-collapsible
2. Middle part is narrow.
3. The lower end is the narrowest part of the gastrointestinal tract (except for the vermiform).

### Boundaries (Figs 14.15 to 14.18)

*Superiorly:* Base of the skull, including the posterior part of the body of the sphenoid and the basilar part of the occipital bone, in front of the pharyngeal tubercle.

*Inferiorly:* The pharynx is continuous with the oesophagus at the level of the sixth cervical vertebra, corresponding to the lower border of the cricoid cartilage.

*Posteriorly:* The pharynx glides freely on the prevertebral fascia which separates it from the cervical vertebral bodies.

*Anteriorly:* It communicates with the nasal cavity, the oral cavity and the larynx. Thus, the anterior wall of the pharynx is incomplete.

*On each side*

- Auditory tube
- Styloid process and the muscles attached to it
- The common carotid, internal carotid, and external carotid arteries
- The last four cranial nerves.

### Parts of the Pharynx

The cavity of the pharynx is divided into (Fig. 14.18):

1. Nasal part—*nasopharynx*
2. Oral part—*oropharynx*
3. Laryngeal part—*laryngopharynx*.

Comparison between nasopharynx, oropharynx and laryngopharynx shown in Table 14.4.

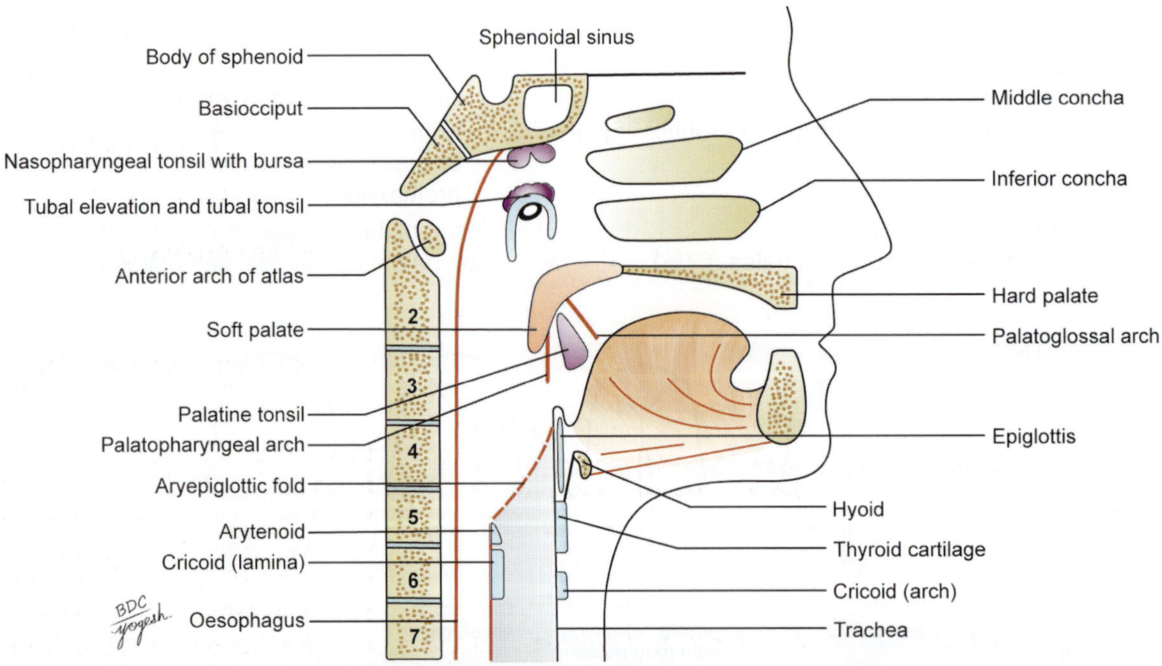


**Fig. 14.15:** Sagittal section through the pharynx, nose, mouth and larynx

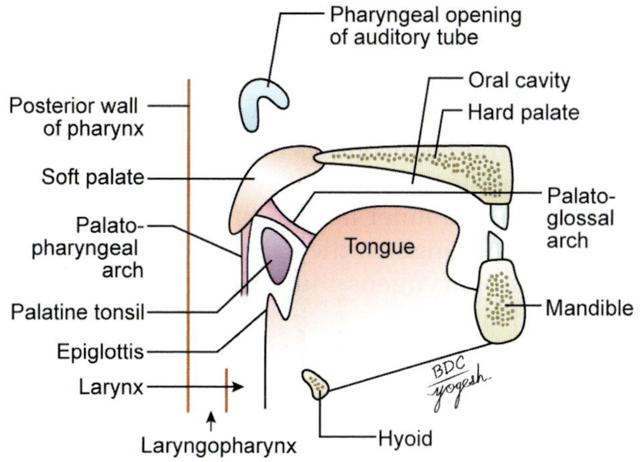


**Fig. 14.16:** Sagittal section through the mouth and pharynx

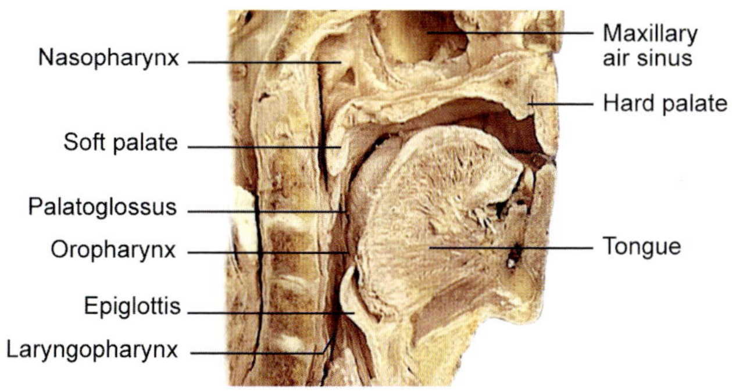


**Fig. 14.17:** Sagittal section of pharynx

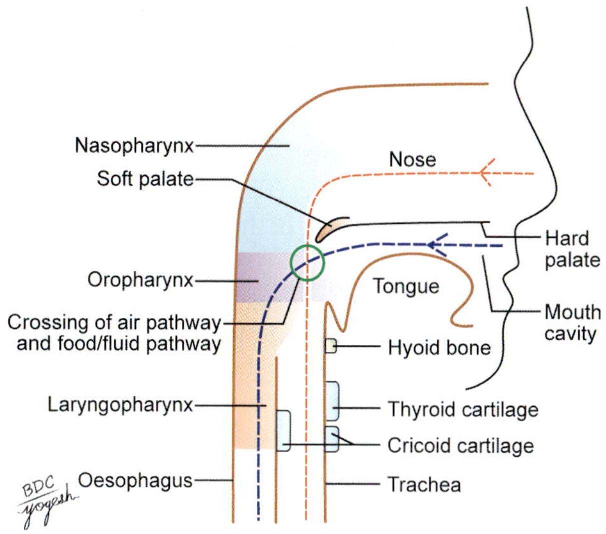


**Fig. 14.18:** Crossing of upper airway and upper food passages

## DISSECTION

Identify the structures in the interior of three parts of pharynx, i.e. nasopharynx, oropharynx and laryngopharynx. Clean the surfaces of buccinator muscle and adjoining superior constrictor muscles by removing connective tissue and buccopharyngeal fascia over these muscles. Detach the medial pterygoid muscle from its origin and reflect it downwards. This will expose the superior constrictor muscle completely.

**TABLE 14.4: Comparison between nasopharynx, oropharynx and laryngopharynx**

| *Particulars* | *Nasopharynx* | *Oropharynx* | *Laryngopharynx* |
|---|---|---|---|
| Situation | Behind nose | Behind oral cavity | Behind larynx |
| Extent | Base of skull (body of sphenoid) to soft palate | Soft palate to upper border of epiglottis (Figs 14.9a and b) | Upper border of epiglottis to lower border of cricoid cartilage |
| Communications | Anteriorly with nose (Fig. 14.9a)<br>Below with oropharynx | 1. Anteriorly with oral cavity<br>2. Above with nasopharynx<br>3. Below with laryngopharynx | Inferiorly with oesophagus<br>Anteriorly with larynx (Fig.14.9b)<br>Above with oropharynx |
| Nerve supply | Pharyngeal branches of pterygopalatine ganglion | IX and X nerves | IX and X nerves |
| *Relations*: | | | |
| i. Anterior | Posterior nasal aperture | Oral cavity | 1. Inlet of larynx<br>2. Posterior surface of cricoid cartilage<br>3. Arytenoid cartilage |
| ii. Posterior and roof | Body of sphenoid bone and basiocciput and anterior arch of atlas<br>Presence of:<br>a. Nasopharyngeal tonsil prominent in children<br>b. Nasopharyngeal bursa—mucus diverticulum | Body of second and third cervical vertebrae | Fourth and fifth cervical vertebrae |
| iii. Lateral wall | Opening of auditory tube above tube is tubal elevation with tubal tonsil | Tonsillar fossa containing palatine tonsils | Piriform fossa on each side of inlet of larynx, bounded by aryepiglottic fold medially and thyroid cartilage laterally. |
| Lining epithelium | Ciliated columnar epithelium | Stratified squamous nonkeratinised epithelium | Stratified squamous nonkeratinised epithelium |
| Function | Passage for air (respiratory function) | Passage for air and food | Passage for food |

### Laryngeal Part of Pharynx (Laryngopharynx)

This is the lower part of the pharynx situated behind the larynx. It extends from the upper border of the epiglottis to the lower border of the cricoid cartilage.

The *anterior wall* presents:

a. The inlet of the larynx (Plate 14.3)
b. The posterior surfaces of the cricoid and arytenoid cartilages.

The *posterior wall* is supported mainly by the fourth and fifth cervical vertebrae, and partly by the third and sixth vertebrae. In this region, the posterior wall of the pharynx is formed by the superior, middle and inferior constrictors of the pharynx (Fig. 14.19).

The *lateral wall* presents a depression called the ***piriform fossa***, one on each side of the inlet of the larynx (Fig. 14.20). The fossa is bounded medially by the aryepiglottic fold, and laterally by the thyroid cartilage and the thyrohyoid membrane. Beneath the mucosa of fossa, there lies the internal laryngeal nerve. Removal of foreign bodies from the piriform fossa may damage the internal laryngeal nerve, leading to anaesthesia in the supraglottic part of the larynx.

### Structure of Pharynx

The wall of the pharynx is composed of the following five layers from within outwards (Fig. 14.21):

1. *Mucosa*
2. *Submucosa*
3. ***Pharyngobasilar fascia*** or pharyngeal aponeurosis. This is a fibrous sheet internal to the pharyngeal muscles. It is thickest in the upper part where it fills the gap between the upper border of the superior constrictor and the base of the skull, and also posteriorly where it forms pharyngeal raphe. Superiorly, the fascia is attached to basiocciput, the petrous temporal bone, the auditory tube, posterior border of the medial pterygoid plate, and pterygomandibular raphe. Inferiorly, it is gradually lost deep to muscles, and hardly extend beyond the superior constrictor.
4. The ***muscular coat*** consists of an outer circular layer made up of the three constrictors (*superior, middle* and *inferior*) and an inner longitudinal layer made up of the stylopharyngeus, the salpingopharyngeus and the palatopharyngeus muscles. These muscles are described later.
5. The ***buccopharyngeal fascia*** covers the outer surface of the constrictors of the pharynx and extends forwards across the pterygomandibular raphe to cover the buccinator. Like the pharyngobasilar fascia, the buccopharyngeal fascia is best developed in the upper part of the pharynx.

Between the buccopharyngeal fascia and the muscular coat, there are the pharyngeal plexuses of veins and nerves (Fig. 14.21).

### Muscles of Pharynx

#### Constrictors of the Pharynx

The muscular basis of the wall of the pharynx is formed mainly by the three pairs of constrictors—superior, middle and inferior (Plate 14.4, Table 14.5 and Flowchart 14.4). The *inferior constrictor* consists of two parts: *thyropharyngeus* and *cricopharyngeus*.

***Median raphe:*** All the constrictors of the pharynx are inserted into a median raphe on the posterior wall of the pharynx. The upper end of the raphe reaches the base of the skull where it is attached to the pharyngeal tubercle on the basilar part of the occipital bone (Fig. 14.22).

*Note*: The origins of the constrictors are situated anteriorly in relation to the posterior openings of the nose—the mouth and the larynx. From here their fibres pass into the lateral and posterior walls of the pharynx, the fibres of the two sides meeting in the midline in a fibrous raphe.

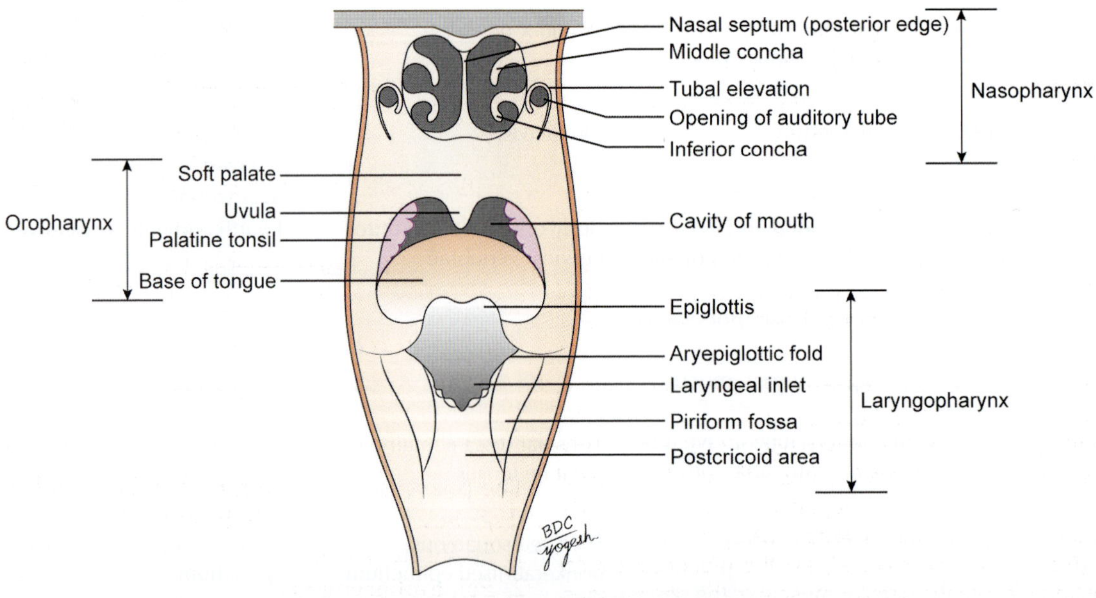


**Fig. 14.19:** Three regions of the pharynx

**Plate 14.3:** Interior of the pharynx (posterior view, the pharynx opened from behind)

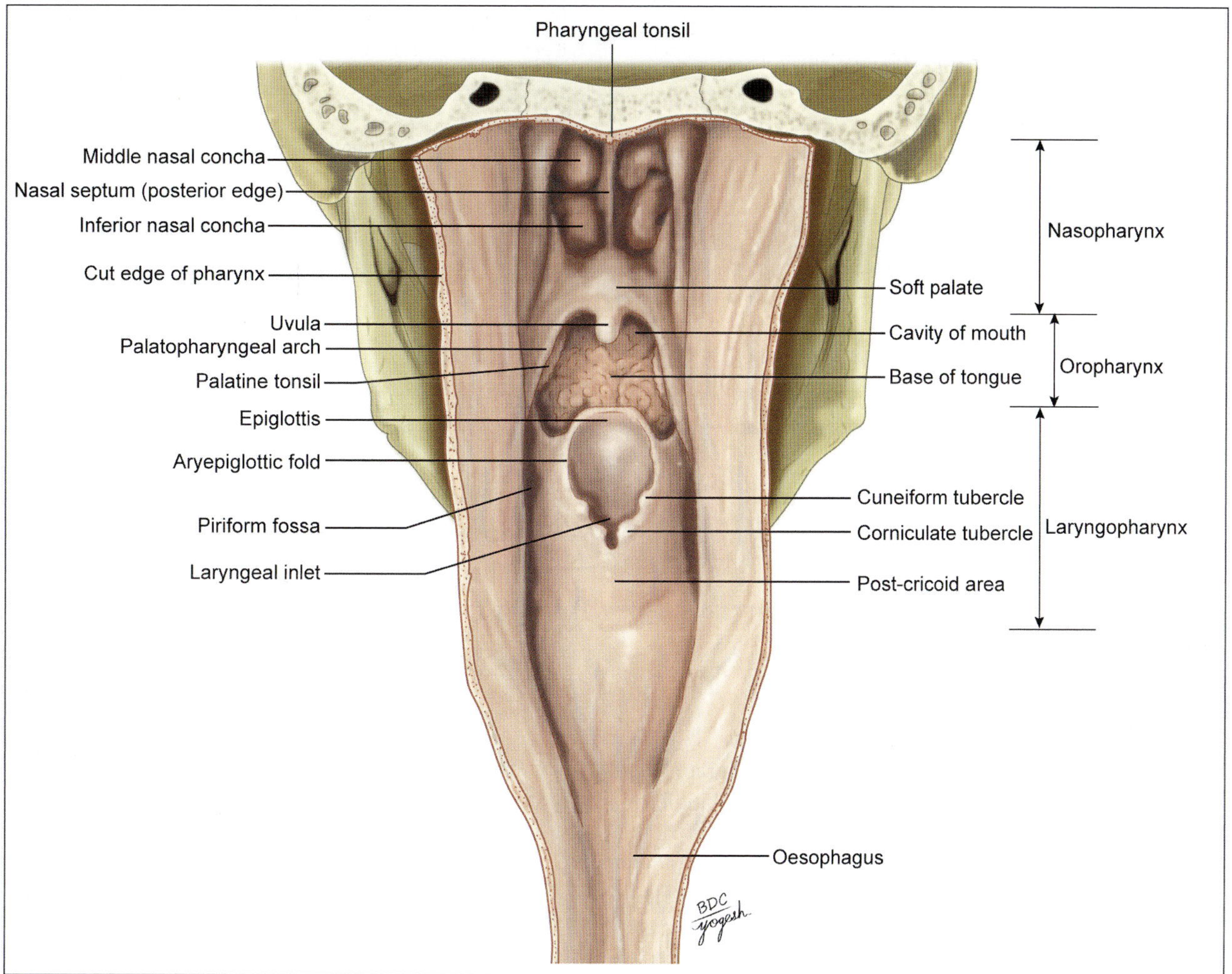


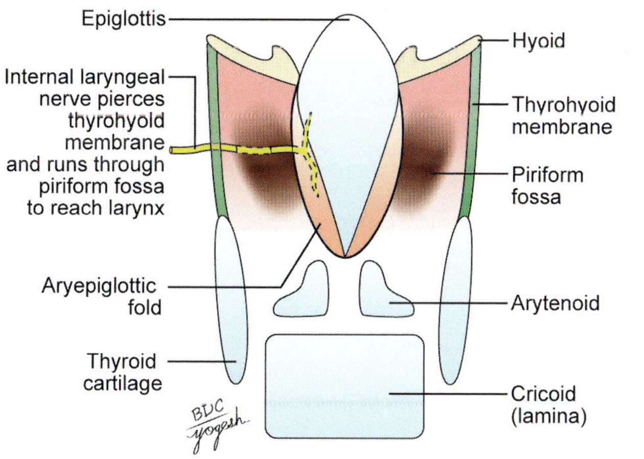


**Fig. 14.20:** Posterior view of the piriform fossa after removal of the tongue: Internal laryngeal nerve is shown only on left side

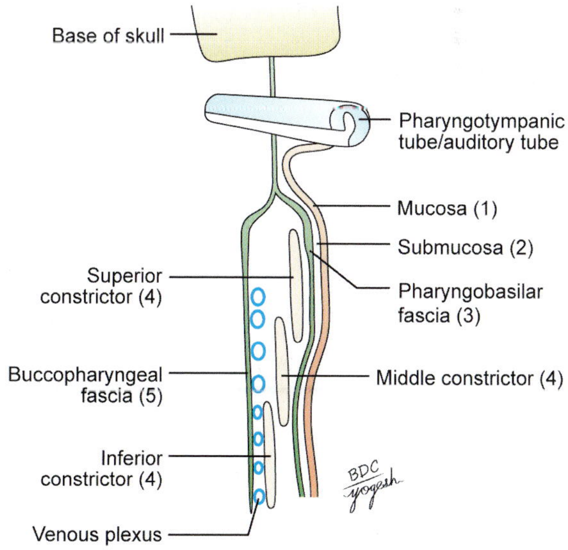


**Fig. 14.21:** Structure of the pharynx

The three constrictors are so arranged that the inferior overlaps middle which in turn overlaps the superior. The fibres of the superior constrictor reach the base of skull posteriorly, in the middle line. On the sides, however, there is a gap between the base of the skull and the upper edge of the superior constrictor. This gap is closed by the ***pharyngobasilar fascia*** which is thickened in this situation (Fig. 14.21). The lower edge of the inferior constrictor becomes continuous with the circular muscle of the oesophagus. These muscles develop from IV arch.

### *Longitudinal Muscle Coat*

The pharynx has three muscles that run longitudinally (Fig. 14.23, Flowchart 14.5, Table 14.6):

1. Stylopharyngeus
2. Palatopharyngeus
3. Salpingopharyngeus

**Plate 14.4:** Constrictors of the pharynx

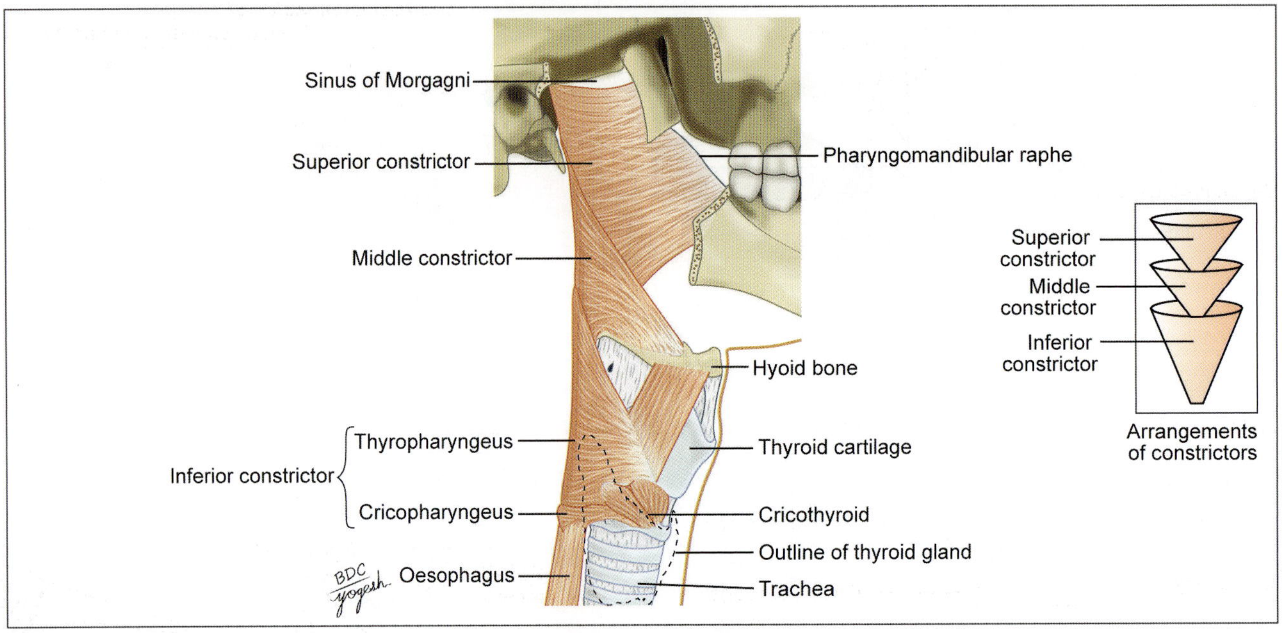


**TABLE 14.5: Constrictor muscles of pharynx**

| *Muscle* | *Origin* | *Insertion* |
|---|---|---|
| Superior constrictor | Pterygoid hamulus<br>Pterygomandibular raphe<br>Medial surface of mandible at the posterior end of mylohyoid line<br>Side of posterior part of the tongue | Pharyngeal tubercle on the base of skull<br>Median fibrous raphe |
| Middle constrictor | Lower part of stylohyoid ligament<br>Lesser cornua of hyoid bone<br>Upper border of greater cornua of hyoid bone | Median fibrous raphe |
| Inferior constrictor: Two parts— | | |
| 1. Thyropharyngeus | Oblique line on lamina of thyroid cartilage<br>Tendinous band between inferior tubercle of thyroid cartilage and cricoid cartilage | Median fibrous raphe |
| 2. Cricopharyngeus | Cricoid cartilage | Median fibrous raphe |

**TABLE 14.6: Longitudinal muscles of pharynx**

| *Muscle* | *Origin* | *Insertion* | *Nerve supply* |
|---|---|---|---|
| Stylopharyngeus | Styloid process | Posterior border of lamina of thyroid cartilage | Glossopharyngeal nerve |
| Palatopharyngeus | Arises by two fasciculi (anterior and posterior) from upper surface of palatine aponeurosis | Posterior border of lamina of thyroid cartilage<br>Few fibres run posteriorly to form *Passavant's ridge* | Cranial root of 11th cranial nerve |
| Salpingopharyngeus | Lower part of the cartilage of auditory tube | Posterior border of lamina of thyroid cartilage | Cranial root of 11th cranial nerve |

*Note: Action of longitudinal muscles of pharynx*: Elevate the larynx and shorten the pharynx during deglutition.

All these muscles are inserted on the *posterior border of lamina of thyroid cartilage*. These muscles elevate the larynx and shorten the pharynx during swallowing.

### Structures in between Pharyngeal Muscles (Fig. 14.24)

1. The *large gap between the upper concave border of the superior constrictor and the base of the skull* is semilunar and is known as the ***sinus of Morgagni***. It is closed by the upper strong part of the pharyngobasilar fascia. The structures passing through this gap are (Fig. 14.24):
   a. Auditory tube
   b. Levator veli palatini muscle
   c. Ascending palatine artery
   d. Palatine branch of ascending pharyngeal artery.

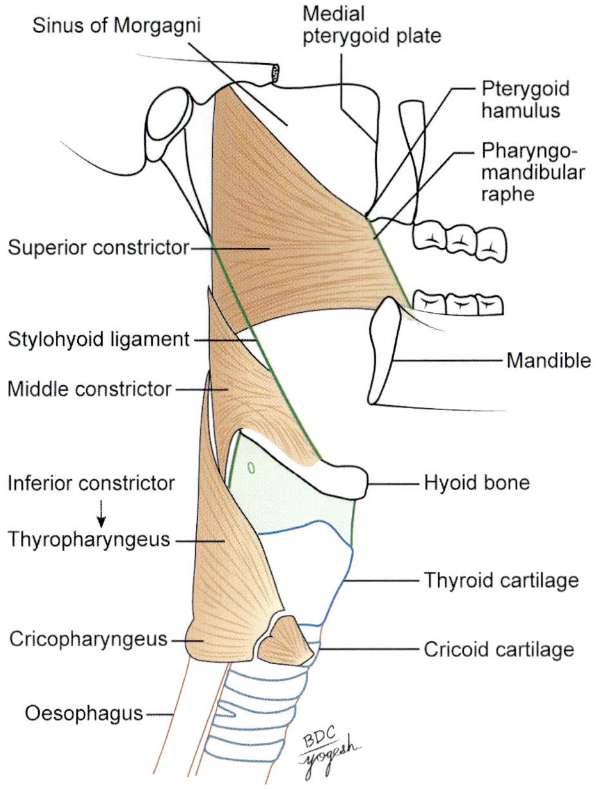


**Fig. 14.22:** Constrictors of the pharynx

**Flowchart 14.4:** Constrictor muscles of pharynx

***Constrictor muscles of pharynx***

| ***Muscle*** | ***Origin*** | ***Insertion*** |
|---|---|---|
| Superior | Pterygoid hamulus<br>Pterygomandibular raphe<br>Mandible at posterior end of mylohyoid line, side of tongue | Pharyngeal tubercle<br>Median raphe |
| Middle | Lower part of stylohyoid ligament<br>Lesser cornua, upper border of greater cornua of hyoid bone | Median raphe |
| Inferior<br>A. Thyro-pharyngeus | Oblique line on lamina of thyroid cartilage | Median raphe |
| B. Crico-pharyngeus | Cricoid cartilage | Median raphe |

***Nerve supply:*** Cranial root of accessory nerve

2. The structures passing through the *gap between the superior and middle constrictors* are:
   a. Stylopharyngeus muscle
   b. Glossopharyngeal nerve.
3. The structures passing through the *gap between the middle and inferior constrictors are:*
   a. Internal laryngeal nerve
   b. Superior laryngeal vessels
4. The structures passing through the *gap between the lower border of the inferior constrictor and the oesophagus* are:
   a. Recurrent laryngeal nerve
   b. Inferior laryngeal vessels.

**Flowchart 14.5:** Longitudinal muscles of pharynx

***Longitudinal muscles of pharynx***

Elevate, shorten the pharynx

| ***Muscle*** | ***Origin*** | ***Insertion*** |
|---|---|---|
| Stylopharyngeus | Styloid process | Posterior border of lamina of thyroid cartilage |
| Palatopharyngeus | Upper surface of palatine aponeurosis | Posterior border of lamina of thyroid cartilage |
| Salpingopharyngeus | Lower part of cartilage of auditory tube | Posterior border of lamina of thyroid cartilage |

***Nerve supply:*** Stylopharyngeus by glossopharyngeal nerve, palatopharyngeus and salpingopharyngeus by cranial root of XI cranial nerve

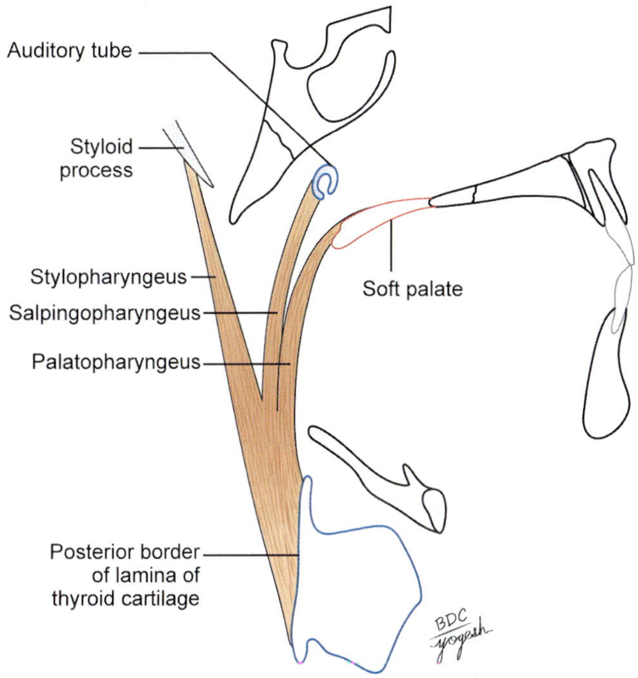


**Fig. 14.23:** Longitudinal muscles of pharynx

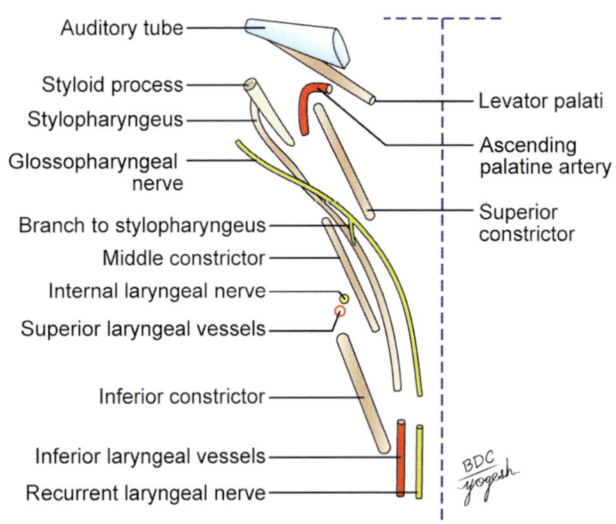


**Fig. 14.24:** Schematic coronal section through the pharynx, showing the gaps between pharyngeal muscles and the structures related to them

## DISSECTION

Define the attachments of middle and inferior constrictors of pharynx, and the structures situated traversing through the gaps between the three constrictor muscles. Identify structures above the superior constrictor muscle and below the inferior constrictor muscle.

Cut through the tensor veli palatini and reflect it downwards. Remove the fascia and identify the mandibular nerve again with otic ganglion medial to it. Identify the branches of the mandibular nerve. Locate the middle meningeal artery at the foramen spinosum, as it lies just posterior to mandibular nerve.

*Competency:*

**AN36.7** Describe the clinical significance of Killian's dehiscence.

### Killian's Dehiscence

***Zenker's diverticulum*** (*hypopharyngeal diverticulum*) or pharyngeal pouch is a diverticulum of pharyngeal mucosa, just above the cricopharyngeus muscle. *Killian dehiscence* is a weak posterior part of the pharyngeal wall that lies between cricopharyngeus and thyropharyngeus parts of the inferior constrictor of pharynx (Figs 14.25a and b and Flowchart 14.6).

In case of the excessive pressure within the lower part of pharynx, the mucosa of the pharyngeal wall balloon out through the Killian dehiscence to form Zenker's diverticulum. It may result due to neuromuscular incoordination or spasm of cricopharyngeus muscle. It occurs because the two parts of the inferior constrictor have different nerve supplies. The propulsive thyropharyngeus is supplied by the pharyngeal plexus and the sphincteric cricopharyngeus is supplied by the recurrent laryngeal nerve. In neuromuscular incoordination, if the cricopharyngeus fails to relax when the thyropharyngeus contracts, the bolus of food is pushed backward and tends to produce a diverticulum.

Signs and symptoms of Zenker's diverticulum:

1. Asymptomatic
2. Dysphagia (difficulty in swallowing)
3. Regurgitation of food
4. Cough.

It can be diagnosed using:

1. Barium swallow radiography
2. Endoscopy.

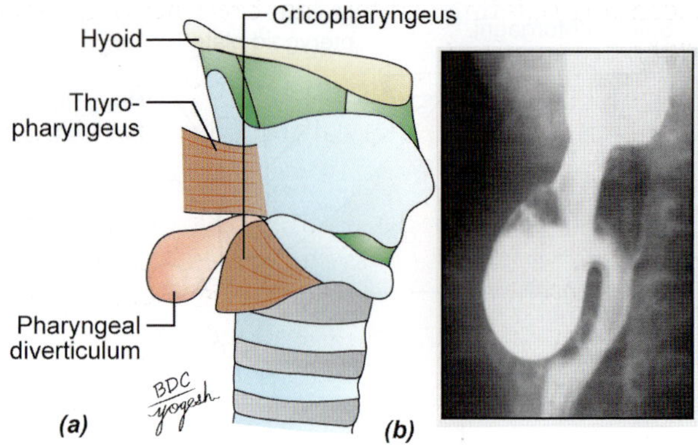


**Figs 14.25a and b:** (a) Pharyngeal diverticulum and (b) pharyngeal diverticulum after barium swallow

### Nerve Supply of Pharynx

The pharynx is supplied by the pharyngeal plexus of nerves which lies chiefly on the middle constrictor. The plexus is formed by:

1. Pharyngeal branch of the vagus carrying fibres of the cranial accessory nerve.
2. Pharyngeal branches of the glossopharyngeal nerve.
3. Pharyngeal branches of the superior cervical sympathetic ganglion.

***Motor fibres*** are derived from the cranial accessory nerve through the branches of the vagus. They supply all muscles of pharynx, except the stylopharyngeus which is supplied by the glossopharyngeal nerve.

The inferior constrictor receives an additional supply from the external and recurrent laryngeal nerves.

***Sensory fibres*** or general visceral afferent from the pharynx travel mostly through the glossopharyngeal nerve, and partly through the vagus. However, the nasopharynx is supplied by the maxillary nerve through the pterygopalatine ganglion; and the soft palate and tonsil by the lesser palatine and glossopharyngeal nerves.

***Taste sensations*** from the vallecula and epiglottic area pass through the internal laryngeal branch of the vagus.

The parasympathetic ***secretomotor fibres*** to the pharynx are derived from the lesser palatine branches of the pterygopalatine ganglion.

### Blood Supply of Pharynx

The pharynx is supplied by:

1. Ascending pharyngeal branch of the external carotid.

**Flowchart 14.6:** Killian dehiscence Zenker's diverticulum

**Zenker's diverticulum**

- ***Definition***
  - Pharyngeal pouch
  - Diverticulum of pharyngeal mucosa
- ***Killian dehiscence***
  - Weak part of posterior pharyngeal wall
  - Lies between cricopharyngeus and thyropharyngeus
- ***Formation***
  - Excessive pressure in pharynx → Balooning of pharyngeal mucosa through Killian dehiscence → Formation of Zenker's diverticulum
- ***Cause***
  - Neuromuscular incoordination
- ***Signs and symptoms***
  1. Asymptomatic
  2. Dysphagia
  3. Regurgitation of food
  4. Cough
- ***Diagnosis***
  1. Barium swallow radiography
  2. Endoscopy

2. Ascending palatine and tonsillar branches of the facial artery.
3. Dorsal lingual branches of the lingual artery.
4. Greater palatine, pharyngeal and pterygoid branches of the maxillary artery.

The veins form a plexus on the posterolateral aspect of the pharynx. The plexus receives blood from the pharynx, the soft palate and the prevertebral region. It drains into the internal jugular and facial veins.

### Lymphatic Drainage of Pharynx

Lymph from the pharynx drains into the retropharyngeal and deep cervical lymph nodes.

### Deglutition (Swallowing)

Swallowing of food occurs in three stages described below. Muscles of pharynx act during swallowing.

#### *First Stage*

1. This stage is voluntary in character.
2. The anterior part of the tongue is raised and pressed against the hard palate by the intrinsic muscles of the tongue, especially the superior longitudinal and transverse muscles. The movement takes place from anterior to the posterior side. This pushes the food bolus (Greek *lump*) into the posterior part of the oral cavity.
3. The soft palate closes down onto the back of the tongue, and helps to form the bolus.
4. Next, the hyoid bone is moved upwards and forwards by the suprahyoid muscles. The posterior part of the tongue is elevated upwards and backwards by the styloglossi; and the palatoglossal arches are approximated by the palatoglossi. This pushes the bolus through the oropharyngeal isthmus to the oropharynx, and the second stage begins.

#### *Second Stage*

1. It is involuntary in character. During this stage, the food is pushed from the oropharynx to the lower part of the laryngopharynx.
2. The nasopharyngeal isthmus is closed by elevation of the soft palate by levator veli palatini and tensor veli palatini and by its approximation to the posterior pharyngeal wall (ridge of Passavant). This prevents the food bolus from entering the nose.
3. The inlet of larynx is closed by approximation of the aryepiglottic folds by aryepiglottic and oblique arytenoid. This prevents the food bolus from entering the larynx.
4. Next, the larynx and pharynx are elevated behind the hyoid bone by the longitudinal muscles of the pharynx. Then the bolus is pushed down over the posterior surface of the epiglottis, the closed inlet of the larynx and the posterior surface of the arytenoid cartilages, by gravity, and by contraction of the superior and middle constrictors and the palatopharyngeus.

#### *Third Stage*

1. This is also involuntary in character. In this stage, food passes from the lower part of the pharynx to the oesophagus.
2. This is brought about by the inferior constrictors of the pharynx.

### Development of Pharynx

The primitive gut extends from the buccopharyngeal membrane cranially, to the cloacal membrane caudally. It is divided into four parts—the pharynx, the foregut, the midgut and the hindgut. The pharynx extends from buccopharyngeal membrane to the tracheobronchial diverticulum. It is divided into upper part, the nasopharynx; middle part, the oropharynx; and the lower part, the laryngopharynx.

***Competency:***
**AN36.4** Describe the components and functions of Waldeyer's lymphatic ring.

### Waldeyer's Lymphatic Ring

In relation to the naso-oropharyngeal isthmus, there are several aggregations of lymphoid tissue that constitute Waldeyer's lymphatic ring (Fig. 14.26). The most important aggregations are the right and left palatine tonsils usually referred to simply as the tonsils. Posteriorly and above, there is the nasopharyngeal tonsil; laterally and above, there are the tubal tonsils, and inferiorly, there is the lingual tonsil over the posterior part of the dorsum of the tongue. [*Mnemonics: Tonsils: The four types "PPLT (people) have tonsils":* **P**haryngeal, **P**alatine, **L**ingual, **T**ubal].

### CLINICAL ANATOMY

1. Hypertrophy or enlargement of the nasopharyngeal tonsil or adenoids may obstruct the posterior nasal aperture and may interfere with nasal respiration and speech leading to mouth breathing. These tonsils usually regress by puberty.
2. Hypertrophy of the tubal tonsil may occlude the auditory or pharyngotympanic tube leading to middle ear problems.

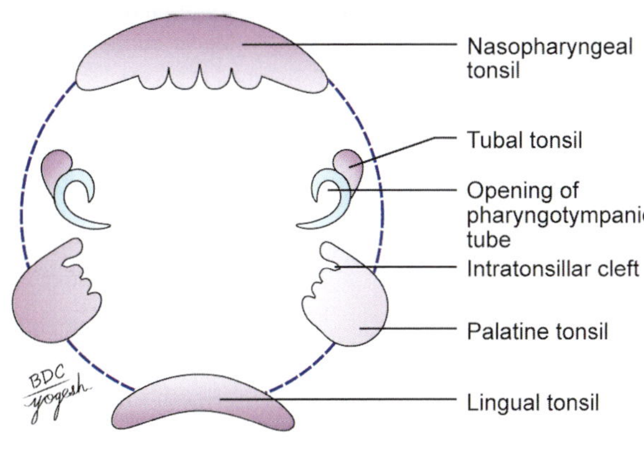


**Fig. 14.26:** Waldeyer's lymphatic ring

**Competencies:**

**AN36.2** Describe the (1) morphology, relations, blood supply and applied anatomy of palatine tonsil, (2) composition of soft palate.

**AN40.2** Describe and demonstrate the boundaries, contents, relations and functional anatomy of middle ear and auditory tube.

## PALATINE TONSIL (THE TONSIL)

The palatine tonsil (Latin *swelling*) occupies the ***tonsillar sinus*** or ***fossa*** between the palatoglossal and palatopharyngeal arches (Fig. 14.27 and Flowchart 14.7). It can be seen through the mouth.

### Features

The tonsil is almond-shaped. It has two surfaces—medial and lateral; two borders—anterior and posterior; and two poles—upper and lower.

1. ***Medial surface*** is covered by stratified squamous epithelium continuous with that of the mouth. This surface has 12 to 15 crypts. The largest of these is called the ***intratonsillar cleft***.
2. ***Lateral surface*** is covered by a sheet of fascia which forms the hemicapsule of the tonsil. The capsule is an extension of the pharyngobasilar fascia. It is only loosely attached to the muscular wall of the pharynx, formed here by the superior constrictor and by the styloglossus, but anteroinferiorly the capsule is firmly adherent to the side of the tongue (suspensory ligament of tonsil) just in front of the insertion of the palatoglossus and the palatopharyngeus muscle. This firm attachment keeps the tonsil in place during swallowing.

The ***bed of the tonsil*** is formed from within outwards by:

a. Pharyngobasilar fascia
b. Superior constrictor and palatopharyngeus muscles
c. Buccopharyngeal fascia
d. In the lower part, the styloglossus
e. Glossopharyngeal nerve.

Still more laterally, there is the facial artery with its tonsillar and ascending palatine branches. The

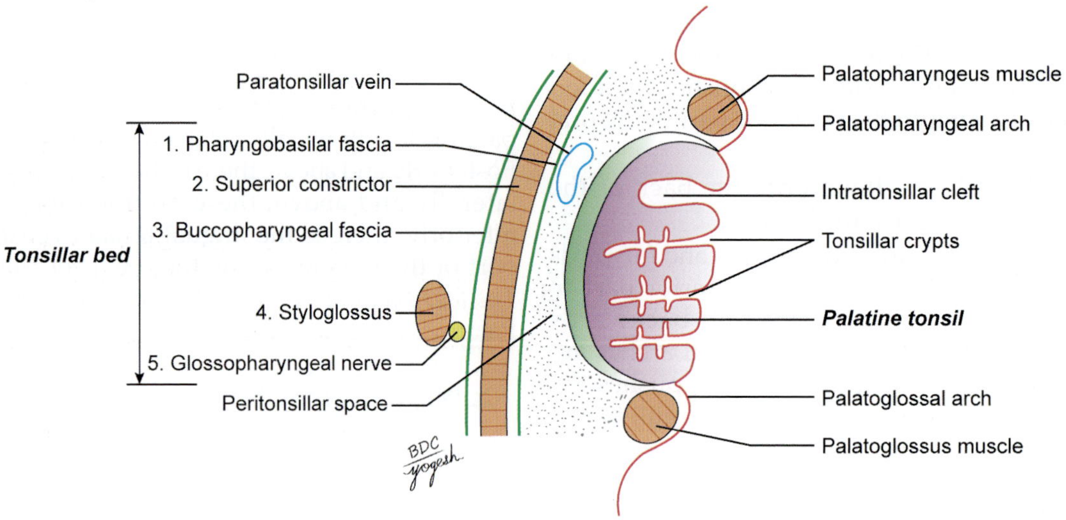


**Fig. 14.27:** Horizontal section through the tonsil showing its deep relations

**Flowchart 14.7:** Palatine tonsil

***Palatine tonsil***

Almond-shaped mass

***Location***
- In the lateral wall of oropharynx
- In tonsillar fossa:
  - Boundaries
  - Anterior: palatoglossal arch
  - Posterior: palatopharyngeal arch
  - Apex: Soft palate
  - Base: Posterior 1/3rd of tongue

***Tonsillar bed***
- Pharyngobasillar fascia
- Superior constrictor
- Buccopharyngeal fascia
- Styloglossus
- Glossopharyngeal nerve

***External features***
- Medial surface
  - Free
  - Lined by nonkeratinized stratified squamous epithelium
- Tonsillar pits (12–15)
- Tonsillar crypts
- Intratonsillar cleft
- Lateral surface
  - covered by capsule
- Anterior border
  - related to palatoglossal arch
- Posterior border
  - related to palatopharyngeal arch
- Upper pole:
  - Reach soft palate
- Lower pole:
  - Suspensory ligament of tonsil

***Supply***
- Arterial supply
  - Tonsillar branches of facial artery
  - Ascending palatine branch of facial artery
  - Dorsal lingual branches of lingual artery
  - Ascending pharyngeal branches of external carotid artery
  - Greater palatine branches of maxillary artery
- ***Venous drainage***
  - Paratonsillar vein
  - Pharyngeal plexus
- ***Lymphatic drainage***
  - Jugulodigastric nodes
- ***Innervation***
  - Glossopharyngeal nerve
  - Greater and lesser palatine branches of pterygopalatine ganglion

***Clinical***
- Tonsillitis
- Tonsillectomy
- Quinsy
- Ear pain in tonsillitis
- Postoperative haemorrhage in tonsillectomy

BDC yogesh

internal carotid artery is 2.5 cm posterolateral to the tonsil.

3. ***Anterior border*** is related to the palatoglossal arch with its muscle.
4. ***Posterior border*** is related to the palatopharyngeal arch with its muscle.
5. ***Upper pole*** is related to the soft palate, and the *lower pole*, to the tongue.
6. ***Plica triangularis*** is a triangular vestigial fold of mucous membrane covering the anteroinferior part of the tonsil.
7. ***Plica semilunaris*** is a similar semilunar fold that may cross the upper part of the tonsillar sinus.
8. ***Intratonsillar cleft*** is the largest crypt of the tonsil. It is present in its upper part. It is sometimes wrongly named the supratonsillar fossa. The mouth of cleft is semilunar in shape and parallel to dorsum of tongue. It represents the internal opening of the second pharyngeal pouch. A peritonsillar abscess or quinsy often begins in this cleft.

### Arterial Supply of Tonsil

1. *Main source*: Tonsillar branch of facial artery (Fig. 14.28).
2. *Additional sources*:
   a. Ascending palatine branch of facial artery
   b. Dorsal lingual branches of the lingual artery
   c. Ascending pharyngeal branch of the external carotid artery
   d. Greater palatine branch of the maxillary artery.

### Venous Drainage

One or more paratonsillar veins leave the lower part of deep surface of the tonsil, pierce the superior constrictor, and join the palatine, pharyngeal, or facial veins.

*Note*: The tonsillar artery enters the tonsil by piercing the superior constrictor just behind the firm attachment.

The palatine vein or external palatine or ***paratonsillar vein*** descends from the palate in the loose areolar tissue on the lateral surface of the capsule, and crosses the tonsil before piercing the wall of the pharynx. The vein may be injured during removal of the tonsil or tonsillectomy.

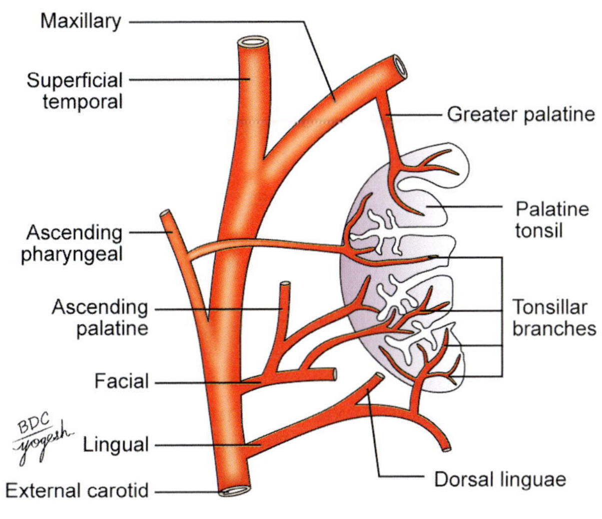


**Fig. 14.28:** Arterial supply of palatine tonsil

### Lymphatic Drainage

Lymphatics pass to *jugulodigastric nodes*. There are no afferent lymphatics to the tonsil.

### Nerve Supply

1. Glossopharyngeal nerve.
2. Greater and lesser palatine nerves from the pterygopalatine ganglion.

***Competencies:***

**AN43.2** Identify, describe and draw the microanatomy of pituitary gland, thyroid, parathyroid gland, tongue, salivary glands, tonsil, cornea, retina.

**AN36.6** Describe the anatomical basis of tonsillitis, tonsillectomy, adenoids and peritonsillar abscess. Microanatomy of tonsil is described here. For the other tissues please see respective chapters.

### Histology of Tonsil

A section of palatine tonsil shows (Plate 14.5):

1. Lining epithelium
2. Tonsillar crypts
3. Lymphatic follicles.

The oral surface of the palatine tonsil is covered by nonkeratinized stratified squamous epithelium. The epithelium invaginates internal surface of tonsil and forms tonsillar crypts. Tonsillar crypts are lined by nonkeratinized stratified squamous epithelium. Epithelium and even the lumen of crypts may show invaginated lymphocytes. It is difficult to find boundary between epithelium and lymphoid tissue.

Laterally, tonsil is bounded by connective tissue capsule and has some efferent lymphatic vessels. Just beneath epithelium, palatine tonsil shows dense aggregation of lymphatic follicles. Lymphatic follicles are supported by meshwork of reticular fibres.

### Development of Tonsil

Palatine tonsil develops from two sources:

1. Endoderm of second pharyngeal pouch
2. Mesoderm (lymphocytes).

#### *Stages of Development*

1. During the 3rd month of development, ventral part of the 2nd pouch proliferates outwards in surrounding mesoderm as several solid cords called tonsillar buds.
2. On degeneration of central cells, tonsillar buds cannulate to form hollow tonsillar crypts.
3. During 3rd to 5th month, lymphocytes aggregate on the mesoderm that surrounds crypts and forms lymphatic follicles.
4. Mesodermal cells condense to form a capsule of the tonsil. Lymphocyte proliferates and forms pharyngeal tonsillar bulging. The remnant of the pouch is represented by an intratonsillar cleft and tonsillar fossa.

**Plate 14.5:** Histology of palatine tonsil

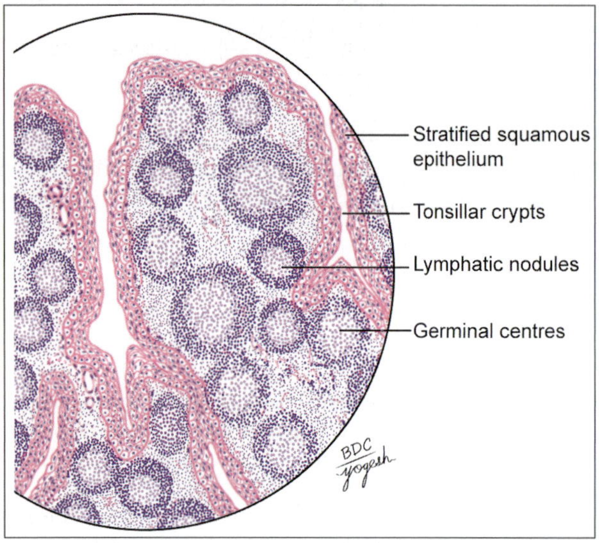


## CLINICAL ANATOMY

1. The tonsils are large in children. They retrogress after puberty.
2. ***Tonsillitis***: The tonsils are frequently sites of infection, especially in children. Infection may spread to surrounding tissue forming a peritonsillar abscess.
3. Enlarged and infected tonsils often require surgical removal. The operation is called ***tonsillectomy***. A knowledge of the relationship of the tonsil is of importance to the surgeon.
4. Tonsillectomy is usually done by the ***guillotine method***. Haemorrhage after tonsillectomy is checked by removal of clot from the raw tonsillar bed. This is to be compared with the method for checking postpartum haemorrhage from the uterus. These are the only two organs in the body where bleeding is checked by removal of clots. In other parts of the body, clot formation is encouraged.
5. Tonsillitis may cause ***referred pain*** in the ear as glossopharyngeal nerve supplies both these areas.
6. Suppuration in the peritonsillar area is called ***quinsy***. A peritonsillar abscess is drained by making an incision in the most prominent point of the abscess.
7. Tonsils are often sites of a septic focus. Such a focus can lead to serious disease like pulmonary tuberculosis, meningitis, etc. and is often the cause of general ill health.

## PHARYNGOTYMPANIC TUBE

Auditory tube is also known as the pharyngotympanic tube or the eustachian tube.

The auditory tube is a trumpet-shaped channel that connects the middle ear cavity with the nasopharynx (Figs 14.29a and b).

### Measurements

It is about 4 cm long, and is directed downwards, forwards and medially. It forms an angle of 45° with the sagittal plane and 30° with the horizontal plane.

### Parts

The tube is divided into bony and cartilaginous parts.

#### *Bony Part*

The bony part forms the posterior and lateral one-third of the tube. It is 12 mm long, and lies in the petrous temporal bone near the tympanic plate. Its lateral end is wide and opens on the anterior wall of the middle ear cavity. The medial end is narrow (isthmus) and is jagged for attachment of the cartilaginous part. The lumen of the tube is oblong being widest from side-toside.

#### *Relations*

1. *Superior:* Canal for the tensor tympani.
2. *Medial:* Carotid canal.
3. *Lateral:* Chorda tympani, spine of sphenoid, auriculotemporal nerve and the temporomandibular joint.

#### *Cartilaginous Part*

The cartilaginous part forms the anterior and medial two-thirds of the tube. It is 25 mm long, and lies in the sulcus tubae, a groove between the greater wing of the sphenoid and the apex of the petrous temporal. It is made up of a triangular plate of cartilage which is curled to form the superior and medial walls of the tube. The lateral wall and floor are completed by a fibrous membrane. The apex of the plate is attached to the medial end of the bony part. The base is free and forms the tubal elevation in the nasopharynx.

#### *Relations*

1. *Anterolaterally:* Tensor veli palatini, mandibular nerve and its branches, otic ganglion, chorda tympani, middle meningeal artery and medial pterygoid plate.
2. *Posteromedially:* Petrous temporal and levator veli palatini.
3. The levator veli palatini is attached to its inferior surface, and the salpingopharyngeus to lower part near the pharyngeal opening.

### Vascular Supply

The arterial supply of the tube is derived from the ascending pharyngeal and middle meningeal arteries and the artery of the pterygoid canal. The veins drain into the pharyngeal and pterygoid plexuses of veins. Lymphatics pass to the retropharyngeal nodes.

### Nerve Supply

1. At the ostium, by the pharyngeal branch of the pterygopalatine ganglion suspended by the maxillary nerve.
2. Cartilaginous part, by the nervus spinosus branch of mandibular nerve.
3. Bony part, by the tympanic plexus formed by glossopharyngeal nerve.

### Functions

1. The tube provides a communication of the middle ear cavity with the exterior, thus ensuring equal air pressure on both sides of the tympanic membrane.
2. The tube is usually closed. It opens during swallowing, yawning and sneezing, by the actions of the tensor and levator veli palatini muscles.

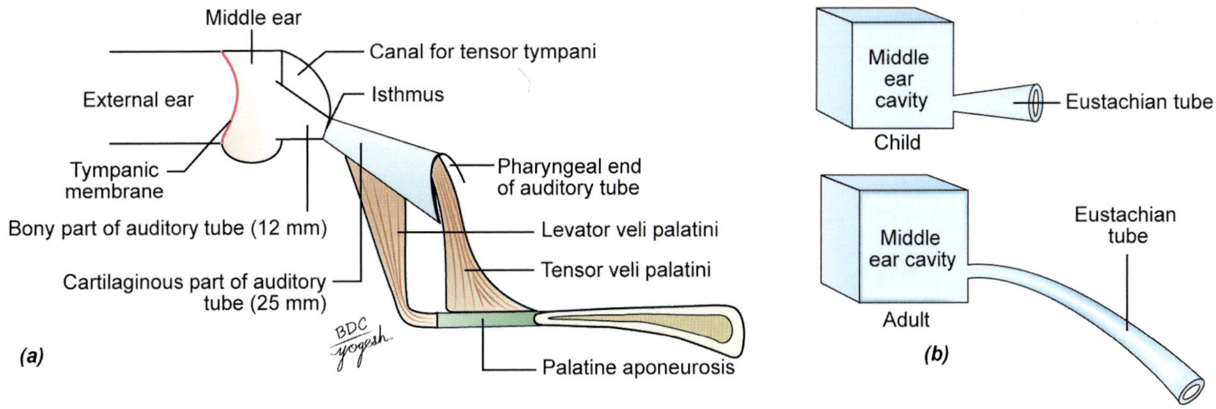


**Figs 14.29a and b:** (a) Scheme showing anatomy of auditory tube and external auditory meatus and (b) differences in Eustachian tube in an adult and a child

## CLINICAL ANATOMY

- Infections may pass from the throat to the middle ear through the auditory tube. This is more common in children because the tube is shorter, wider and straighter in them.
- Inflammation of the auditory tube (Eustachian catarrh) is often secondary to an attack of common cold, or of sore throat. This causes pain in the ear which is aggravated by swallowing, due to blockage of the tube. Pain is relieved by instillation of decongestant drops in the nose, which help to open the ostium. The ostium is commonly blocked in children by enlargement of the tubal tonsil.

VIDEO

**Video 3.14 Pharynx:** Introduction, Muscles of pharynx, Palate

## *Facts to Remember*

- Upper teeth are supplied by branches of maxillary nerve.
- Lower teeth are supplied by branches of mandibular nerve.
- All the 3 constrictors and 2 longitudinal muscles of pharynx are supplied by vagoaccessory complex, only stylopharyngeus is supplied by IX nerve.
- All the muscles of soft palate are supplied by vagoaccessory complex except tensor veli palatini, supplied by V3 nerve.
- Tonsils have only efferent lymph vessels but no afferent lymph vessel.
- Killian's dehiscence is a potential gap between thyropharyngeus and cricopharyngeus.
- Waldeyer's ring consists of lingual tonsil, palatine tonsils, tubal tonsils and nasopharyngeal tonsils.
- Tonsillar branch of facial artery is the main artery of the palatine tonsil.
- Common source of bleeding after tonsillectomy is paratonsillar vein.
- Quinsy is the chronic infection of peritonsillar space.

## BDC's Anatomy e-book

1. Molecular regulation of tooth development
2. Morphology of palatopharyngeus
3. Further reading
4. Viva voce questions

Chapter

# 15

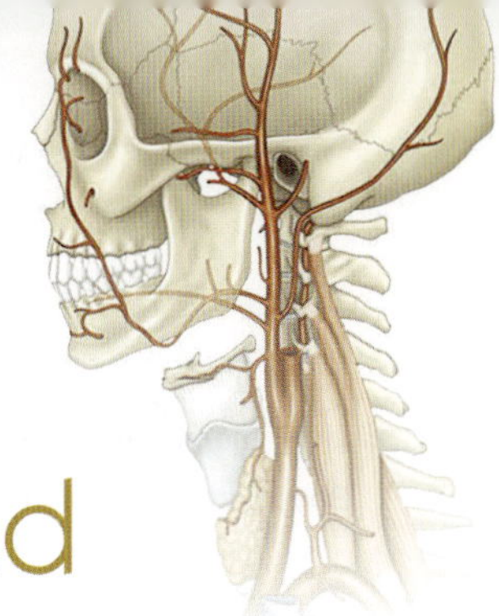

# Nose, Paranasal Sinuses and Pterygopalatine Fossa

## NOSE

The nose performs two functions. It is a respiratory passage. It is also the organ of smell. The receptors for smell are placed in the upper one-third of the nasal cavity. This part is lined by olfactory mucosa. The rest of the nasal cavity is lined by respiratory mucosa. The respiratory mucosa is highly vascular and warms the inspired air.

For descriptive purposes, the nose is divided into two main parts, the external nose and nasal cavity.

### EXTERNAL NOSE

The external nose presents the following features:

1. *Tip* or apex is lower free end.
2. *Root* or bridge is an upper narrow part which is continuous with the forehead.
3. *Dorsum* is a rounded border between the tip and root.
4. *Nostrils* or nares are two piriform apertures at the lower ends of the nose.
5. *Ala* is a lower flared part on the side of nose.
6. *Nasal septum* separates the nostrils.

The external nose has a skeletal framework that is partly bony and partly cartilaginous. The bones are the nasal bones, which form the bridge of the nose, and the frontal processes of the maxillae. The cartilages are the superior and inferior nasal cartilages, the septal cartilage, and small alar cartilages (Fig. 15.1).

The ***skin over the external nose*** is supplied by the external nasal, infratrochlear and infraorbital nerves.

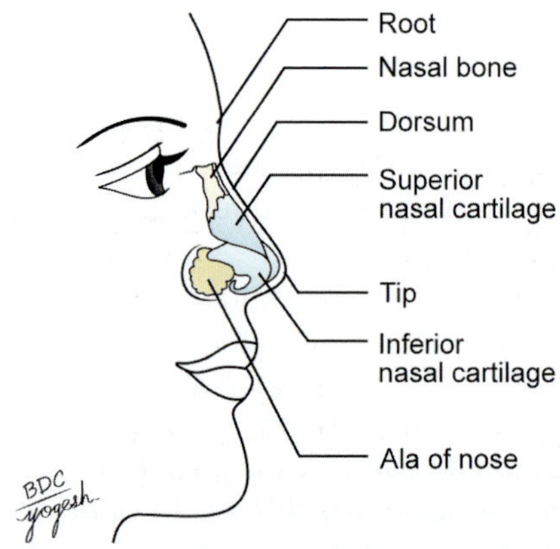


**Fig. 15.1:** Skeleton of the external nose

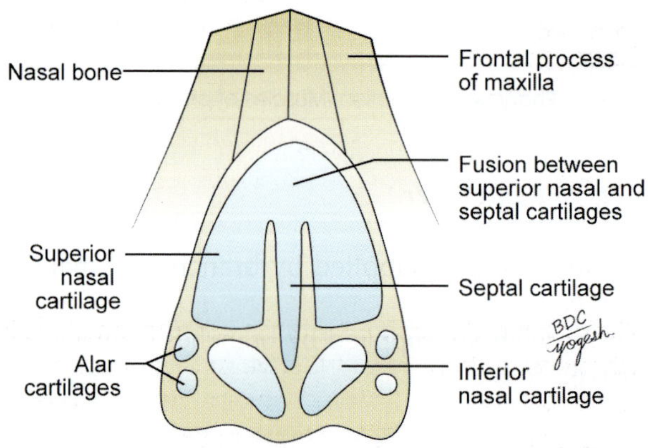


**Fig. 15.2:** Osseocartilaginous framework of the external nose

### NASAL CAVITY

The nasal cavity extends from the external nares or nostrils to the posterior nasal apertures, and is subdivided into right and left halves by the nasal septum (Figs 15.2 and 15.3).

#### *Divisions*

Each cavity is divided into two parts:

1. *Vestibule*: It is a small anterior part lined by skin.
2. *Nasal cavity proper*: It is large posterosuperior part lined by nasal mucosa.

#### Vestibule of Nose

The vestibule of nose is a small anteroinferior part of nasal cavity. It is lined by skin which contains sebaceous glands and hairs. ***Vibrissae*** are stiff interlacing hairs of the vestibule. ***Limen nasi*** is a ridge between the vestibule and the nasal cavity proper. ***Columella*** is a median lower part of the nose separating the right and left vestibules of nose.

#### Nasal Cavity Proper

##### *Boundaries*

Each half has a roof, a floor, and medial and lateral walls. Each half measures about 5 cm in height, 5–7 cm

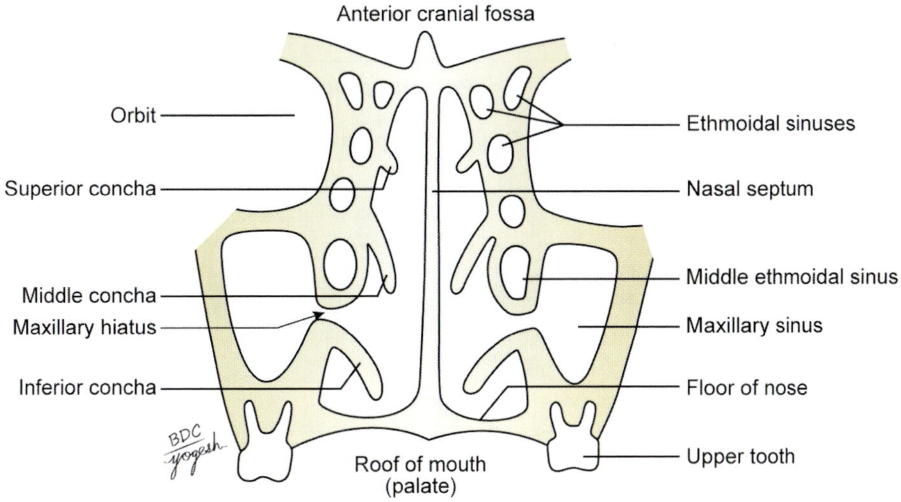


**Fig. 15.3:** Coronal section through the nasal cavity and the maxillary air sinuses

in length, and 1.5 cm in width near the floor. The width near the roof is only 1–2 mm.

1. ***Roof*** is about 7 cm long and 2 mm wide. It slopes downwards, both in front and behind. The middle horizontal part is formed by the cribriform plate of the ethmoid. The anterior slope is formed by the nasal part of the frontal bone, nasal bone, and the nasal cartilages. The posterior slope is formed by the inferior surface of the body of the sphenoid bone.
2. ***Floor*** is about 5 cm long and 1.5 cm wide. It is formed by the palatine process of the maxilla and the horizontal plate of the palatine bone. It is concave from side-to-side and is slightly higher anteriorly than posteriorly (Fig. 15.2).
3. ***Medial wall*** is formed by the nasal septum.
4. ***Lateral wall*** of nose is irregular and has shelf-like projections called conchae or turbinate.

## CLINICAL ANATOMY

- ***Common cold or rhinitis*** is the commonest infection of the nose. It may be infective or allergic or both. It commonly occurs during change of the seasons.
- Fracture of cribriform plate of ethmoid with tearing off of the meninges may tear the olfactory nerve rootlets (Fig. 15.4). In such cases, CSF may drip from the nasal cavity. It is called ***CSF rhinorrhoea***.

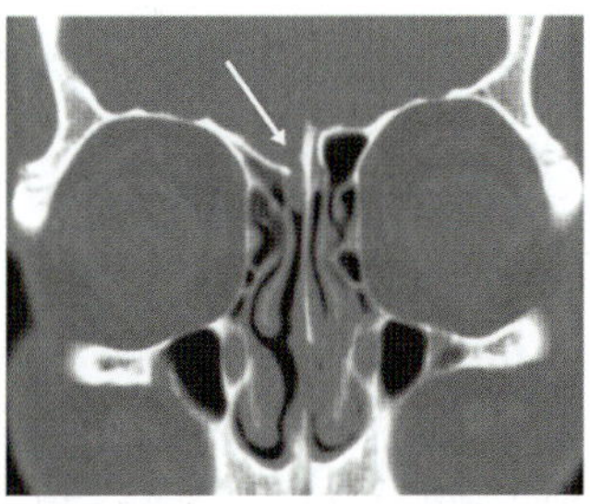

Fracture of cribriform plate of ethmoid
↓
Tearing off of meninges
↓
CSF drips from nasal cavity
↓
CSF rhinorrhoea

**Fig. 15.4:** CSF rhinorrhoea

*Competency:*
**AN37.1** Describe and demonstrate features of nasal septum, lateral wall of nose, their blood supply and nerve supply.

## NASAL SEPTUM

The *nasal septum* is a median osseocartilaginous partition between the two halves of the nasal cavity. On each side, it is covered by mucous membrane and forms the medial wall of both nasal cavities (Plate 15.1 and Fig. 15.5, Flowchart 15.1).

### Formation

***Bony part*** is formed almost entirely by:
a. Vomer
b. Perpendicular plate of ethmoid.

***Cartilaginous part*** is formed by:
a. Septal cartilage
b. Septal processes of the inferior nasal cartilages.

***Cuticular part*** or lower end is formed by fibrofatty tissue covered by skin. The lower margin of the septum is called the ***columella***.

*Note*: The nasal septum is rarely strictly median. Its central part is usually *deflected* to one or the other side. The deflection is produced by overgrowth of one or more of the constituent parts.

### Arterial Supply

1. *Anterosuperior part* is supplied by the anterior and posterior ethmoidal artery (Fig. 15.6).
2. *Anteroinferior part* is supplied by the septal branch of superior labial branch of facial artery.
3. *Posterior part* is supplied by the sphenopalatine artery. *It is the main artery*.
4. Braches of greater palatine artery.

***Kiesselbach's plexus:*** The anteroinferior part or vestibule of the septum contains anastomoses between all branches, e.g. the septal branch of the superior labial branch of the facial artery, sphenopalatine artery, and anterior ethmoidal artery. These form a large capillary

**Plate 15.1:** Formation of the nasal septum

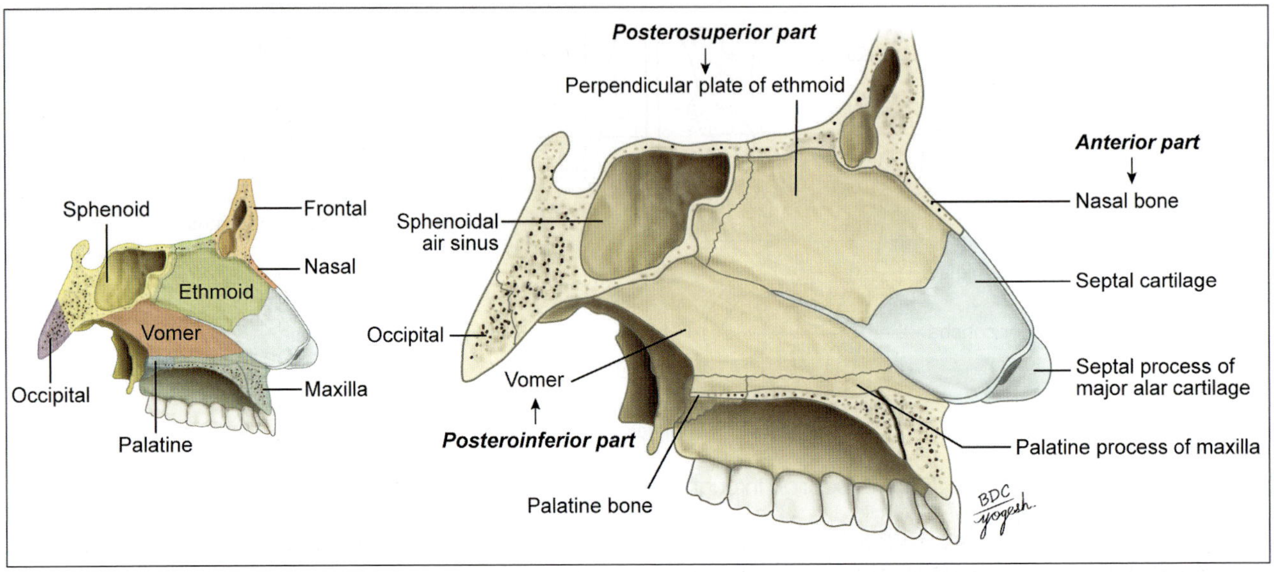


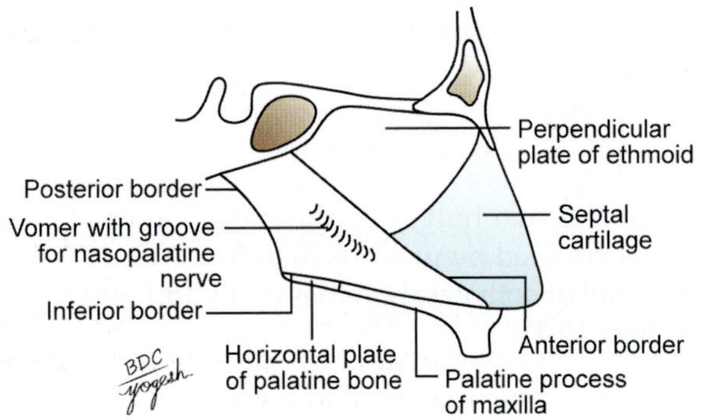


**Fig. 15.5:** Formation of the nasal septum

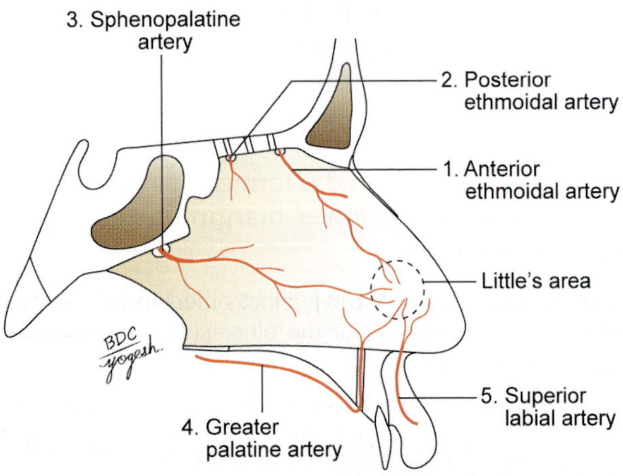


**Fig. 15.6:** Arterial supply of nasal septum

**Flowchart 15.1:** Kiesselbach plexus

***Kiesselbach plexus***

- ***Location***: Lies at little area at the antero-inferior part of nasal septum
- ***Definition***: Arterial anastomosis at Little's area
- ***Arteries***: Septal branches of: Sphenopalatine artery, Anterior ethmoid artery, Greater palatine artery, Superior labial artery

***Clinical intergation:*** Epistaxis

network called the *Kiesselbach's plexus*. This is a common site of bleeding from the nose or epistaxis, and is known as ***Little's area***.

## Venous Drainage

The veins form a plexus which is more marked in the lower part of septum or Little's area. The plexus drains anteriorly into the facial vein, and posteriorly through the sphenopalatine vein to pterygoid venous plexus.

## Nerve Supply

1. ***General sensory nerves***, arising from trigeminal nerve, are distributed to whole of the septum (Fig. 15.7).
   a. The anterosuperior part of the septum is supplied by the internal nasal branches of the anterior ethmoidal nerve.
   b. The posteroinferior part is supplied by the nasopalatine branch of the pterygopalatine ganglion. *It is the main nerve.*
2. ***Special sensory nerves or olfactory*** nerves are confined to the upper part or olfactory area.

## Lymphatic Drainage

*Anterior half* to the submandibular nodes.
*Posterior half* to the retropharyngeal and deep cervical nodes.

## CLINICAL ANATOMY

- Sphenopalatine artery is the artery of ***epistaxis***.
- Little's area on the septum is a common site of bleeding from the nose or epistaxis (Fig. 15.5).
- Pathological ***deviation of the nasal septum*** is often responsible for repeated attacks of common cold, allergic rhinitis, sinusitis, etc. It requires surgical correction (Fig. 15.8).

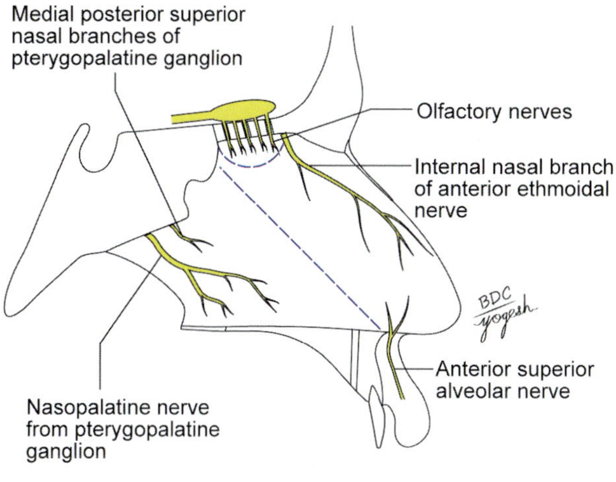


**Fig. 15.7:** Nerve supply of the nasal septum

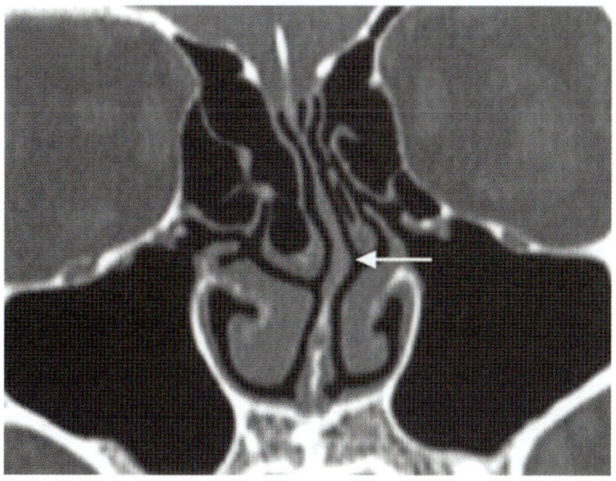

**Fig. 15.8:** Deviated nasal septum

**DISSECTION**

Take the sagittal section of head and neck. Dissect and remove mucous membrane of the septum of nose in small pieces. The mucous membrane is covering both surfaces of the septum of the nose.

Dissect and preserve the nerves lying in the mucous membrane. Remove the entire mucous membrane to see the details in the interior of the nasal cavity.

## LATERAL WALL OF NOSE

The lateral wall of the nose is irregular owing to the presence of three shelf-like bony projections called *conchae.* The conchae increase the surface area of the nose for effective air-conditioning of the inspired air (Plate 15.2).

### Parts

The lateral wall can be subdivided into three parts:

a. A small depressed area in the anterior part is called the ***vestibule***. It is lined by modified skin containing short, stiff, curved hairs called ***vibrissae***.
b. The middle part is known as the ***atrium*** of the middle meatus.
c. The posterior part contains the ***conchae***. Spaces separating the conchae are called meatuses (Fig. 15.9).

**Plate 15.2:** Bony formation of the lateral wall of the nasal cavity

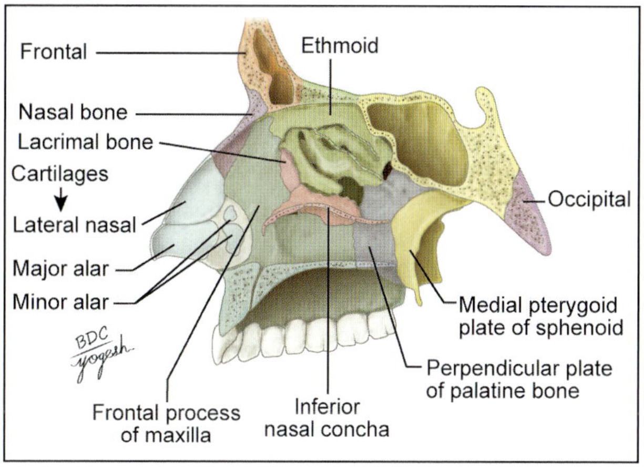


### Formation

The *skeleton of the lateral wall* is partly bony, partly cartilaginous, and partly made up only of soft tissues (Plate 15.3, Fig. 15.9).

1. ***Bony part*** is formed from before backwards by the following bones:
   a. Nasal
   b. Frontal process of maxilla
   c. Lacrimal
   d. Labyrinth of ethmoid with superior and middle conchae
   e. Inferior nasal concha, made up of spongy bone only
   f. Perpendicular plate of palatine bone together with its orbital and sphenoidal processes
   g. Medial pterygoid plate.
2. ***Cartilaginous part*** is formed by:
   a. Superior nasal cartilage
   b. Inferior nasal cartilage
   c. 3 or 4 small cartilages of the ala.
3. ***Cuticular lower part*** is formed by fibrofatty tissue covered with skin.

### Features of Conchae and Meatuses

#### *Nasal Conchae*

These are curved bony projections directed downwards and medially. The following three conchae are usually found:

1. ***Inferior concha*** (Latin *shell*) is an independent bone.
2. ***Middle concha*** is a projection from the medial surface of ethmoidal labyrinth.
3. ***Superior concha*** is also a projection from the medial surface of the ethmoidal labyrinth. This is the smallest concha situated just above the posterior part of the middle concha.

#### *Meatuses of the Nose*

These are passages beneath the overhanging conchae. Each meatus communicates freely with the nasal cavity proper (Fig. 15.9 and Flowchart 15.2).

1. ***Inferior meatus*** lies underneath the inferior concha, and is the largest of the three meatuses. The nasolacrimal

**Plate 15.3:** Formation of the lateral wall of the nasal cavity (bony formation and openings, 1: Superior concha and 2: inferior concha of ethmoid bone)

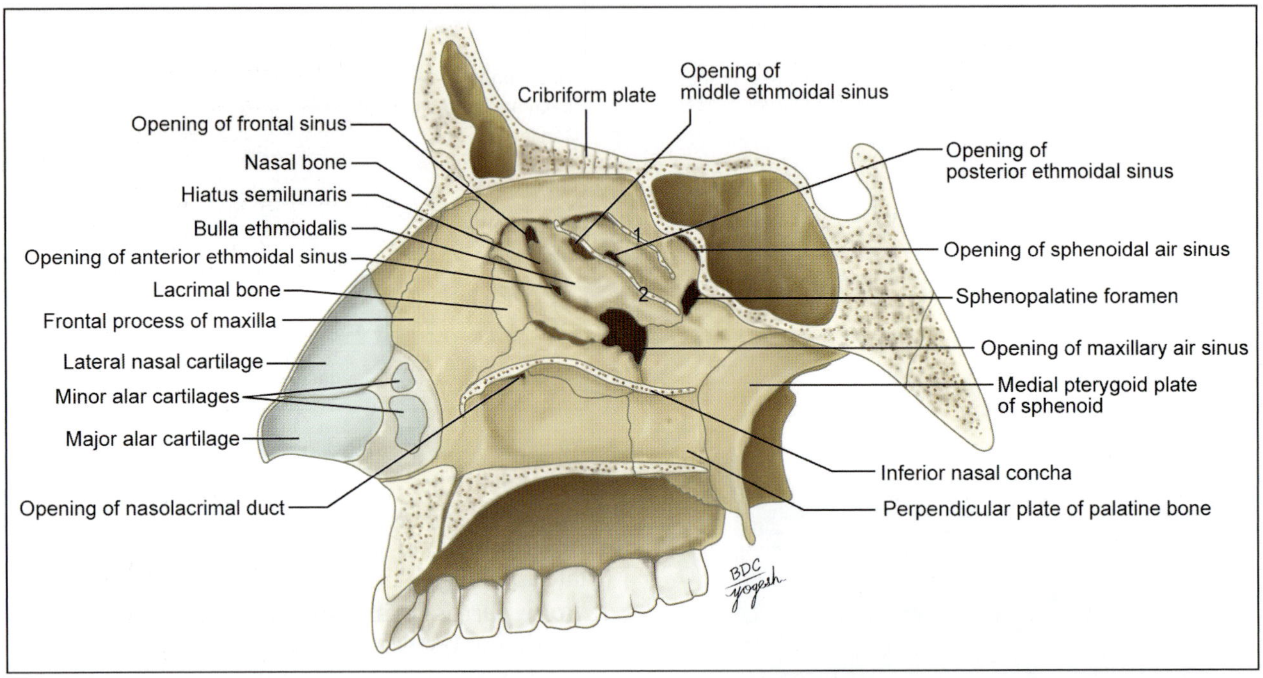


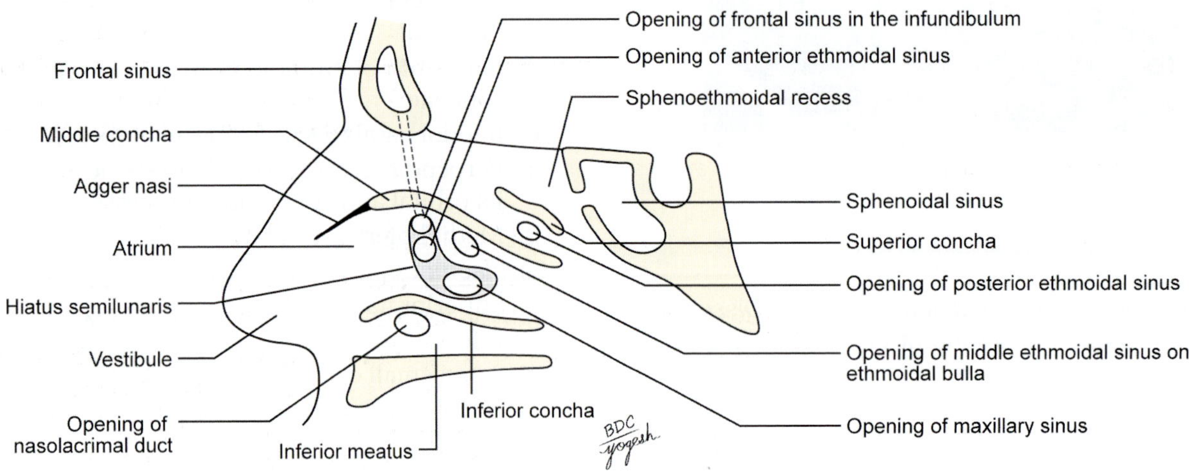


**Fig. 15.9:** Lateral wall of the nasal cavity seen after removing the conchae

**Flowchart 15.2:** Openings in lateral wall of nose

***Openings in lateral wall of nose***

- ***Sphenoethmoidal recess***
  - Sphenoid sinus
- ***Superior meatus***
  - Posterior ethmoidal sinus
- ***Middle meatus***
  - ***On bulla ethmoidalis***
    - Middle ethmoidal sinus
  - ***Hiatus semilunaris***
    - Frontal sinus
    - Anterior ethmoidal sinus
    - Maxillary sinus
- ***Inferior meatus***
  - Nasolacrimal duct

duct opens into it at the junction of its anterior one-third and posterior two-thirds. The opening is guarded by the lacrimal fold, or ***Hasner's valve***.

2. ***Middle meatus*** lies underneath the middle concha. It presents the following features:
   a. *Ethmoidal bulla* is a rounded elevation produced by the underlying middle ethmoidal sinuses which open at upper margin of bulla.
   b. *Hiatus semilunaris* is a deep semicircular sulcus below the bulla.
   c. *Infundibulum* is a short passage at the anterior end of the hiatus.
   d. *Openings*:
   Opening of *frontal air sinus* is seen in the anterior part of hiatus semilunaris.
   Opening of *the anterior ethmoidal air sinus* is present behind the opening of frontal air sinus.
   Opening of *maxillary air sinus* is located in posterior part of the hiatus semilunaris. It is often represented by two openings.

3. ***Superior meatus*** lies below the superior concha. This is the shortest and shallowest of the three meatuses. It receives the *openings of the posterior ethmoidal air sinuses.*
4. ***Sphenoethmoidal recess*** is a triangular fossa just above the superior concha. It receives the *opening of the sphenoidal air sinus.*

*Note*: The ***atrium of the middle meatus*** is a shallow depression just in front of the middle meatus and above the vestibule of the nose. It is limited above by a faint ridge of mucous membrane, the ***agger nasi***, which runs forwards and downwards from the upper end of the anterior border of the middle concha (Fig. 15.8).

## Arterial Supply (Fig. 15.10)

1. *Anterosuperior quadrant* is supplied by the anterior ethmoidal artery assisted by the posterior ethmoidal artery.
2. *Anteroinferior quadrant* is supplied by branches from the facial artery.
3. *Posterosuperior quadrant* is supplied by a few branches of the sphenopalatine artery.
4. *Posteroinferior quadrant* is supplied by branches from greater palatine artery which pierce the perpendicular plate of palatine bone to run on the hard palate and passes up in the nose through the incisive fossa.

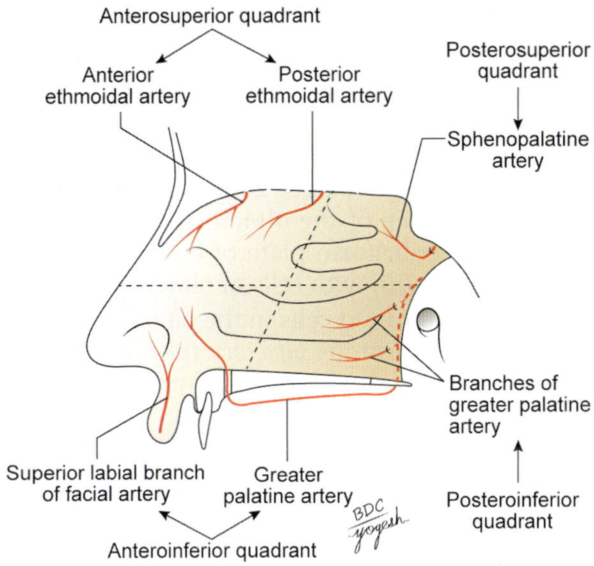


**Fig. 15.10:** Arteries supplying lateral wall of the nasal cavity

## Venous Drainage

The veins form a plexus which drains anteriorly into the facial vein; posteriorly, into the pharyngeal plexus of veins; and from the middle part, to the pterygoid plexus of veins.

## Nerve Supply

***General sensory nerves:*** They derived from the branches of trigeminal nerve are distributed to whole of the lateral wall (Fig. 15.11):

1. *Anterosuperior quadrant* is supplied by the anterior ethmoidal nerve branch of ophthalmic nerve.
2. *Anteroinferior quadrant* is supplied by the anterior superior alveolar nerve, branch of infraorbital, continuation of maxillary nerve.
3. *Posterosuperior quadrant* is supplied by the lateral posterior superior nasal branches from the pterygopalatine ganglion.
4. *Posteroinferior quadrant* is supplied by the anterior palatine branch from the pterygopalatine ganglion.

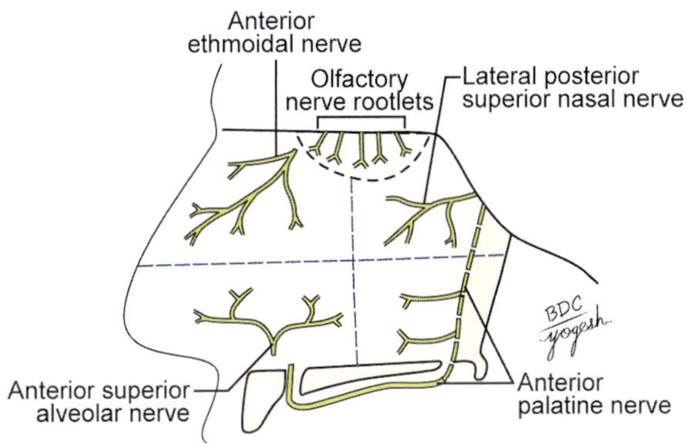


**Fig. 15.11:** Nerve supply of lateral wall of the nasal cavity

***Special sensory nerves or olfactory nerves:*** They are distributed to the upper part of the lateral wall just below the cribriform plate of the ethmoid up to the superior concha.

Note that the olfactory mucosa lies partly on the lateral wall and partly on the nasal septum.

## Lymphatic Drainage

Lymphatics from the anterior half of the lateral wall pass to the submandibular nodes, and from the posterior half, to the retropharyngeal and upper deep cervical nodes.

## CLINICAL ANATOMY

Hypertrophy of the mucosa over the inferior nasal concha is a common feature of allergic rhinitis, which is characterised by sneezing, nasal blockage and excessive watery discharge from the nose.

## DISSECTION

Remove with scissors the anterior part of inferior nasal concha. This will reveal the opening of the nasolacrimal duct. Pass a thin probe upwards through the nasolacrimal duct into the lacrimal sac at the medial angle of the eye. Remove all the three nasal conchae to expose the meatuses lying below the respective concha. This will expose the openings of the sinuses present there.

Trace the nasopalatine nerve till the sphenopalatine foramen. Try to find a few nasal branches of the greater palatine nerve.

Gently break the perpendicular plate of palatine bone to expose the greater or anterior palatine nerve, branch of the pterygopalatine ganglion. Follow the nerve and its accompanying vessels to the hard palate. Identify the lesser or middle palatine nerves and trace them till the soft palate.

## OLFACTORY NERVE—1ST NERVE

1. The *olfactory cells* (16–20 million in man) are bipolar neurons. They lie in the olfactory part of the nasal mucosa and serve both as receptors as well as the first neurons in the olfactory pathway.
2. The *olfactory nerves*, about 20 in number, represent central processes of the olfactory cells. They pass through the cribriform plate of ethmoid and make synaptic glomeruli with cells of olfactory bulb.
3. The mitral and tufted cells in the olfactory bulb give off fibres that form the *olfactory tract* and reach the anterior perforated substance and uncus.

### CLINICAL ANATOMY

- Anosmia: Loss of olfactory fibres with ageing.
- Sense of smell is tested separately in each nostril.
- Allergic rhinitis causes temporary olfactory impairment.

***Competency:***
**AN37.2** Describe location and functional anatomy of paranasal sinuses.

## PARANASAL SINUSES

Paranasal sinuses are air-filled spaces present within some bones around the nasal cavities. The sinuses are *frontal, maxillary, sphenoidal and ethmoidal.* All of them open into the nasal cavity through its lateral wall (Fig. 15.12 and Flowchart 15.3).

### *Functions*

The *function* of the sinuses is to make the skull lighter, warm up and humidify the inspired air. These also add resonance to the voice. In infections of the sinuses or *sinusitis*, the voice is altered.

*Note*: The sinuses are rudimentary, or even absent at birth. They enlarge rapidly during the ages of 6 to 7 years, i.e. time of eruption of permanent teeth and then after puberty. From birth to adult life, the growth of the sinuses is due to enlargement of the bones; in old age, their size may increase. It is due to resorption of the surrounding cancellous bone.

### Frontal Sinus

1. The frontal sinus lies in the frontal bone deep to the superciliary arch. It extends upwards above the medial end of the eyebrow, and backwards into the medial part of the roof of the orbit.
2. It *opens* into the middle meatus of nose at the anterior end of the hiatus semilunaris either through the infundibulum or through the frontonasal duct.
3. The right and left sinuses are usually unequal in size; and rarely one or both may be absent. Their *average* height, width and anteroposterior depth are each about 2.5 cm. The sinuses are better developed in males than in females.
4. They are rudimentary or absent at birth. They are well developed between 7 and 8 years of age, but reach full size only after puberty.

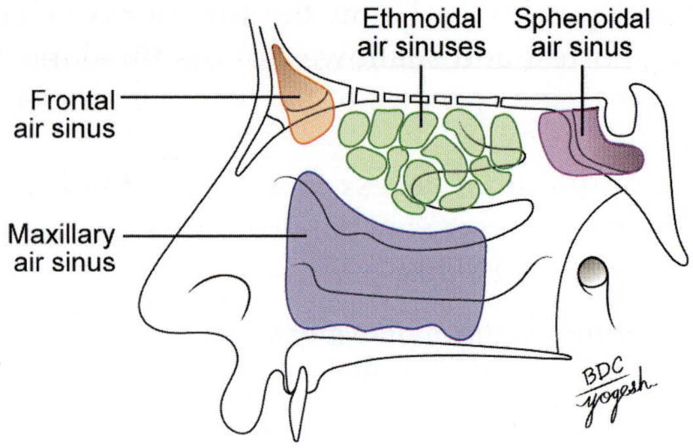


**Fig. 15.12:** Lateral wall of nasal cavity with location of paranasal sinuses

**Flowchart 15.3:** Paranasal air sinuses

***Paranasal air sinuses***
Air-filled spaces within bone

| ***Features*** | ***Functions*** | ***Classification*** |
|---|---|---|
| - Open in lateral wall of nose<br>- Develop as mucosal diverticulum<br>- Lined by pseudostratified ciliated columnar epithelium | Maintain temperature and humidity in inspired air<br>Make the skull lighter<br>Add resonance to voice<br>Secrete mucus | Frontal<br>Ethmoidal:<br>Anterior<br>Middle<br>Posterior<br>Maxillary<br>Sphenoidal |

***Arterial supply:*** Supraorbital artery.

***Venous drainage:*** Into the supraorbital and superior ophthalmic veins.

***Lymphatic drainage:*** To submandibular nodes.

***Nerve supply:*** Supraorbital nerve.

### Maxillary Sinus (Fig. 15.13 and Flowchart 15.4)

1. The maxillary sinus lies in the body of the maxilla, and is the largest of all the paranasal sinuses. It is pyramidal in shape, with its base directed medially towards the lateral wall of the nose, and the apex directed laterally in the zygomatic process of the maxilla.
2. It *opens* into the middle meatus of the nose in the lower part of the hiatus semilunaris. *The opening/hiatus is nearer the roof.*
3. In an isolated maxilla, the opening or hiatus of the maxillary sinus is large. However, in the intact skull, the size of opening is reduced to 3 or 4 mm as it is overlapped by the following:
   a. From above, by the uncinate process of the ethmoid, and the descending part of lacrimal bone.
   b. From below, by lacrimal and ethmoidal processes of inferior nasal concha.
   c. From behind, by perpendicular plate of palatine bone and by the ethmoidal process of inferior nasal concha. It is further reduced in size by the thick mucosa of nose.
4. The size of sinus is variable. Average measurements are: Height—3.5 cm, width—2.5 cm and anteroposterior depth—3.5 cm.

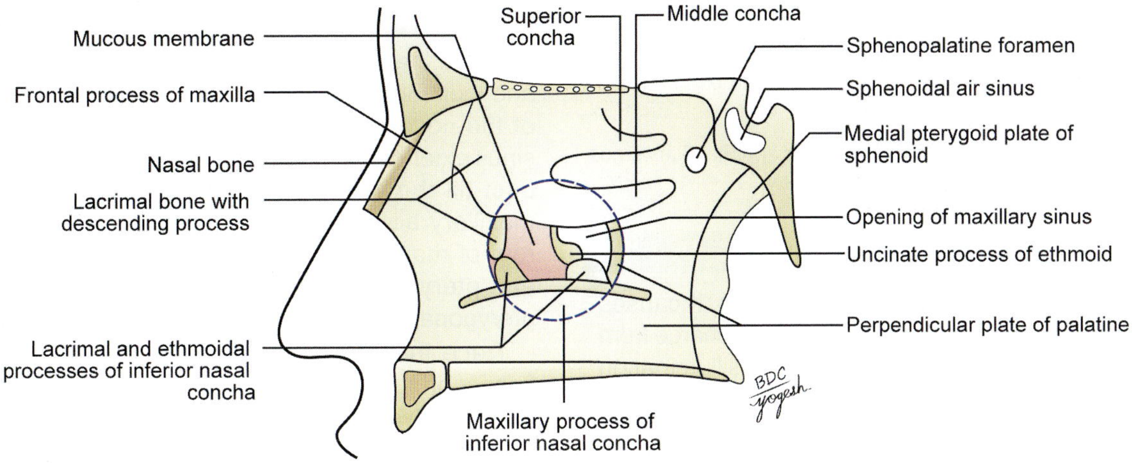


**Fig. 15.13:** Reduced size of maxillary air sinus

**Flowchart 15.4:** Maxillary sinuses

***Maxillary sinus (atrium of Highmore)***

***Introduction***
- Largest air sinus
- Lies in the body of maxilla
- Opening: In hiatus semilunaris in middle meatus
- Size: 3.5 x 2.5 x 3.25 cm
- Pyramidal-shaped

***Boundaries***
- Apex: Zygomatic process of maxilla
- Base: Nasal cavity, maxillary hiatus
- Roof: Orbital plate of maxilla
- Floor: Alveolar process of maxilla
- Anteriorly: Body of maxilla
- Posteriorly: Infratemporal surface of maxilla

***Supply***
- Arterial supply: Anterior, middle, and posterior superior alveolar arteries
- Lymphatic drainage: Submandibular nodes
- Innervation: Anterior, middle, and posterior superior alveolar nerves

***Clinical integration:*** Maxillary sinusitis, referred pain of maxillary sinus, drainage of sinus (antrostomy), carcinoma

5. Its *roof* is formed by the floor of orbit, and is traversed by the infraorbital nerve. The *floor* is formed by the alveolar process of maxilla, and lies about 1 cm below the level of floor of the nose. The level corresponds to the level of lower border of the ala of nose. The floor is marked by several conical elevations produced by the roots of upper molar and premolar teeth. The roots may even penetrate the bony floor to lie beneath the mucous lining. The canine tooth may project into the anterolateral wall.
6. The maxillary sinus is the first paranasal sinus to *develop*.

***Arterial supply:*** Facial, infraorbital and greater palatine arteries.

***Venous drainage*** into the facial vein and the pterygoid plexus of veins.

***Lymphatic drainage*** into the submandibular nodes.

***Nerve supply:*** Posterior superior alveolar branches from maxillary nerve and anterior and middle superior alveolar branches from infraorbital nerve.

## Sphenoidal Sinus

1. The right and left sphenoidal sinuses lie within the body of sphenoid bone. They are separated by a septum. The two sinuses are usually unequal in size. Each sinus opens into the sphenoethmoidal recess of corresponding half of the nasal cavity.
2. Each sinus is related superiorly to the optic chiasma and the hypophysis cerebri; and laterally to the internal carotid artery and the cavernous sinus.

***Arterial supply:*** Posterior ethmoidal and internal carotid arteries.

***Venous drainage:*** Into pterygoid venous plexus and cavernous sinus.

***Lymphatic drainage:*** To the retropharyngeal nodes.

***Nerve supply:*** Posterior ethmoidal nerve and orbital branches of pterygopalatine ganglion.

## Ethmoidal Sinuses

Ethmoidal sinuses are numerous small intercommunicating spaces which lie within the labyrinth of the ethmoid bone. They are completed from above by the orbital plate of the frontal bone, from behind by the sphenoidal conchae and the orbital process of the palatine bone, and anteriorly by the lacrimal bone. The sinuses are divided into anterior, middle and posterior groups.

A. ***Anterior ethmoidal sinus*** is made up of 1 to 11 air cells, opens into the anterior part of the hiatus semilunaris of the nose. It is supplied by the anterior ethmoidal nerve and vessels. Its lymphatics drain into the submandibular nodes.
B. ***Middle ethmoidal sinus*** consisting of 1 to 7 air cells open into the middle meatus of the nose. It is supplied by the anterior ethmoidal nerve and vessels and the orbital branches of the pterygopalatine ganglion. Lymphatics drain into the submandibular nodes.
C. ***Posterior ethmoidal sinus*** consisting of 1 to 7 air cells open into the superior meatus of the nose. It is supplied by the posterior ethmoidal

nerve and vessels and the orbital branches of the pterygopalatine ganglion. Lymphatics drain into the retropharyngeal nodes.

*Competency:*
**AN37.3** Describe anatomical basis of sinusitis and maxillary sinus tumours.

## CLINICAL ANATOMY

- Infection of a sinus is known as ***sinusitis***. It causes headache and persistent, thick, purulent discharge from the nose. Diagnosis is assisted by transillumination and radiography. A diseased sinus is opaque.
- Openings of anterior ethmoidal, frontal and maxillary sinuses in middle meatus is known as ***ostiomeatal complex***.
- ***Anterior ethmoiditis*** narrows the ostiomeatal complex preventing proper drainage from the sinuses. Hence, anterior ethmoiditis is also common cause of chronic sinusitis.
- ***Frontal sinusitis*** and ***ethmoiditis*** can cause oedema of the lids secondary to infection of the sinuses.
- Pain from ethmoid air sinus may be referred to forehead, as both are supplied by ophthalmic division of trigeminal nerve.
- Opening of maxillary air sinus is near the roof of sinus. It cannot drain properly. So ***maxillary sinusitis*** is the commonest cause of chronic sinusitis.
- The maxillary sinus may be infected from the nose or from a caries tooth. Drainage of the sinus is difficult because its ostium lies at a higher level than its floor. Hence, the sinus is drained surgically by:
  - ***Antrum puncture*** can be done by breaking the lateral wall of the inferior meatus and pushing in fluid and letting it drain through the natural orifice with head in dependent position (Fig. 15.14).
- ***Carcinoma of the maxillary sinus*** arises from the mucosal lining.
- Pain of maxillary sinusitis may be referred to upper teeth and infraorbital skin as all these are supplied by the maxillary nerve.

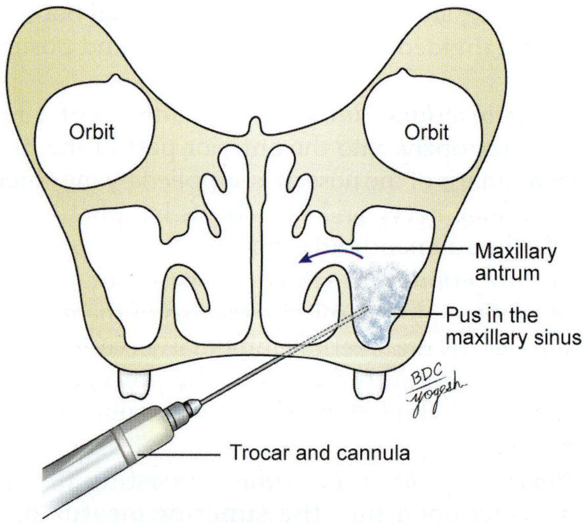


**Fig. 15.14:** Antrum puncture

## DISSECTION

Remove the thin medial walls of the ethmoidal air cells, and look for the continuity with the mucous membrane of the nose. Remove the medial wall of maxillary air sinus extending anteriorly from opening of nasolacrimal duct till the greater palatine canal posteriorly. Now maxillary air sinus can be seen. Remove part of the roof of maxillary air sinus so that the maxillary nerve and pterygopalatine ganglion are identifiable in the pterygopalatine fossa.

Trace the infraorbital nerve in infraorbital canal in floor of orbit. Try to locate the sinuous course of anterior superior alveolar nerve into the upper incisor teeth.

## PTERYGOPALATINE FOSSA

This is small pyramidal space situated deeply, below the apex of the orbit (Fig. 15.15 and Flowchart 15.5).

### Boundaries

*Anterior:* Superomedial part of the posterior surface of the maxilla.

*Posterior:* Root of the pterygoid process and adjoining part of the anterior surface of the greater wing of the sphenoid.

*Medial:* Upper part of the perpendicular plate of the palatine bone. The orbital and sphenoidal processes of the bone also take part.

*Lateral:* The fossa opens into the infratemporal fossa through the pterygomaxillary fissure

*Superior:* Undersurface of the body of sphenoid.

*Inferior:* Closed by the pyramidal process of the palatine bone in the angle between the maxilla and the pterygoid process.

### Communications

*Anteriorly:* With the orbit through the medial end of the inferior orbital fissure.

*Posteriorly:*

1. Middle cranial fossa through the foramen rotundum.
2. Foramen lacerum through the pterygoid canal.
3. Pharynx through the palatinovaginal canal.

*Medially:* With the nose through sphenopalatine foramen.

*Laterally:* With the infratemporal fossa through the pterygomaxillary fissure.

*Inferiorly:* With the oral cavity through the greater and lesser palatine canals.

### Contents

1. Third part of the maxillary artery and its branches which bear the same names as the branches of the pterygopalatine ganglia and accompany all of them.
2. Maxillary nerve and its branches—ganglionic, zygomatic and posterior superior alveolar.
3. Pterygopalatine ganglion with its roots and its numerous branches containing fibres of the maxillary nerve mixed with autonomic nerves (described below).

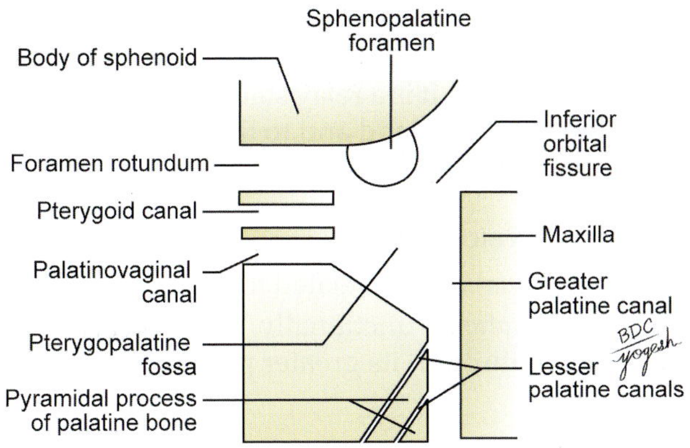


**Fig. 15.15:** Scheme to show the pterygopalatine fossa and its communications

**Flowchart 15.5:** Pterygopalatine fossa

***Pterygopalatine fossa***

- ***Boundaries***
  - Anterior: Posterior surface of maxilla
  - Posterior: Root of pterygoid process, greater wing of sphenoid
  - Medial: Perpendicular plate of palatine bone
  - Lateral: Pterygomaxillary fissure
  - Superior: Body of sphenoid
  - Inferior: Pyramidal process of palatine bone
- ***Communications***
  - Anteriorly: Inferior orbital fissure
  - Posteriorly
    - Foramen rotundum
    - Pterygoid canal
    - Palatovaginal canal
  - Medially:
    - Sphenopalatine foramen
  - Laterally:
    - Pterygomaxillary fissure
  - Inferiorly:
    - Greater and lesser palatine canals
- ***Contents***
  - Third part of maxillary artery
  - Maxillary nerve
  - Pterygopalatine ganglion

## Maxillary Nerve

It arises from the trigeminal ganglion, runs forwards, and leaves the middle cranial fossa by passing through the foramen rotundum. Next, the nerve crosses the upper part of pterygopalatine fossa, beyond which it is continued as the infraorbital nerve (Fig. 15.16 and Flowchart 15.6).

**Flowchart 15.6:** Maxillary nerve

***Maxillary nerve***

- ***Beginning***
  - Branch of trigeminal nerve
  - Arises from trigeminal ganglion
- ***Course***
  - 4 parts
  - 1st: In the middle cranial fossa
  - 2nd: In pterygopalatine fossa
  - 3rd: In infraorbital canal
  - 4th: On the face
- ***Branches***
  - Meningeal branch
  - Ganglionic branches
  - Posterior superior alveolar n.
  - Zygomatic nerve
  - Middle superior alveolar n.
  - Anterior superior alveolar n.
  - Palpebral branch
  - Nasal branch
  - Superior labial branch

In the middle cranial fossa, maxillary nerve gives a meningeal branch.

In the pterygopalatine fossa, the nerve is related to the pterygopalatine ganglion, and gives off the ganglionic, posterior superior alveolar and zygomatic nerves.

### Ganglionic Branches

The pterygopalatine ganglion is suspended by the ganglionic branches.

### Posterior Superior Alveolar Nerve

It enters the posterior surface of the body of the maxilla, and supplies the three upper molar teeth and the adjoining part of the gum.

### Zygomatic Nerve

It is a branch of the maxillary nerve, given off in the pterygopalatine fossa. It enters the orbit through the lateral end of the inferior orbital fissure, and runs along the lateral wall, outside the periosteum, to enter the zygomatic bone. Just before or after entering the bone, it divides into two terminal branches, the *zygomaticofacial* and *zygomaticotemporal nerves* which supply the skin of the face and of the anterior part of the temple. The communicating branch to the lacrimal nerve, which contains secretomotor fibres to the lacrimal gland, arises from the zygomaticotemporal nerve, and runs in the lateral wall of the orbit.

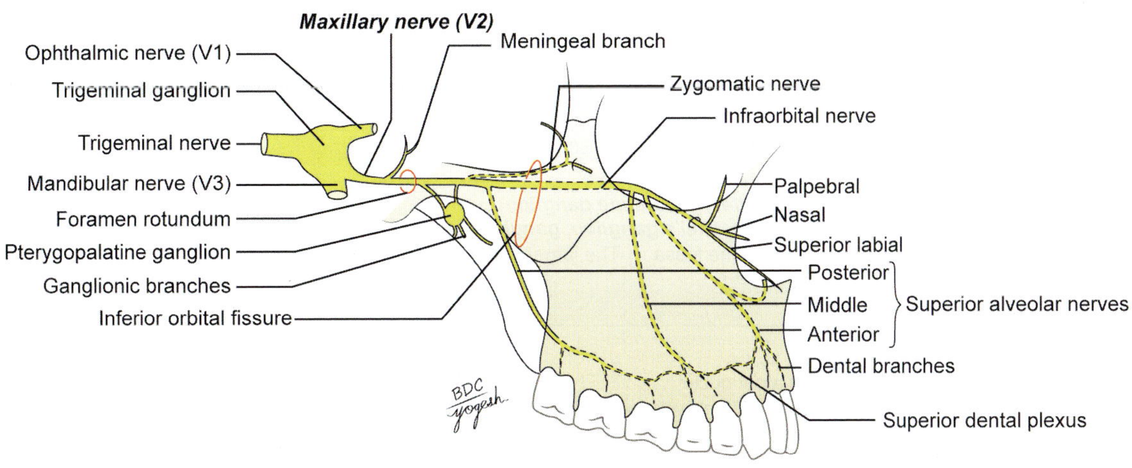


**Fig. 15.16:** Branches of maxillary nerve

### Infraorbital Nerve

It is the continuation of the maxillary nerve. It enters the orbit through the *inferior orbital fissure*. It then runs forwards on the floor of the orbit or the roof of the maxillary sinus, at first in the *infraorbital groove* and then in the *infraorbital canal* remaining outside the periosteum of the orbit. It emerges on the face through the *infraorbital foramen* and terminates by dividing into palpebral, nasal and labial branches. The nerve is accompanied by the infraorbital branch of the third part of the maxillary artery and the accompanying vein.

#### Branches

1. *Middle superior alveolar nerve* arises in the infraorbital groove, runs in the lateral wall of the maxillary sinus, and supplies the upper premolar teeth.
2. *Anterior superior alveolar nerve* arises in the infraorbital canal, and runs in a sinuous canal having a complicated course in the anterior wall of the maxillary sinus. It supplies the upper incisor and canine teeth, the maxillary sinus, and the anteroinferior part of the nasal cavity.
3. *Terminal branches—palpebral, nasal and labial* supply a large area of skin on the face. They also supply the mucous membrane of the upper lip and cheek.

## PTERYGOPALATINE GANGLION

*Synonyms*: Sphenopalatine ganglion, ganglion of Hay fever, or Meckel's ganglion (Figs 15.17a and b, Flowchart 15.7).

### Features

The pterygopalatine is the largest parasympathetic peripheral ganglion. It is a relay station for secretomotor fibres to the lacrimal gland and to the mucous glands of the nose, paranasal sinuses, palate and pharynx.

#### Neurological Relationship

- *Topographic relation*: It is related to the maxillary nerve.
- *Functional relation*: Functionally, it is connected to the facial nerve through its greater petrosal branch.

### Location

The flattened ganglion lies on the pterygopalatine fossa just below the maxillary nerve, in front of the pterygoid canal and lateral to the sphenopalatine foramen.

### Connections

It has three roots as follows:

1. ***Parasympathetic* or *secretomotor root*:** It consists of pre- and post-ganglionic fibres:

   *Preganglionic fibres* arise from *superior salivatory* and *lacrimatory nuclei* in pons and pass through the *nervous intermedius*, the *facial nerve*, the *geniculate ganglion*, the *greater petrosal nerve*, and the *nerve of the pterygoid canal* to reach and relay in the *ganglion*.

   *Postganglionic fibres* arise in the ganglion to supply secretomotor nerves to the lacrimal gland and the

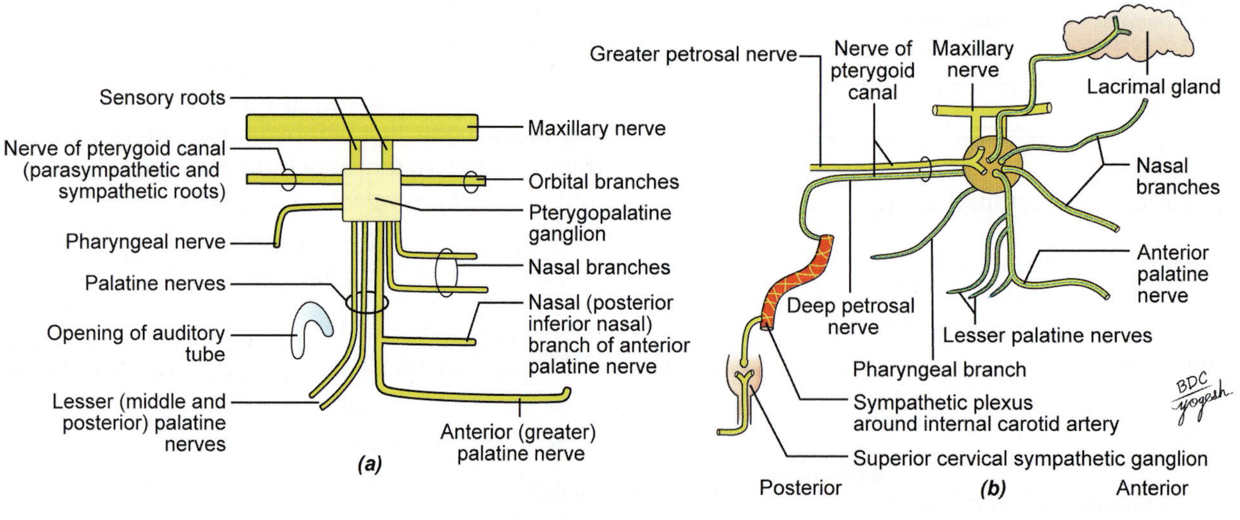


**Figs 15.17a and b:** Pterygopalatine ganglion: (a) Connections and branches and (b) roots and branches

**Flowchart 15.7:** Pterygopalatine ganglion

***Pterygopalatine ganglion***
***(Sphenopalatine/Meckel's ganglion, ganglion of Hay fever)***
Lies in pterygopalatine fossa | The largest peripheral parasympathetic ganglion

***Neurological connection***
Topographic: Maxillary nerve
Functional: Facial nerve

***Roots***

***Parasympathetic***
Superior salivatory and lacrimatory nuclei in pons → nervous intermedius → VII nerve → geniculate ganglion → greater petrosal nerve → nerve to pterygoid canal → relay in ganglion → lacrimal gland, mucous gland of nose, paranasal sinuses, palate, nasopharynx

***Sympathetic***
Lateral horn cells of T1 → superior cervical ganglion → relay → plexus around ICA → deep petrosal nerve → nerve to pterygoid canal → pterygopalatine ganglion (no relay) → vasomotor to nose, paranasal sinuses, palate, nasopharynx

***Sensory***
Maxillary nerve

BDC yogesh

mucous glands of the nose, the paranasal sinuses, the palate, and the nasopharynx.

2. ***Sympathetic root***: The lateral horn cells of T1 segment of spinal cord give rise to the preganglionic sympathetic fibres. They traverse to T1 nerve, sympathetic chain, and relay in superior cervical sympathetic ganglion. Postganglionic fibres pass through internal carotid plexus, the *deep petrosal nerve*, and the *nerve of the pterygoid canal* to reach the ganglion. The fibres pass through the ganglion without relay, supply vasomotor nerves to the mucous membrane of the nose, the paranasal sinuses, the palate, and the nasopharynx.
3. ***Sensory roots***: These are the fibres of maxillary nerve. Its fibres pass through the ganglion without relay. They emerge in the branches.

### Branches

1. *Orbital branches* pass through the inferior orbital fissure, and supply the periosteum of the orbit, and the orbitalis muscle which is involuntary (Table 15.1).
2. *Palatine branches*: *Greater or anterior palatine nerve* descends through the greater palatine canal, and supplies the hard palate and the labial aspect of the upper gums. The *lesser or posterior palatine nerves* supply the soft palate and the tonsil.
3. *Nasal branches* enter the nasal cavity through the sphenopalatine foramen.
   a. *Lateral posterior superior nasal branches* (six in number) supply the posterior parts of the superior and middle conchae.
   b. *Medial posterior superior nasal branches*, two or three in number, supply the posterior part of the roof of the nose and of the nasal septum. The largest of these nerves is known as the *nasopalatine nerve* which descends up to the anterior part of the hard palate through the incisive foramen.

**TABLE 15.1: Branches of pterygopalatine ganglion**

| ***Branch*** | ***Functions*** |
|---|---|
| Orbital branches | Periosteum of the orbit, orbitalis muscle |
| Palatine branches | |
| a. Greater or anterior palatine nerve | Hard palate, labial aspect of the upper gums |
| b. Lesser or posterior palatine nerve | Soft palate and the tonsil |
| Nasal branches | |
| a. Lateral posterior superior nasal branches (6) | Posterior parts of the superior and middle conchae |
| b. Medial posterior superior nasal branches (2–3) | Posterior part of the roof of the nose and of the nasal septum<br>Nasopalatine nerve (largest branch) – anterior part of the hard palate |
| Pharyngeal branch | Part of the nasopharynx behind the auditory tube |
| Lacrimal branch | Parasympathetic supply of lacrimal gland |

4. *Pharyngeal branch* passes through the palatinovaginal canal and supplies the part of the nasopharynx behind the auditory tube.
5. *Lacrimal branch*: The postganglionic fibres pass back into the maxillary nerve to leave it through its zygomatic nerve and its zygomaticotemporal branch, a communicating branch to lacrimal nerve to supply the secretomotor fibres to the lacrimal gland.

### DISSECTION

Trace the connections, and branches of pterygopalatine ganglion. It is responsible for supplying secretomotor fibres to the glands of nasal cavity, palate, pharynx, and the lacrimal gland. It is also called *hay fever ganglion* as inflammation of the ganglion causes allergic sinusitis.

### CLINICAL ANATOMY

- The pterygopalatine ganglion, if irritated or infected, causes congestion of the glands of palate and nose including the lacrimal gland producing running nose and lacrimation. The condition is called hay fever. The ganglion is called '***ganglion of hay fever***.
- Maxillary nerve carries the afferent limb fibres of the sneeze reflex as it carries general sensation from the nasal mucous membrane.

VIDEO

Video 3.15 **Nose**

### *Facts to Remember*

- Artery of epistaxis is sphenopalatine.
- Upper few mm of lateral wall of nose and septum of nose are lined by olfactory epithelium with bipolar neurons in it.
- Most of the nerves and blood vessels to the lateral wall of nose and septum of nose are common. The difference is in their magnitude.
- Maxillary sinusitis is the commonest chronic sinusitis.
- Into the middle meatus of nose drain 4 sets of air sinuses.
- Sinusitis may occur due to air pollution.
- Pterygopalatine ganglion is the ganglion of 'hay fever'. It gives secretomotor fibres to lacrimal, nasal, palatal and pharyngeal glands.
- Pain of maxillary sinusitis is referred to upper teeth; of ethmoidal sinusitis to medial side of orbit and of frontal sinusitis to forehead.

### BDC's Anatomy *e*-book

1. Summary of pterygopalatine fossa
2. Further reading
3. Viva voce questions

Chapter

16

# Larynx

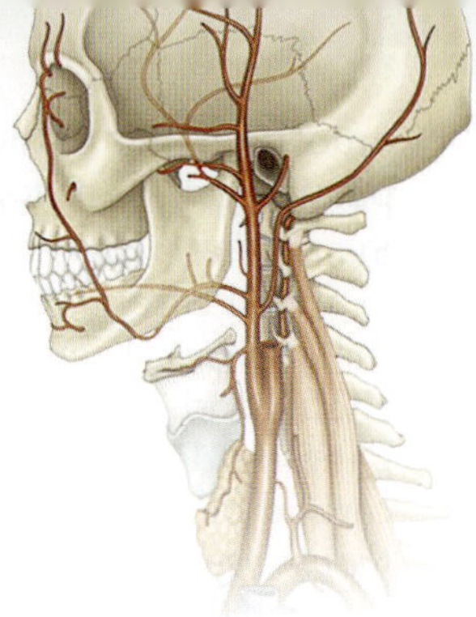

Larynx is a part of upper respiratory tract (Latin *wind pipe)*. It is an organ of phonation or voice box. It acts as a sphincter that protects the lower respiratory tract from entry of foreign bodies.

### *Functions of larynx*

1. Air passage
2. Phonation
3. Protective sphincter
4. Deglutition.

*Note*: The upper respiratory passages include the nose, the nasopharynx and the oropharynx.
One speaks during the expiratory phase of respiration.

**Plate 16.1:** Skeleton of the larynx (lateral view)

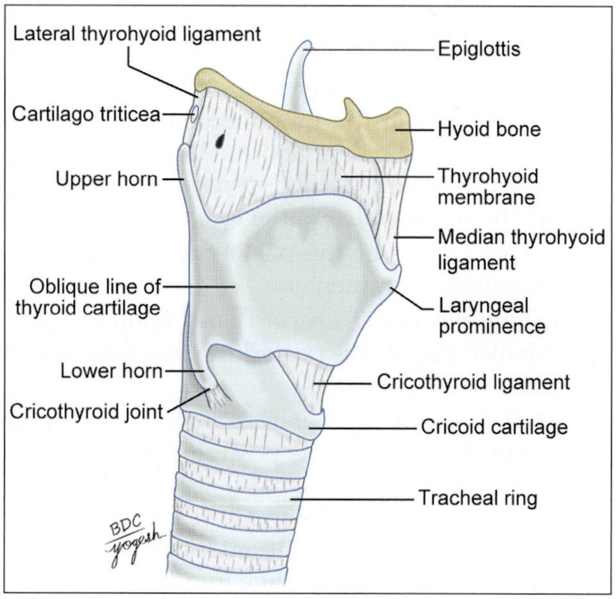


## Location and Extent

The larynx lies in the anterior midline of the neck, extending from the root of the tongue to the trachea. In the adult male, it lies in front of the 3rd to 6th cervical vertebrae, but in children and in the adult female, it lies at a little higher level (at C1–C4 level) (Plate 16.1, Flowchart 16.1).

## Size

The measurements of larynx are as follows:

*Length* (vertical): 44 mm in males and 36 mm in females
*Transverse*: 43 mm in males and 41 mm in females
*Anteroposterior*: 36 mm in males and 26 mm in females.

*Note*: At puberty, the male larynx grows rapidly and becomes larger, seen as prominent angle of thyroid cartilage (Adam's apple); which makes his voice louder and low pitched. The pubertal growth of the female larynx is negligible, and her voice is high pitched. Internal diameter—up to 3 years, it is 3 mm; and in an adult, it is 12 mm.

***Competency:***
**AN38.1** Describe the morphology, identify structure of the wall, nerve supply, blood supply and actions of intrinsic and extrinsic muscles of the larynx.

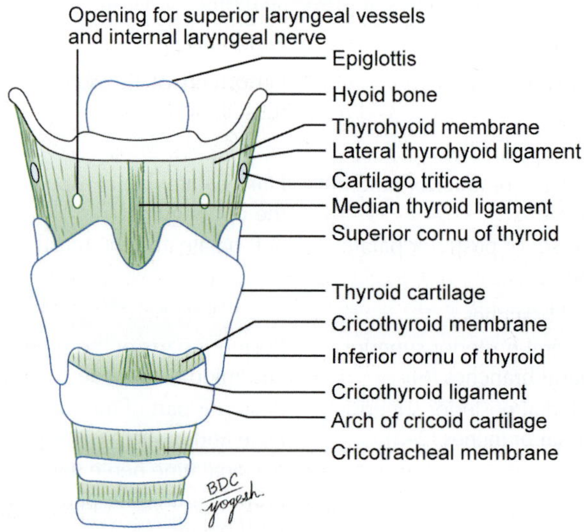


**Fig. 16.1:** Cartilages and skeleton of larynx (anterior view)

## CONSTITUTION OF LARYNX

The larynx is made up of a skeletal framework of cartilages (Plate 16.1 and Fig. 16.1). The cartilages are connected by joints, ligaments and membranes; and are moved by a number of muscles. The cavity of the larynx is lined by mucous membrane.

**Flowchart 16.1:** Larynx

- ***Larynx***
  - ***Location***
    - Anterior midline of neck
    - Extent:
      - From root of tongue to trachea
    - C3–C6 vertebral level
  - ***Size***
    - Length: 36–44 mm
    - Transverse: 41–43 mm
    - Anteroposterior: 26–36 mm
  - ***Skeleton of larynx***
    - ***9 cartilages***
      - Unpaired:
        - Thyroid
        - Cricoid
        - Epiglottis
      - Paired:
        - Arytenoid
        - Corniculate
        - Cuneiform
    - ***Joints***
      - Cricothyroid joint
        - Plane synovial
      - Cricoarytenoid joint
        - Plane synovial
      - Arytenocorniculate joint
        - Synovial/cartilagenous
    - ***Ligaments***
      - Extrinsic ligaments
        - Thyrohyoid membrane and ligaments
        - Cricotracheal ligament
        - Thyroepiglottic ligament
        - Hyoepiglottic ligament
        - Cricothyroid ligament
      - Intrinsic ligaments
        - Cricovocal membrane
        - Vocal ligament
        - Quadrangular membrane
        - Vestibular ligaments
    - ***Intrinsic muscles***
      - Cricothyroid
      - Posterior cricoarytenoid
      - Lateral cricoarytenoid
      - Transverse arytenoid
      - Oblique arytenoid
      - Aryepiglotticus
      - Thyroarytenoid
      - Thyroepiglotticus
      - Vocalis

## CARTILAGES OF LARYNX

The larynx contains nine cartilages, of which three are unpaired and three are paired (Plate 16.1 and Fig. 16.1).

### *Unpaired cartilages*

1. Thyroid (Greek *shield-like*)
2. Cricoid (Greek *ring-like*)
3. Epiglottis (Greek *leaf-like*)

### *Paired cartilages*

1. Arytenoid (Greek *cup-shaped*)
2. Corniculate (Latin *horn-shaped*)
3. Cuneiform (Latin *wedge-shaped*)

### Thyroid Cartilage

1. This cartilage is V-shaped in cross-section. It consists of right and left laminae (Plate 16.2 and Fig. 16.1).
2. Each lamina is roughly quadrilateral. The laminae are placed obliquely relative to the midline, their posterior borders are far apart, but the anterior borders approach each other at an angle that is about 90° in the male and about 120° in the female.
3. The lower parts of the anterior borders of the right and left laminae fuse and form a median projection called the ***laryngeal prominence*** or ***Adam's apple***. The upper parts of the anterior borders are separated by the ***thyroid notch***.
4. The posterior borders are free. They are prolonged upwards and downwards as the ***superior and inferior cornua*** or horns. The *inferior cornua* articulates with the cricoid cartilage to form the ***cricothyroid joint*** (Fig. 16.2).
5. The ***outer surface*** of each lamina is marked by an ***oblique line***.

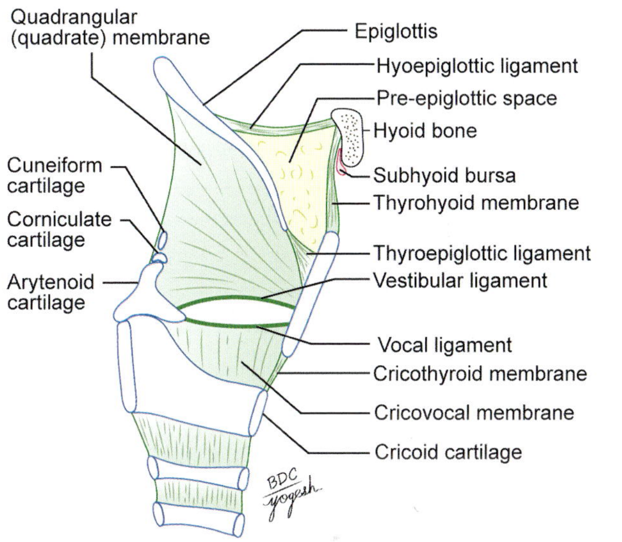


**Fig. 16.2:** Ligaments and membranes of larynx (sagittal section)

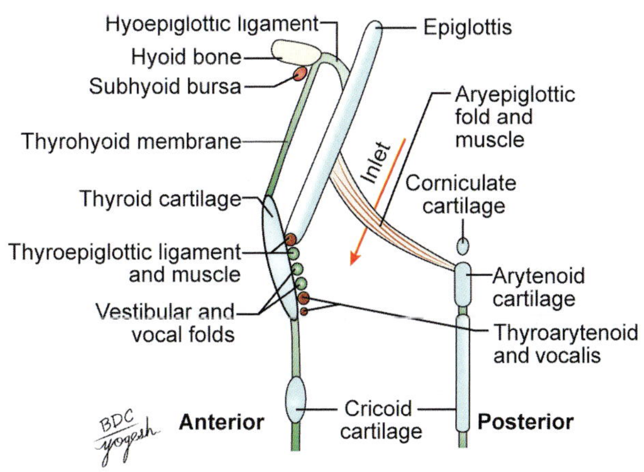


**Fig. 16.3:** Cartilages of the larynx as seen in sagittal section

#### Attachments (Figs 16.2 and 16.3)

1. Oblique line on the outer surface gives attachments to the following muscles:
   a. *Thyrohyoid*
   b. *Sternothyroid*
   c. Thyropharyngeus part of *inferior constrictor* of pharynx
2. Lower border and inferior cornua give insertion to triangular *cricothyroid*.
3. Along the posterior border connecting superior and inferior cornua are the insertion of the following muscles:
   a. *Palatopharyngeus*

**Plate 16.2:** Thyroid cartilage

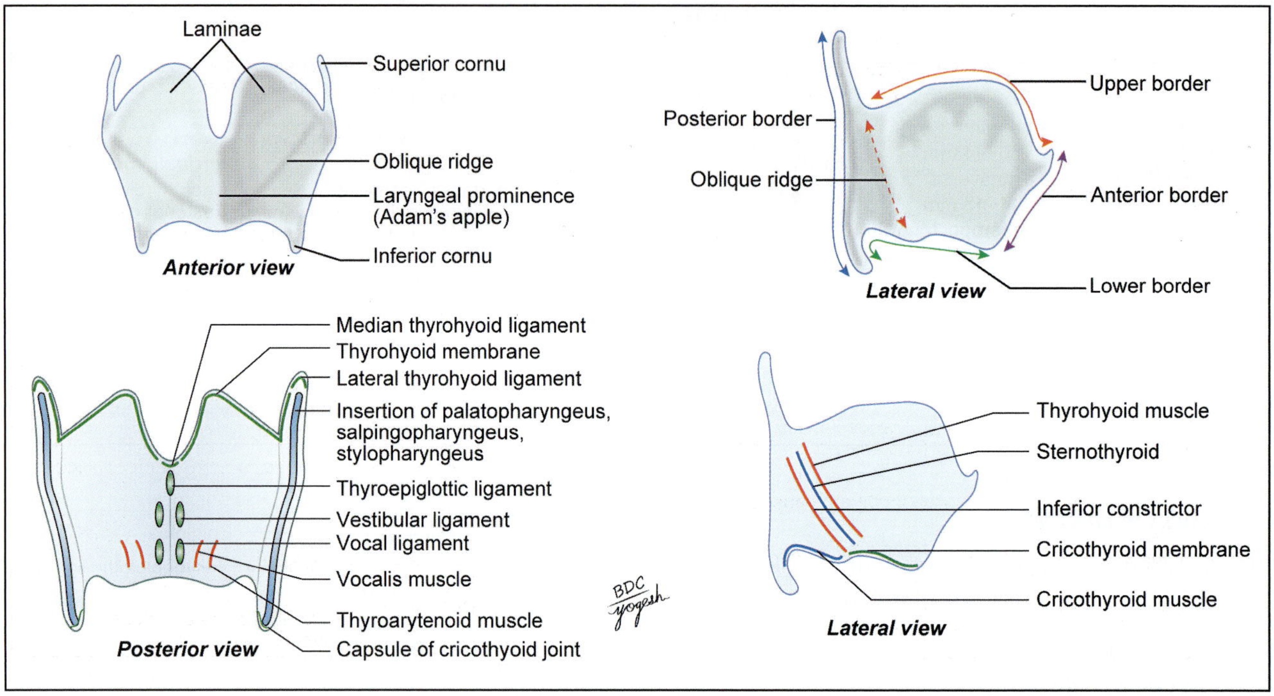


   b. *Salpingopharyngeus*
   c. *Stylopharyngeus*.
4. On inner aspect are attached:
   a. Thyroepiglottic ligament
   b. Thyroepiglottic muscle on each side
   c. Vestibular ligament/fold on each side
   d. Vocal ligament/fold on each side
   e. Thyroarytenoid muscle
   f. Vocalis muscle on each side.
5. The *superior cornua* is connected with the greater cornua of the hyoid bone by the lateral *thyrohyoid ligament*. Thyrohyoid ligament contains 2 nodules of elastic cartilage known as "***cartilage tritiate***" which may strengthen this connection (refer to Gray's Anatomy, 42nd edition).
6. In the median plane, ***inferior cornua*** is connected to the cricoid cartilage by the ***conus elasticus***.

## Cricoid Cartilage

1. Cricoid cartilage is ring-shaped. The ring has a narrow anterior part called the *arch*, and a broad posterior part, called the *lamina* (Plate 16.3).
2. The ***lamina*** projects upwards behind the thyroid cartilage, and articulates superiorly with the arytenoid cartilages.
3. The inferior cornua of the thyroid cartilage articulates with the side of the cricoid cartilage at the junction of the arch and lamina.

### Attachments

1. Anterior part of arch of cricoid gives origin to triangular *cricothyroid muscle*, a tensor of vocal cord.
2. Anterolateral aspect of arch gives origin to *lateral cricoarytenoid muscle*, an adductor of vocal cord.
3. Lamina of cricoid cartilage on its outer aspects gives origin to a very important 'safety muscle', the *posterior cricoarytenoid* muscle. *Cricothyroid* and *quadrate membranes* are also attached.

## Epiglottic Cartilage/Epiglottis

1. This is a *leaf-shaped* cartilage placed in the anterior wall of the upper part of the larynx (Plate 16.4).
2. Its *upper end* is broad and free, and projects upwards behind the hyoid bone and the tongue.
3. The *lower end* is pointed and is attached to the upper part of the angle between the two laminae of the thyroid cartilage by *thyroepiglottic ligament*.

### Attachments

1. The right and left margins of the cartilage provide attachment to the ***aryepiglottic folds***.
2. Its *anterior surface* is connected:
   a. To the tongue by a median ***glossoepiglottic fold***
   b. To the hyoid bone by the *hyoepiglottic ligament*.
3. The *posterior surface* is covered with mucous membrane, and presents a tubercle in the lower part.
4. *Thyroepiglottic muscle* is attached between thyroid cartilage and margins of epiglottis. It keeps the inlet of larynx patent for breathing.
5. *Aryepiglottic muscle* closes inlet during swallowing.

## Arytenoid Cartilage

1. These are two small *pyramid-shaped* cartilages lying on the upper border of the lamina of the cricoid cartilage (Plate 16.5).
2. The *apex* of the arytenoid cartilage is curved posteromedially and articulates with the corniculate cartilage.

Plate 16.3: Cricoid cartilage

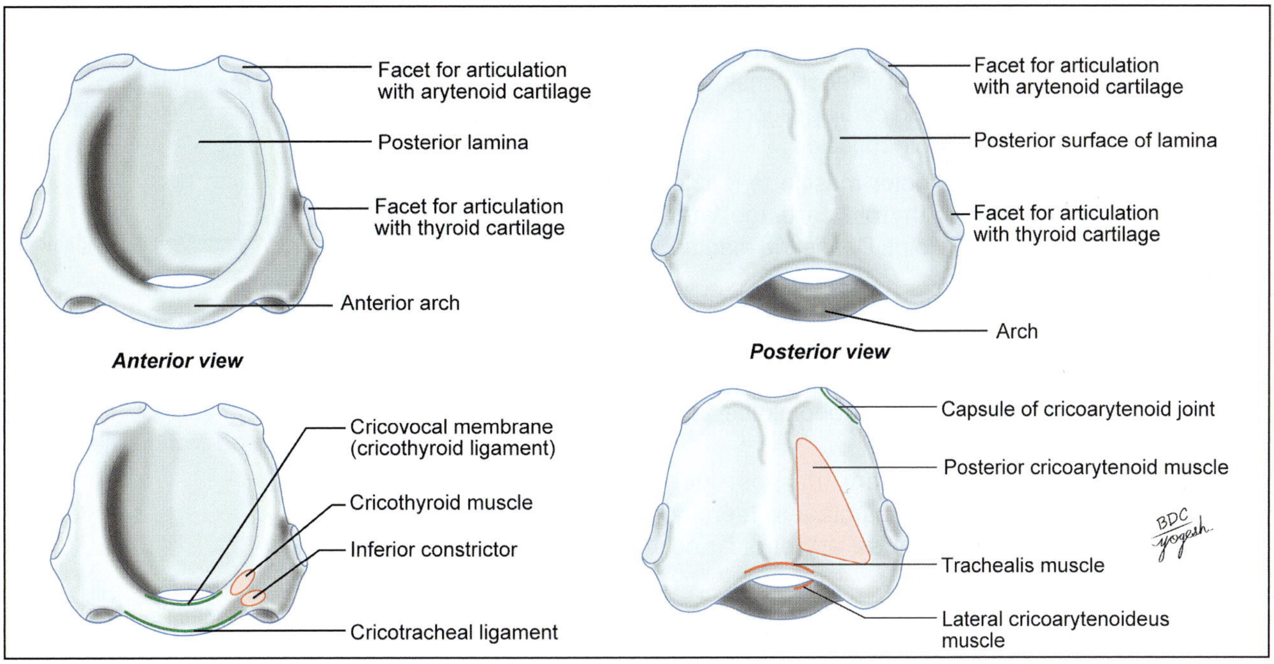


Plate 16.4: Epiglottic cartilage

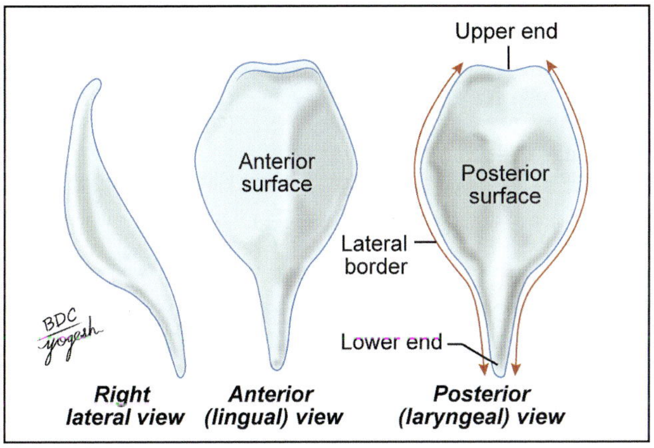


3. Its *base* is concave and articulates with the lateral part of the upper border of the cricoid lamina. Base is prolonged anteriorly to form the ***vocal process***, and laterally to form the ***muscular process***.
4. The *surfaces* of the cartilage are anterolateral, medial and posterior (Plate 16.5).

### Attachments

1. ***Vocal process:*** Vocal fold and vocalis muscle is attached.
2. ***Above vocal process:*** Vestibular fold attached.
3. ***Muscular process:*** Posterior aspect gives insertion to *posterior cricoarytenoid*.
4. Anterior aspect gives insertion to lateral *cricoarytenoid*.
5. ***Posterior surface:*** Transverse arytenoid across the two cartilages.
6. Between base and apex of arytenoid is *oblique arytenoid* which continues as *aryepiglottic muscle* into two sides of epiglottis.

Plate 16.5: Arytenoid cartilage

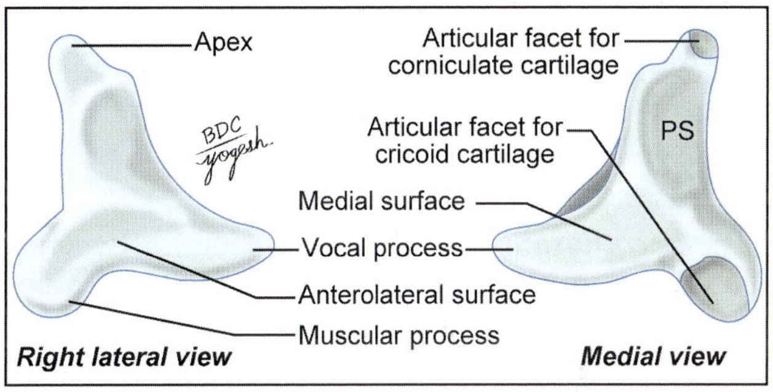


(PS: Posterior surface)

7. Quadrangular or *quadrate membrane* is attached between arytenoid, epiglottis and thyroid cartilages.

### Corniculate/Santorini Cartilages

These are two small conical nodules which articulate with the apex of the arytenoid cartilages, and are directed posteromedially. They lie in the posterior parts of the aryepiglottic folds.

### Cuneiform/Wrisberg Cartilages

These are two small rod-shaped pieces of cartilage placed in the aryepiglottic folds just ventral to the corniculate cartilages.

## TYPES OF LARYNGEAL CARTILAGES

The thyroid, cricoid cartilages, and the basal parts of the arytenoid cartilages are made up of the hyaline cartilage. They may ossify after the age of 25 years. The other cartilages of the larynx, e.g. epiglottis, corniculate, cuneiform and processes of the arytenoid are made of the elastic cartilage and do not ossify.

## DISSECTION

Identify sternothyroid muscle in the sagittal section of head and neck and define its attachments on the thyroid cartilage. Define the attachments of inferior constrictor muscle from both cricoid and thyroid cartilages including the fascia overlying the cricothyroid muscle.

Cut through the inferior constrictor muscle to locate articulation of inferior horn of thyroid cartilage with cricoid cartilage, i.e. cricothyroid joint. Define the median cricothyroid ligament.

Identify thyrohyoid muscle. Remove this muscle to identify thyrohyoid membrane. Identify superior laryngeal vessels and internal laryngeal nerve piercing this membrane. Identify epiglottis, thyroepiglottic and hyoepiglottic ligaments.

Strip the mucous membrane from the posterior surfaces of arytenoid and cricoid cartilages. Identify posterior cricoarytenoid, transverse arytenoid and oblique arytenoid muscles.

Recurrent laryngeal nerve was seen to enter larynx deep to the inferior constrictor muscle.

Identify cricothyroid muscle, which is the only intrinsic muscle of larynx placed on the external aspect of larynx. Remove the lower half of lamina of thyroid cartilage including the inferior horn of thyroid cartilage. Visualise the thyroarytenoid muscle in the vocal fold.

## LARYNGEAL JOINTS

1. The ***cricothyroid joint*** is a *synovial* joint between the inferior cornua of the thyroid cartilage and the side of the cricoid cartilage. It permits rotatory movements around a transverse axis passing through both cricothyroid joints permitting tension and relaxation of vocal cords. There are some gliding movements also in different directions.
2. The ***cricoarytenoid joint*** is also a *synovial* joint between the base of the arytenoid cartilage and the upper border of the lamina of the cricoid cartilage. It permits rotatory movements around a vertical axis permitting adduction and abduction of the vocal cords and also gliding movements in all directions.

## LARYNGEAL LIGAMENTS AND MEMBRANES

**Extrinsic** (Figs 16.2, 16.4 and 16.5)

1. ***Thyrohyoid membrane*** connects the thyroid cartilage to the hyoid bone. Its median and lateral parts are thickened to form the ***median and lateral thyrohyoid ligaments***.

*Note:*

The membrane is pierced by the internal laryngeal nerve, and by the superior laryngeal vessels.

***Tritiate cartilages*** are small nodules of elastic cartilage present in the free posterior edge of thyrohyoid membrane. These serve to strengthen the connection between superior cornua of thyroid cartilage and tip of greater cornua of hyoid bone.

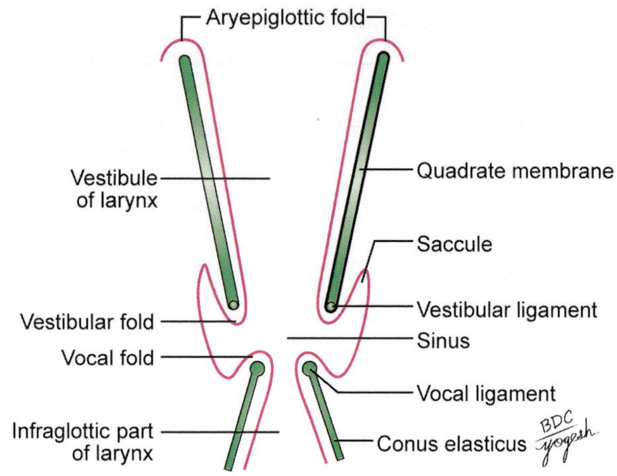


**Fig. 16.4:** Coronal section showing parts of cavity of the larynx

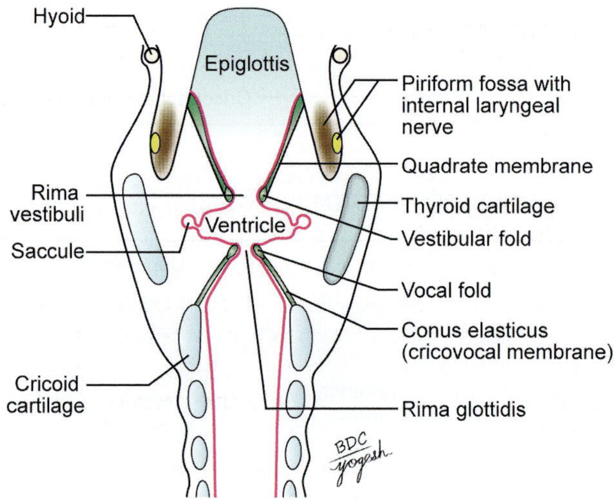


**Fig. 16.5:** Cavity of larynx and position of piriform fossa

2. ***Hyoepiglottic ligament*** connects the upper end of the epiglottic cartilage to the hyoid bone.
3. ***Cricotracheal ligament*** connects the cricoid cartilage to the upper end of the trachea.

**Intrinsic** (Figs 16.2, 16.4 and 16.5)

1. The intrinsic ligaments are part of a broad sheet of fibroelastic tissue, known as the ***fibroelastic membrane of the larynx***. This membrane is placed just outside the mucous membrane. It is interrupted on each side by the sinus of the larynx. The part of the membrane above the sinus is known as the ***quadrate membrane***, and the part below the sinus is called the ***conus elasticus*** (Fig. 16.4).
2. ***Quadrate membrane*** extends from the arytenoid cartilage to the epiglottis. It has a lower free border which forms the *vestibular fold* and an upper border which forms the *aryepiglottic fold*.
3. ***Conus elasticus*** or ***cricovocal membrane*** extends upwards and medially from the arch of the cricoid cartilage. The anterior part is thick and is known as the ***cricothyroid ligament***. The upper free border of the conus elasticus forms the *vocal fold* (Fig. 16.5).

## CAVITY OF LARYNX

The cavity of the larynx extends from the inlet of larynx to the lower border of the cricoid cartilage (Plate 16.6 and Flowchart 16.2).

### Communications

1. Above the larynx, communicates with laryngopharynx through the *laryngeal inlet*. Below the larynx, continues with the trachea at the lower border of cricoid cartilage.
2. *Laryngeal inlet* is placed obliquely, sloping downward and backwards.

   *Boundaries*

   *Anterior*: Epiglottis

   *Posterior*: Interarytenoid fold of mucous membrane

   *Lateral (on each side)*: Aryepiglottic fold of mucous membrane.
3. *Vestibular and vocal folds:* The cavity of larynx shows two mucosal folds on each side as follows:
   i. Upper *vestibular (false vocal) folds* are produced by vestibular ligaments.
   ii. Lower *vocal (true vocal) folds* are produced by vocal ligament and vocalis muscle. They extend from the middle of the thyroid angle to the vocal process of arytenoid cartilage.
4. *Rima vestibuli* and *rima glottidis: The rima vestibuli* is a space (gap) between the right and left vestibular folds. *The rima glottidis* is a space (gap) between the right and left vocal folds. It is the narrowest part of larynx.

### Subdivisions of Laryngeal Cavity

The laryngeal cavity is divided into three parts by two pairs of vestibular and vocal folds:

1. *Vestibule (supraglottic compartment)*: It extends from the laryngeal inlet to the vestibular folds.
2. *Ventricle or sinus of larynx (glottic compartment)*: It is an elliptical space that extends from vestibular folds to vocal folds.
3. *Infraglottic compartment*: It extends from vocal folds to the lower border of cricoid cartilage.

### Saccule of Larynx

The anterior part of sinus of larynx extends upward as a diverticulum between the vestibular folds and lamina of thyroid cartilage. This extension is known as *saccule of larynx* (Plate 16.6).

*Note*: **Oil can of larynx:** The saccule contains mucous glands which lubricates the vocal folds. Hence, the saccule is also termed as oil can of larynx.

## MUCOUS MEMBRANE OF LARYNX

1. The anterior surface and upper half of the posterior surface of the epiglottis, the upper parts of the aryepiglottic folds, and the vocal folds are lined by the *stratified squamous epithelium*. The rest of the laryngeal mucous membrane is covered with the *ciliated columnar epithelium.*
2. The mucous membrane is loosely attached to the cartilages of the larynx except over the vocal ligaments and over the posterior surface of the epiglottis where it is thin and firmly adherent.
3. The *mucous glands* are absent over the vocal cords, but are plentiful over the anterior surface of the epiglottis, around the cuneiform cartilages and in the vestibular folds. The glands are scattered over the rest of the larynx.

**Plate 16.6:** Interior of the larynx (coronal section of the laryngeal cavity)

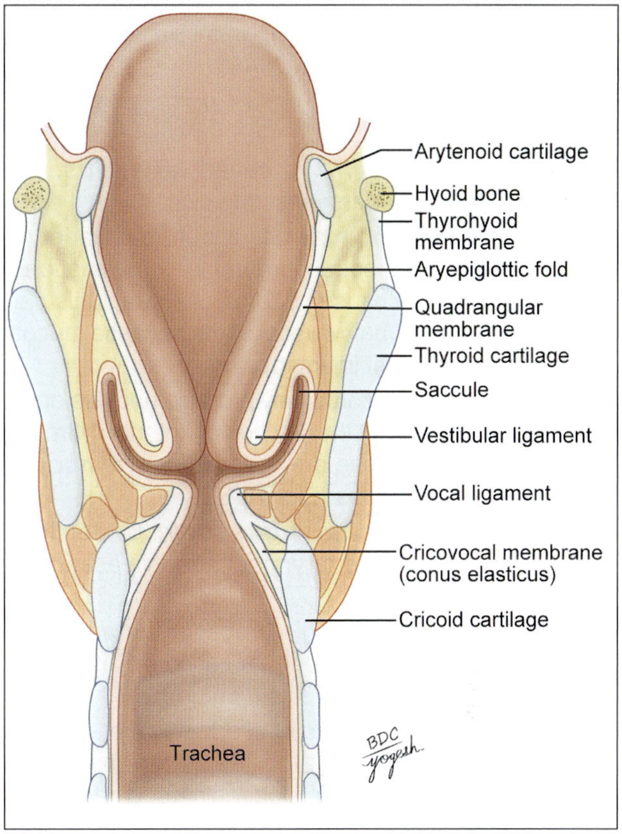


**Flowchart 16.2:** Cavity of larynx

***Cavity of larynx***

| ***Extent*** | ***Laryngeal inlet*** | ***Other features*** | ***Subdivisions*** |
|---|---|---|---|
| From inlet of larynx to lower border of cricoid cartilage | Anterior: Epiglottis<br>Posterior: Interarytenoid fold of mucous membrane<br>Lateral: Aryepiglottic fold of mucous membrane | Vestibular fold<br>Vocal fold<br>Rima vestibuli<br>Rima glottidis | Vestibule<br>- Above vestibular folds<br>Ventricle or sinus of larynx<br>- Between vestibular and vocal folds<br>Infraglottic compartment<br>- Below vocal folds |

***Saccule of larynx:*** Upward extension of anterior part of sinus of larynx, oil can of larynx (contains mucous glands)

BDC yogesh

*Competencies:*

**AN36.5** Describe the pharyngeal spaces. Also describe the boundaries and clinical significance of pyriform fossa.

**AN38.2** Describe the anatomical aspects of laryngitis.

## CLINICAL ANATOMY

- Infection of the larynx is called ***laryngitis***. It is characterized by hoarseness of voice.
- ***Laryngeal oedema*** may occur due to a variety of causes. This can obstruct breathing. Inflammation of upper larynx may cause oedema of supraglottis part. It does not extend below vocal cords because mucosa is adherent to vocal ligament.
- Misuse of the vocal cords may produce nodules on the vocal cords mostly at the junction of anterior 1/3rd and posterior 2/3rd. These are called ***Singer's nodules*** or ***Teacher's nodules*** (Fig. 16.6).
- *Fibreoptic flexible* ***laryngoscopy:*** Under local anaesthesia, flexible laryngoscope is passed and larynx well visualised.
- ***Microlaryngoscopy:*** This procedure is performed under operating microscope. Vocal cord tumours and diseases are excised by this method.
- ***Foreign body in larynx:*** Since the larynx or glottis is the narrowest part of the respiratory passages, ***foreign bodies*** are usually lodged here. Large foreign bodies may block laryngeal inlet leading to suffocation.
- At times fish bones may get impacted in the vallecula or piriform fossa. Often these bones just scratch the mucosa on their way down, and the person gets a feeling of foreign body sensation, due to a dull visceral pain caused by the scratch.
- ***Piriform fossa*** lies between quadrate membrane and medial side of thyroid cartilage. It is traversed by internal laryngeal nerve. Piriform fossa is used to smuggle out precious stones, diamonds, etc. It is called ***smuggler's fossa***.
- The mucous membrane of the larynx is supplied by X nerve through superior laryngeal or recurrent laryngeal nerves. So laryngeal tumours may also cause referred pain in the ear partly supplied by auricular branch of X nerve.

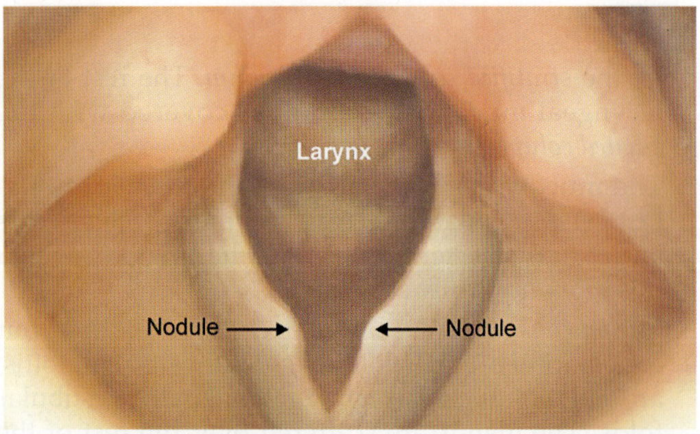


**Fig. 16.6:** Indirect laryngoscopic examination

## MUSCLES OF LARYNX

The muscles of the larynx are grouped as extrinsic and intrinsic muscles (Tables 16.1 and 16.2).

### Extrinsic Muscles

These are paired muscles and move the larynx as a whole. They are:

1. Palatopharyngeus
2. Salpingopharyngeus
3. Stylopharyngeus
4. Thyrohyoid
5. Sternothyroid.

These are attached to one of the laryngeal cartilages and adjacent bones.

### Intrinsic Muscles

These muscles extend between laryngeal cartilages. They include (Plate 16.7 and Figs 16.7 to 16.9):

1. Cricothyroid
2. Posterior cricoarytenoid
3. Lateral cricoarytenoid
4. Transverse arytenoid
5. Oblique arytenoid
6. Aryepiglotticus
7. Thyroarytenoid
8. Thyroepiglotticus
9. Vocalis.

The intrinsic muscle of larynx:

1. Opens or closes the laryngeal inlet
2. Adducts or abducts the vocal cords
3. Lengthens or shortens the vocal cords
4. Increases or decreases the tension in vocal cords.

### Nerve Supply

All intrinsic muscles of the larynx are supplied by the ***recurrent laryngeal nerve*** *except* for the cricothyroid which is supplied by the external laryngeal nerve.

*Note*:

The vocal and muscular processes move in opposite directions. Any muscle which pulls the muscular process medially, pushes the vocal process laterally, resulting in abduction of vocal cords. This is done by only one pair of muscle, the posterior cricoarytenoid.

Muscles which pull the muscular process forward and laterally will push the vocal process medially causing adduction of vocal cords. This is done by lateral cricoarytenoid and transverse arytenoid.

The cricothyroid causes rocking movement of thyroid forwards and downwards at cricothyroid joints, thus tensing and lengthening the vocal cords.

Muscles which abduct the vocal cords: Only posterior crico-arytenoids (safety muscle of larynx).

## MOVEMENTS OF VOCAL FOLDS

Movements of the vocal folds affect the shape and size of the rima glottidis (Figs 16.10 to 16.15).

1. During quiet breathing or condition of rest, the intermembranous part of the rima is triangular, and the intercartilaginous part is quadrangular (Fig. 16.8).

Plate 16.7: Intrinsic muscles of larynx

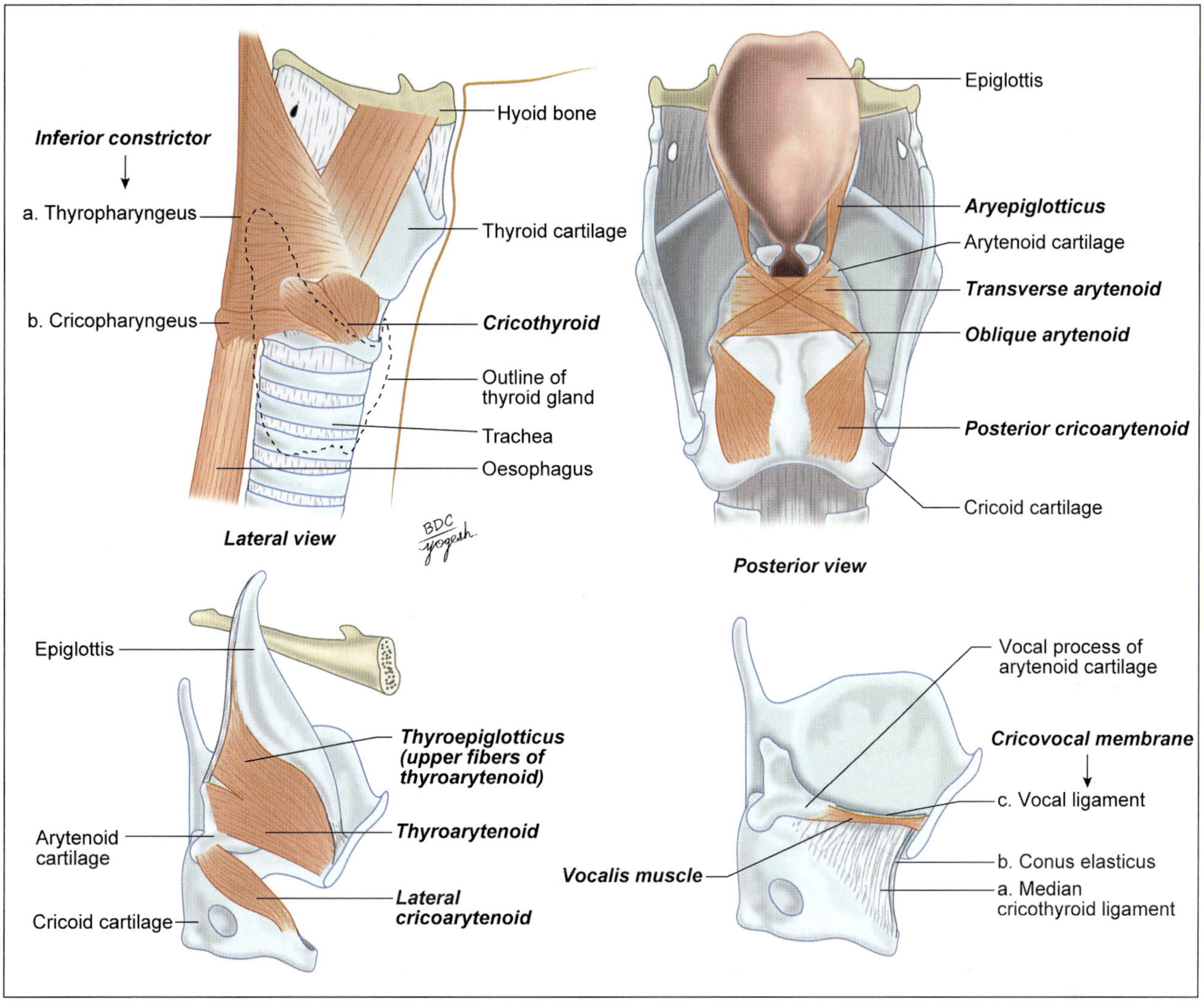


**TABLE 16.1: Origin, fibres and insertion of intrinsic muscles of the larynx** (Plate 16.7 and Figs 16.7 to 16.9)

| *Muscle* | *Origin* | *Fibres* | *Insertion* |
|---|---|---|---|
| 1. **Cricothyroid**<br>The only muscle outside the larynx<br>It is called 'tuning fork of larynx' | Lower border and lateral surface of cricoid cartilage | Fibres pass backwards and upwards | Inferior cornua and lower border of thyroid cartilage |
| 2. **Posterior cricoarytenoid**<br>Triangular | Posterior surface of the lamina of cricoid cartilage | Upwards and laterally | Posterior aspect of muscular process of arytenoid cartilage |
| 3. **Lateral cricoarytenoid** | Upper border of arch of cricoid cartilage | Upwards and backwards | Anterior aspect of muscular process of arytenoid cartilage |
| 4. **Transverse arytenoid**<br>Unpaired muscle | Posterior surface of one arytenoid cartilage | Transverse | Posterior surface of another arytenoid cartilage |
| 5, 6. **Oblique arytenoid** and **aryepiglottic** | Muscular process of one arytenoid cartilage | Oblique | Apex of the other arytenoid. Some fibres are continued as *aryepiglottic* muscle to the edge of the epiglottis |
| 7, 8. **Thyroarytenoid** and **thyroepiglotticus** | Thyroid angle and adjacent cricothyroid ligament | Backwards and upwards | Anterolateral surface of arytenoid cartilage<br>Some of the upper fibres of thyroarytenoid curve upwards into the aryepiglottic fold to reach the edge of epiglottis, known as *thyroepiglotticus* |
| 9. **Vocalis** | Vocal process of arytenoid cartilage | Pass forwards | Vocal ligament and thyroid angle |

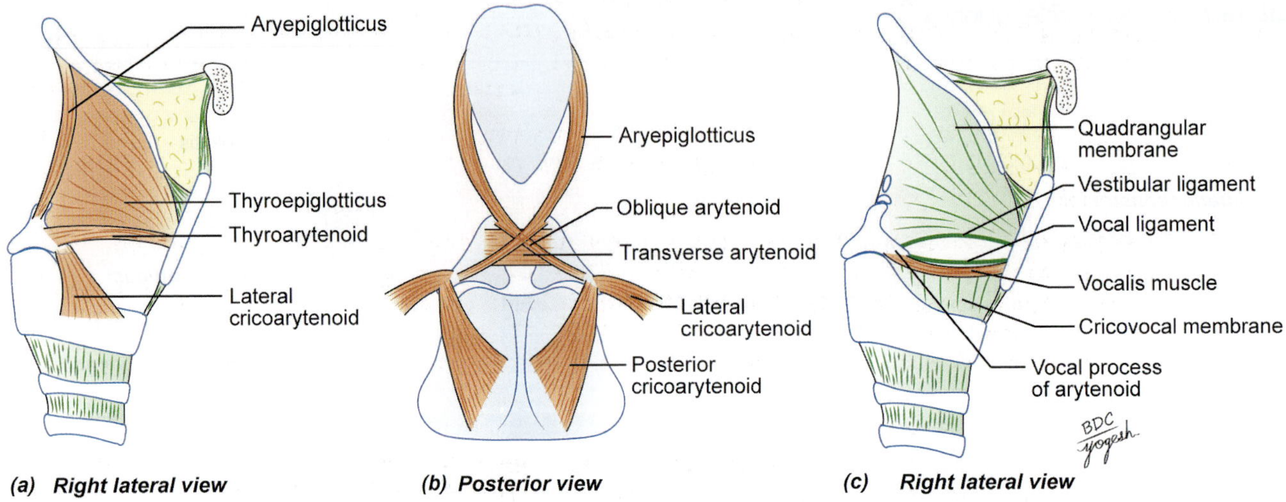


**Figs 16.7a to c:** Intrinsic muscles of the larynx

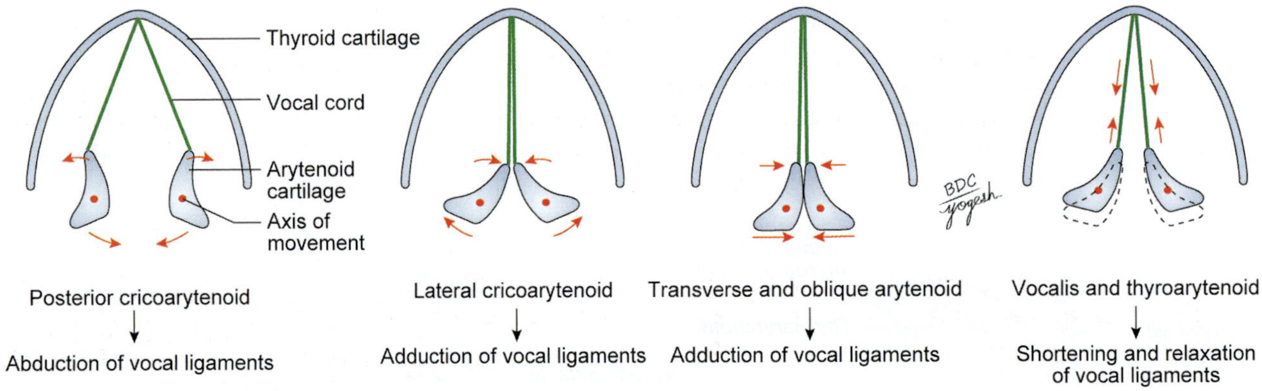


**Fig. 16.8:** Actions of intrinsic muscles of larynx

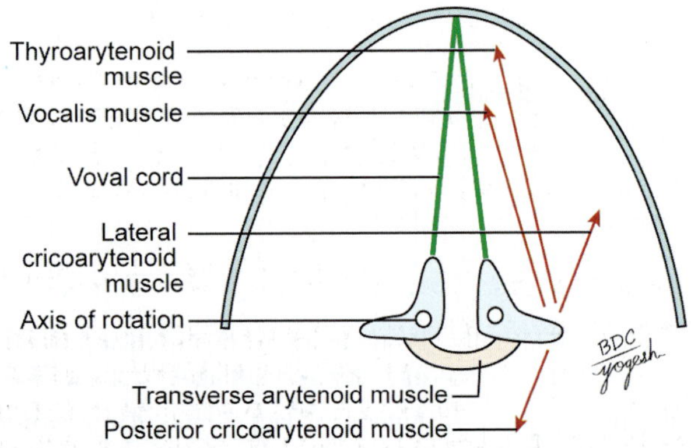


**Fig. 16.9:** Scheme to show the direction of pull of some intrinsic muscles of the larynx

**TABLE 16.2: Muscles acting on the larynx**

| *Movement* | *Muscle* |
|---|---|
| Elevation of larynx | Thyrohyoid, mylohyoid |
| Depression of larynx | Sternothyroid, sternohyoid |
| Opening inlet of larynx | Thyroepiglotticus |
| Closing inlet of larynx | Aryepiglotticus |
| Abductor of vocal cords | Posterior cricoarytenoid only |
| Adductor of vocal cords | Lateral cricoarytenoid, transverse and oblique arytenoids |
| Tensor of vocal cords and modulation of voice (lengthening of vocal cord) | Cricothyroid |
| Relaxor and adjust tension of vocal cords | Thyroarytenoid and vocalis |

2. During phonation or speech, the glottis is reduced to a chink by the adduction of the vocal folds.
3. During forced inspiration, both parts of the rima are triangular, so that the entire rima is lozenge-shaped; the vocal folds are fully abducted (i.e. diamond-shaped glottis).
4. During whispering, the intermembranous part of the rima glottidis is closed, but the intercartilaginous part is widely open(i.e. funnel-shaped glottis).

## BLOOD SUPPLY, NERVE SUPPLY AND LYMPHATIC DRAINAGE OF LARYNX

### Arterial Supply and Venous Drainage

#### *Up to the Vocal Folds*

By the superior laryngeal artery, a branch of the superior thyroid artery. The superior laryngeal vein drains into the superior thyroid vein.

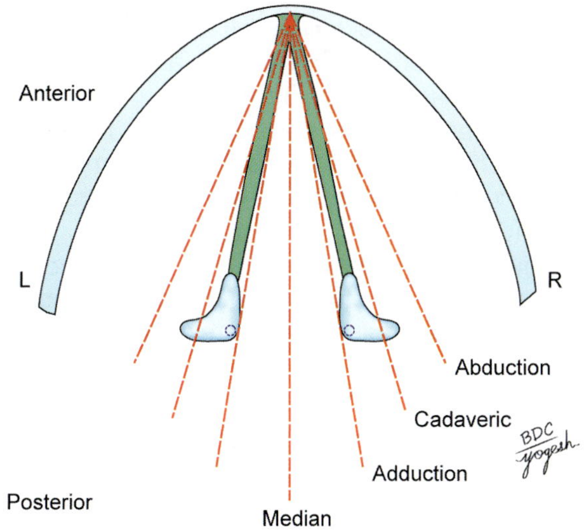


**Fig. 16.10:** Various positions of the vocal cords

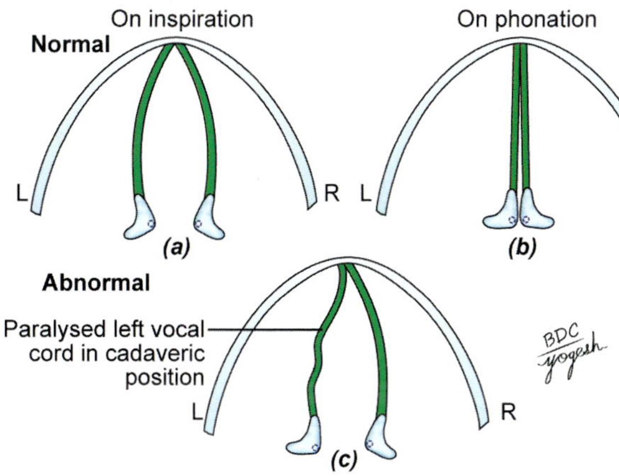


**Figs 16.11a to c:** Position of vocal cords: (a) Inspiration, (b) phonation and (c) abnormal

### *Below the Vocal Folds*

By the inferior laryngeal artery, a branch of the inferior thyroid artery. The inferior laryngeal vein drains into the inferior thyroid vein.

## Nerve Supply

### *Motor Nerves*

Recurrent laryngeal nerve supplies posterior cricoarytenoid, lateral cricoarytenoid, transverse and oblique arytenoid, aryepiglottic, thyroarytenoid, thyroepiglottic

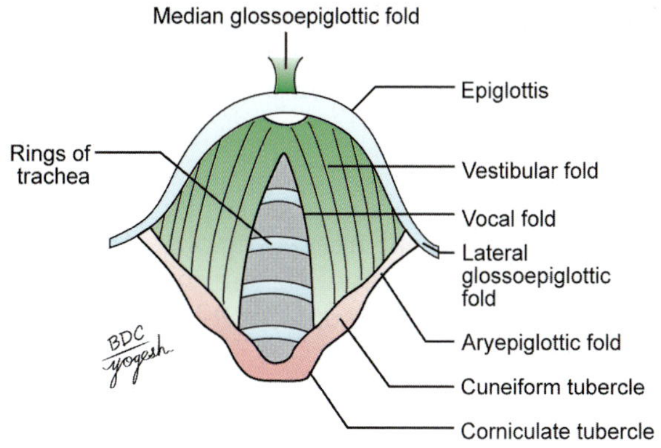


**Fig. 16.12:** Parts of larynx seen by indirect laryngoscopy

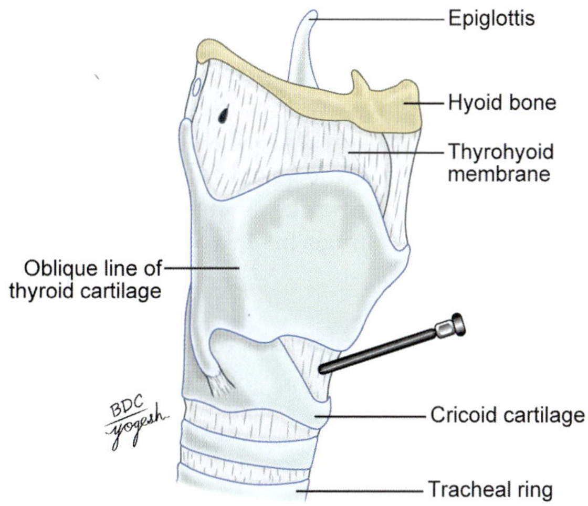


**Fig. 16.13:** Laryngotomy

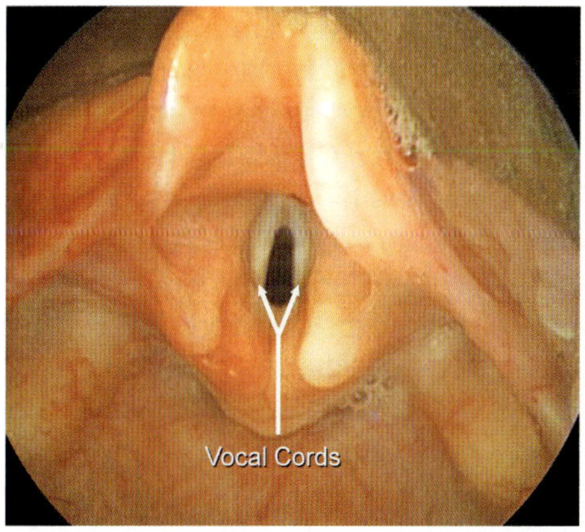


**Fig. 16.14:** Direct laryngoscopic view of vocal cords in adducted position

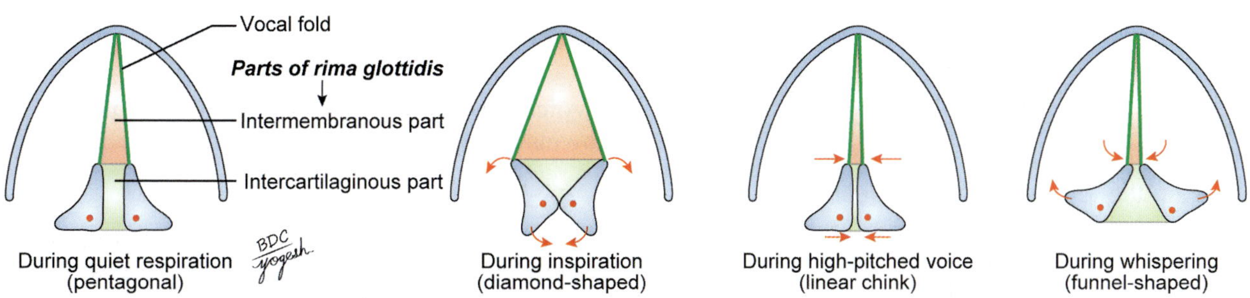


**Fig. 16.15:** Rima glottidis during different movements of the vocal cords

muscles. It supplies all intrinsic muscles except crico-thyroid.

External laryngeal nerve only supplies cricothyroid muscle.

### Sensory Nerves

The internal laryngeal nerve supplies the mucous membrane up to the level of the vocal folds. The recurrent laryngeal nerve supplies it below the level of the vocal folds.

### Lymphatic Drainage

Lymphatics from the part above the vocal folds drain along the superior thyroid vessels to the anterosuperior group of deep cervical nodes by piercing thyrohyoid membrane.

Those from the part below the vocal folds drain to the posteroinferior group of deep cervical nodes. A few of them drain into the prelaryngeal nodes by piercing cricothyroid. True vocal folds, i.e. glottis acts as watershed for lymphatics. It has 'no' lymphatics. Carcinoma of glottis carries best prognosis.

*Competency:*
**AN38.3** Describe anatomical basis of recurrent laryngeal nerve injury.

## CLINICAL ANATOMY

- When any foreign object enters the larynx severe protective coughing is excited to expel the object. However, damage to the internal laryngeal nerve produces anaesthesia of the mucous membrane in the supraglottic part of the larynx breaking the reflex arc so that foreign bodies can readily enter it.
- Damage to the external laryngeal nerve causes some weakness of phonation due to loss of the tightening effect of the cricothyroid on the vocal cord.
- When both recurrent laryngeal nerves are interrupted, the vocal cords lie in the cadaveric position in between abduction and adduction, and phonation is completely lost. Deep breathing also becomes difficult through the partially opened glottis.
- When only one recurrent laryngeal nerve is paralysed, the opposite vocal cord compensates for it and phonation is possible but there is hoarseness of voice. There is failure of forceful explosive part of voluntary and reflex coughing.
- Tumours in the piriform fossa cause dysphagia. These also cause referred pain in the ear. Pain of pharyngeal tumours may be referred to the ear, as X nerve carries sensation both from the pharynx and the external auditory meatus and the tympanic membrane.
- *Recurrent laryngeal nerve:* Mediastinal tumours may press on the left recurrent laryngeal nerve, as it is given off in the thorax. The pressure on the nerve may present as alteration in the voice. Right recurrent laryngeal nerve is given off in the neck, so it is not affected by mediastinal tumours.
- The larynx can be examined either directly through a laryngoscope or indirectly through a laryngeal mirror (indirect laryngoscopy) (Fig. 16.14).
- By laryngoscopy, one can inspect the base of the tongue, the valleculae, the epiglottis, the aryepiglottic folds, the piriform fossae, the vestibular folds, and the vocal folds.
- Tumours of the vocal cords can be diagnosed early, because there are changes in the voice. Tumours in subglottic area present late so are diagnosed late and have poor prognosis.
- ***Laryngotomy:*** The needle is inserted in the midline of cricothyroid membrane, below the thyroid prominence. This is done as an emergency procedure.

## INFANT'S LARYNX

Cavity of infant's larynx is short and funnel-shaped.

- Size is one-third of an adult. Lumen is very narrow.
- Position is higher than in adult.
- Epiglottis lies at C2 and during elevation, it reaches C1, so that infant can use nasal airway for breathing while suckling.
- Laryngeal cartilages are softer, more pliable than in adult.
- Thyroid cartilage is shorter and broader.
- Vocal cords are only 4–4.5 mm long, shorter than in childhood and in adult.
- Supraglottic and subglottic mucosa are lax, swelling results in respiratory obstruction.
- One must be careful while giving anaesthesia to an infant (birth to one year).

## MECHANISM OF SPEECH

The mechanism of speech involves the following four processes:

- Expired air from lungs
- Vibrators
- Resonators
- Articulators

### Expired Air

As the air is forced out of lungs and larynx, it produces voice. Loudness or intensity of voice depends on the force of expiration of air.

### Vibrators

The expired air causes vibrations of the vocal cords. Pitch of voice depends on the rate of vibration of vocal cords. Vowels are produced in the larynx.

### Resonators

The column of air between vocal cords and nose and lips act as resonators. Quality of sound depends on resonators. One can make out change of quality of voice even on the telephone.

### Articulators

These are formed by palate, tongue, teeth and lips. These narrow or stop the exhaled air. Vowels are produced due to vibrations of vocal cords. Many of the consonants are produced by the intrinsic muscles of tongue. Consonants produced by lips are:

Pa, Pha, Ba, Bha, Ma

Labiodental—Ta, Tha, Da, Dha, Na

Lingual—Cha, Ja, Jha

Palatal—Ka, Kha, Ga, Gha.

VIDEO

**Video 3.16** Larynx

### *Facts to Remember*

- Only intrinsic muscle of larynx placed on the outer aspect of laryngeal cartilages is cricothyroid.
- Cricothyroid is the only muscle supplied by external laryngeal nerve.
- External laryngeal nerve runs with superior thyroid artery. Near the apex of the lobe, it deviates medially to supply inferior constrictor and cricothyroid muscles.
- Posterior cricoarytenoid is the only abductor of vocal cord and so it is a life-saving muscle.
- Tuning fork of larynx (chief tensor of vocal cords) is cricothyroid.
- Piriform fossa is called smuggler's fossa as precious stones, etc. can be hidden here.
- The primary function of larynx is to protect the lower respiratory tract. Phonation has developed with evolution and is related to motor speech area of the cerebral cortex.
- Singer's or teacher's nodules are inflammatory nodules on the vocal cords at the junction of anterior one-third and posterior two-third.
- Rima glottidis is the narrowest region of the laryngeal cavity.

### BDC's Anatomy *e*-book

1. Cricothyroid – tuning fork of larynx
2. Posterior cricoarytenoid – safety muscle of larynx
3. Further reading
4. Viva voce questions

Chapter

17

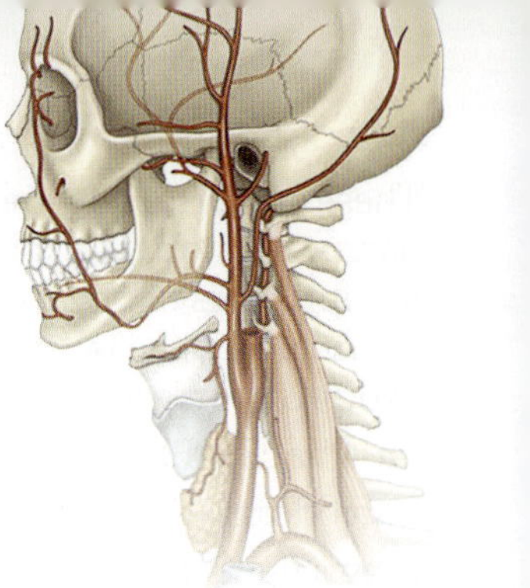

# Tongue

The tongue is a muscular organ situated in the floor of the mouth. It is associated with the functions of taste, speech, chewing, deglutition, and cleansing of mouth. The tongue comprises voluntary skeletal muscles.

## PARTS OF TONGUE

The tongue has:
1. Root
2. Tip
3. Body

### Root

The *root* is a fixed part. It is attached to the styloid process and soft palate above, and to mandible and the hyoid bone below. In between the mandible and hyoid bones, it is related to the geniohyoid and mylohyoid muscles.

### Tip

The *tip* of the tongue forms the anterior free end which, at rest, lies behind the upper incisor teeth.

### Body

The body of the tongue has:
a. A curved upper surface or *dorsum* (Fig. 17.1), and
b. An inferior surface confined to the oral part only.

The *dorsum* of the tongue (Fig. 17.1) is convex in all directions. It is divided into:
- An *oral part* or anterior two-thirds.
- A *pharyngeal part* or posterior one-third, by a faint V-shaped groove, the ***sulcus terminalis***. The two limbs of the 'V' meet at a median pit, named the ***foramen caecum***. They run laterally and forwards up to the palatoglossal arches.

  *Note*: The foramen caecum represents the site from which the thyroid diverticulum grows down in the embryo. The oral and pharyngeal parts of the tongue differ in their development, topography, structure, and function.
- Small posteriormost part.

### *Oral Part*

The ***oral or papillary part*** of the tongue is placed on the floor of the mouth. Its *margins* are free and in contact with the gums and teeth. Just in front of the circumvallate papillae, each margin shows 4 to 5 vertical folds, named the ***foliate papillae***.

The *superior surface* of the oral part shows a median furrow and is covered with papillae which make it rough (Fig. 17.1).

The ***inferior surface*** is covered with a smooth mucous membrane, which shows a median fold called the ***frenulum linguae***.

On either side of the frenulum, there is a prominence produced by the deep lingual veins. More laterally, there is a fold called the ***plica fimbriata*** that is directed forwards and medially towards the tip of the tongue (Fig. 17.2).

### *Pharyngeal Part*

The ***pharyngeal or lymphoid part*** *of the tongue* lies behind the palatoglossal arches and the sulcus terminalis. Its posterior surface, sometimes called the base of the tongue, forms the anterior wall of the oropharynx. The mucous membrane has no papillae, but has many *lymphoid follicles* that collectively constitute the ***lingual tonsil***. Mucous glands are also present.

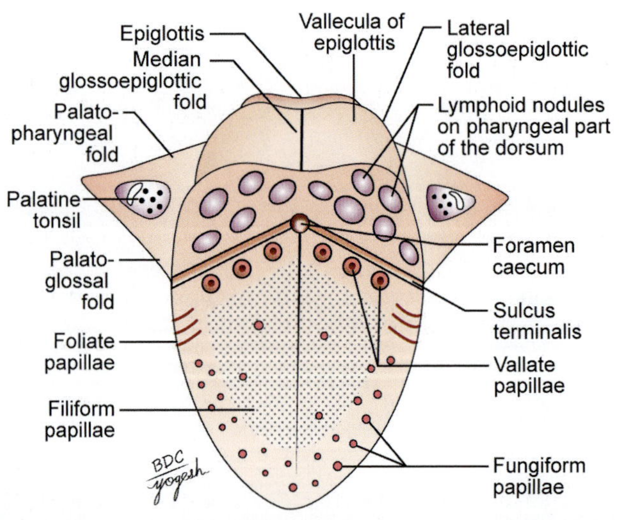


**Fig. 17.1:** Dorsum of the tongue, epiglottis and palatine tonsil

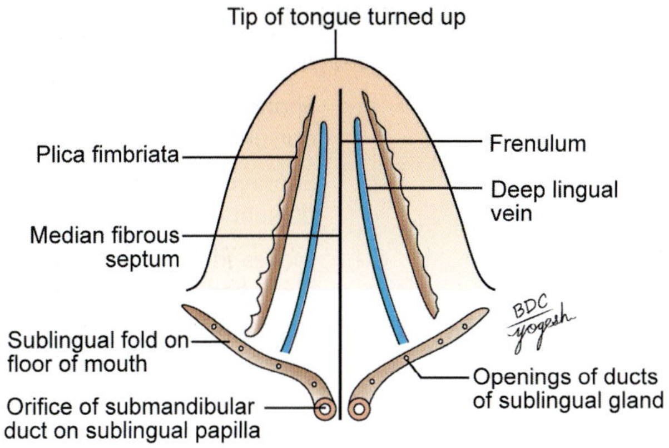


**Fig. 17.2:** Inferior surface of tongue and the floor of the mouth

### *Posteriormost Part*

The ***posteriormost part*** *of the tongue* is connected to the epiglottis by three folds of mucous membrane. These are the median glossoepiglottic fold and the right and left lateral glossoepiglottic folds. On either side of the median fold, there is a depression called the ***vallecula*** (Fig. 17.1). The lateral folds separate the vallecula from the piriform fossa.

## CLINICAL ANATOMY

- ***Glossitis*** is usually a part of generalized ulceration of the mouth cavity or stomatitis. In certain anaemias, the tongue becomes smooth due to atrophy of the filiform papillae.
- The presence of a rich network of lymphatics and of loose areolar tissue in the substance of tongue is responsible for enormous swelling of tongue in ***acute glossitis***. The tongue fills up the mouth cavity and then protrudes out of it.
- The undersurface of the tongue is a good site along with the bulbar conjunctiva for observation of ***jaundice***.
- In unconscious patients, the tongue may fall back and obstruct the air passages. This can be prevented either by lying the patient on one side with head down (the 'tonsil position') or by keeping the tongue out mechanically.
- Lingual tonsil in the posterior one-third of the tongue forms part of Waldeyer's ring.

***Competency:***

**AN43.2** Identify, describe and draw the microanatomy of pituitary gland, thyroid, parathyroid gland, tongue, salivary glands, tonsil, epiglottis, cornea, retina.

Microanatomy of tongue is given here. For the rest of tissues, please see the appropriate chapters.

## PAPILLAE OF THE TONGUE

These are projections of mucous membrane or corium which give roughness the anterior two-thirds of the tongue. These are of the following four types (Fig. 17.3 and Flowchart 17.1).

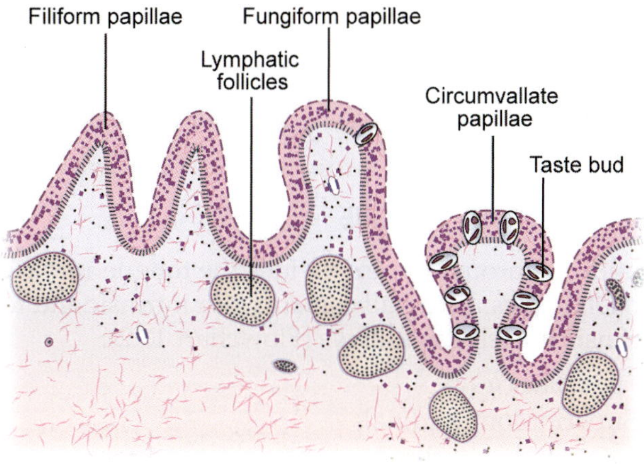


**Fig. 17.3:** Types of papillae

**Flowchart 17.1:** Papillae of tongue

***Papillae of tongue***
Surface projections

| ***Filiform*** | ***Fungiform*** | ***Circumvallate*** | ***Foliate*** |
|---|---|---|---|
| Most numerous<br>Smallest<br>Minute conical projections<br>No taste buds | Mushroom-shaped<br>Small pink spots<br>Contains apical taste buds | 8–12 papillae<br>Dome-shaped<br>Located anterior to suclus terminalis<br>Contains lateral wall taste buds | Parallel rows of ridges near the margin of tongue<br>Rudimentary<br>No taste buds |

1. ***Vallate*** or ***circumvallate papillae:*** They are large in size, 1–2 mm in diameter and are 8–12 in number. They are situated immediately in front of the sulcus terminalis. Each papilla is a cylindrical projection surrounded by a circular sulcus. The walls of the papilla have taste buds.
2. ***Fungiform papillae*** are numerous near the tip and margins of the tongue, but some of them are also scattered over the dorsum. These are smaller than the vallate papillae but larger than the filiform papillae. Each papilla consists of a narrow pedicle and a large rounded head. They are distinguished by their bright red colour.
3. ***Filiform papillae*** or *conical papillae* cover the presulcal area of the dorsum of the tongue, and give it a characteristic velvety appearance. They are the smallest and most numerous of the lingual papillae. Each is pointed and covered with keratin; the apex is often split into filamentous processes.
4. ***Foliate papillae*** are present at the lateral border just in front of circumvallate papillae. They are leaf shaped.

## DISSECTION

In the sagittal section, identify fan-shaped genioglossus muscle. Cut the attachments of buccinator, superior constrictor muscles and the intervening pterygomandibular raphe and reflect these downwards exposing the lateral surface of the tongue.

**Competency:**

**AN39.1** Describe and demonstrate the morphology, nerve supply, embryological basis of nerve supply, blood supply, lymphatic drainage and actions of extrinsic and intrinsic muscles of tongue.

## MUSCLES OF THE TONGUE

A middle fibrous septum divides the tongue into right and left halves. Each half contains four intrinsic and four extrinsic muscles as follows (Flowchart 17.2):

*Intrinsic muscles*

1. Superior longitudinal
2. Inferior longitudinal
3. Transverse
4. Vertical

*Extrinsic muscles*

1. Genioglossus
2. Hyoglossus
3. Styloglossus
4. Palatoglossus.

### Intrinsic Muscles

They occupy the upper part of the tongue, and are attached to the submucous fibrous layer and to the median fibrous septum. They alter the shape of the tongue (Fig. 17.4, Table 17.1).

***Superior longitudinal:*** It arises from the fibrous tissue deep to the mucous membrane on the dorsum of the tongue and the midline lingual septum. It passes longitudinally back from the tip of the tongue to its root posteriorly. It inserts into the overlying mucous membrane. The superior longitudinal muscles act to elevate the tip and sides of the tongue superiorly. This shapes the dorsum of tongue into a concavity and it shortens the tongue.

***Inferior longitudinal:*** It originates from the fibrous tissue beneath the mucous membrane stretching from tip of tongue longitudinally back to the root of the tongue and the hyoid bone. It is inserted into the mucous membrane of the dorsum of tongue. It lies between the genioglossus and the hyoglossus. The inferior longitudinal muscles act to curl the tip of the tongue inferiorly. This makes the dorsum of the tongue convex in shape and shortens the tongue.

**TABLE 17.1: The actions of intrinsic muscles of tongue**

| *Intrinsic muscles* | *Actions* |
|---|---|
| Superior longitudinal | Shortens the tongue, makes its dorsum concave |
| Inferior longitudinal | Shortens the tongue, makes its dorsum convex |
| Transverse | Makes the tongue narrow and elongated |
| Vertical (Fig. 17.4) | Makes the tongue broad and flattened |

**Flowchart 17.2:** Muscles of tongue

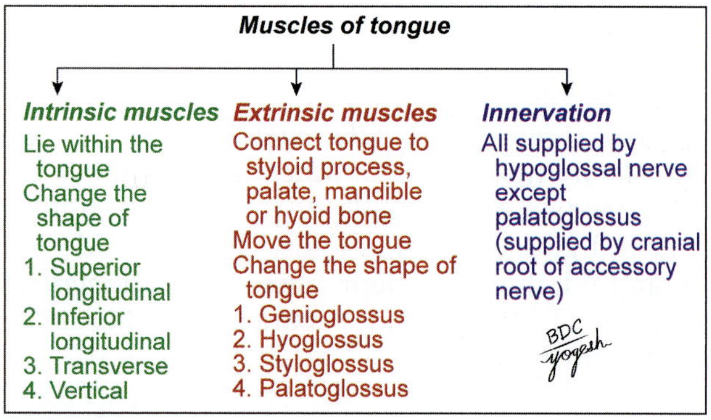


***Transverse:*** It lies as a sheet on either side of the midline in a plane that is deep to the superior longitudinal muscles but superficial to genioglossus.

Each runs transversely from its origin at the fibrous lingual septum to insert into the submucous fibrous tissue at the lateral margins of the tongue.

Contraction of the transverse muscles acts to narrow and increases the thickness of the tongue.

***Vertical:*** It is found at the borders of the anterior part of the tongue. It makes the tongue broad.

### Extrinsic Muscles

These include genioglossus, hyoglossus, styloglossus, and palatoglossus (Plate 17.1, Figs 17.5 and 17.6 and Table 17.2).

The *extrinsic muscles* connect the tongue to the mandible via genioglossus; to the hyoid bone through

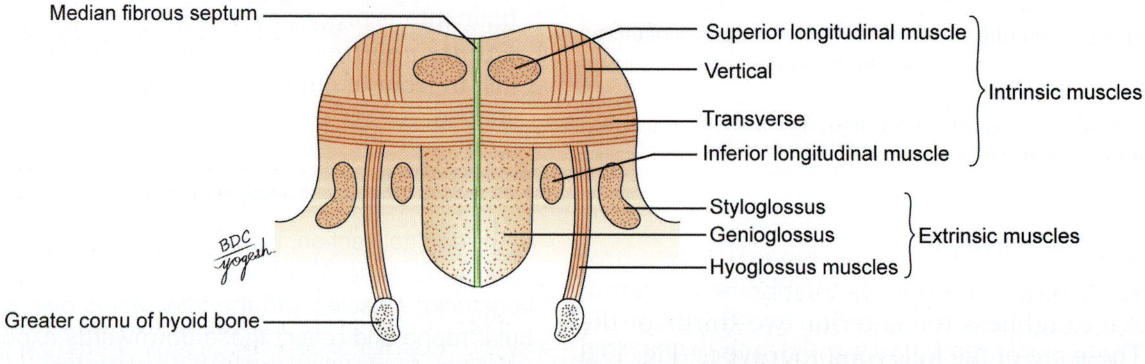


**Fig. 17.4:** Coronal section of the tongue showing arrangement of the intrinsic and extrinsic muscles

**Plate 17.1:** Extrinsic muscles of the tongue (cut section, right lateral view showing muscles of right side)

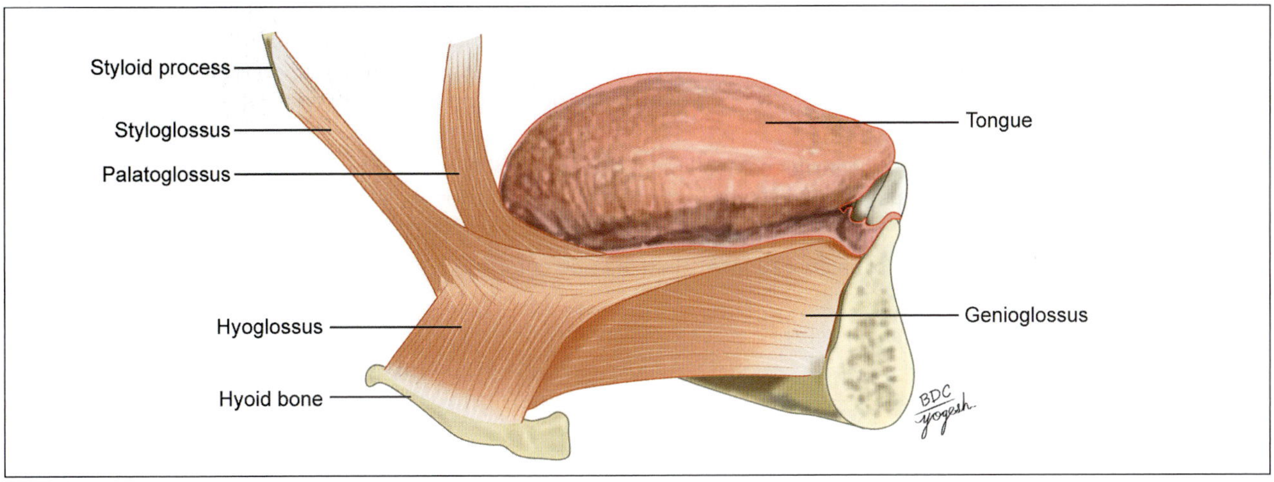


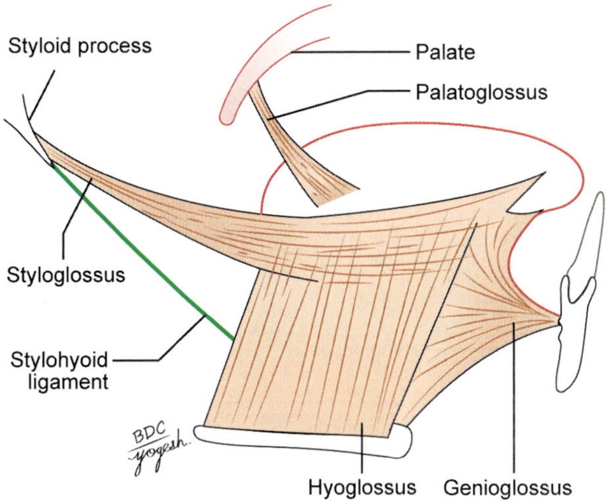


**Fig. 17.5:** Extrinsic muscles of the tongue

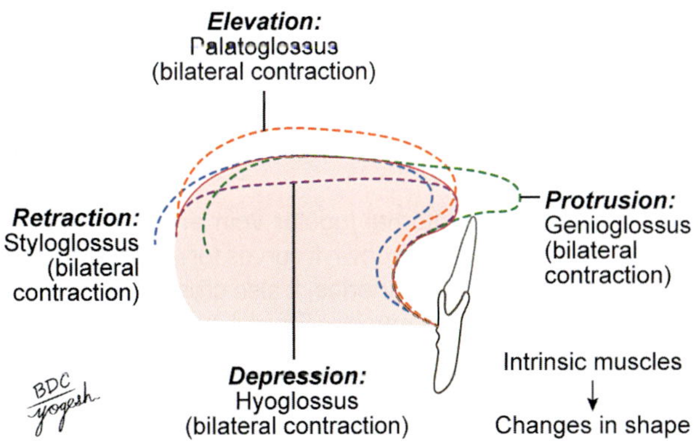


**Fig. 17.6:** Movements of tongue

hyoglossus; to the styloid process via styloglossus, and the palate via palatoglossus.

## Arterial Supply

It is derived from the tortuous ***lingual artery***, a branch of the external carotid artery. The root of the tongue is also supplied by the tonsillar artery, a branch of facial artery, and ascending pharyngeal branch of external carotid artery (Fig. 17.7).

## Venous Drainage

1. *Deep lingual vein:* The chief vein of tongue, seen on the inferior surface of tongue near median plane.
2. *Venae comitantes*, accompany lingual artery. They are joined by dorsal lingual veins.
3. *Venae comitantes* accompanying the hypoglossal nerve.

These veins unite at the posterior border of the hyoglossus to form the ***lingual vein*** which ends in the internal jugular vein.

## Lymphatic Drainage

The lymphatic drainage of tongue can be divided into three main regions: Marginal, central, and dorsal (*Reference*: Grey's Anatomy, 42nd edn.) (Figs 17.8a and b and Flowchart 17.3).

1. *Marginal vessels* drain the marginal area of anterior part of the tongue.
   a. The lymphatics from the tip of the tongue and lingual frenulum drains bilaterally into:
      - Submental nodes
      - Submandibular nodes
      - Jugulo-omohyoid nodes.
   b. The lymphatics from the rest of margin of the tongue drain into:
      - Submandibular nodes
      - Digastric nodes.
2. *Central vessels* drain the central region of the anterior two-thirds of tongue. They drain into jugulodigastric and jugulo-omohyoid nodes and submandibular nodes.
3. *Dorsal vessels* drain the circumvallate papillae and posterior one-third of tongue into jugulo-omohyoid and jugulodigastric nodes.

*Note*: The lymphatics near the median plane pass bilaterally.
The most of the lymph from the tongue finally drains to the ***jugulo-omohyoid nodes***. These are known as the ***lymph nodes of the tongue***.

## Nerve Supply

### *Motor Nerves*

All the muscles of tongue (intrinsic and extrinsic) are supplied by *hypoglossal nerve* except palatoglossus

**TABLE 17.2: Origin, insertion and actions of extrinsic muscles of tongue**

| *Muscle* | *Origin* | *Insertion* | *Actions* |
|---|---|---|---|
| **Palatoglossus** | Oral surface of ***palatine aponeurosis*** | Descends in the palatoglossal arch to the side of tongue at the junction of oral and pharyngeal parts | Pulls up the root of tongue, approximates the palatoglossal arches and thus closes the oropharyngeal isthmus |
| **Hyoglossus** | Whole length of greater cornua and lateral part of ***hyoid bone*** | Side of tongue between styloglossus and inferior longitudinal muscle of tongue | Depresses tongue, makes dorsum convex, retracts the protruded tongue |
| **Styloglossus** | Tip and part of anterior surface of ***styloid process*** | Into the side of tongue | Pulls tongue upwards and backwards, i.e. retracts the tongue |
| **Genioglossus**<br>Fan-shaped bulky muscle | Upper genial tubercle of ***mandible*** | *Upper fibres* into the tip of tongue<br>*Middle fibres* into the dorsum<br>*Lower fibres* into the hyoid bone | Retracts the tongue<br>Depresses the tongue<br>Pulls the posterior part of tongue forwards and protrudes the tongue. It is a ***life-saving muscle*** |

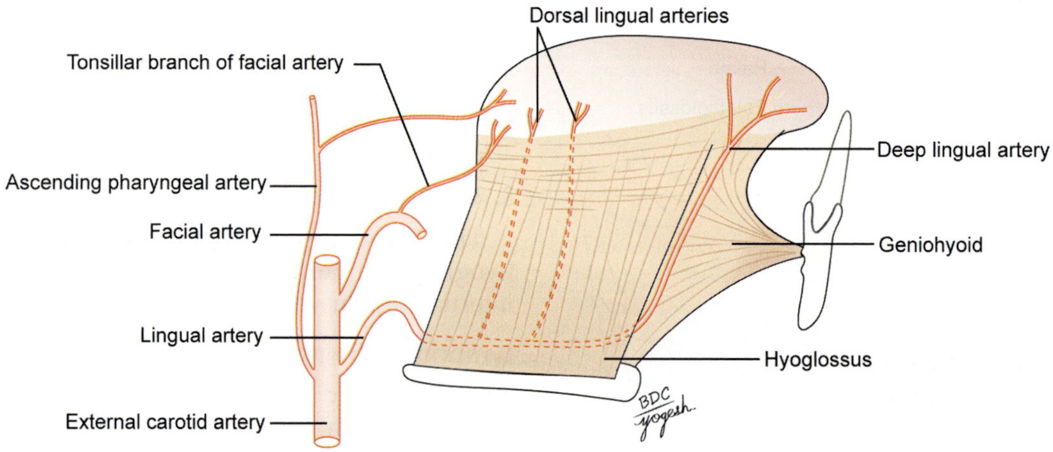


**Fig. 17.7:** Arterial supply and extrinsic muscles of the tongue

**Flowchart 17.3:** Lymphatic drainage of tongue

***Lymphatic drainage of tongue***

***Marginal vessels***
Drain marginal area of anterior part of tongue to:
- Submental LN
- Submandibular LN
- Jugulo-omohyoid LN
- Digastric LN

***Central vessels***
Drain central region of anterior 2/3rd of tongue to:
- Jugulodigastric LN
- Jugulo-omohyoid LN

***Dorsal vessels***
Drain circumvallate papillae and posterior 1/3rd of tongue to:
- Jugulodigastric LN
- Jugulo-omohyoid LN

***Note:*** Lymphatics from the tip and the central part of tongue drain bilaterally.

which is supplied by the *cranial root of accessory nerve* via pharyngeal plexus (Fig. 17.9).

### *Sensory Supply*

1. Anterior two-thirds of tongue without circumvallate papillae:
   - General sensations are carried by *lingual nerve*
   - Taste sensation are carried by *chorda tympani.*
2. Posterior one-third of tongue with circumvallate papillae:
   Both general and special sensation are carried by *glossopharyngeal nerve.*
3. Posterior most part is supplied by *internal laryngeal branch of superior laryngeal nerve* (branch of vagus nerve).

*Note*:

***Hypoglossal nerve (XII* nerve)** is the nerve of muscles of the tongue. It leaves the cranial cavity through anterior condylar/hypoglossal canal.

*Course*: Lies between internal jugular vein and internal carotid artery in front of vagus. Lower down it curves forwards to cross both internal and external carotid arteries. It also crosses loop of lingual artery to lie on hyoglossus muscle. Finally, it enters substance of tongue. It supplies 3 extrinsic muscles and all 4 intrinsic muscles of tongue (details can be read from Chapter 6, *BD Chaurasia's Human Anatomy, Volume 4*.

*Competency:*
**AN39.2** Explain the anatomical basis of hypoglossal nerve palsy.

## CLINICAL ANATOMY

- ***Carcinoma of the tongue*** is quite common. The affected side of the tongue is removed surgically. All the deep cervical lymph nodes are also removed, i.e. block dissection of neck because recurrence of malignant disease occurs in lymph nodes.

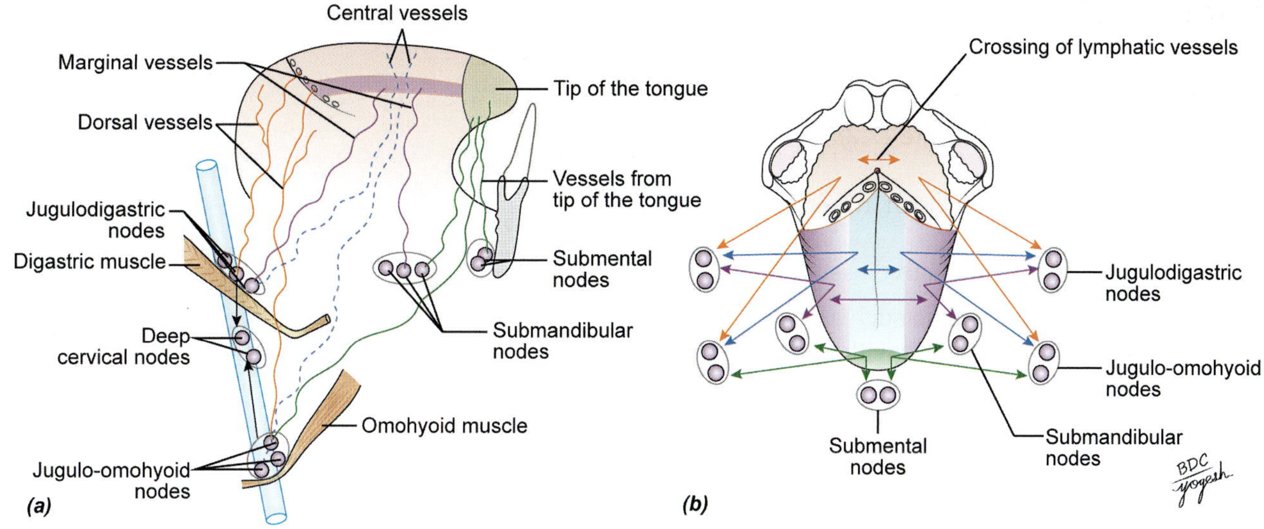


**Figs 17.8a and b:** Lymphatic drainage of the tongue: (a) Side view and (b) superior view showing midline crossing of lymphatic vessels

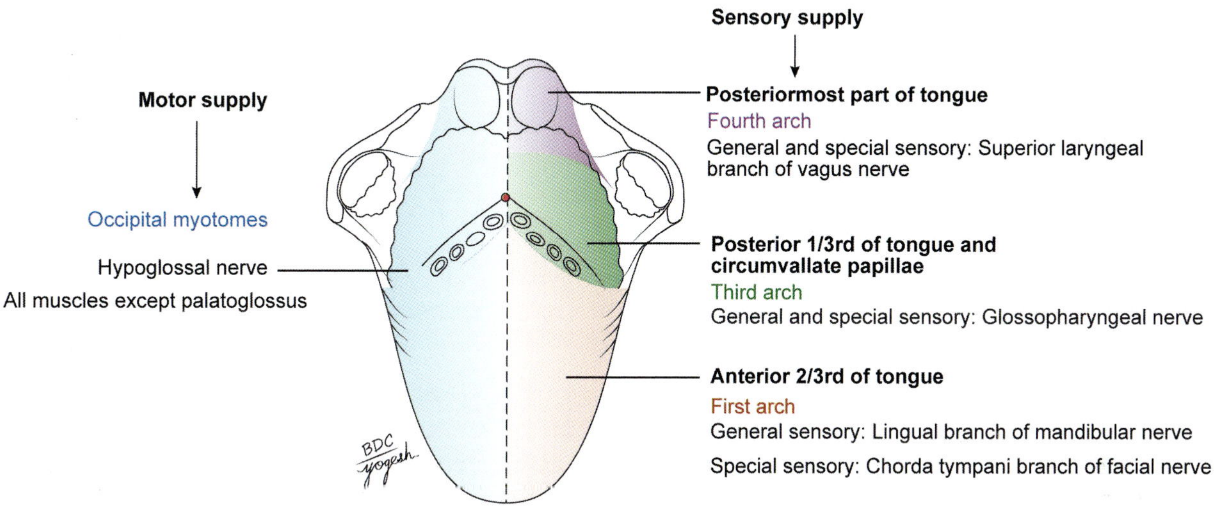


**Fig. 17.9:** Nerve supply of tongue

- ***Sorbitrate*** is taken sublingually for immediate relief from angina pectoris. It is absorbed fast because of rich blood supply of the tongue and bypassing of portal circulation.
- Genioglossus is called the '***safety muscle of the tongue***' because if it is paralysed, the tongue will fall back on the oropharynx and block the air passage. During anaesthesia, the tongue is pulled forwards to clear the air passage.
- Genioglossus is the only muscle of the tongue that protrudes it forwards. It is used for testing the integrity of hypoglossal nerve. If hypoglossal nerve of right side is paralysed, the tongue on protrusion will deviate to the right side. Normal left genioglossus will pull the base to left side and apex will get pushed to right side (apex and base lie at opposite ends) (Fig. 17.10).

*Note*: The lymphatic crossing is more profound in the posterior one-third of tongue; hence, cancer in the posterior one-third of tongue has poor prognosis.

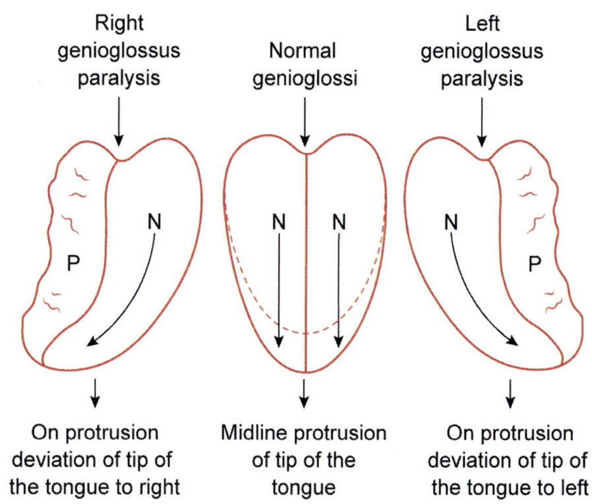


**Fig. 17.10:** Action and unilateral paralysis of genioglossus muscle (*Note*: The tip of the tongue deviates to the paralysed side due to unopposed action of contralateral genioglossus, N: normal genioglossus, P: Paralysed genioglossus)

## HISTOLOGY

### Anterior Two-thirds of Tongue

The tongue consists of mucous membrane that covers core of skeletal muscle fibres (Plate 17.2).

*Mucous membrane* has:

- Lining epithelium – nonkeratinized stratified squamous epithelium
- Lamina propria – loose connective tissue.

Mucosa shows projecting papillae such as:

1. Filiform: Small, conical projections with keratinized tips
2. Fungiform: Mushroom-shaped projections
3. Circumvallate: Dome-shaped papillae surrounded by circular sulcus
4. Foliate: Rudimentary papillae.

*Taste buds:* Fungiform and circumvallate papillae have taste buds that open as taste pores. Taste buds have receptor, supporting, and basal cells (Fig. 17.11).

Skeletal muscle fibres in tongue are arranged longitudinally, transversely, and vertically.

Tongue also shows mucous lingual salivary glands and von Ebner's serous salivary glands.

### Posterior One-third of Tongue

The posterior one-third of tongue consists of mucous membrane (nonkeratinized stratified squamous epithelium and lamina propria) that covers the following structures (Plate 17.3):

1. Numerous mucous lingual salivary glands and their ducts
2. Lymphatic follicles
3. Core of skeletal muscle fibres (arranged longitudinally, transversely, and vertically).

**Competency:**

**AN43.4** Describe the development and developmental basis of congenital anomalies of face, palate, tongue, branchial apparatus, pituitary gland, thyroid gland and eye. (Development of tongue is described here. For the development of other organs please see the appropriate chapters.)

## DEVELOPMENT OF TONGUE

Tongue develops in the floor of primitive pharynx and developing mouth (Fig. 17.12 and Flowchart 17.4).

### Mucous Membrane

Mandibular arches show three swellings: Single midline swelling as tuberculum impar and two lateral lingual swellings. In the 4th week, two lingual swellings and tuberculum impar become visible. Caudal to tuberculum impar, proliferating epithelium forms thyroglossal duct and its pharyngeal site is marked by a depression called *foramen caecum*.

The ***lingual swellings*** grow and fuse with each other and with ***tuberculum impar***. These combined swellings form anterior two-thirds of the tongue. The developing alveololingual sulcus gradually separates tongue from floor of mouth.

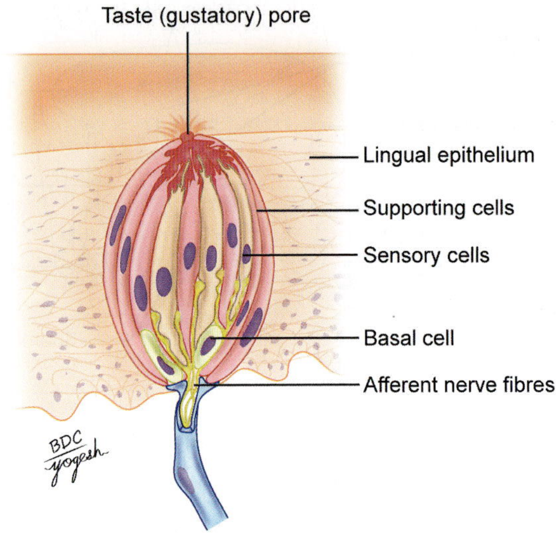


**Fig. 17.11:** Structure of taste bud

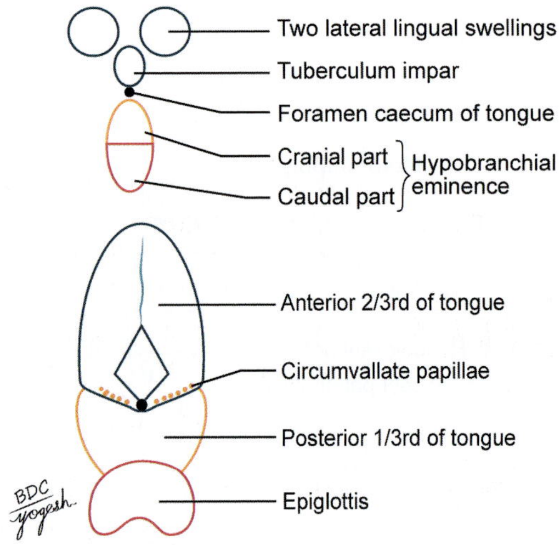


**Fig. 17.12:** Development of tongue

**Flowchart 17.4:** Development of tongue

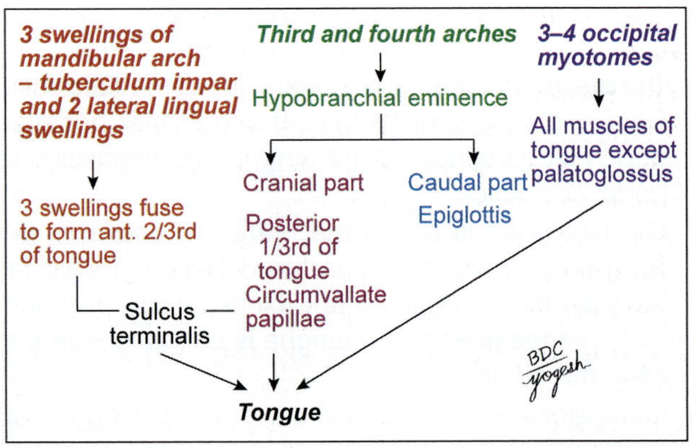


In relation to 3rd and 4th arches, pharyngeal surface shows a midline swelling called ***hypobranchial eminence*** or copula of His. In 5th week, hypobranchial eminence becomes visible. The hypobranchial eminence is divided into ventral and dorsal parts. Ventral part expands to form posterior one-third of the tongue. Fusion of anterior and posterior part is represented by sulcus terminalis. Caudal part of the hypobranchial eminence forms

**Plate 17.2:** Histology of anterior two-thirds of the tongue

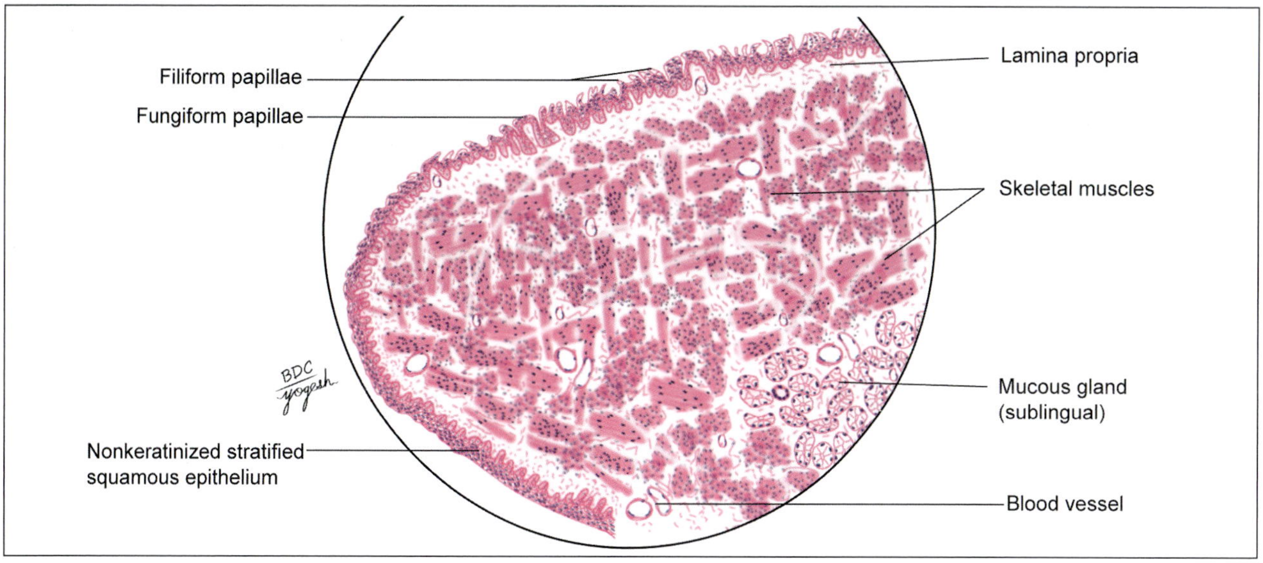


**Plate 17.3:** Histology of posterior one-third of tongue

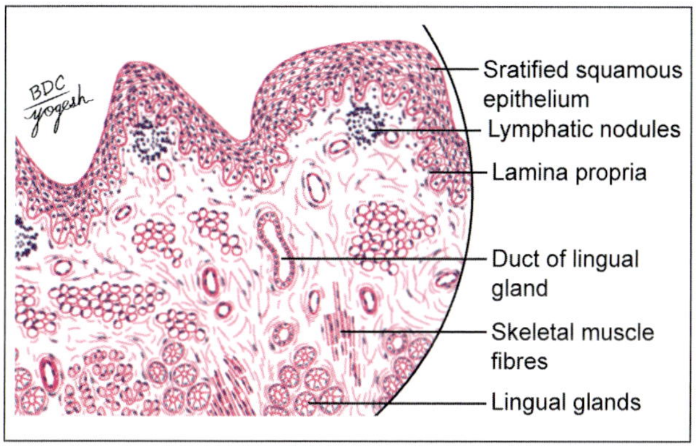


(*Noto*: Lingula tonsils are not shown in this figure to avoid the confusion with the histology of palatine tonsil)

epiglottis. Some cells migrate from posterior one-third of tongue and cross sulcus terminalis to form *circumvallate papillae.*

The 3rd arch overgrows over the second arch and fuses with the first arch; thus the 2nd arch mesoderm gets buried in the substance of the tongue.

## Muscles of Tongue

About 3–4 occipital myotomes migrate ventrally to the mesenchyme of the tongue and form all extrinsic and intrinsic muscles of tongue. The occipital myotomes pull their nerve (hypoglossal nerve) during migration; hence, hypoglossal nerve crosses both external and internal carotid arteries, superficially.

Table 17.3 has the comparison of parts of the tongue.

## TASTE PATHWAY

- The taste from anterior 2/3rd of tongue, except from vallate papillae, is carried by *chorda tympani* branch of facial nerve till the geniculate ganglion. The central processes go to the *tractus solitarius* in the medulla.
- Taste from posterior 1/3rd of tongue including the circumvallate papillae is carried by cranial nerve IX till the inferior ganglion. The central processes also reach the *tractus solitarius* (Fig. 17.13).
- Taste from posteriormost part of tongue and epiglottis travels through *vagus* nerve till the inferior ganglion of vagus. These *central* processes also reach *tractus solitarius.*

**TABLE 17.3: Comparison of the parts of the tongue**

| | *Anterior two-thirds* | *Posterior one-third* | *Posteriormost part and vallecula* |
|---|---|---|---|
| Situation | Lies in mouth cavity | Oropharynx | Oropharynx |
| Structure | Contains papillae | Contains lymphoid tissue | — |
| Function | Chewing | Deglutition | Deglutition |
| Sensory nerve | Lingual (post-trematic branch of 1st arch) | Glossopharyngeal nerve of 3rd arch | Internal laryngeal branch of vagus (nerve of 4th arch) |
| Sensation of taste | Chorda tympani except circum-vallate papillae (pre-trematic branch of 2nd arch) | Glossopharyngeal including the vallate papillae | Internal laryngeal branch of vagus |
| Development of epithelium from endoderm | Lingual swellings of 1st arch Tuberculum impar which soon disappears | Third arch which forms large ventral part of hypobranchial eminence | Fourth arch which forms small dorsal part of hypobranchial eminence |

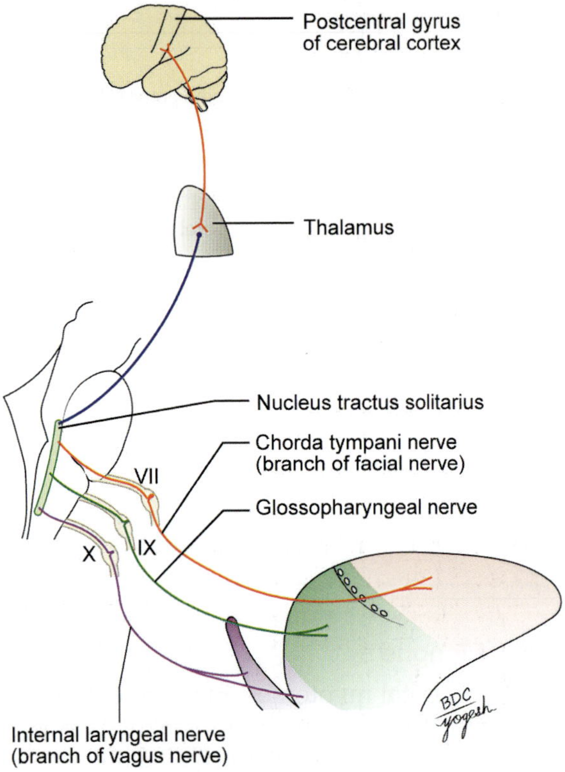


**Fig. 17.13:** Taste pathways

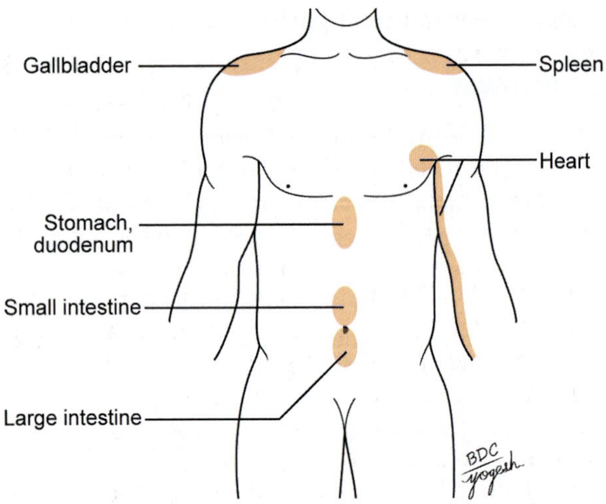


**Fig. 17.14:** Examples of referred pain

- After a relay in tractus solitarius, the *solitariothalamic tract* is formed which becomes a part of *trigeminal lemniscus* and reaches posteroventromedial nucleus of thalamus of the opposite side. Another relay here takes them to *lowest part of postcentral gyrus*, which is the area for taste.

## CLINICAL ANATOMY

- Injury to any part of the pathway causes abnormality in appreciation of taste.
- Referred pain is felt in the ear in diseases of posterior part of the tongue, as 9th and 10th nerves are common supply to both the regions. Other examples of referred pain are seen in Fig. 17.14.

VIDEO

**Video 3.17 Tongue**

### *Facts to Remember*

- All four intrinsic muscles of tongue are supplied by XII nerve.
- Out of four extrinsic muscles of tongue, three are supplied by XII nerve. Only palatoglossus is supplied by vagoaccessory complex.
- Lingual artery is a tortuous artery as it moves up and down with movements of pharynx.
- Tongue is kept in position by its attachment to neighbouring structures through the 4 pairs of extrinsic muscles.
- Nerve supply correlates with development. Anterior two-thirds develop from 1st arch, the nerves being lingual and chorda tympani. Chorda tympani is pre-trematic branch of the 2nd arch.
- Genioglossus is the life-saving muscle as it protrudes the tongue forwards.
- Jugulo-omohyoid nodes are considered as principal lymph nodes of the tongue.

### BDC's Anatomy *e*-book

1. Chondroglossus
2. Anatomical basis of referred pain of cancer of tongue
3. Further reading
4. Viva voce questions

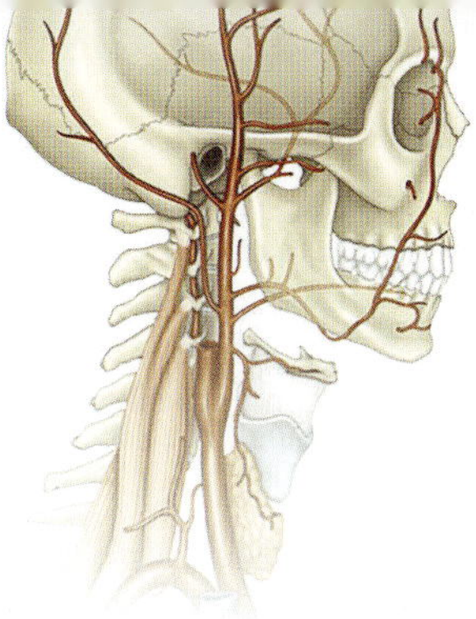

Chapter

18

# Ear

The ear is an organ of hearing. It is also concerned in maintaining the equilibrium of the body (Figs 18.1 and 18.2). It consists of three parts:

1. External ear
2. Middle ear
3. Internal ear.

The *tympanic membrane* separates external ear from middle ear. Mastoid antrum lies in the petrous part of temporal bone. Mastoid air cells are situated in the mastoid process.

### Features of the Temporal Bone

1. *External auditory meatus* is for air waves.
2. *Internal auditory meatus* is for passage of VII, VIII nerves and labyrinthine vessels.
3. *Suprameatal triangle* is the landmark for mastoid antrum. It is bounded by supramastoid crest, posterosuperior margin of external acoustic meatus and a tangent drawn from the crest to the margin. Mastoid antrum lies about 15 mm deep to the suprameatal triangle in adult.
4. *Tympanic canaliculus* lies on the inferior surface of petrous temporal bone between carotid canal and jugular fossa.
5. *Petrotympanic fissure* gives passage to anterior tympanic artery, anterior ligament of malleus and chorda tympani nerve.
6. *Stylomastoid foramen* gives passage to stylomastoid branch of posterior auricular artery for middle ear and facial nerve.
7. Hiatus for greater petrosal nerve gives passage to nerve of the same name and a branch of middle meningeal artery.
8. *Tegmen tympani* on the anterior face of petrous temporal bone forms roof of the middle ear, mastoid antrum and canal for tensor tympani muscle.
9. The aqueduct of vestibule opens on posterior aspect of petrous temporal bone. It is plugged by ductus endolymphaticus.
10. *Organ of Corti* is the end organ for hearing, situated in the cochlear duct. *Crista* is an end organ in the semicircular canal. These are kinetic balance receptors. *Macula* are end organs in the utricle and saccule and are static balance receptors.

***Competency:***
**AN40.1** Describe and identify the parts, blood supply and nerve supply of external ear.

## EXTERNAL EAR

The external ear consists of:

- Auricle or pinna
- External acoustic meatus.

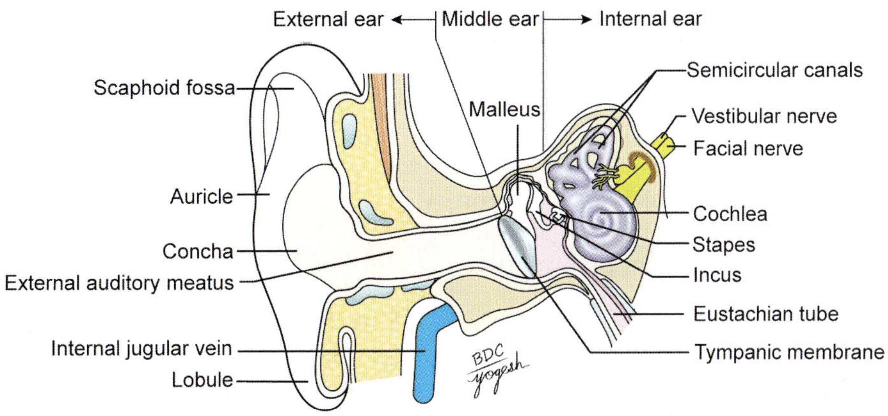


**Fig. 18.1:** The ear and its subdivisions (external, middle, and internal ear)

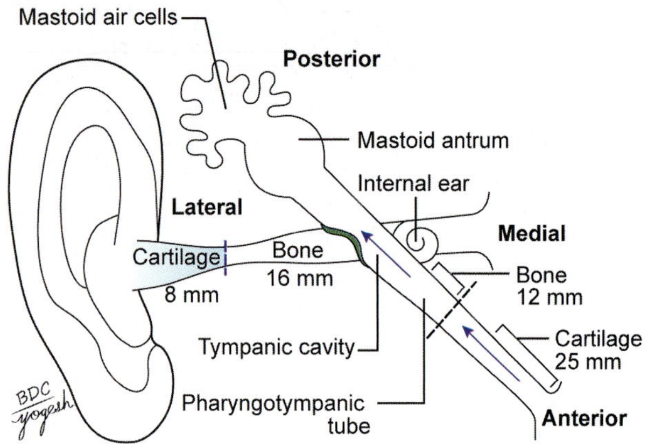


**Fig. 18.2:** Parts of external ear, middle ear, and mastoid antrum (schematic representation)

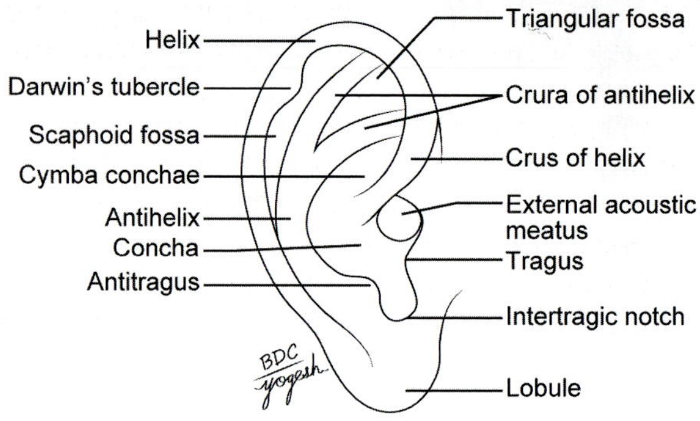


**Fig. 18.3:** Features of auricle

## AURICLE/PINNA

The auricle is the part seen on the surface.

### Features

1. The greater part of it is made up of a single crumpled plate of ***elastic cartilage*** which is lined on both sides by skin. It supports the spectacles (Fig. 18.3).
2. The lowest part of the auricle is soft and consists only of fibrofatty tissue covered by skin: This part is called the ***lobule*** for wearing the ear rings.
3. The rest of the auricle is divided into a number of parts. These are helix, antihelix, concha, tragus, and scaphoid fossa. In particular, note the large depression called the ***concha;*** it leads into the external acoustic meatus.
4. In relation to the auricle, there are a number of muscles. These are all vestigeal in man. In lower animals, the *intrinsic* muscles alter the shape of the auricle, while the *extrinsic* muscles move the auricle as a whole.

### Nerve Supply

1. *Lateral surface*: The upper two-thirds of the lateral surface of the auricle are supplied by the auriculotemporal nerve; and the lower one-third by the great auricular nerve (Fig. 18.4).
2. *Medial surface:* The upper two-thirds of the medial surface are supplied by the lesser occipital nerve; and the lower one-third by the great auricular nerve.
3. The *root* of the auricle is supplied by the auricular branch of the vagus. The auricular muscles are supplied through branches of the facial nerve.

### Blood Supply

The blood supply of the auricle is derived from the posterior auricular and superficial temporal arteries (Fig. 18.5). The *lymphatics* drain into the preauricular, and postauricular lymph nodes.

## EXTERNAL ACOUSTIC MEATUS (EAM)

The external auditory meatus conducts sound waves from the concha to the tympanic membrane.

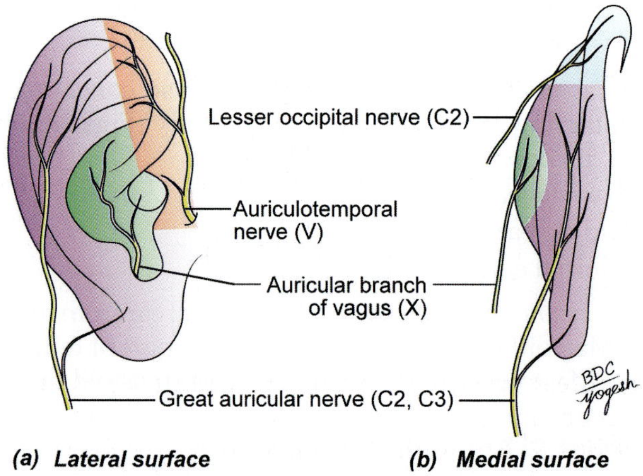


**Figs 18.4a and b:** Pinna of the ear: (a) Nerve supply of the lateral surface; (b) Nerve supply of the medial surface

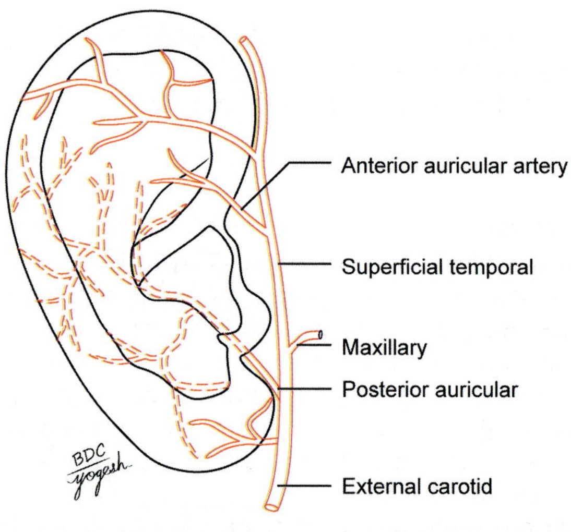


**Fig. 18.5:** Blood supply of the auricle

### Features

1. Its canal is S-shaped. Its outer part is directed medially, forwards and upwards. The middle part is directed medially, backwards and upwards. The inner part is directed medially, forwards and downwards.
2. The meatus can be straightened for examination by pulling the auricle *upwards, backwards and slightly laterally*.

3. The meatus or canal is about 24 mm long, of which the medial two-thirds or 16 mm is bony, and the lateral one-third or 8 mm is cartilaginous. Due to the obliquity of the tympanic membrane, the anterior wall and floor are longer than the posterior wall and roof.
4. The canal is oval in section. The greatest diameter is vertical at the lateral end, and anteroposterior at the medial end. The bony part is narrower than the cartilaginous part. The narrowest point, the *isthmus*, lies about 5 mm from the tympanic membrane.
5. The ***bony part*** is formed by the tympanic plate of the temporal bone which is C-shaped in cross-section. The posterosuperior part of the plate is deficient. Here the wall of the meatus is formed by a part of the squamous temporal bone. The meatus is lined by thin skin, firmly adherent to the periosteum.
6. The ***cartilaginous part*** is also C-shaped in section; and the gap of the 'C' is filled with fibrous tissue. The lining skin is adherent to the perichondrium, and contains hairs, sebaceous glands, and ceruminous or wax glands. *Ceruminous glands* are modified sweat glands. EAM protects tympanic membrane from blows. It maintains humidity and proper temperature.

### Blood Supply

The outer part of the canal is supplied by the superficial temporal and posterior auricular arteries, and the inner part, by the deep auricular branch of the maxillary artery.

### Lymphatics

The lymphatics pass to preauricular, postauricular and superficial cervical lymph nodes.

### Nerve Supply

The skin lining the anterior half of the meatus is supplied by the auriculotemporal nerve, and that lining the posterior half, by the auricular branch of the vagus.

## CLINICAL ANATOMY

- ***Painful boils***: The skin of the external ear is adherent to the underlying bone and cartilage. Hence, infection of hair follicles or boils in the external ear is very painful.
- ***Ear cough***: The floor and posterior wall of the external acoustic meatus is supplied by the auricular branch of vagus nerve. Irritation of this area by ear wax or cold or hot water (used in syringing) may induce ear cough, vomiting or death due to sudden cardiac arrest by vagus nerve.
- ***Alderman's nerve***: The Alderman community of ancient Rome were used to increase appetite by dropping cold water or spirit behind the ear stimulation of this area supplied by vagus nerve, in reflex, it enhances peristalsis of intestine and acid secretion in stomach.
- ***Ear wax***: Accumulation of secretions of ceruminous glands in the external ear forms ear wax. It may cause itching, irritation, and ear pain.
- ***Syringing and Waxsol eardrop***: The wax from the ear should be removed carefully using earbuds, Waxsol eardrop, or syringing (Fig. 18.6).

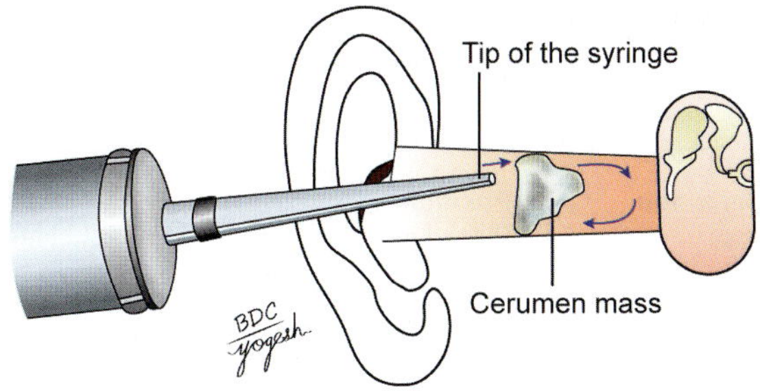


**Fig. 18.6:** Syringing of the ear

## DISSECTION

Expose the external auditory meatus by cutting the tragus of the auricle. Put a probe into the external auditory meatus and remove the anterior wall of cartilaginous and bony parts of the external auditory meatus with the scissors. Be slow and careful not to damage the tympanic membrane.

## TYMPANIC MEMBRANE

The tympanic membrane or *eardrum* is an oval semi-transparent membrane that separates the external ear from the middle ear (Figs 18.7 to 18.9 and Flowchart 18.1).

### Size and Shape

- The tympanic membrane is oval.
- *Diameter*: 8 mm

### Position

The tympanic membrane is placed obliquely at an angle of about 55° with the floor of external acoustic meatus. Thus, the tympanic membrane faces downward, forward, and laterally (*mnemonic*: DFL).

*Tympanic membrane in newborn*: The tympanic membrane in the newborn is almost horizontal.

### Structure

The tympanic membrane consists of three layers:

1. Outer cuticular layer of stratified squamous epithelium (skin)
2. Middle fibrous layer
3. Inner mucosal layer of low columnar epithelium.

The inner surface of tympanic membrane provides attachment to the handle of malleus which extends up to its center. It makes the tympanic membrane convex, internally.

***Umbo:*** It is a point of maximum convexity of the tympanic membrane. It lies at the tip of the handle of malleus.

### Parts

The tympanic membrane has two parts (Fig. 18.8):

1. Pars tensa
2. Pars flaccida

***Pars tensa*** forms the greater part of the tympanic membrane. It is tightly stretched, hence called pars tensa.

**Flowchart 18.1:** Tympanic membrane

**Tympanic membrane (eardrum)**

- ***Definition***
  - Oval semitransparent membrane
  - Separates external ear from middle ear
  - Size: 8 mm diameter
- ***Position***
  - Placed obliquely 55° angle with floor of external acoustic meatus
  - Looks downward, forward, and laterally
  - In newborn: Lies horizontally
- ***Structure***
  - Outer cuticular layer (skin)
  - Middle fibrous layer
  - Inner mucosal layer
  - Umbo – point of maximum convexity
- ***Parts***
  - Pars tensa
  - Pars flacida
  - Annulus tympanicus
  - Anterior and posterior malleolar folds
- ***Blood supply***
  - Arterial supply
    - Deep auricular branch of maxillary artery
    - Anterior tympanic branch of maxillary artery
    - Posterior tympanic branch of stylomastoid artery
  - Venous drainage
    - External jugular vein
    - Transverse sinus
- ***Innervation***
  - Outer surface:
    - Auriculotemporal branches of vagus nerve
    - Auricular branch of vagus nerve
  - Inner surface:
    - Tympanic branch of glossopharyngeal nerve

***Clinical integration:*** Clinical examination, otoscopy, myringotomy

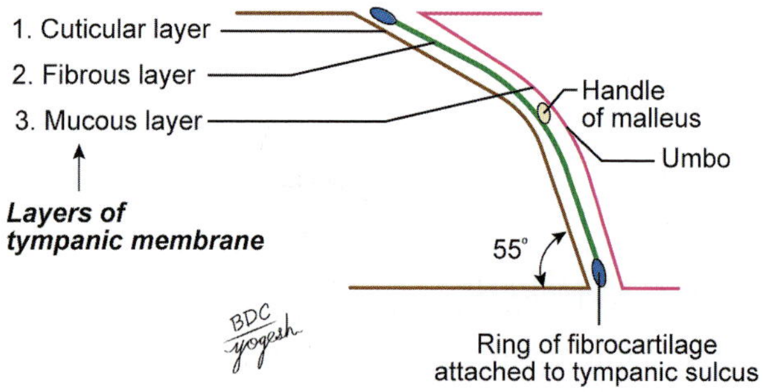


**Fig. 18.7:** Layers of the tympanic membrane

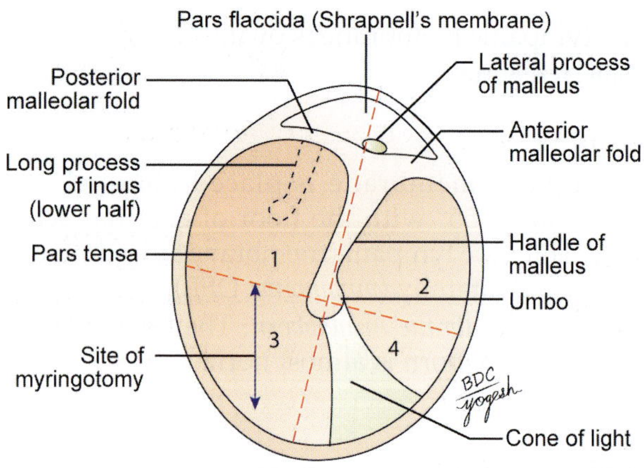


**Fig. 18.8:** Tympanic membrane seen through the external acoustic meatus. (1) Posterosuperior quadrant; (2) Anterosuperior quadrant; (3) Posteroinferior quadrant; (4) Anteroinferior quadrant

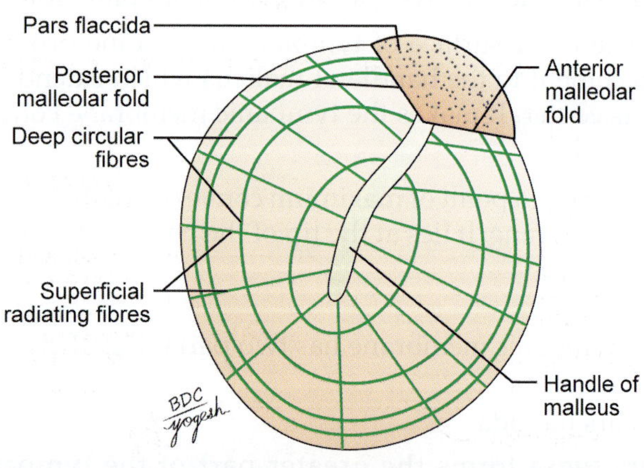


**Fig. 18.9:** Fibres of tympanic membrane

***Pars flaccida*** (*Sharpnell's membrane*) is a small triangular area above the lateral process of malleus. It is loose, hence called pars flaccida.

***Annulus tympanicus*** is a thick peripheral part of the tympanic membrane which fits the tympanic membrane into the tympanic sulcus.

***Malleolar folds*** are anterior and posterior malleolar folds that run from the tympanic sulcus to the handle of malleus. They separate pars faccida from pars tensa.

## Blood Supply

### *Arterial Supply*

1. Outer surface is supplied by deep auricular branch of the maxillary artery.
2. Inner surface is supplied by:
   a. Anterior tympanic branch of maxillary artery
   b. Posterior tympanic branch of stylomastoid branch of posterior auricular artery.

### *Venous Drainage*

1. Outer surface is drained into external jugular vein.
2. Inner surface is drained into transverse sinus and venous plexus around the auditory tube.

## Lymphatic Drainage

Preauricular and retropharyngeal lymph nodes.

## Innervation

1. *Outer surface:*

   Anteroinferior part – auriculotemporal branches of mandibular nerve.

   Posterosuperior part – auricular branch of vagus nerve (fibers of facial nerve).
2. *Inner surface* – tympanic branch of glossopharyngeal nerve.

***Competency:***

**AN40.5** Explain anatomical basis of myringotomy.

## CLINICAL ANATOMY

- Clinical examination of tympanic membrane: To visualize the tympanic membrane, the auricle should be pulled upward, backward, and slightly laterally in adults.

- ***Otoscope*** is useful to visualize the tympanic membrane (Fig. 18.10). It shows:
  1. Semitransparent oval tympanic membrane
  2. Concavity of the membrane directed medially
  3. *Umbo* – maximum point of convexity
  4. Handle of malleus – visualized as yellow streak extending upward and forward from umbo.
  5. Long process of incus – visualized as white prominence in the upper part of handle of malleus.
  6. Cone of light – reflected light produces cone of light in anteroinferior quadrant at 5'o clock position.
  7. Pus or blood, hole in tympanic membrane can also be visualized.
- ***Myringotomy*** is a surgical procedure to drain pus from the middle ear by giving a small incision in the tympanic membrane.

  *Procedure*: The incision for myringotomy is usually given in the posteroinferior quadrant of the tympanic membrane at the most bulging point and temporary ear tube is inserted. It will avoid injury to chorda tympani nerve.
- ***Injury to chorda tympani nerve*** in myringotomy: The chorda tympani nerve passes downward and forward across the inner surface of the tympanic membrane, lateral to the long process of incus and medial to the handle of malleus (Fig. 18.11). Injury to chorda tympani nerve results into:
- Loss of taste sensation over anterior two-thirds of tongue.
- Loss of salivation from submandibular and sublingual glands.

## MIDDLE EAR

The middle ear is also called the tympanic cavity, or tympanum.

The middle ear is a narrow air-filled space situated in the petrous part of the temporal bone between the external ear and the internal ear (Fig. 18.12 and Flowchart 18.2).

### Shape and Size

The middle ear is shaped like a cube. Its lateral and medial walls are large, but the other walls are narrow, because the cube is compressed from side-to-side.

### *Measurements* (Fig. 18.13)

- Vertical diameter: 15 mm
- Anteroposterior diameter: 15 mm
- Transverse diameters: 6 mm at roof, 2 mm in the centre, 4 mm at the floor.

*Note*: The middle ear assumes full adult size at birth. On coronal section, the middle ear resembles biconcave disc (cube compressed from side-to-side).

### Communications

The middle ear has two communications as follows:

1. Anterior with nasopharynx through *pharyngotympanic/ auditory tube*.

**Flowchart 18.2:** Middle ear: Introduction

**Middle ear**

| *Definition* | *Measurement* | *Communication* | *Contents* |
|---|---|---|---|
| Tympanic cavity<br>Narrow slit within the petrous part of temporal bone | Vertical: 15 mm<br>Anteroposterior: 15 mm<br>Transverse:<br>6 mm at roof<br>2 mm in center<br>4 mm at floor | Anteriorly with nasopharynx through auditory tube<br>Posteriorly with mastoid antrum through aditus to antrum | Air<br>Ear ossicles<br>Muscles:<br>Tensor tympani<br>Stapedius<br>Chorda tympani<br>Tympanic plexus |

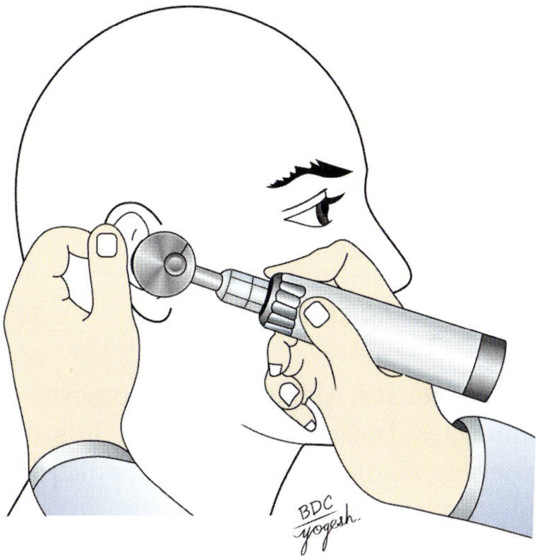

**Fig. 18.10:** Otoscopic examination

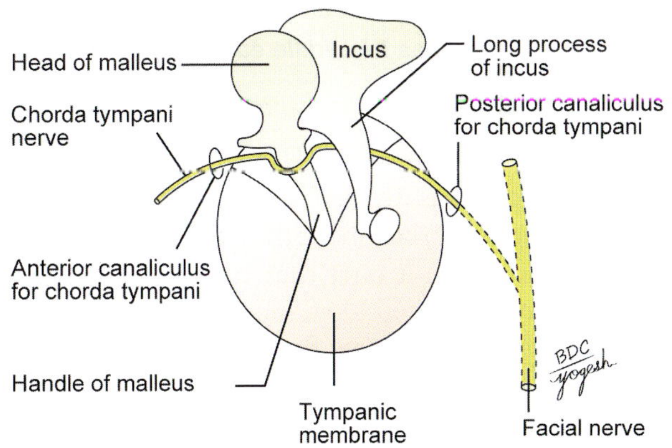


**Fig. 18.11:** Internal surface of the right tympanic membrane

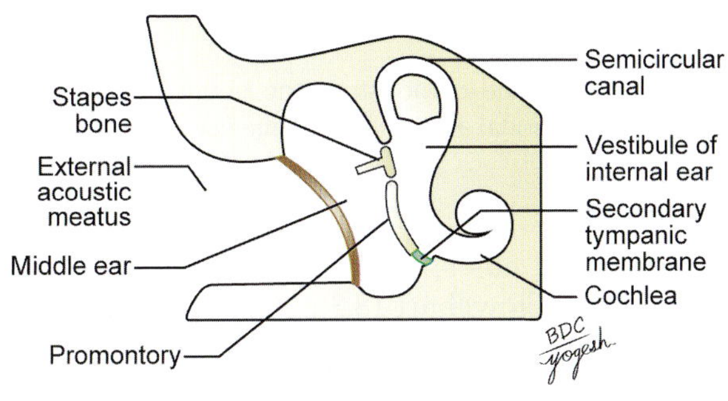


**Fig. 18.12:** Scheme to show the three parts of the ear

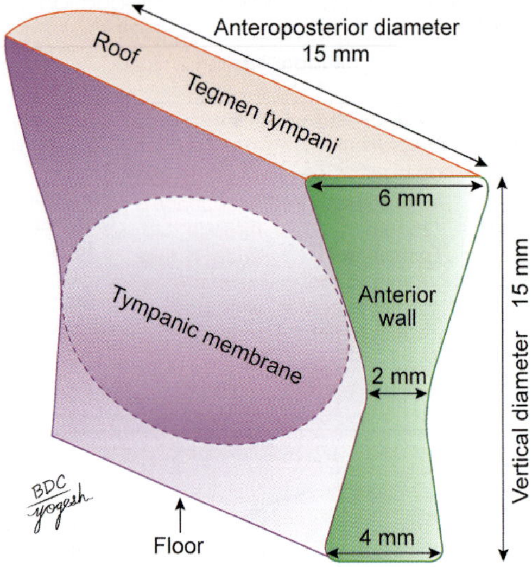


**Fig. 18.13:** Measurements of middle ear

2. Posterior with mastoid antrum and mastoid air cells through *aditus to antrum*.

## Contents of Middle Ear

1. Air
2. Three ear ossicles: Malleus, incus, stapes
3. Two muscles: Tensor tympani, stapedius
4. Two nerves: Chorda tympani, tympanic plexus
5. Blood vessels
6. Ligaments of ear ossicles.

*Note*: The mucous membrane lining the middle ear cavity invests all the contents and forms several vascular folds which project into the cavity. This gives the cavity, a honeycombed appearance.

[***Mnemonics*: *Ear: Bones of middle ear MISs:*** **M**–Malleus, **I**–Incus, **Ss**–Stapes]

## Subdivisions of Middle Ear (Fig. 18.14)

The tympanic cavity is divided into three parts as follows:

1. *Epitympanum* (*attic*) lies above the tympanic membrane.
2. *Mesotympanum* is a part that lies opposite to the tympanic membrane.
3. *Hypotympanum* lies below the tympanic membrane.

*Note*: The middle ear is linked to a pistol in the sloping course of the aditus to the epitympanic recess and the auditory tube (Figs 18.15a and b). The trigger of pistol is tympanic cavity. Outlet is auditory tube. Handle is aditus to mastoid antrum and mastoid air cells.

***Competency:***
**AN40.2** Describe and demonstrate the boundaries, contents, relations and functional anatomy of middle ear and auditory tube

## Boundaries

The middle ear has six walls (similar to matchbox) (Fig. 18.16 and Flowchart 18.3):

1. Roof
2. Floor
3. Lateral wall

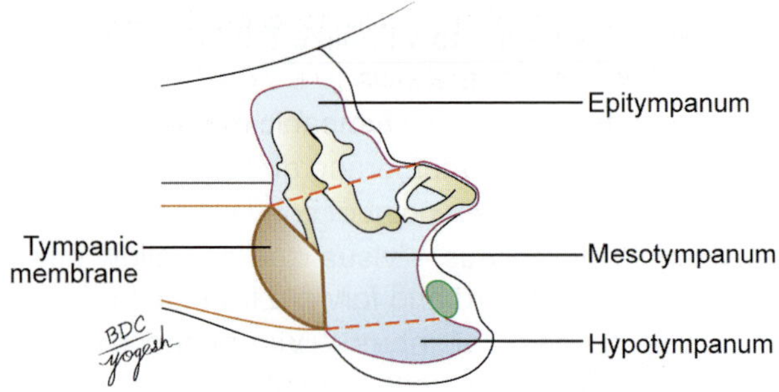


**Fig. 18.14:** Subdivisions of the middle ear

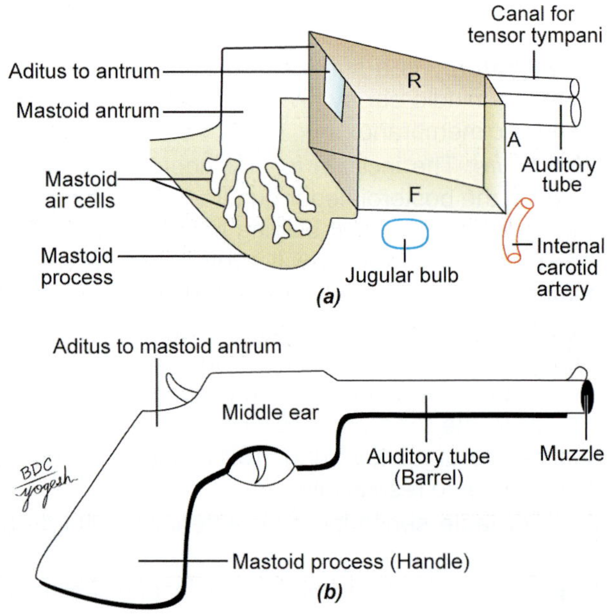


**Figs 18.15a and b:** (a) Scheme to show some relationships of the middle ear cavity and (b) note that the cavity resembles a pistol

4. Medial wall
5. Anterior wall
6. Posterior wall.

### Roof or Tegmental Wall

The roof separates the middle ear from the middle cranial fossa. It is formed by a thin plate of bone called the ***tegmen tympani***. This plate is prolonged forwards as the roof of the canal for the tensor tympani and posteriorly as the roof of the mastoid antrum (Fig. 18.16).

*Note*: In young children, the roof presents a gap at the unossified petrosquamous suture where the middle ear is in direct contact with the meninges. In adults, the suture is ossified and transmits a vein from the middle ear to the superior petrosal sinus.

### Floor or Jugular Wall

1. The floor is formed by a thin plate of bone which separates the middle ear from the superior bulb of the internal jugular vein. This plate is a part of the temporal bone.
2. Near the medial wall, the floor presents the ***tympanic canaliculus*** which transmits the tympanic branch of the glossopharyngeal nerve to the medial wall of the middle ear.

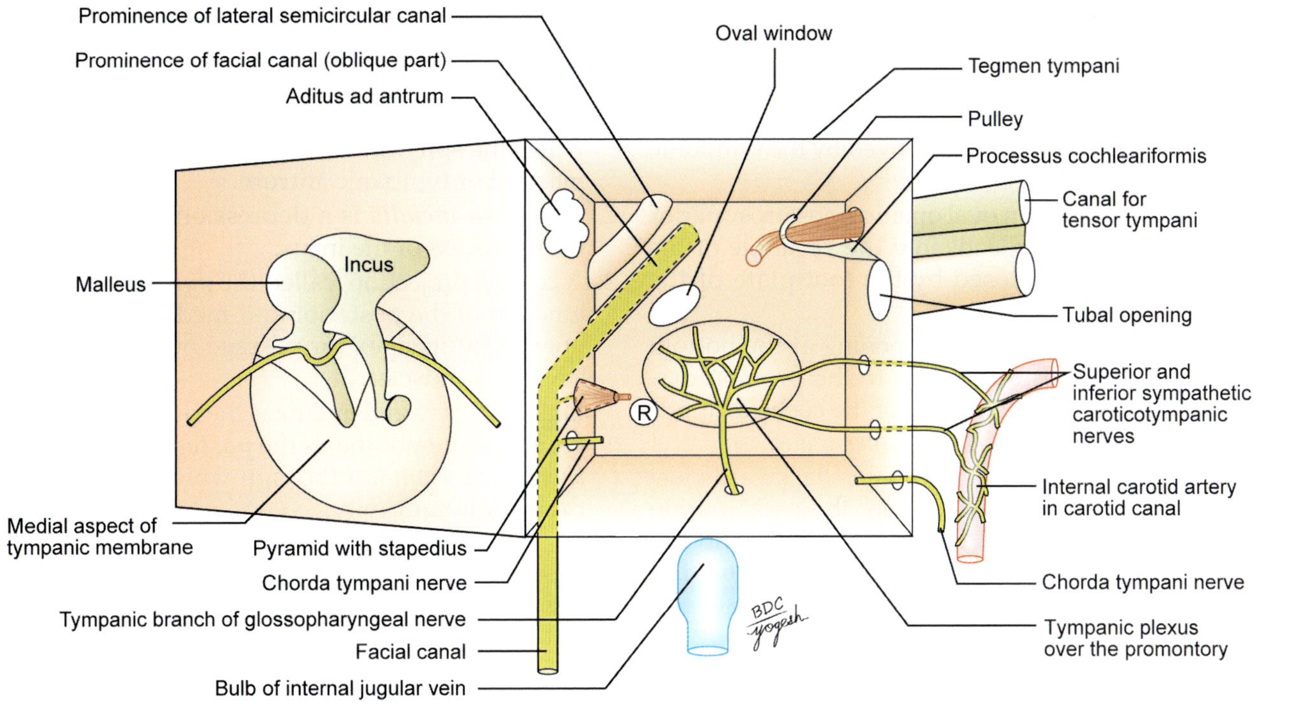


**Fig. 18.16:** Walls of middle ear (right middle ear, right lateral view, lateral wall is reflected to show interior or right middle ear, R: round window)

**Flowchart 18.3:** Boundaries of middle ear

***Boundaries of middle ear***

***Roof***
- Tegmental wall
- Formed by tegmen tympani
- Continue
  - anteriorly as roof of canal for tensor tympani
  - posteriorly as roof of mastoid antrum

***Floor***
- Jugular wall
- Formed by thin, convex plate of temporal bone
- Separates from superior bulb of IJV
- Tympanic canaliculus for tympanic branch of glossopharyngeal nerve

***Lateral wall***
- Tympanic membrane
- Temporal bone in epitympanum
- Petrotympanic fissure
- Anterior canal for chorda tympani nerve

***Medial wall***
- Labyrinthine wall
- Promontory
- Oval window
- Round window
- Sinus tympani
- Prominence of facial canal
- Prominence of lateral semicircular canal

***Anterior wall***
- Narrow
- Openings of canal for tensor tympani, auditory tube
- Bony plate separates it from carotid canal
- Processus cochleariformis

***Posterior wall***
- Aditus to mastoid antrum
- Pyramid:
  - Origin of stapedius
- Vertical part of facial canal
- Posterior canaliculus for chorda tympani
- Fossa incudis

***Clinical integration:*** Otitis media, chronic suppurative otitis media.

## *Lateral or Membranous Wall*

1. The lateral wall separates the middle ear from the external acoustic meatus. It is formed (Fig. 18.17):
   a. Mainly by the ***tympanic membrane*** along with the tympanic ring and sulcus (described earlier).
   b. Partly by the squamous temporal bone, in the region of the epitympanic recess.
2. Near the tympanic notch, there are following small apertures:
   a. ***Petrotympanic fissure*** lies in front of the upper end of the bony rim. It lodges the anterior process of the malleus and transmits the tympanic branch of the maxillary artery.
   b. ***Anterior canaliculus for the chorda tympani*** nerve lies either in the fissure or just in front of it. The nerve leaves the middle ear through this canaliculus to emerge at the base of the skull.

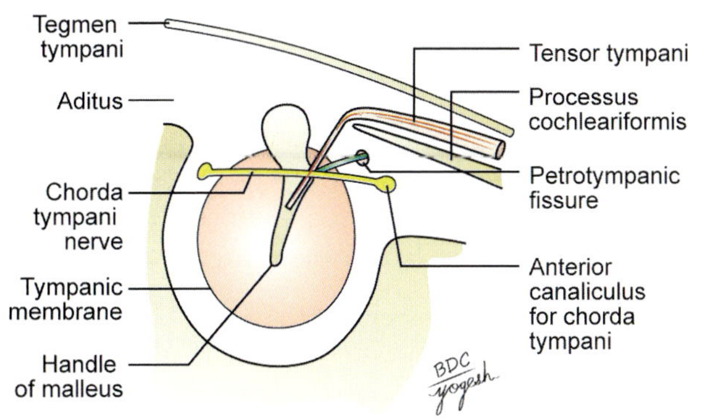


**Fig. 18.17:** Lateral wall of the middle ear viewed from the medial side

   c. ***Posterior canal for chorda tympani nerve*** is situated behind the tympanic membrane at the junction of the posterior and lateral walls.

### Medial or Labyrinthine Wall

The medial wall separates the middle ear from the internal ear. It presents the following features:

1. ***Promontory*** is a rounded bulging produced by the first turn of the cochlea. It is grooved by the tympanic plexus (Fig. 18.18).
2. ***Fenestra vestibuli*** is an oval opening posterosuperior to the promontory. It leads into the vestibule of the internal ear and is closed by the foot-plate of the stapes.
3. ***Fenestra cochleae*** is a round opening at the bottom of a depression posteroinferior to the promontory. It opens into the scala tympani of the cochlea, and is closed by the *secondary tympanic membrane.*
4. ***Prominence of the facial canal*** runs backwards just above the fenestra vestibuli, to reach the lower margin of the aditus. The canal then descends behind the posterior wall to end at the stylomastoid foramen.
5. Prominence of lateral semicircular canal above the facial canal.
6. ***Sinus tympani*** is a depression behind the promontory, opposite the ampulla of the posterior semicircular canal.

### Anterior or Carotid Wall

1. The anterior wall is narrow. It has two openings (Fig. 18.18):
   a. Opening of canal for tensor tympani above
   b. Opening of auditory tube below.
2. Below the opening of auditory tube, the anterior wall is formed by a thin plate of bone which separates the middle ear from the carotid canal and internal carotid artery. This plate is perforated by:
   a. Superior and inferior sympathetic caroticotympanic nerves and
   b. Tympanic branch of internal carotid artery.
3. ***Processus cochleariformis*** is a curved bony lamina that is extending from the bony plate separating canal for tensor tympani and auditory tube.
4. The posterior end of processus cochleariformis forms a *pulley* around which the tendon of the tensor tympani turns laterally to reach the upper part of the handle of the malleus.

### Posterior or Mastoid Wall

The posterior wall presents these features from above downwards (Fig. 18.18):

1. Superiorly, there is an opening or ***aditus*** through which the epitympanic recess communicates with the mastoid or tympanic antrum.
2. The ***fossa incudis*** is a depression which lodges the short process of the incus.
3. A conical projection, called the ***pyramid,*** lies near the junction of the posterior and medial walls. It has an opening at its apex for passage of the tendon of the stapedius muscle.
4. Lateral to pyramid and near the posterior edge of the tympanic membrane, is the ***posterior canaliculus for the chorda tympani*** through which the nerve enters the middle ear cavity.

**Competency:**
**AN40.4** Explain anatomical basis of otitis externa and otitis media.

## CLINICAL ANATOMY

- ***Otitis media*** is a suppurative infection of the middle ear. It is common in infants and children due to horizontally placed auditory tubes and short external ear. The infection may reach to the middle ear from nasopharynx through auditory tube or from external ear (Fig. 18.21).
- ***Chronic suppurative otitis media*** is a persistent infection of middle ear leading to persistent perforation of tympanic membranes and hearing impairment.
- ***Myringoplasty*** is a surgical procedure in which a graft is used to support healing of tympanic membrane perforation. Temporal fascia is commonly used as a graft in myringoplasty.

### Ear Ossicles (Plate 18.1, Fig. 18.19)

### Malleus

The malleus (Latin *hammer*) is so-called because it resembles a hammer. It is the largest, and the most laterally placed ossicle. It has the following parts:

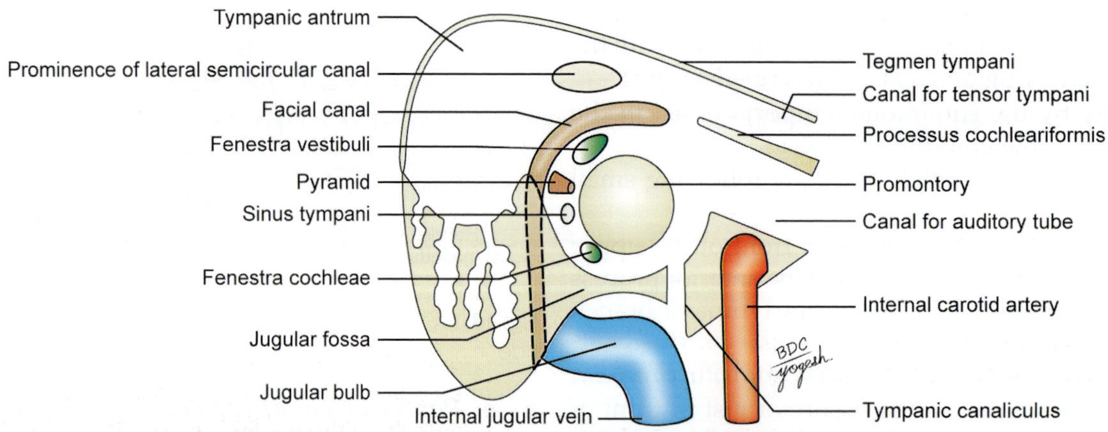


**Fig. 18.18:** Medial wall of the middle ear and adjacent structures

Plate 18.1: Parts of ear ossicles

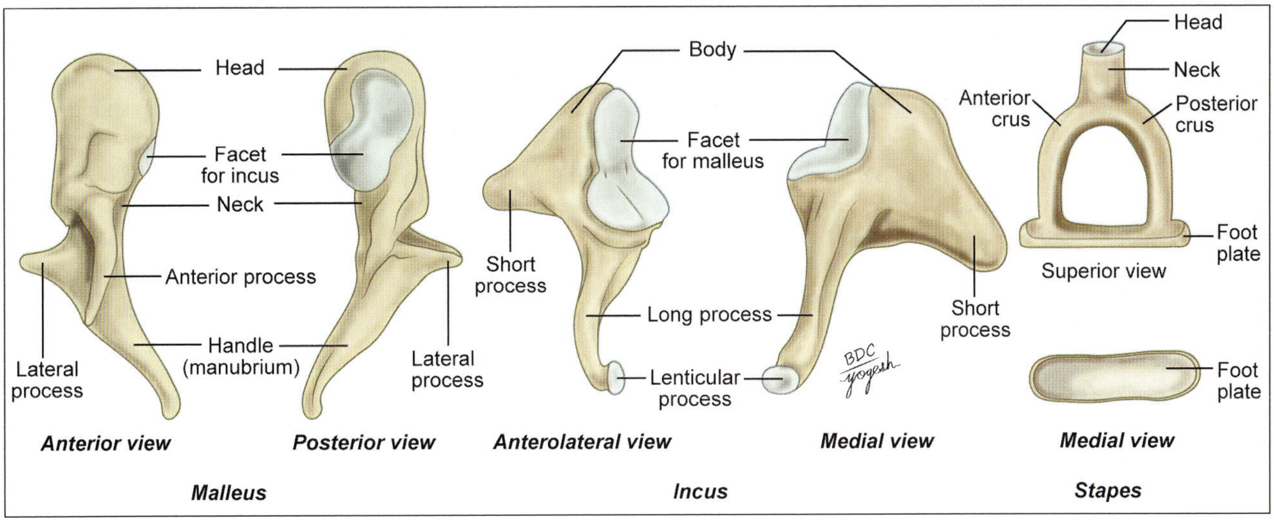


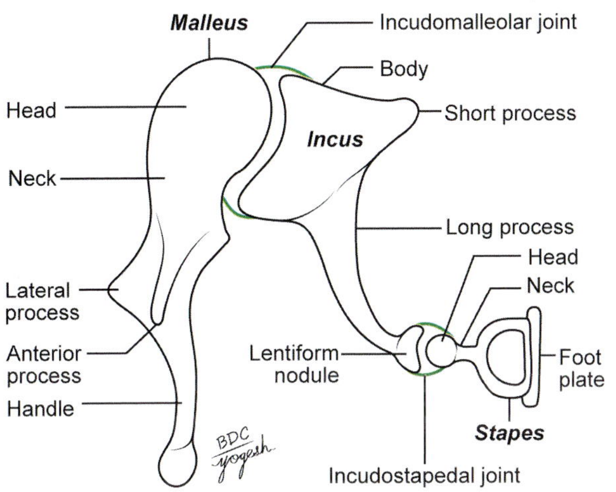


Fig. 18.19: Ear ossicles

1. The rounded ***head*** lies in the epitympanic recess. It articulates posteriorly with the body of the incus. It provides attachment to the superior and lateral ligaments.
2. The *neck* lies against the pars flaccida and is related medially to the chorda tympani nerve.
3. The ***anterior process*** is connected to the petrotympanic fissure by the anterior ligament.
4. The ***lateral process*** projects from the upper end of the handle and provides attachment to the malleolar folds.
5. The ***handle*** extends downwards, backwards and medially, and is attached to the upper half of the tympanic membrane.

### Incus or Anvil

It is so-called because it resembles an anvil, used by blacksmiths. It resembles a molar tooth and has the following parts:

1. The ***body*** is large and bears an articular surface that is directed forwards. It articulates with the head of the malleus.
2. The ***long process*** projects downwards just behind and parallel with the handle of the malleus. Its tip bears a lentiform nodule directed medially which articulates with the head of the stapes.

### Stapes

This bone is so-called because it is shaped like a stirrup. It is the smallest, and the most medially placed ossicle of the ear.

It has the following parts:

a. The small ***head*** has a concave facet which articulates with the lentiform nodule of the incus.
b. The narrow ***neck*** provides insertion, posteriorly, to the thin tendon of the stapedius.
c. ***Two limbs*** or crura; anterior, the shorter and less curved; and posterior, the longer which diverge from the neck and are attached to the footplate.
d. The ***footplate***, a *footpiece* or *base*, is oval in shape, and fits into the fenestra vestibuli.

## Joints of the Ossicles

1. The ***incudomalleolar joint*** is a saddle joint.
2. The ***incudostapedial joint*** is a ball and socket joint. Both of them are synovial joints. They are surrounded by capsular ligaments. Accessory ligaments are three for the malleus, and one each for the incus and the stapes which stabilize the ossicles. All ligaments are extremely elastic (Fig. 18.19).

## Muscles of the Middle Ear

There are two muscles—the tensor tympani and the stapedius. Both act simultaneously to damp down the intensity of high-pitched sound waves and thus protect the internal ear (Table 18.1).

Tensor tympani is derived from the 1st branchial arch, whereas the stapedius from 2nd branchial arch.

## CLINICAL ANATOMY

- ***Otosclerosis*** is a bony fusion between the footplate of stapes and the margin of oval window. It leads to deafness. The condition of deafness or otosclerosis can be treated with prosthesis (Figs 18.20a and b).

**TABLE 18.1: Muscles of middle ear (intratympanic muscles)**

| *Muscle* | *Origin* | *Insertion* | *Innervation* | *Actions* |
|---|---|---|---|---|
| ***Tensor tympani*** Long, slender muscle lies in the bony canal | Cartilaginous part of auditory tube Greater wing of sphenoid | Tendon bends sharply around the *processus cochleariformis* to insert at the handle of malleus | Mandibular nerve (V3) | Tenses the tympanic membrane To damp sound vibrations |
| ***Stapedius*** | Internal walls of pyramidal eminence that lie on the posterior wall of middle ear Its tendon emerges through the tip of pyramid | Posterior aspect of neck of stapes | Facial nerve (VII) | Draw stapes laterally To damp excessive sound vibrations |

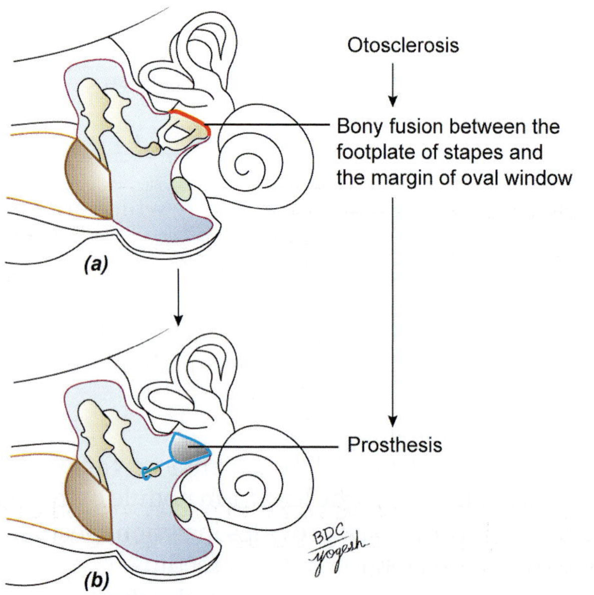


**Figs 18.20a and b:** (a) Otosclerosis and (b) treated by a prosthesis

- ***Stapedectomy*** is a surgical removal of stapes in case of otosclerosis.
- ***Stapedotomy***: Some surgeons refixed same stapes instead of its removal. This method is called stapedotomy.
- ***Hyperacusis***: Tensor tympani and stapedius dampen very loud sounds and protect the internal ear. Paralysis of these muscles result in hyperacusis.

### Arterial Supply

The middle ear is supplied by six arteries:

1. Anterior tympanic branch of maxillary artery
2. Stylomastoid branch of posterior auricular artery
3. Petrosal branch of middle meningeal artery
4. Superior tympanic branch of middle meningeal artery
5. Branch from artery of pterygoid canal
6. Tympanic branch of internal carotid artery.

*Note*: The anterior tympanic branch of the maxillary artery which enters the middle ear through the petrotympanic fissure. The posterior tympanic branch of the stylomastoid branch of the posterior auricular artery which enters through the stylomastoid foramen.

### Venous Drainage

Veins from the middle ear drain into the superior petrosal sinus and the pterygoid plexus of the veins.

### Lymphatic Drainage

Lymphatics pass to the preauricular and retropharyngeal lymph nodes.

### Nerve Supply

The nerve supply is derived from the tympanic plexus which lies over the promontory. The plexus is formed by the following.

1. The tympanic branch of the glossopharyngeal nerve. Its fibres are distributed to the mucous membrane of the middle ear, auditory tube, mastoid antrum and air cells. It also gives off the lesser petrosal nerve.
2. The superior and inferior caroticotympanic nerves arise from the sympathetic plexus around the internal carotid artery. These fibres are vasomotor to the mucous membrane.

## CLINICAL ANATOMY

***Otalgia*** (*ear pain*): The pain of the middle ear and external ear gets referred to:

1. Tongue, tonsil and pharynx, through glossopharyngeal nerve
2. Teeth through mandibular nerve.

## FUNCTIONS OF THE MIDDLE EAR

1. It transmits sound waves from the external ear to the internal ear through the chain of ear ossicles, and thus transforms the air-borne vibrations from the tympanic membrane to liquid-borne vibrations in the internal ear.
2. The intensity of the sound waves is increased ten times by the ossicles. It may be noted that the frequency of sound does not change.

## DISSECTION

Remove the dura mater and endosteum from the floor of the middle cranial fossa. Identify greater petrosal nerve emerging from a canaliculus on the anterior surface of petrous temporal bone. Trace it as it passes inferior to trigeminal ganglion to reach the carotid canal.

Carefully break the roof of the middle ear formed by tegmen tympani which is a thin plate of bone situated parallel and just lateral to the greater petrosal nerve. Cavity of the middle ear can be visualised. Try to put a probe in the anteromedial part of the cavity of middle ear till it appears at the opening in the lateral wall of nasopharynx. Identify the posterior wall of the middle ear which has an opening in its upper part. This is the aditus to mastoid antrum, which in turn, connects the cavity to the mastoid air cells.

***Ear ossicles***

Identify the bony ossicles. Locate the tendon of tensor tympani muscle passing from the malleus towards the medial wall of the cavity where it gets continuous with the muscle. Trace the tensor tympani muscle traversing in a semicanal above the auditory tube. Break one wall of the pyramid to visualise the stapedius muscle. Just superior to the attachment of tendon of tensor tympani, look for chorda tympani traversing the tympanic membrane.

## TYMPANIC OR MASTOID ANTRUM

### Features

Mastoid antrum is a small, circular, air-filled space situated in the posterior part of the petrous temporal bone. It is of adult size at birth, size of a small pea, or 1 cm in diameter and has a capacity of about 1 ml (Fig. 18.21).

### Boundaries

*Superiorly:* Tegmen tympani, and beyond it the temporal lobe of the cerebrum.

*Inferiorly:* Mastoid process containing the mastoid air cells.

*Anteriorly:* It communicates with the epitympanic recess through the aditus. The aditus is related medially to the ampullae of the superior and lateral semicircular canals, and posterosuperiorly to the facial canal.

*Posteriorly:* It is separated by a thin plate of bone from the sigmoid sinus. Beyond the sinus there is the cerebellum.

*Medially:* Petrous temporal bone.

*Laterally:* It is bounded by part of the squamous temporal bone.

*Note*: The lateral wall of mastoid antrum corresponds to the *suprameatal triangle* seen on the surface of the bone. This wall is 2 mm thick at birth, but increases in thickness at the rate of about 1 mm per year up to a maximum of about 12 to 15 mm.

### Mastoid Air Cells

Mastoid air cells are a series of intercommunicating spaces of variable size present within the mastoid process. Their number varies considerably. Sometimes there are just a few, and are confined to the upper part of the mastoid process. Occasionally, they may extend beyond the mastoid process into the squamous or petrous parts of the temporal bone.

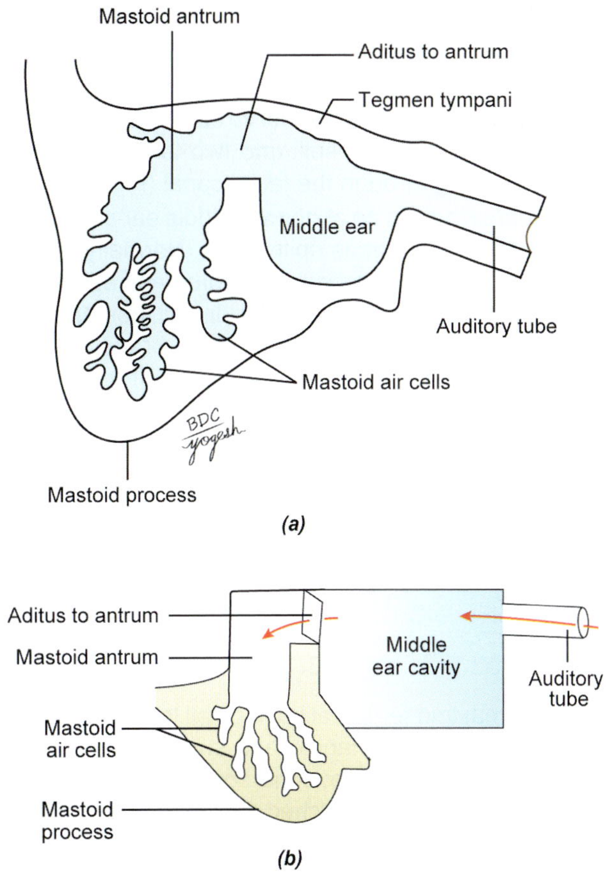


**Figs 18.21a and b:** (a) Mastoid antrum and mastoid air cells (section through long axis of the petromastoid bone) and (b) schematic representation

### Vessels, Lymphatics and Nerves

The mastoid antrum and air cells are supplied by the *posterior tympanic artery* derived from the stylomastoid branch of the posterior auricular artery. The *veins* drain into the mastoid emissary vein, the posterior auricular vein and the sigmoid sinus.

*Lymphatics* pass to the postauricular and upper deep cervical lymph nodes.

*Nerves* are derived from the tympanic plexus formed by the glossopharyngeal nerve and from the meningeal branch of the mandibular nerve.

## CLINICAL ANATOMY

- Fracture of the middle cranial fossa breaks the roof of the middle ear, ruptures the tympanic membrane, and thus causes bleeding through the ear along with discharge of CSF.
- Throat infections commonly spread to the middle ear through the auditory tube and cause ***otitis media***. The pus from the middle ear may erode the floor and spread downwards, causing thrombosis of the sigmoid sinus and the internal jugular vein (Fig. 18.22).
- ***Bezold's abscess*** is subperiosteal postauricular abscess. The spread of infection of mastoiditis may cause Bezold's abscess.

- Mastoiditis is a potentially dangerous and life-threatening condition as it can easily spread to cranial cavity.
- ***Dehiscence of the facial nerve canal***: Occasionally, the facial nerve may split into two-to-three strands while passing through the facial canal (Fig. 18.23).
- ***Cholesteatoma*** is an abnormal middle ear cavity lined by stratified squamous epithelium. (Normally, middle ear cavity is lined by ciliated columnar epithelium except over ear ossicles, posterior wall, posterior part of medial wall, parts of tympanic membrane, mastoid antrum, and mastoid air cells where it is lined by nonciliated flat epithelium.)
- Glands are absent in mucosa of tympanic cavity, but goblet cells are abundant.
- ***Mastoid abscess*** is secondary to otitis media.
- In surgical drainage of mastoid abscess, facial nerve should be protected carefully.

### DISSECTION

Clean the mastoid temporal bone off all the muscles and identify suprameatal triangle and supramastoid crest. Use a fine chisel to remove the bone of the triangle till the mastoid antrum is reached. Examine the extent of mastoid air cells.

Remove the posterior and superior walls of external auditory meatus till the level of the roof of mastoid antrum. Identify the chorda tympani nerve at the posterosuperior margin of tympanic membrane.

Look for arcuate eminence on the anterior face of petrous temporal bone. Identify internal acoustic meatus on the posterior face of petrous temporal bone, with the nerves in it. Try to break off the superior part of petrous temporal bone above the internal acoustic meatus. Identify the facial nerve as it passes towards the aditus. Identify the sharp bend of the facial nerve with the geniculate ganglion.

Identify the facial nerve turning posteriorly into the medial wall. Trace it above the fenestra vestibuli till it turns inferiorly in the medial wall of aditus.

Identify facial nerve at the stylomastoid foramen. Try to break the bone vertically along the lateral edge of the foramen to expose the whole of facial nerve canal.

Break off more of the superior surface of the petrous temporal bone. Remove the bone gently. Examine the holes in the bone produced by semicircular canals and look for the semicircular ducts lying within these canals. Note the branches of vestibulocochlear nerve entering the bone at the lateral end of the meatus. Study the internal ear from the models in the museum.

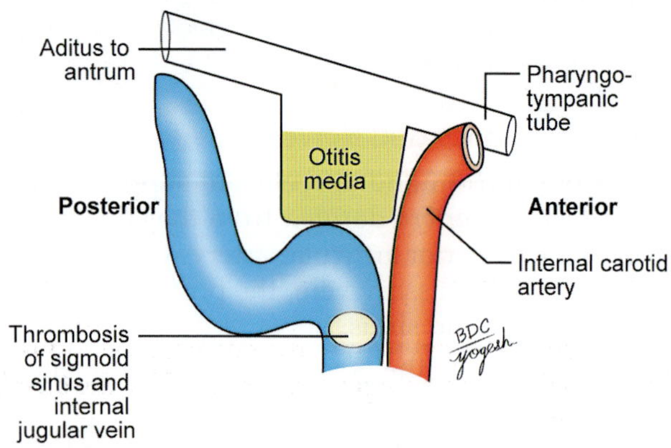


**Fig. 18.22:** Otitis media causing thrombosis of the sigmoid sinus and the internal jugular vein

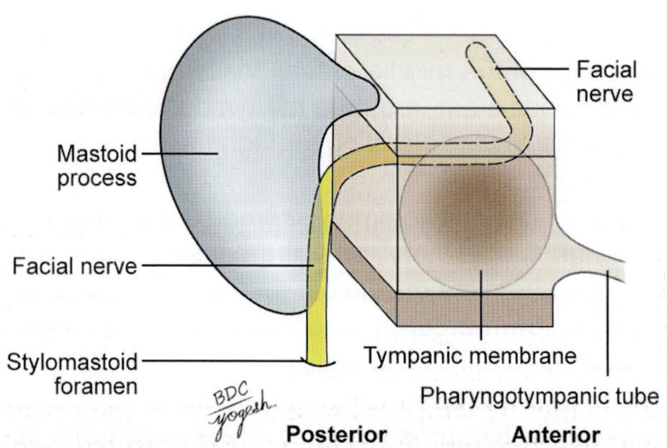


**Fig. 18.23:** Site of injury to facial nerve during mastoid operation

***Competency:***
**AN40.3** Describe the features of internal ear.

## INTERNAL EAR

The internal ear, or labyrinth, lies in the petrous part of the temporal bone. It consists of:

1. *Bony labyrinth* within which there is a membranous labyrinth.
2. *Membranous labyrinth* is filled with a fluid called *endolymph*. It is separated from the bony labyrinth by another fluid called the *perilymph*.

### BONY LABYRINTH

The bony labyrinth consists of three parts (Plate 18.2 and Flowchart 18.4):

1. Cochlea, anteriorly
2. Vestibule, in the middle
3. Semicircular canals, posteriorly.

#### Cochlea

1. The bony cochlea resembles the shell of a common snail. It forms the anterior part of the labyrinth. It has a conical central axis known as the ***modiolus*** around which the cochlear canal makes two and three quarter turns (Fig. 18.24).
2. The modiolus is directed forwards and laterally. Its apex points towards the anterosuperior part of the medial wall of the middle ear and the base towards the fundus of the internal acoustic meatus.

**Plate 18.2:** Right bony labyrinth and interior of vestibule (medial view, ASC, LSC, PSC: Anterior, lateral and posterior semicircular canals)

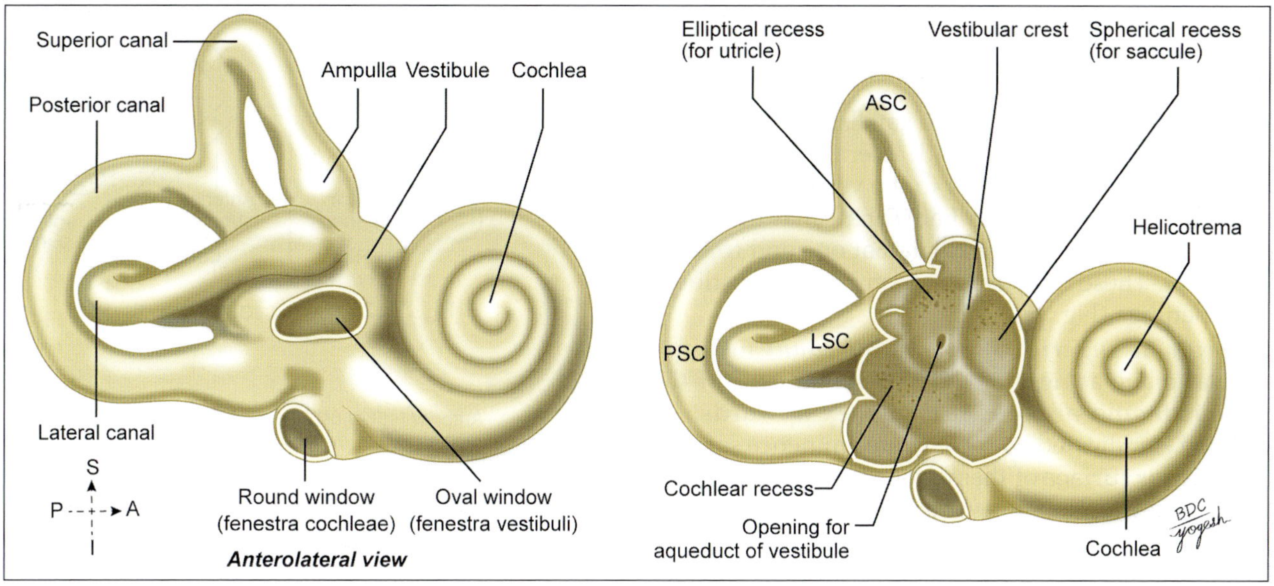


**Flowchart 18.4:** Bony and membranous labyrinth

***Bony labyrinth***

***Cochlea***
- Resembles shell of snail
- Cone-shaped
- Spirally arranged bony canal
- Modiolus:
  - Central axis
- Spiral lamina
- Scala vestibuli
- Helicotrema
- Aqueduct of cochlea

***Vestibule***
- Central ovoid cavity
- 2 openings
  - Oval window
  - Round window
- Interior:
  - Spherical recess
  - Elliptical recess
  - Cochlear recess
  - Openings of aqueduct of vestibule
  - 5 openings of semicircular canals

***Semicircular canals***
- Three canals
  - Superior (anterior)
  - Posterior
  - Lateral
- Each canal
  - two-thirds of circle
- Ampulla – dilated ends

***Membranous labyrinth filled with endolymph***

***Duct of cochlea***
- Scala media
- Occupies middle part of cochlear canal
- 3 walls
  - Floor – basilar membrane
  - Roof – vestibular membrane
  - Outer wall – bony
- Organ of Corti lies on basilar membrane

***Saccule and utricle***
- Lies in vestibule
- Dilated sacs
- Reuniens duct: Connects cochlear duct with saccule
- Utriculosaccular duct: Connects saccule with utricle
- Maculae: Thickening of saccule and utricle
- Ductus endolymphaticus

***Semicircular ducts***
- Three ducts
  - Superior/anterior
  - Posterior
  - Lateral
- Ampulla – dilated terminal part
- Ampullary crest/ cupola

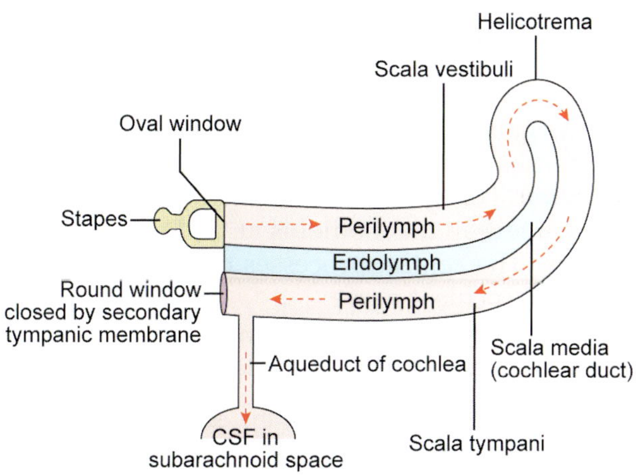


**Fig. 18.24:** Cochlear duct, scala vestibulli, and scala tympani (CSF: Cerebrospinal fluid)

3. A spiral ridge of the bone, the ***spiral lamina***, projects from the modiolus and partially divides the cochlear canal into the scala vestibuli above, and the scala tympani below. These relationships apply to the lowest part or basal turn of the cochlea. The division between the two passages is completed by the ***basilar membrane***.
4. The scala vestibuli communicates with the scala tympani at the apex of the cochlea by a small opening, called the ***helicotrema***.

## Vestibule

1. This is the central part of the bony labyrinth. It lies medial to the middle ear cavity. Its lateral wall opens into the middle ear at the fenestra vestibuli which is closed by the footplate of the stapes.
2. Three semicircular canals open into its posterior wall. The medial wall is related to the internal acoustic meatus, and presents the ***spherical recess*** in front, and the ***elliptical recess*** behind. The two recesses are separated by a ***vestibular crest*** which splits inferiorly to enclose the ***cochlear recess***.
3. Just below the elliptical recess, there is the opening of a diverticulum, the *aqueduct of the vestibule* which opens at a narrow fissure on the posterior aspect of the

petrous temporal bone, posterolateral to the internal acoustic meatus. It is plugged in life by the *ductus endolymphaticus* and a vein; no perilymph escapes through it.

### Semicircular Canals

There are three bony semicircular canals: (1) An anterior or superior, (2) posterior, and (3) lateral; each has two ends. They lie posterosuperior to the vestibule, and are set at right angles to each other. Each canal describes two-thirds of a circle, and is dilated at one end to form the ***ampulla***. These three canals open into the vestibule by *five* openings (Fig. 18.25).

1. ***Anterior* or *superior semicircular canal*** lies in a vertical plane at right angles to the long axis of the petrous temporal bone. It is convex upwards. Its position is indicated by the arcuate eminence seen on the anterior surface of the petrous temporal bone. Its ampulla is situated anterolaterally. Its posterior end unites with the upper end of the posterior canal to form the ***crus commune*** which opens into the medial wall of the vestibule.
2. ***Posterior semicircular canal*** also lies in a vertical plane parallel to the long axis of the petrous temporal bone. It is convex backwards. Its ampulla lies at its lower end. The upper end joins the anterior canal to form the crus commune.
3. ***Lateral semicircular canal*** lies in the horizontal plane with its convexity directed posterolaterally. The ampulla lies anteriorly, close to the ampulla of the anterior canal.

*Note:* The lateral semicircular canals of the two sides lie in the same plane. The anterior canal of one side lies in the plane of the posterior canal of the other side.

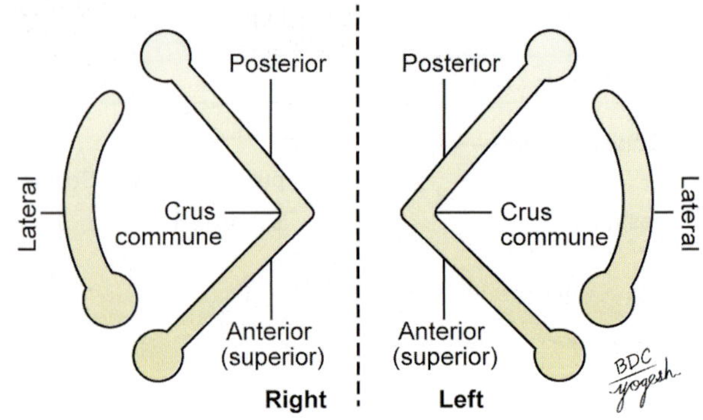


**Fig. 18.25:** Semicircular canals

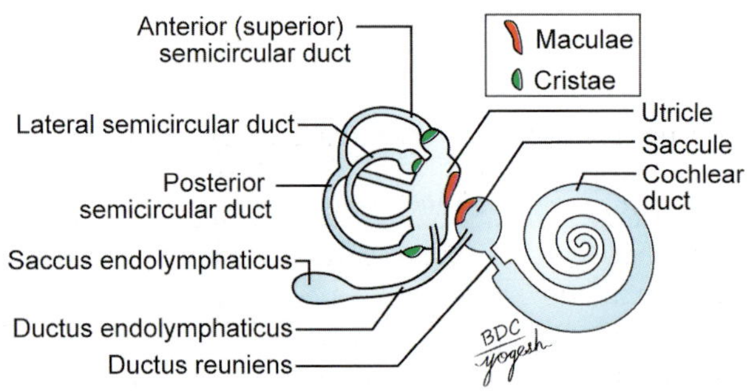


**Fig. 18.26:** Parts of the membranous labyrinth (as seen from the lateral side)

## MEMBRANOUS LABYRINTH

It is a membrane-bound cavity filled with ***endolymph***.

The epithelium of the membranous labyrinth is specialized to form the following receptors:

1. For sound, i.e. ***organ of Corti***
2. For static balance, the ***maculae***
3. For kinetic balance, the ***cristae***.

Like the bony labyrinth, the membranous labyrinth also consists of three main parts:

1. Spiral duct of the cochlea or organ of Corti, anteriorly.
2. Utricle and saccule with maculae, the organs of static balance, within the vestibule.
3. Semicircular ducts with cristae, the organs of kinetic balance, posteriorly (Fig. 18.26).

***Competency:***
**AN43.3** Identify, describe and draw microanatomy of olfactory epithelium, eyelid, lip, sclerocorneal junction, optic nerve, cochlea—organ of Corti, pineal gland.

Microanatomy of cochlea and organ of corti is given here. For microanatomy of other structures please refer to appropriate chapters.

### Duct of the Cochlea or the Scala Media

1. The spiral duct occupies the middle part of the cochlear canal between the scala vestibuli and the scala tympani (Fig. 18.27).
2. It is triangular in cross-section. It has three walls:
   - *Floor* is formed by the *basilar membrane*
   - *Roof* by the *vestibular* or *Reissner's membrane*
   - Outer wall by the bony wall of the cochlea.
3. The ***basilar membrane*** supports the spiral ***organ of Corti*** which is the end organ for hearing. It comprises rods of Corti and hair cells. Hair is embedded in a gelatinous membrane called the ***membrana tectoria***. The organ of Corti is innervated by peripheral processes of bipolar cells located in the ***spiral ganglion***. This ganglion is located in the spiral canal present within the modiolus at the base of the spiral lamina. The central processes of the ganglion cells form the cochlear nerve.
4. Posteriorly, the duct of the cochlea is connected to the saccule by a narrow ***ductus reunions***.

*Note*: The sound waves reaching the endolymph through the vestibular membrane make appropriate parts of the basilar membrane vibrate, so that different parts of the organ of Corti are stimulated by different frequencies of sound. The loudness of the sound depends on the amplitude of vibration.

### Saccule and Utricle

1. The ***saccule*** lies in the anteroinferior part of the vestibule, and is connected to the basal turn of the cochlear duct by the ductus reunions.

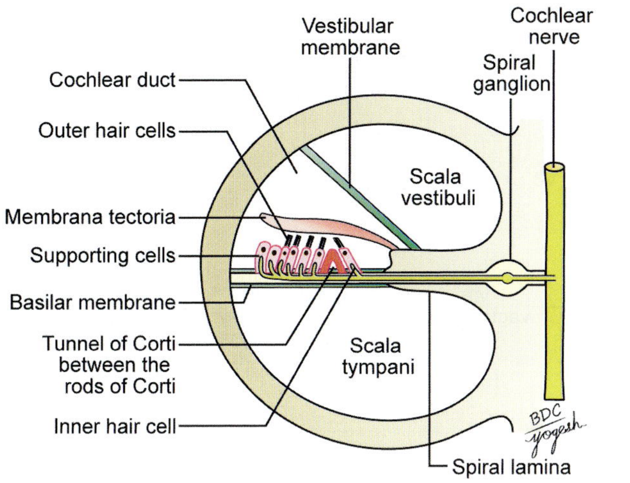


**Fig. 18.27:** Schematic section through one turn of the cochlea

2. The ***utricle*** is larger than the saccule and lies in the posterosuperior part of the vestibule. It receives *the ends of three* semicircular ducts through *five openings*. The duct of the saccule unites with the duct of the utricle to form the ***ductus endolymphaticus***. The ductus endolymphaticus ends in a dilatation, the ***saccus endolymphaticus***. The ductus and saccus occupy the aqueduct of the vestibule.
3. The medial walls of the saccule and utricle are thickened to form a ***macula*** in each chamber. The maculae are end organs that give information about the position of the head. They are static balance receptors. They are supplied by peripheral processes of neurons in the vestibular ganglion.
4. Saccule gets stimulated by vertical linear motions, e.g. going in 'lift'. Utricle gets stimulated by horizontal linear motion, e.g. going in car.

### Semicircular Ducts

1. The three semicircular ducts lie within the corresponding bony canals. Each duct has an ampulla corresponding to that of the bony canal.
2. In each ampulla, there is an end organ called the ampullary crest or ***crista*** or cupola. Cristae respond to pressure changes in the endolymph caused by movements of the head.

### Blood Supply of Labyrinth

The arterial supply is derived mainly from the labyrinthine branch of the basilar artery which accompanies the vestibulocochlear nerve; and partly from the stylomastoid branch of the posterior auricular artery.

The labyrinthine vein drains into the superior petrosal sinus or the transverse sinus. Other inconstant veins emerge at different points and open separately into the superior and inferior petrosal sinuses and the internal jugular vein.

## VESTIBULOCOCHLEAR NERVE

### Cochlear Pathway

Vestibulocochlear nerve comprises hearing and vestibular parts. The first neurons of the pathway are located in the spiral ganglion. They are bipolar. Their peripheral processes innervate the spiral organ of Corti, while central processes form the cochlear nerve. This nerve terminates in the dorsal and ventral cochlear nuclei. From cochlear nuclei, fibres travel through pons, midbrain, thalamus and internal capsule to reach auditory area in temporal pole (Fig. 18.28).

### Vestibular Pathway

The vestibular receptors are the maculae of the saccule and utricle (for static balance) and in the crista of the ampullaris of semicircular ducts (for kinetic balance).

Fibres from cristae of anterior and lateral semicircular canals and some fibres from the two maculae lie in superior vestibular area of internal acoustic meatus.

Fibres of crista of posterior semicircular canal lie in foramen singulare.

Most of the fibres from maculae of utricle and saccule lie in inferior vestibular area.

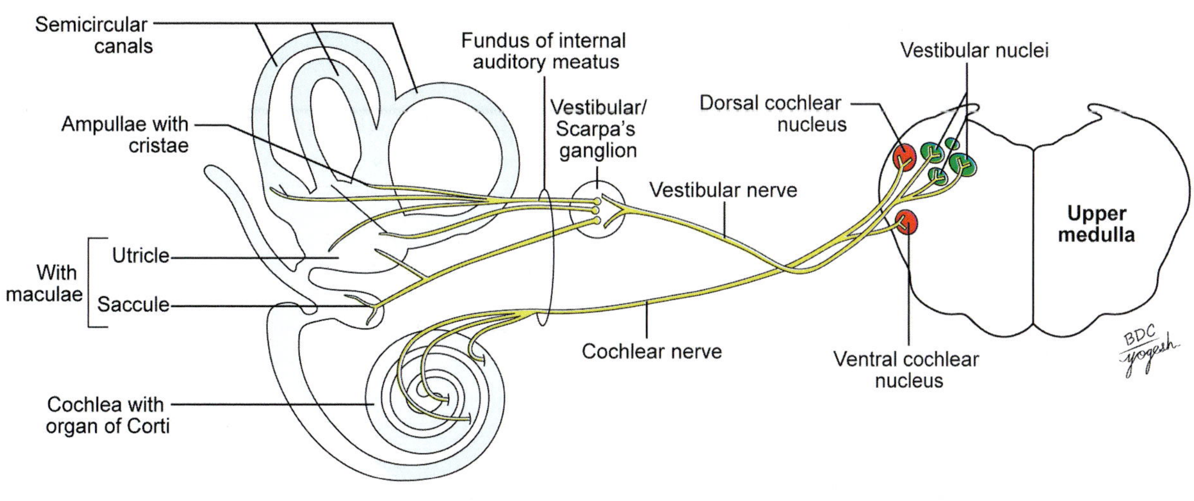


**Fig. 18.28:** Course of vestibulocochlear nerve

**Flowchart 18.5:** Reasons of earache

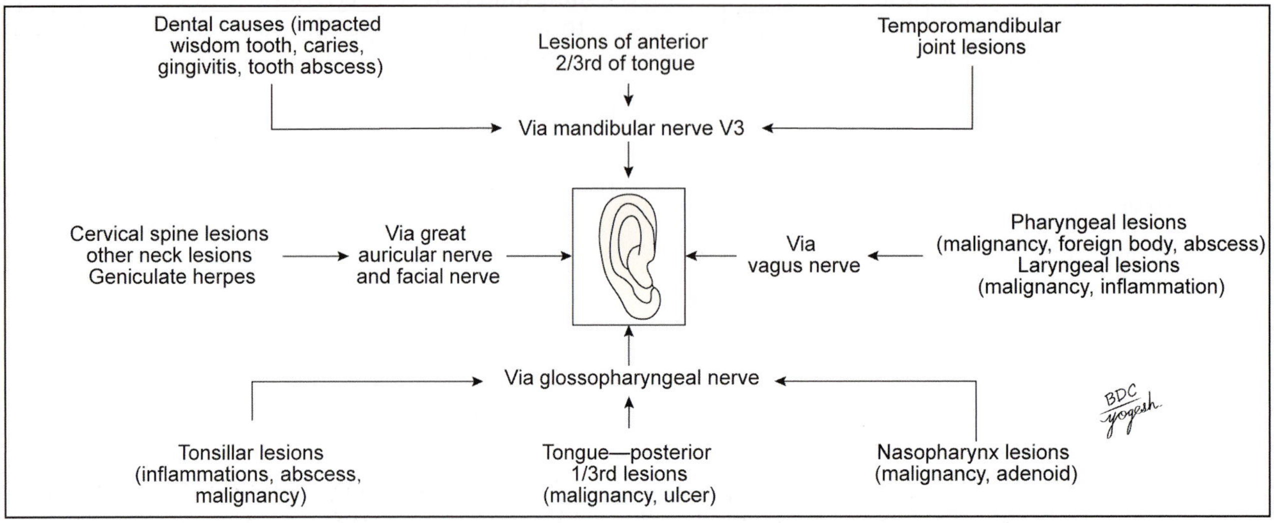


These three nerve divisions are peripheral processes of bipolar neurons of the vestibular ganglion. This ganglion is situated in the internal acoustic meatus. The central processes arising from the neurons of the ganglion form the vestibular nerve which ends in the vestibular nuclei.

These nuclei send fibres:

a. To the archicerebellum through the inferior cerebellar peduncle.
b. To the motor nuclei of the brainstem (chiefly of the III, IV, VI and XI nerves)

Through the vestibular pathway, the impulses arising in the labyrinth can influence the movements of the eyes, the head, the neck and the trunk.

## CLINICAL ANATOMY

- Endolymph is produced by striae vascularis. This process requires melanocytes. The disorders of melanocytes, i.e. albinism, are associated with deafness.
- Acoustic neuroma is a tumour of Schwann cells of VIII nerve. If neuroma extends into internal auditory meatus, VII nerve will get pressed. There will be VIII nerve paralysis and VII nerve paralysis as well.
- Reasons of earache are depicted in Flowchart 18.5.

## DEVELOPMENT

***External auditory meatus:*** Dorsal part of 1st ectodermal cleft.

***Auricle:*** Tubercles appearing on 1st and 2nd branchial arches around the opening of external auditory meatus.

***Middle ear cavity and auditory tube:*** Tubotympanic recess.

***Ossicles***

a. *Malleus and incus:* From *1st arch cartilage.*
b. *Stapes:* From *2nd arch cartilage.*

***Muscles***

a. *Tensor tympani:* From *1st pharyngeal arch mesoderm.*
b. *Stapedius:* From *2nd pharyngeal arch mesoderm.*

***Membranous labyrinth:*** From ectodermal vesicle on each side of hindbrain vesicle. Organ of Corti—ectodermal.

VIDEO

**Video 3.18 Ear**

### *Facts to Remember*

- Tympanic membrane develops from ectoderm, mesoderm and endoderm.
- Outer aspect of tympanic membrane is supplied by part of V and X nerves.
- Malleus and incus develop from 1st pharyngeal arch, while stapedius develops from second pharyngeal arch.
- Tensor tympani develops from 1st arch and is supplied by V3, while stapedius develops from 2nd arch and is supplied by VII nerve.
- Eustachian tube equalizes the pressure on both sides of the tympanic membrane. This tube connects the nasopharynx to the anterior wall of middle ear.
- Malleus, incus and stapes are *bone within bone*, as these 3 bony ossicles lie within the petrous temporal bone.
- There are 2 synovial joints between these three bony ossicles, which are fully developed at birth.
- One may slowly become deaf to soft sounds, if one is continuously exposed to a lot of loud sounds.

### BDC's Anatomy *e*-book

1. Noise pollution - poem
2. Organ of Corti
3. Macula
4. Ampullary crests
5. Molecular regulation
6. Further reading
7. Viva voce questions

# RIGHT MIDDLE EAR

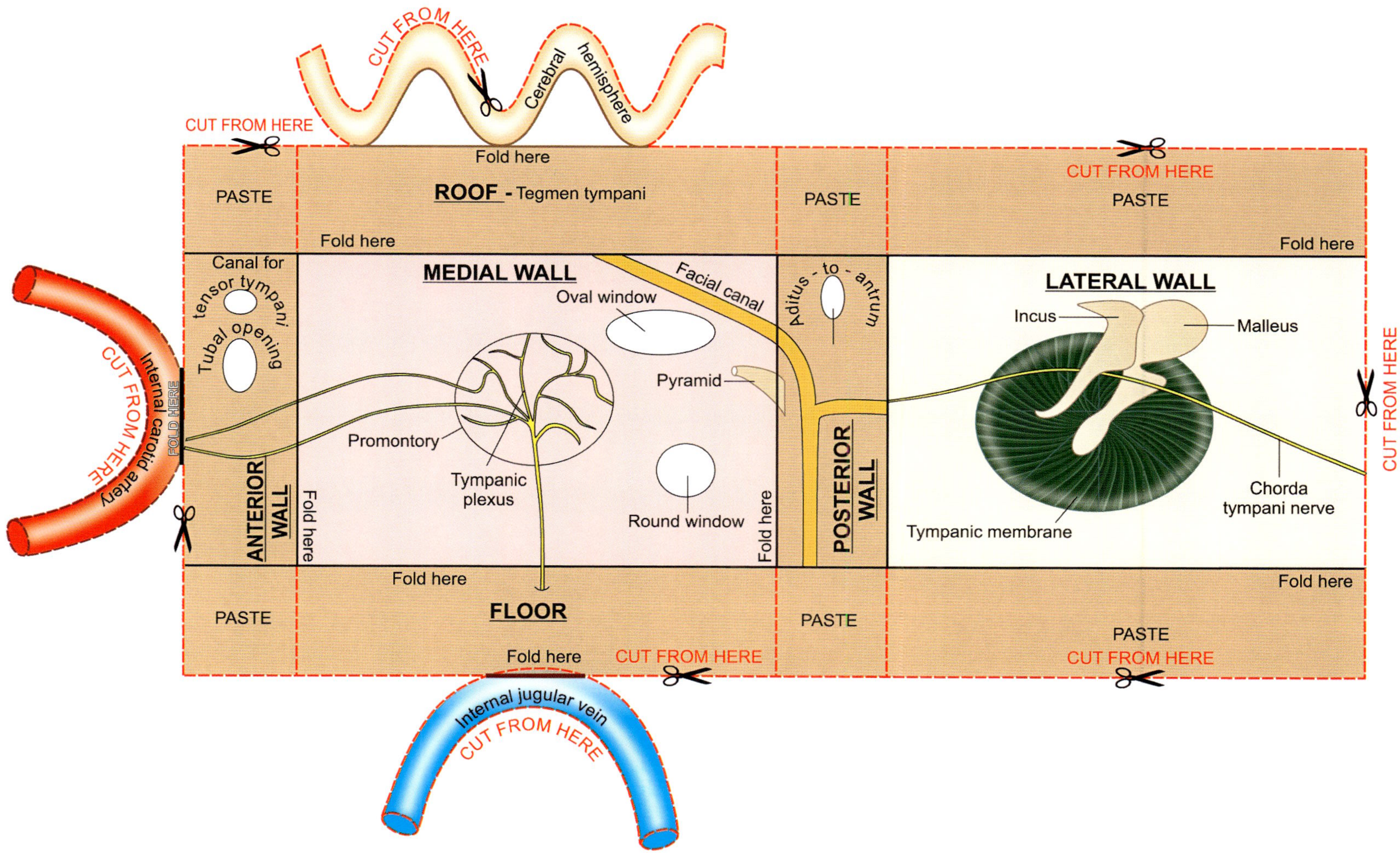

Chapter

19

# Eyeball

Eye is a peripheral organ of vision located in the bony orbit. The eye is spherical in shape (25 mm in diameter). Its movements are facilitated by six extraocular muscles.

### Tunics of Eyeball

The wall of eyeball consists of three structural layers (Fig. 19.1):

1. Outer fibrous layer – sclera and cornea
2. Middle vascular coat/uvea – choroid, ciliary body and iris
3. Inner nervous coat – retina.

The eyeball (= *oculus* in Latin and *ophthalmos* in Greek) has three chambers as follows:

1. Anterior chamber: Space between cornea and iris (Fig. 19.1)
2. Posterior chamber: Space between iris and anterior surface of lens
3. Vitreous chamber: Space between posterior surface of lens and retina.

The anterior and posterior chambers contain aqueous humour (watery fluid), whereas posterior compartment contains gel-like vitreous body. The cornea, lens, aqueous humour, and vitreous body are transparent refractive media of eyeball.

*Competency:*
**AN41.1** Describe and demonstrate parts and layers of eyeball.

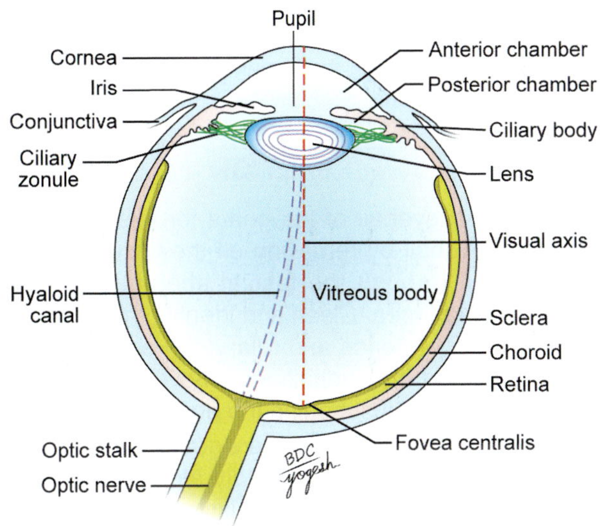


**Fig. 19.1:** Sagittal section through the eyeball

## OUTER COAT

### SCLERA

The sclera (*skleros* = hard) is opaque and forms the posterior five-sixths of the eyeball.

### Structure

1. It is composed of dense fibrous tissue which is firm and maintains the shape of the eyeball.
2. It is thickest behind, near the entrance of the optic nerve, and thinnest about 6 mm behind the ***sclerocorneal junction*** where the recti muscles are inserted. However, it is weakest at the entrance of the optic nerve. Here the sclera shows numerous perforations for passage of fibres of the optic nerve. Because of its sieve-like appearance, this region is called the ***lamina cribrosa*** (*crib* = sieve).
3. The *outer surface* of the sclera is white and smooth, it is covered by Tenon's capsule. Its anterior part is covered by conjunctiva through which it can be seen as the white of the eye.
4. The *inner surface* is brown and grooved for the ciliary nerves and vessels. It is separated from the choroid by the ***perichoroidal space*** which contains a delicate cellular tissue, termed the ***suprachoroidal lamina*** or *lamina fusca of the sclera.*
5. The sclera is continuous anteriorly with the cornea at the *sclerocorneal junction or limbus* (Fig. 19.1). The deep part of the limbus contains a circular canal, known as the *sinus venosus sclerae or the* ***canal of Schlemm***. The aqueous humour drains into the anterior scleral or ciliary veins through this sinus.
6. The sclera is fused posteriorly with the *dural sheath of the optic nerve.* It provides insertion to the extrinsic muscles of the eyeball: The recti in front of the equator, and the oblique muscles behind the equator.

### Functions of Sclera

1. *Support*: It helps to maintain the shape of the eyeball.
2. *Protection*: It protects internal structures.
3. *Attachments*: It provides attachment to muscles that move the eyeball.

### Structures Piercing Sclera

The sclera is pierced by a number of structures:

a. *Optic nerve* pierces it a little inferomedial to the posterior pole of the eyeball.
b. *Ciliary nerves and arteries* pierce it around the entrance of the optic nerve.
c. *Anterior ciliary arteries*, derived from muscular arteries to the recti, pierce it near the limbus.
d. Four *venae vorticosae* or the choroid veins pass out through the sclera just behind the equator (Fig. 19.2).

*Note*: The sclera is almost avascular. However, the loose connective tissue between the conjunctiva and sclera called as the *episclera* is vascular.

### DISSECTION

Use the fresh eyeball of the goats for this dissection. Clean the eyeball by removing all the tissues from its surface. Cut through the fascial sheath around the margin of the cornea. Clean and identify the nerve with posterior ciliary arteries and ciliary nerves close to the posterior pole of the eyeball. Identify venae vorticosae piercing the sclera just behind the equator.

Incise only the sclera at the equator and then cut through it all around and carefully strip it off from the choroid. Anteriorly, the ciliary muscles are attached to the sclera, offering some resistance. As the sclera is steadily separated, the aqueous humour will escape from the anterior chamber of the eye. On dividing the optic nerve fibres, the posterior part of sclera can be removed.

## CORNEA

The cornea is transparent. It replaces the sclera over the anterior one-sixth of the eyeball. Its junction with the sclera is called the *sclerocorneal junction or limbus* (Fig. 19.1).

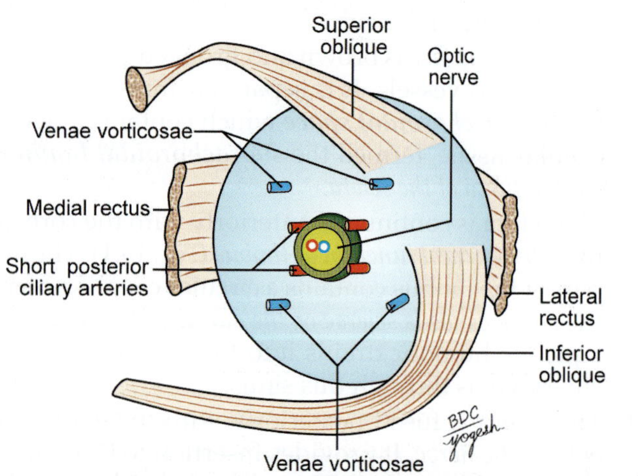


**Fig. 19.2:** Structures piercing the posterior aspect of the eyeball

### Structure

1. The cornea is more convex than the sclera, but the curvature diminishes with age. It is separated from the iris by a space called the *anterior chamber of the eye*.
2. The cornea is avascular and is nourished by lymph which circulates in the numerous corneal spaces and by the lacrimal fluid.
3. It is supplied by branches of the ophthalmic nerve and the short ciliary nerves (through the ciliary ganglion). Pain is the only sensation aroused from the cornea.

*Competency*:

**AN43.2** Identify, describe and draw the microanatomy of pituitary gland, thyroid, parathyroid gland, tongue, salivary glands, tonsil, epiglottis, cornea, retina.

Microanatomy of cornea is described here. For the other organs, please see appropriate chapters.

### Histology/Microanatomy

Cornea is a transparent, colourless, avascular structure that has five layers, before backwards (Plate 19.1 and Flowchart 19.1):

1. *Corneal epithelium* consists of nonkeratinized stratified squamous epithelium.
2. *Bowman's membrane*/anterior limiting lamina is thickened basal lamina of corneal epithelium.
3. *Corneal stroma* consists of layers of collagen fibrils having orthogonal array and few fibroblasts.
4. *Descemet's membrane*/posterior limiting lamina is the thickened basal lamina of corneal endothelium.
5. *Posterior endothelium* consists of simple squamous (low cuboidal) epithelium.

### CLINICAL ANATOMY

- After the injury, swelling of cornea causes disruption of orthogonal array of cornea. This leads to corneal opacity.
- In corneal inflammation, lymphocytes enter corneal stroma from blood vessels that lie at sclerocorneal junction (Plate 19.2).
- Bowman's membrane cannot regenerate but Descemet's membrane can regenerate.
- As cornea is an avascular structure, severely damaged cornea can be easily treated with corneal transplantation.
- ***Corneal opacity***: The injury to cornea may cause opacity that may interfere with vision.
- *Corneal transplantation*: The lack of vascularity and lymph vessels make the corneal grafting suitable. The cornea is successfully grafted from one person to the other.
- ***Corneal reflex***: The cornea is highly sensitive to touch and pain.
  *Procedure to elicit*: Touch gently the cornea with wisp of cotton wool and observe the blinking of eyelids.

**Plate 19.1:** Histology of cornea

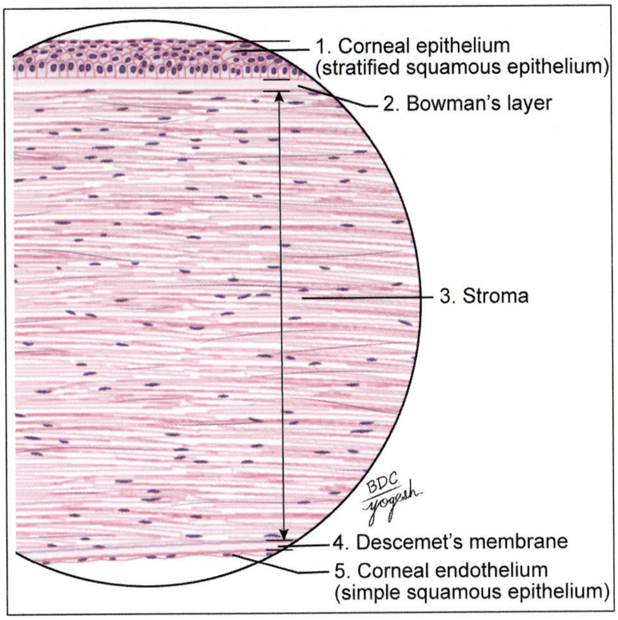


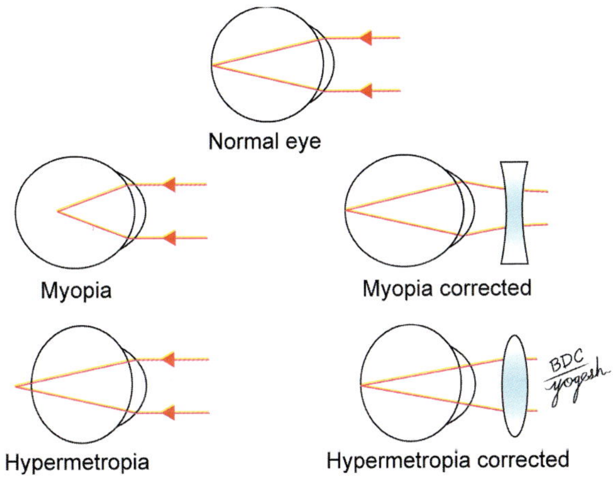


**Fig. 19.3:** Optical defects

*Pathway*: Ophthalmic nerve (afferent neurons) → main sensory nucleus of trigeminal nerve in midbrain → reticular formation → both the facial nerves (efferent neurons).

- The anteroposterior diameter of the eyeball and shape and curvature of the cornea determine the focal point. Changes in these result in myopia or shortsightedness, hypermetropia or longsightedness (Fig. 19.3).

## DISSECTION

Identify the cornea. Make an incision around the corneoscleral junction and remove the cornea so that the iris is exposed for examination. Identify the middle coat comprising choroid, ciliary body and iris deep to the sclera. Lateral to iris is the ciliary body with ciliary muscles and ciliary processes.

Strip off the iris, ciliary processes, anterior part of choroid. Remove the lens and put it in water. As the lens is removed, the vitreous body also escapes. Only the posterior part of choroid and subjacent retina is left.

## MIDDLE COAT (VASCULAR COAT OR UVEA)

Deep to sclera, there is a vascular coat of eyeball. It consists of:

1. Choroid
2. Ciliary body, and
3. Iris.

## CHOROID

Choroid is a thin pigmented layer which separates the posterior part of the sclera from the retina.

### Structure

The choroid consists of two layers: Choriocapillary layer and Bruch's membrane.

1. ***Choriocapillary layer:*** It lies superficial to Bruch's membrane. It consists of a network of blood vessels and supportive collagen fibres. It also contains many pigmented cells that give dark colour to choroid. The outer vascular lamina of choriocapillary layer has larger vessels, whereas inner capillary lamina (choroidocapillaries) contains a network of capillaries. Choriocapillary layer is externally supported by a nonvascular connective tissue coat called suprachoroid lamina or lamina fusca.
2. ***Bruch's membrane (lamina vitrea):*** It lies between choriocapillary layer and retina. It is a thin amorphous refractive layer. It consists of layers of elastic and collagen fibres. The choroid extends from optic nerve to ***ora serrata***.

### Blood Supply

1. *Arteries*: Choroid is supplied by short ciliary arteries, which pierce the sclera around the optic nerve.

**Flowchart 19.1:** Histology of cornea

*Cornea*

- ***Corneal epithelium***: Stratified squamous epithelium
- ***Bowman's membrane***: Basal lamina of corneal epithelium
- ***Corneal stroma***: Orthogonal array of collagen fibrils; Few fibroblasts
- ***Descemet's membrane***: Thick basal lamina of corneal endothelium
- ***Corneal endothelium***: Simple squamous or low cuboidal epithelium

**Plate 19.2:** Sclerocorneal junction, ciliary body and suspensory ligament of lens

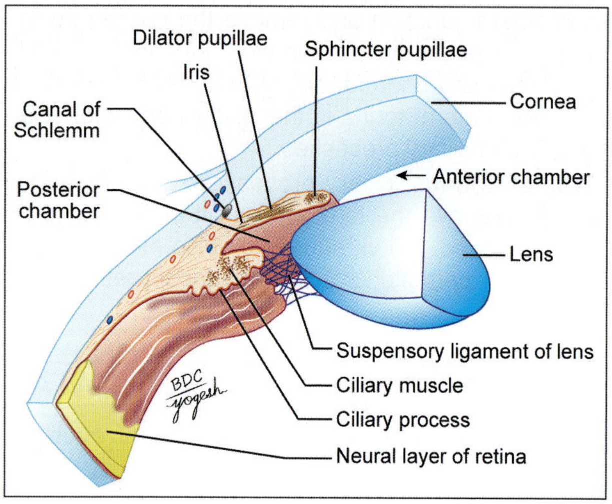


2. *Veins*: They are arranged in the form of whorls. These veins converge to form 4 or 5 venae vorticosae, which pierce the sclera just behind the equator to open into the ophthalmic veins.

***Competencies:***

**AN41.3** Describe the position, nerve supply and actions of intraocular muscles.

**AN43.3** Identify, describe and draw microanatomy of olfactory epithelium, microanatomy of iridio eyelid, lip, sclerocorneal junction, optic nerve, cochlea— organ of Corti, pineal gland.

## CILIARY BODY

The ciliary body is the thickened circular anterior portion of vascular coat of eyeball. It posteriorly continues with the choroid and anteriorly with iris. It is connected to lens by suspensory ligaments.

### Parts of Ciliary Body

1. The ciliary body consists of *ciliaris* muscles and vascular connective tissue (Plate 19.2). Ciliaris muscle consists of three functional groups of smooth muscle fibres as follows:
   - Longitudinal portion that helps to open iridocorneal angle and facilitate drainage of aqueous humour.
   - Oblique portion that causes flattening of lens during distant vision.
   - Circular portion that reduces tension of lens during accommodation for near vision.
2. *Ciliary processes*: These are approximately 75 thickenings of ciliary body that are covered by double layers of columnar epithelium cells (ciliary epithelium). Ciliary epithelium secretes aqueous humour and maintains blood–aqueous barrier. Outer cell layer of epithelium is pigmented, whereas inner cell layer secretes aqueous humour. Zonular fibres arise from suspensory ligament of the lens. *Ciliary ring* is an outer fibrous ring, which is continuous with the choroid.

### Functions

1. *Accommodation*: The main function of ciliary body is to focus the lens for near vision.
   *Mechanism*: The ciliary muscle as a whole acts as a sphincter, therefore, when its muscle fibres, both radial and circular contract, the choroid is pulled toward the lens reducing the tension on the suspensory ligaments. This allows the lens to assume a more spherical form because of its own elastic nature. Thus, the lens can cause more refraction needed for accommodation.
2. Production of aqueous humour.
3. Maintenance of blood – aqueous barrier.

## IRIS

1. The iris is the anteriormost part of vascular coat of eyeball. Iris is attached peripherally to sclera, at about 2 mm posterior to corneoscleral junction.
2. *Pupil*: Central aperture of the iris is called pupil.
3. Iris forms a contractile diaphragm in front of lens that controls entry of light in the eyeball.

### Structure of Iris

1. Iris consists of two parts:
   - Posterior pigmented epithelium
   - Anterior connective tissue stroma
2. Posterior pigmented epithelium consists of two layers: Posterior densely pigmented epithelium and anterior pigmented myoepithelial cells.
3. Stroma of iris consists of smooth muscle fibres, fibroblasts, melanocytes, connective tissue fibres, and blood vessels.
4. Smooth muscle fibres are arranged as:
   a. Circumferentially oriented *sphincter pupillae* muscle
   b. Longitudinally (radially) oriented *dilator pupillae* muscle
5. Numerous melanocytes are present in the stroma of iris. These melanocytes decide the colour of iris.

### CLINICAL ANATOMY

- While looking at infinite far, the light rays run parallel; ciliary muscle is relaxed, suspensory ligament is tense and lens is flat (Fig. 19.4a).
- While reading a book, the ciliary muscles contract and suspensory ligament is relaxed making the lens more convex (Fig. 19.4b).
- Human vision is coloured, binocular and three dimensional. Normally, right and left eyes are focused on one object (Fig. 19.5a). In squinting, fixing eye (F) focuses on the object, but the squinting eye (S) is 'turned inwards' resulting in a convergent squint (Fig. 19.5b).

## INNER COAT/RETINA

1. This is the thin, delicate innermost layer of the eyeball. It is continuous posteriorly with the optic nerve. The outer surface of the retina (formed by pigment cells) is attached to the choroid, while the inner surface is in

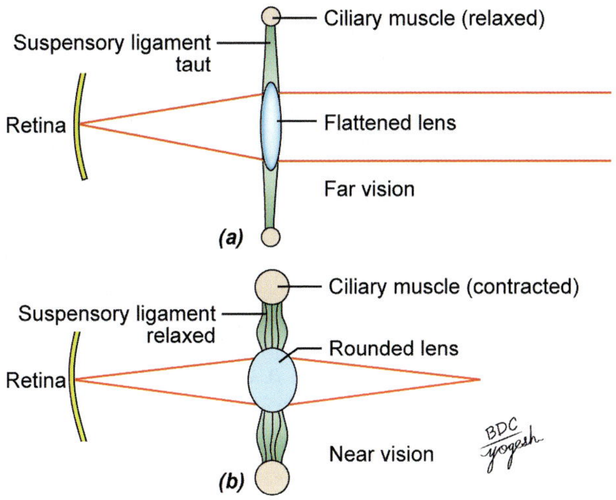


**Figs 19.4a and b:** (a) Relaxed ciliary muscles with flattened lens and (b) contracted ciliary muscles with round lens

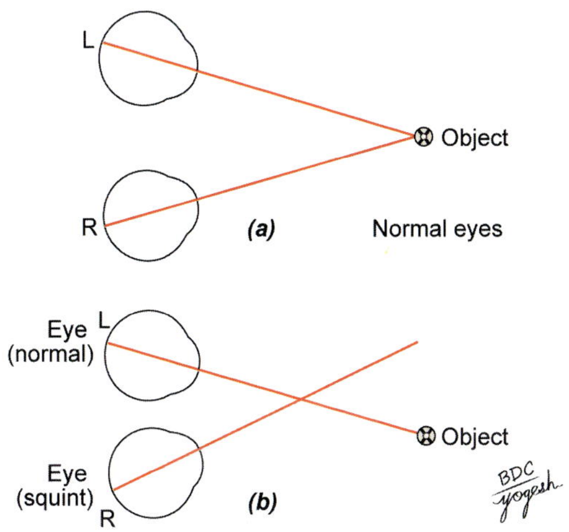


**Figs 19.5a and b:** (a) Normal eyes and (b) in squinting eyes

contact with the hyaloid membrane (of the vitreous). Opposite the entrance of the optic nerve (inferomedial to the posterior pole), there is a circular area known as the ***optic disc***. It is 1.5 mm in diameter.

2. The retina diminishes in thickness from behind forwards and is divided into optic, ciliary and iridial parts. The ***optic part of the retina*** contains nervous tissue and is sensitive to light. It extends from the optic disc to the posterior end of the ciliary body. The anterior margin of the optic part of the retina forms a wavy line called the **ora serrata**.
3. Beyond the ora serrata, the retina is continued forwards as a thin, non-nervous insensitive layer that covers the ciliary body and iris, forming the ***ciliary and iridial parts of the retina***. These parts are made up of two layers of epithelial cells.
4. The depressed area of the optic disc is called the ***physiological cup***. It contains no rods or cones and is, therefore, insensitive to light, i.e. it is the ***physiological blind spot***. At the posterior pole of the eye 3 mm lateral to the optic disc, there is another depression of similar size, called the ***macula lutea***. It is avascular and yellow in colour. The centre of the macula is further depressed to form the ***fovea centralis***. This is the thinnest part of the retina. It contains cones only, and is the site of maximum acuity of vision.
5. The rods and cones are the light receptors of the eye.

   *Note*: The *rods* contain a pigment called ***visual purple***. They can respond to dim light (*scotopic vision*). The periphery of the retina contains only rods, but the fovea has none at all. The *cones* respond only to bright light (*photopic vision*) and are sensitive to colour. The fovea centralis has only cones. Their number diminishes towards the periphery of the retina.

6. The retina is composed of ten layers (Plate 19.3):
   i. Retinal pigmented epithelium (RPE)
   ii. Layer of rods and cones
   iii. Outer limiting membrane
   iv. Outer nuclear layer
   v. Outer/external plexiform layer
   vi. Inner nuclear layer
   vii. Inner plexiform layer
   viii. Ganglion cell layer
   ix. Layer of optic nerve fibers
   x. Inner limiting membrane.
7. ***Blood supply***: The retina is supplied by the ***central artery***. This is an end artery. In the optic disc, it divides into an upper and a lower branch, each giving off nasal and temporal branches. The artery supplies the deeper layers of the retina up to the bipolar cells. The rods and cones are supplied by diffusion from the capillaries of the choroid. The retinal veins run with the arteries (Fig. 19.6).

***Competency:***

**AN43.2** Identify, describe and draw the microanatomy of pituitary gland, thyroid, parathyroid gland, tongue, salivary glands, tonsil, epiglottis, cornea, retina.

Microanatomy of retina is given here. For rest of the topics, please see respective chapters.

## CLINICAL ANATOMY

- ***Retinal detachment*** occurs between outer single pigmented layer and inner nine nervous layers. Actually, it is an inter-retinal detachment. Silicone sponge is put over the detached retina, which is kept in position by a 'band' (Figs 19.7a and b).
- The central artery of retina is an end-artery. Blockage of the artery leads to sudden blindness.

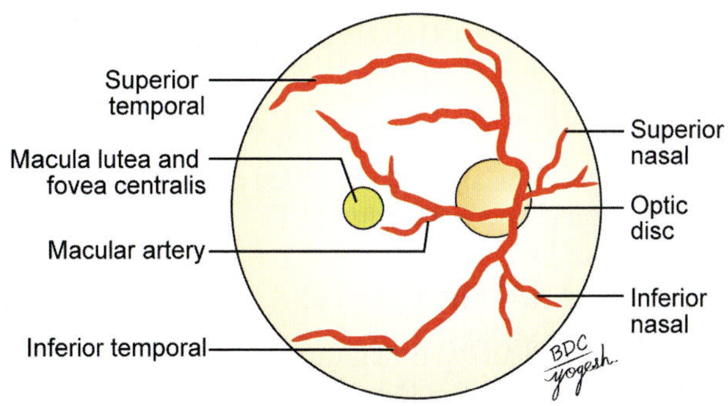


**Fig. 19.6:** Distribution of central artery of the retina

Plate 19.3: Histological layers of the retina

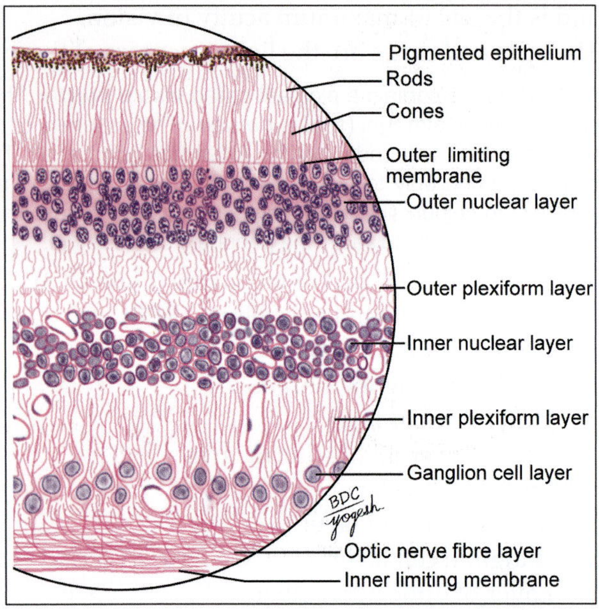


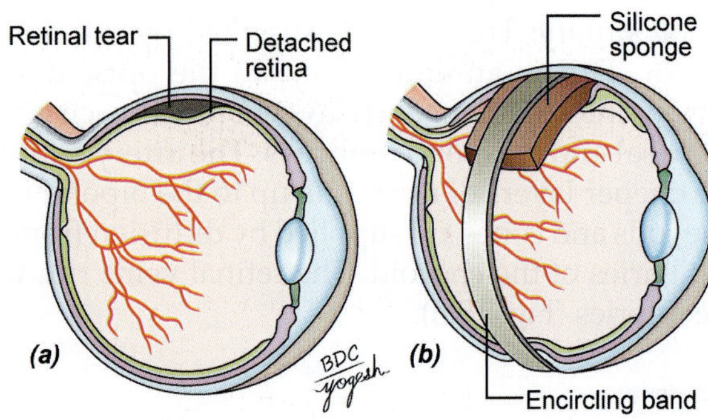


**Figs 19.7a and b:** (a) Detached retina and (b) banding of the retina

## AQUEOUS HUMOUR

1. This is a clear fluid which fills the space between the cornea in front and the lens behind. It is called the anterior segment. This segment is divided by the iris into anterior and posterior chambers which freely communicate with each other through the pupil.
2. The aqueous humour is secreted into the posterior chamber from the capillaries in the ciliary processes. It passes into the anterior chamber through the pupil. From the anterior chamber, it is drained into the anterior ciliary veins through the spaces of the iridocorneal angle or angle of anterior chamber (located between the fibres of the ligamentum pectinatum) and the canal of Schlemm.

***Competency:***
**AN41.2** Describe the anatomical aspects of cataract, glaucoma and central retinal artery occlusion.

### CLINICAL ANATOMY

- Interference with the drainage of the aqueous humour into the canal of Schlemm results in an increase of intraocular pressure (***glaucoma***). This produces cupping of the optic disc and pressure atrophy of the retina causing blindness.
- The intraocular pressure is due chiefly to the aqueous humour which maintain the constancy of the optical dimensions of the eyeball. The aqueous is rich in ascorbic acid, glucose and amino acids, and nourishes the avascular tissues of the cornea and lens.

## LENS

The crystalline lens of eye is a transparent, biconvex, avascular structure. Lens is suspended from ciliary body by zonular fibres (Fig. 19.8). Lens lies between aqueous humour and vitreous humour.

### Structure

The lens has the following three components:

1. **Lens capsule:** It capsule is a transparent homogenous basal lamina of lens epithelium. The capsule consists of type IV collagen fibres and glycoproteins. It is produced by lens epithelium.
2. **Lens epithelium:** Deep to capsule, anterior surface of lens is covered by a layer of *cuboidal epithelium*. This is also called *anterior lens epithelium* or subcapsular epithelium. Towards periphery, cells of epithelium become progressively longer and ultimately get converted into long fibres that form substance of the lens.
3. **Lens fibres (lens fibre cells):** The lens epithelium develops to form lens fibres. These are composed of soluble proteins called *crystallins*.

*Note*:

- The lens is circular in outline and has a diameter of 1 cm. The central points of the anterior and posterior surfaces are called the anterior and posterior *poles* (Fig. 19.8). The line connecting the poles constitutes the *axis* of the lens, while the marginal circumference is termed the *equator.* The chief advantage of the lens is that it can vary its dioptric power. It contributes about 15 dioptres to the total of 58 dioptric power of the eye.
- A dioptre is the inverse of the focal length in meters. A lens having a focal length of half meter has a power of two dioptres.
- The posterior surface of the lens is more convex than the anterior. The anterior surface is kept flattened by the tension of the suspensory ligament. When the ligament is relaxed by contraction of the ciliary muscle, the anterior surface becomes more convex due to elasticity of the lens substance.
- The *suspensory ligament of the lens* (or the zonule of Zinn) retains the lens in position and its tension keeps the anterior surface of the lens flattened. The ligament is made up of a series of fibres which are attached peripherally to the ciliary processes, to the furrows between the ciliary processes, and to the ora serrata. Centrally, the fibres are attached to the lens, mostly in front, and a few behind the equator (Fig. 19.5).

### DISSECTION

Give an incision in the anterior surface of lens and with a little pressure of fingers and thumb press the body of lens outside from the capsule.

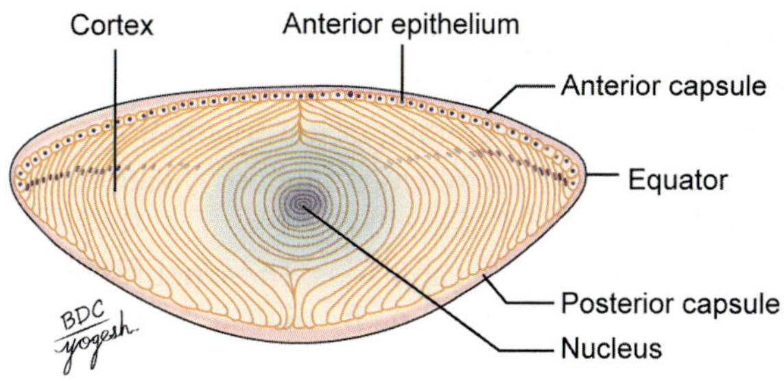


**Fig. 19.8:** The lens

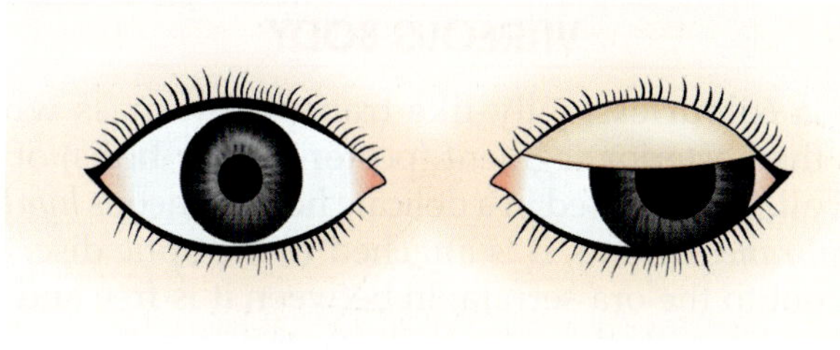

**Fig. 19.9:** Left third nerve paralysis

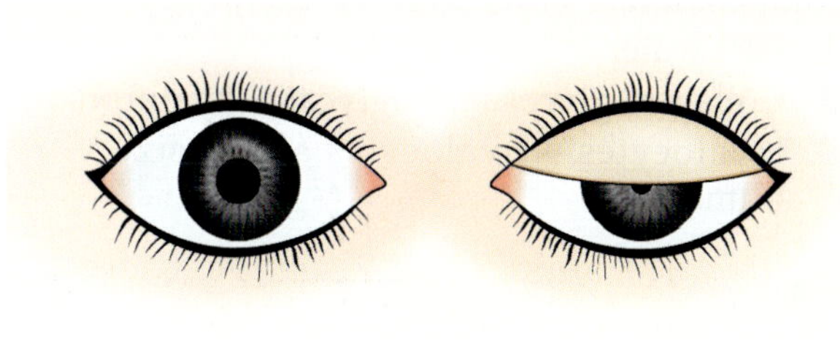

**Fig. 19.10:** Horner's syndrome in left eye

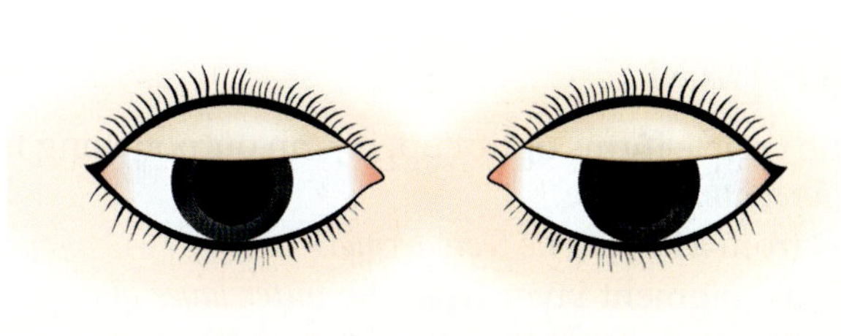

**Fig. 19.11:** Brainstem death

*Competency:*

**AN41.2** Describe the anatomical aspects of cataract, glaucoma and central retinal artery occlusion.

## CLINICAL ANATOMY

- Lens becomes opaque with increasing age (***cataract***). Since the opacities cause difficulty in vision, lens has to be replaced.
- ***Presbyopia:*** With increasing age, crystalline lens loses its elasticity and power of accommodation for near vision (reading). These changes are more evident by the age of 40 to 45 years and the condition is called presbyopia. It can be corrected with convex lens.
- Left third nerve paralysis causes partial ptosis and dilated pupil. The cornea is turned downwards and outwards (Fig. 19.9).
- Horner's syndrome results in partial ptosis and miosis (Fig. 19.10).
- In brainstem death, both the pupils are dilated and fixed (Fig. 19.11).
- ***Fundoscopy*** (*fundoscopic examination*): It is a visualization of the retina and the interior of the eyeball using an *ophthalmoscope*. It is useful for examination of the posterior region of retina (fundus).

  Structures visualized (Figs 19.12a and b):
  - *Macula lutea*: It is a pale yellowish area near the posterior pole. It is approximately 4 mm in diameter.
  - *Fovea*: It is a small pit (1.5 mm in diameter) in centre of macula lutea. It is called fovea centralis, which is the point where light is normally focused.
  - The fovea is the portion of retina with maximum concentration of cone receptors, hence the site of the greatest visual acuity.
  - *Optic disc* (1.5 mm in diameter): It is a white spot about 3 mm medial to the macula. The nerve fibres from retina converge and pass through the optic disc of the eyeball to form the optic nerve. The blood vessels of retina also pass through the optic disc.
  - *Central artery of the retina*: It enters the eye through the centre of the optic disc. It divides into superior and inferior branches. Each of them further divides into temporal and nasal branches.

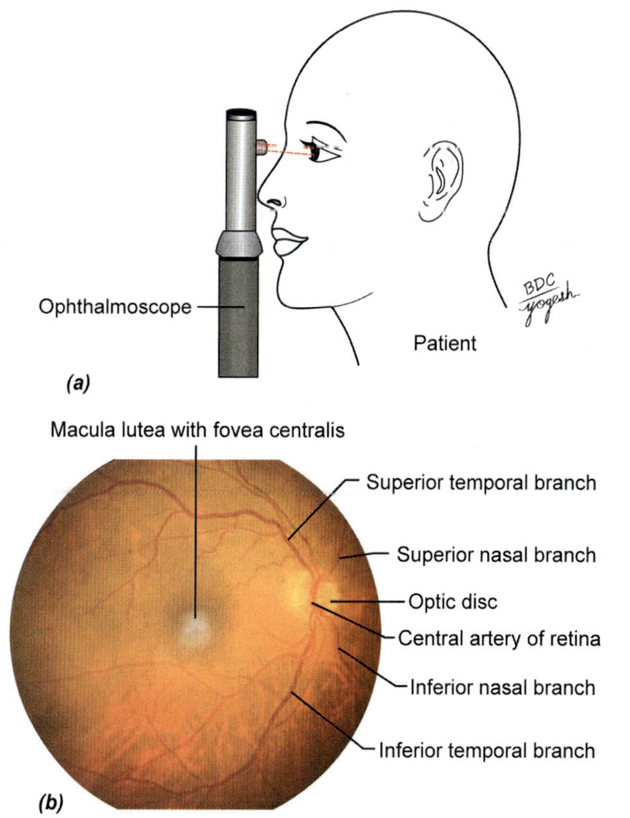


**Figs 19.12a and b:** (a) Procedure for ophthalmoscopy and (b) retina as seen by ophthalmoscope (*Image courtesy*: Dr Rohit Rao)

## VITREOUS BODY

It is a colourless, jelly-like transparent mass which fills the posterior segment (posterior four-fifths) of the eyeball. It is enclosed in a delicate homogeneous ***hyaloid membrane***. Behind, it is attached to the optic disc, and in front to the ora serrata; in between it is free and lies in contact with the retina. The anterior surface of the vitreous body membrane is indented by the ciliary processes to form ciliary zonule.

Composition of vitreous body:

1. 99% water
2. Collagen, glycosaminoglycans (hyaluronan)
3. Hyalocytes – hyalocytes synthesize vitreous humour.

*Competency:*

**AN43.4** Describe the development and developmental basis of congenital anomalies of face, palate, tongue, branchial apparatus, pituitary gland, thyroid gland and eye.

## DEVELOPMENT

Optic vesicle forms optic cup. It is an outpouching from the *forebrain* vesicle.

Lens from *lens placode (ectodermal)*

Retina—pigment layer from the *outer layer of optic cup;* nervous layers from the *inner layer of optic cup.*

Choroid, sclera—*mesoderm*

Cornea—*surface ectoderm forms the epithelium, other layers develop from mesoderm.*

VIDEO

**Video 3.19 Eyeball**

### *Facts to Remember*

- Cornea is used for grafting or transplantation.
- Tenon's capsule is a thin membranous sheath enclosing the eyeball
- Choroid contains big capillaries. These nourish the layer of rods and cones of retina by diffusion.
- Ciliary body contains ciliary muscles supplied by short ciliary nerves. These contract to relax the suspensory ligament of lens, so that the anterior surface of lens can become more convex for accommodation.
- Iris contains a weak dilator pupillae at the periphery, supplied by sympathetic fibres. It also contains a strong constrictor or sphincter pupillae near the pupillary margin. This is supplied by parasympathetic fibres relayed through ciliary ganglion.
- Uvea (vascular coat) = choroid + ciliary body + iris.
- Canal of Schlemm is a circular vascular channel within sclera just behind the corneoscleral junction.
- Lamina cribrosa is the weakest site of sclera.
- Central artery of retina is an 'end artery'.
- Optic disc is the blind spot of the retina.
- Fundoscopy is a visualisation of the retina and the interior of the eyeball using an ophthalmoscope.

### BDC's Anatomy *e*-book

1. Structures piercing the eyeball seen in a sagittal section
2. Differences between rod and cone cells
3. Molecular regulation of eye development
4. Further reading
5. Viva voce questions

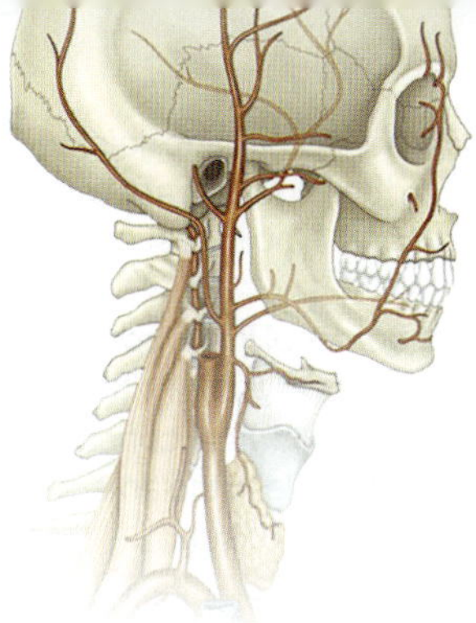

Chapter

20

# Surface Marking and Radiological Anatomy

***Competency:***

**AN43.5** Demonstrate: (1) Testing of muscles of facial expression, extraocular muscles, muscles of mastication, (2) Palpation of carotid arteries, facial artery, superficial temporal artery, (3) Location of internal and external jugular veins, (4) Location of hyoid bone, thyroid cartilage and cricoid cartilage with their vertebral levels.

*Surface anatomy* is the study of outline of organs and important internal structures on the surface of body. The surface anatomy or ***living surface anatomy*** of head, neck and face is very essential in clinical practice. It is a useful guide for visual inspection, palpation (feeling of internal structures through skin), for determination of size, consistency, and borders of structures (such as parotid gland, lymph nodes, and so on), and surgical procedures. These landmarks include bony and soft tissue landmarks.

## SURFACE LANDMARKS

1. *Supraorbital margin* lies beneath the upper margin of the eyebrow.
2. *Supraorbital notch* is palpable at the junction of the medial 1/3rd with the lateral 2/3rd of the supraorbital margin, except in those cases in which the notch is converted into a foramen.
3. *Superciliary arch* is a curved bony ridge situated immediately above the medial part of each supraorbital margin.
4. *Glabella* is the median elevation connecting the two superciliary arches and corresponds to the elevation between the two eyebrows.
5. *Nasion* is the point where the internasal and frontonasal sutures meet. It lies a little above the floor of the depression at the root of the nose, below the glabella.
6. *Chin* is an anterior median area just above the centre of the lower border of mandible.
7. *Lower border or base of the mandible* demarcates face from neck.
8. *Body of the U-shaped hyoid bone* can be felt in the median plane just below and behind the chin, at the junction of the neck with the floor of the mouth. On each side, the body of hyoid bone is continuous posteriorly with the *greater cornua* which is overlapped in its posterior part by the sternocleidomastoid muscle.
9. *Thyroid cartilage of the larynx* forms a sharp protuberance in the median plane just below the hyoid bone. This protuberance is called the *laryngeal prominence or Adam's apple.* It is more prominent in males than in females.
10. *Suprasternal notch* is present above the upper border of manubrium sterni in between the medial ends of clavicle. It lies at the level of lower border of T2 vertebra.
11. *Trachea* is commonly palpated in the *suprasternal notch.* In certain diseases, the trachea may shift to one side from the median plane. This indicates a shift in the mediastinum.
12. *Sternocleidomastoid muscle* becomes prominent when the face is turned to the opposite side.
13. *Lesser supraclavicular fossa* is a small triangular depression above the medial end of the clavicle between the sternal and clavicular heads of sternocleidomastoid muscle. The internal jugular vein lies deep to this fossa.
14. *Greater supraclavicular fossa* is a depression above the middle one-third of the clavicle. The cervical part of brachial plexus and the third part of the subclavian artery are situated deep to this fossa.
15. *External ear* or *pinna* is a prominent feature of the lateral aspect of the head (for details, *see* Chapter 18).
16. *Zygomatic bone* is a prominent bar at the inferolateral corner of the orbit. The *zygomatic arch* bridges the gap between the eye and the ear.
17. *Preauricular point* lies on the posterior root of the zygoma immediately in front of the upper part of the tragus.
18. *Head of the mandible* can be felt in front of the tragus, during movements of the lower jaw.
19. *Ramus of the mandible* can be felt through the skin. The outer surface of the ramus is covered by the masseter which becomes prominent when the teeth are clenched. The lower border of the mandible can be traced posteriorly into the *angle* of the mandible.

20. *Parietal eminence* is the most prominent part of the parietal bone, situated far above and a little behind the auricle.
21. *Mastoid process* is a large bony prominence situated behind the lower part of the auricle.
22. *Supramastoid crest* is about 2.5 cm long, begins immediately above the external acoustic meatus and soon curves upward and backward.
23. *Temporal line*: The upper margin of the contracted temporalis muscle demarcates the temporal line. This line extends from the zygomatic process of the frontal bone, arches posterosuperiorly across the coronal suture, passes a little below the parietal eminence, and turns downward to become continuous with the supramastoid crest. The area of the temporal fossa on the side of the head, above the zygomatic arch, is called the *temple* or temporal region.
24. *Pterion*: It is the area in the temporal fossa. It is the meeting point of four bones: Frontal, parietal, temporal and sphenoid. It is a H-shaped suture. *Surface marking*: The centre of the pterion is marked by a point 4 cm above the midpoint of the zygomatic arch, falling 3.5 cm behind the frontozygomatic suture.

    *Note*: Deep to the pterion lie the anterior branch of the middle meningeal artery, the middle meningeal vein, and deeper still the stem of the lateral sulcus of the cerebral hemisphere (at the Sylvian point) dividing into three rami. The pterion is a common site for trephining (making a hole in the skull) during operation.
25. *External occipital protuberance* is a median bony prominence at the junction of the back of the head with the neck.
26. *Superior nuchal lines* are indistinct curved ridges which extend from the external occipital protuberance to the mastoid processes.
27. *Inion* is the most prominent median point situated on the external occipital protuberance.
28. *Transverse process of the atlas vertebra* can be felt on deep pressure midway between the angle of the mandible and the mastoid process, immediately anteroinferior to the tip of the mastoid process.
29. The *4th cervical transverse process* is just palpable at the level of the upper border of the thyroid cartilage; and the *6th cervical transverse process* at the level of the cricoid cartilage.
30. The anterior tubercle of the *transverse process of the 6th cervical vertebra* is the largest of all such processes and is called the *carotid tubercle* (of Chassaignac). The common carotid artery can be best pressed against this tubercle, deep to the anterior border of the sternocleidomastoid muscle.

*Note*:

***Other important landmarks***

- *Frontozygomatic suture* can be felt as a slight depression in the upper part of the lateral orbital margin.
- *Marginal tubercle* lies a short distance below the frontozygomatic suture along the posterior border of the frontal process of the zygomatic bone.
- *Frankfurt's plane* is represented by a horizontal line joining the infraorbital margin to the centre of the external acoustic meatus. Posteriorly, the line passes through a point just below the external occipital protuberance.
- *Jugal point* is the anterior end of the upper border of the zygomatic arch where it meets the frontal process of the zygomatic bone.
- *Mandibular notch* is represented by a curved line concave upwards, extending from the head of the mandible to the anterior end of the zygomatic arch. The notch is 1–2 cm deep.

***Competency:***

**AN43.6** Demonstrate surface projection of: Thyroid gland, parotid gland and duct, pterion, common carotid artery, internal jugular vein, subclavian vein, external jugular vein, facial artery in the face and accessory nerve.

## SURFACE MARKING OF VARIOUS STRUCTURES

### ARTERIES

#### Facial Artery

It is marked on the face by joining these three points (Fig. 20.1):

- Point 1: On the base of the mandible at the anterior border of the masseter muscle.
- Point 2: 1.2 cm lateral to the angle of the mouth.
- Point 3: At the medial angle of the eye.

The artery is tortuous in its course and is more so between the first two points (Fig. 20.1).

#### Common Carotid Artery

It is marked by a broadline along the anterior border of the sternocleidomastoid muscle by joining the following two points (Fig. 20.2):

- Point 1: On the sternoclavicular joint.
- Point 2: On the anterior border of the sternocleidomastoid muscle at the level of upper border of the thyroid cartilage (Fig. 20.2).

The thoracic part of the left common carotid artery is marked by a broadline extending from a point a little to the left of the centre of the manubrium to the left sternoclavicular joint.

#### Internal Carotid Artery

It is marked by a broadline joining these two points (Fig. 20.2).

- Point 2: On the anterior border of the sternocleidomastoid muscle at the level of the upper border of the thyroid cartilage.
- Point 3: On the posterior border of the condyle of the mandible.

#### External Carotid Artery

The artery is marked by joining these two points (Fig. 20.3).

- Point 2: On the anterior border of the sternocleidomastoid muscle at the level of the upper border of the thyroid cartilage.
- Point 4: On the posterior border of the neck of the mandible.

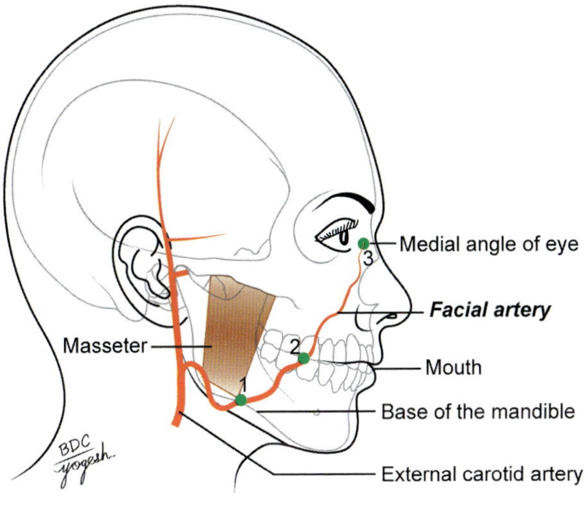


Fig. 20.1: Facial artery

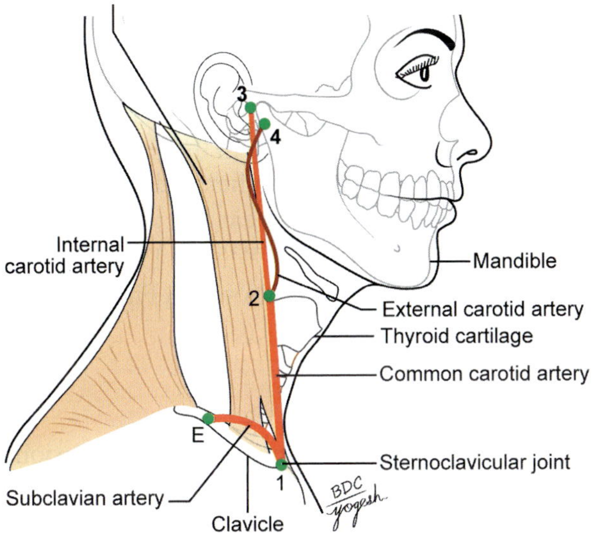


Fig. 20.2: Surface marking of common, external and internal carotid arteries

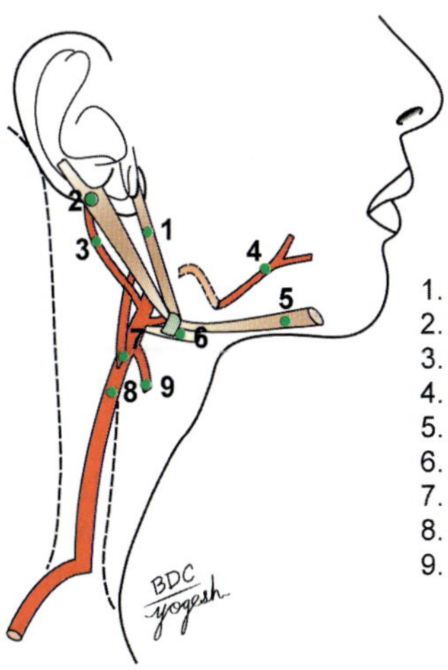


Fig. 20.3: Some branches of external carotid artery

The artery is slightly convex forwards in its lower half and slightly concave forwards in its upper half.

Branches of external carotid artery are shown in Fig. 20.3.

## Subclavian Artery

It is marked by a broad curved line, convex upwards, by joining these two points (Fig. 20.2).

- Point 1: On the sternoclavicular joint.
- Point 5: At the middle of the lower border of the clavicle.

The artery rises about 2 cm above the clavicle.

The thoracic part of the left subclavian artery is marked by a broad vertical line along the left border of the manubrium a little to the left of the left common carotid artery.

## Middle Meningeal Artery

It is marked by joining these points (Fig. 20.4):

- Point 1: Immediately above the middle of the zygoma. The artery enters the skull opposite this point.
- Point 2: 3 cm above the first point. The artery divides deep to this point.
- Point 3: At the centre of pterion, that is, 3.5 cm behind and 1.5 cm above the frontozygomatic suture.
- Point 4: Midway between the nasion and inion.
- Point 5: At the superior attachment of auricle.
- Point 6: At lambda, that is, 6 cm above the external occipital protuberance.

The line joining points 1 and 2 represents the stem of the middle meningeal artery inside the skull.

The line joining points 2, 3 and 4 represents the anterior (frontal) branch. It first runs upwards and forwards and then upwards and backwards, towards the point 4.

The line joining points 2, 5 and 6 represents the posterior (parietal) branch. It runs backwards and upwards, towards the point 5.

# VEINS/SINUSES

## External Jugular Vein

The vein is usually visible through the skin and can be made more prominent by blowing with the mouth and nostrils closed (Fig. 20.5).

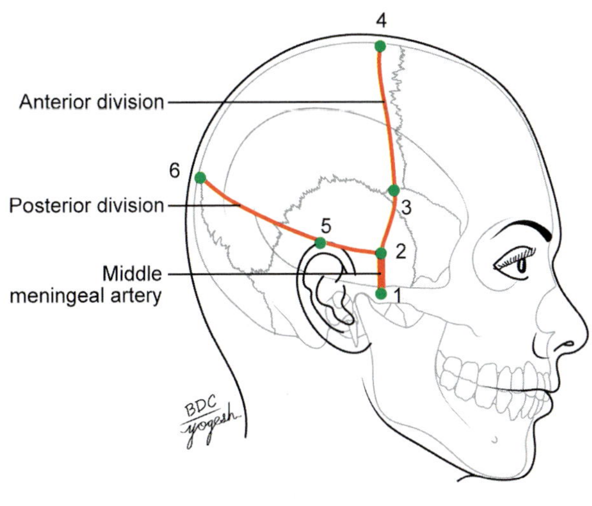


Fig. 20.4: Surface marking of middle meningeal artery

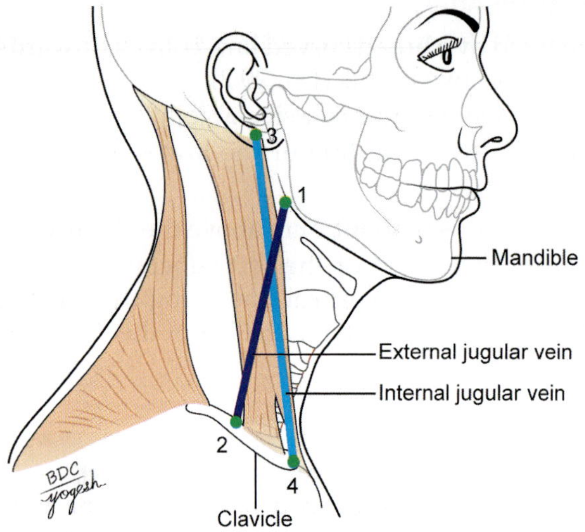


Fig. 20.5: Surface marking of internal and external jugular veins

It can be marked, if not visible, by joining these points:

- Point 1: A little below and behind the angle of the mandible.
- Point 2: On the clavicle just lateral to the posterior border of the sternocleidomastoid.

### Internal Jugular Vein

Internal jugular vein is marked by a broadline by joining these two points (Fig. 20.5):

- Point 3: On the neck medial to the lobule of the ear.
- Point 4: At the medial end of the clavicle (Fig. 20.5).

The lower bulb of the vein lies beneath the lesser supraclavicular fossa between the sternal and clavicular heads of the sternocleidomastoid muscle.

### Subclavian Vein

Subclavian vein is represented by a broadline along the clavicle extending from a little medial to its midpoint to the medial end of the bone (Fig. 20.2).

### Superior Sagittal Sinus

Superior sagittal sinus is marked by two lines (diverging posteriorly) joining these two points (Fig. 20.6):

- Point A: At the glabella.
- Point B: At the inion, two dots situated side-by-side, 1.2 cm apart (Fig. 20.6).

### Transverse Sinus

Transverse sinus is marked by two parallel lines, 1.2 cm apart extending between the following points (Fig. 20.6):

- Point B: Two dots, at the inion, situated one above the other and 1.2 cm apart.
- Point C: Two dots, at asterion 3.75 cm behind external auditory meatus and 1.25 cm above this point (Fig. 20.6).
- Point D: Two dots, at the base of the mastoid process, situated one in front of the other and 1.2 cm apart.

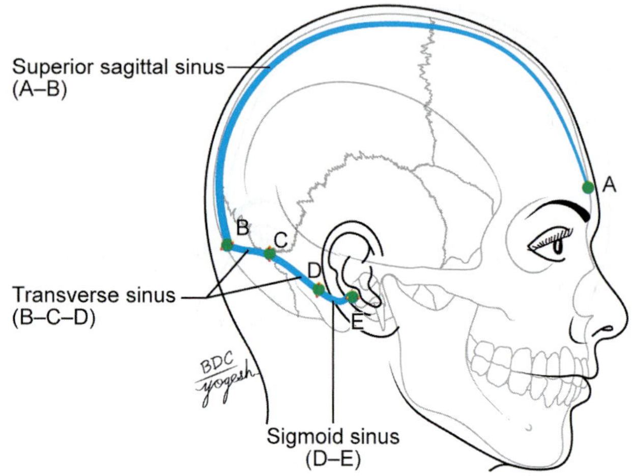


Fig. 20.6: Surface marking of superior, transverse, and sigmoid sinuses

### Sigmoid Sinus

Sigmoid sinus is marked by two parallel lines situated 1.2 cm apart and extending between the following two points (Fig. 20.6):

- Point D: Two dots, at the base of the mastoid process, situated one in front of the other and 1.2 cm apart.
- Point E: Two similar dots, near the posterior border and 1.2 cm above the tip of mastoid process.

Veins of face and neck are shown in Fig. 20.7.

## NERVES

### Facial Nerve

Facial nerve is marked by a short horizontal line joining the following two points (Fig. 20.8):

- Point 1: At the middle of the anterior border of the mastoid process. The stylomastoid foramen lies 2 cm deep to this point.
- Point 2: Behind the neck of mandible. Here the nerve divides into its five branches to the facial muscles (Fig. 20.8).

### Mandibular Nerve

Mandibular nerve (point 1 to point 2) is marked by a short vertical line (2 cm) in the posterior part of the mandibular notch just in front of the head of the mandible (Fig. 20.9).

### Auriculotemporal Nerve

Auriculotemporal nerve is marked by a line drawn first backwards from the posterior part of the mandibular notch (point 2) (site of mandibular nerve) across the neck of the mandible, and then upwards across the preauricular point 3 (Fig. 20.9).

### Lingual and Inferior Alveolar Nerves

Lingual nerve is marked by a curved line running downwards and forwards by joining these points (Fig. 20.9):

- Point 2: On the posterior part of the mandibular notch, in line with the mandibular nerve.

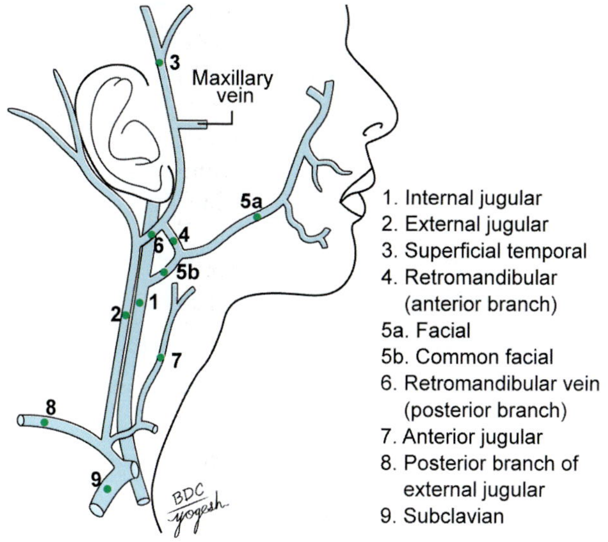


**Fig. 20.7:** Veins of the face and neck

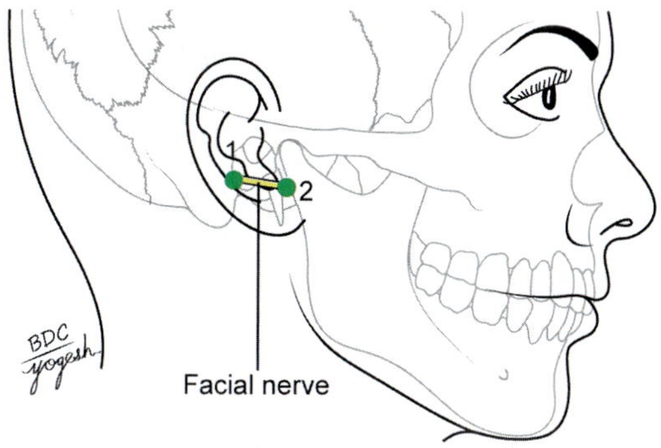


**Fig. 20.8:** Surface marking of facial nerve

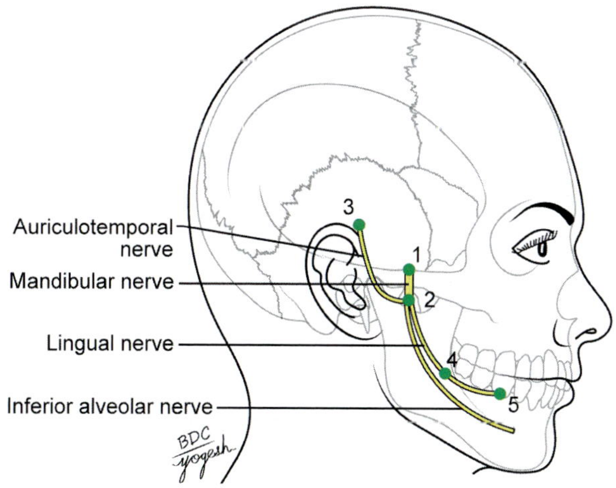


**Fig. 20.9:** Surface marking of mandibular, auriculotemporal, lingual and inferior alveolar nerves

- Point 4: A little below and behind the last lower molar tooth.
- Point 5: Opposite the first lower molar tooth.

The concavity in the course of the nerve is more marked between the 4 and 5 points and is directed upwards.

Inferior alveolar nerve lies a little below and parallel to the lingual nerve.

### Glossopharyngeal Nerve

Glossopharyngeal nerve is marked by joining the following points (Fig. 20.10):

- Point A: On the anteroinferior part of the tragus.
- Point B: Anterosuperior to the angle of the mandible.

From point B, the nerve runs forwards for a short distance above the lower border of the mandible.

The nerve describes a gentle curve in its course (Fig. 20.10).

### Vagus Nerve

The nerve runs along the medial side of the internal jugular vagus vein. It is marked by joining these two points (Fig. 20.10):

- Point A: At the anteroinferior part of the tragus.
- Point C: At the medial end of the clavicle (Fig. 20.10).

### Accessory Nerve (Spinal Part)

Accessory nerve (spinal part) is marked by joining the following four points (Fig. 20.10):

- Point A: At the anteroinferior part of the tragus.
- Point D: At the tip of the transverse process of the atlas.
- Point E: At the middle of the posterior border of the sternocleidomastoid muscle.
- Point F: On the anterior border of the trapezius 6 cm above the clavicle.

### Hypoglossal Nerve

Hypoglossal nerve is marked by joining these points (Fig. 20.10):

- Point A, at the anteroinferior part of the tragus.
- Point G, posterosuperior to the tip of the greater cornua of the hyoid bone.
- Point H, midway between the angle of the mandible and the symphysis menti.

The nerve describes a gentle curve in its course.

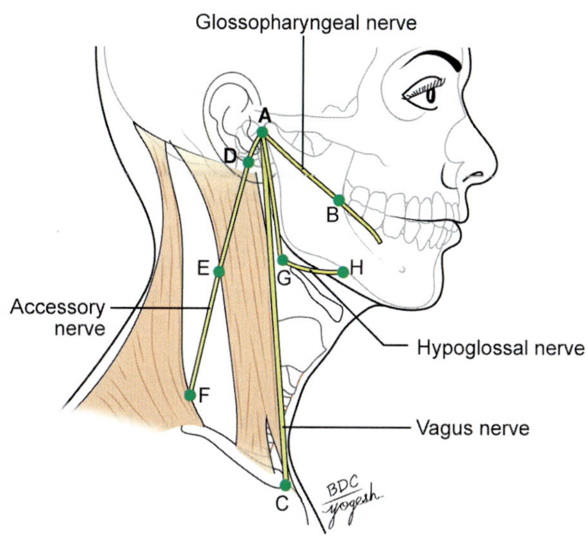


**Fig. 20.10:** Position of last four cranial nerves

### Phrenic Nerve

Phrenic nerve is marked by a line joining the following points (Fig. 20.11):

- Point A: On the side of the neck at the level of the upper border of the thyroid cartilage and 3.5 cm from the median plane.
- Point B: At the medial end of the clavicle (Fig. 20.11).

### Cervical Sympathetic Chain

Cervical sympathetic chain is marked by a line joining the following points (Fig. 20.11):

- Point C: At the sternoclavicular joint.
- Point D: At the posterior border of the condyle of the mandible.

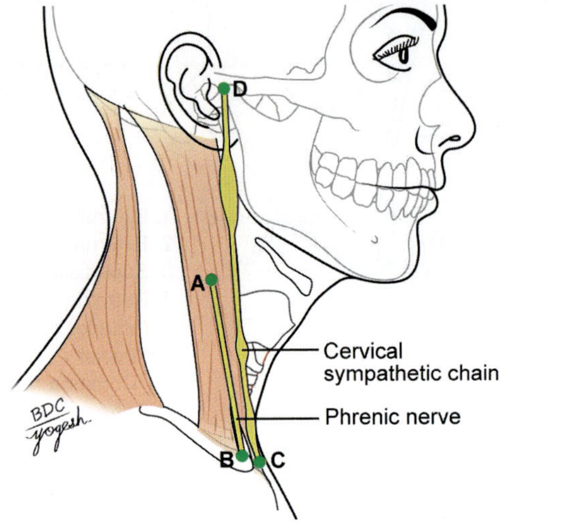


**Fig. 20.11:** Position of phrenic nerve and sympathetic trunk

## GLANDS

### Parotid Gland

Parotid gland is marked by joining these four points with each other (Fig. 20.12):

- Point A: At the upper border of the head of the mandible.
- Point B: Just above the centre of the masseter muscle.
- Point C: At the posteroinferior to the angle of the mandible.
- Point D: On the upper part of the anterior border of the mastoid process.

The anterior border of the gland is obtained by joining the points A, B, C; the posterior border, by joining the points C, D; and the superior curved border with its concavity directed upwards and backwards, by joining the points A, D across the lobule of the ear (Fig. 20.12).

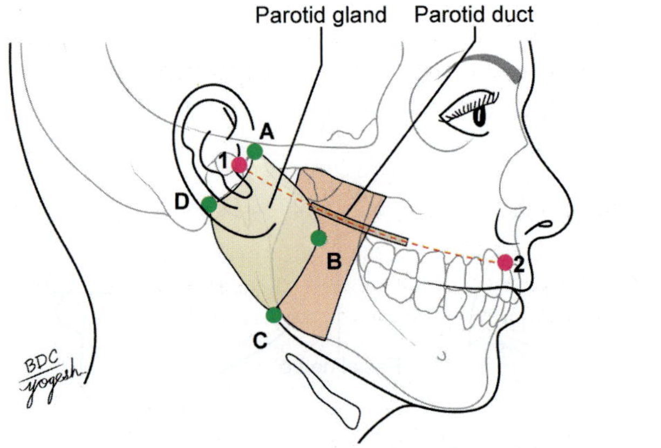


**Fig. 20.12:** Surface marking of parotid gland and parotid duct

### Parotid Duct

To mark this duct, first draw a line joining the following two points (Fig. 20.12):

- Point 1: At the lower border of the tragus.
- Point 2: Midway between the ala of the nose and the red margin of the upper lip.

The middle-third of this line represents the parotid duct (Fig. 20.12).

### Submandibular Gland

The submandibular salivary gland is marked by an oval area joining the following points (Fig. 20.13):

- Point A: A point below the angle of mandible.
- Point B: Midway between the angle of mandible and the symphysis menti.
- Point C: About 1.5 cm above the angle of mandible.
- Point D: Near the posterior end of the tip of the greater cornua of the hyoid bone.

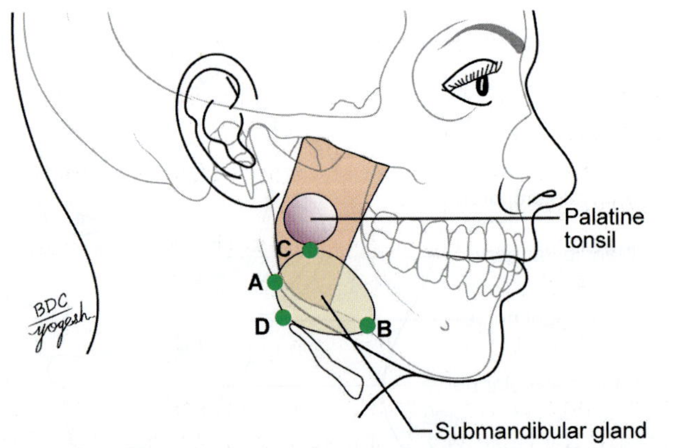


**Fig. 20.13:** Surface marking of submandibular gland and palatine tonsil

### Thyroid Gland

The isthmus of thyroid gland is marked by two transverse parallel lines (each 1.2 cm long) on the trachea, the upper 1.2 cm and the lower 2.5 cm below the arch of the cricoid cartilage.

Each lobe extends up to the middle of the thyroid cartilage, below to the clavicle, and laterally to be overlapped by the anterior border of sternocleidomastoid muscle. The upper pole of the lobe is pointed, and the lower pole is broad and rounded (Fig. 20.14).

### Palatine Tonsil

Palatine tonsil is marked by an oval (almond-shaped) area over the masseter just anterosuperior to the angle of the mandible.

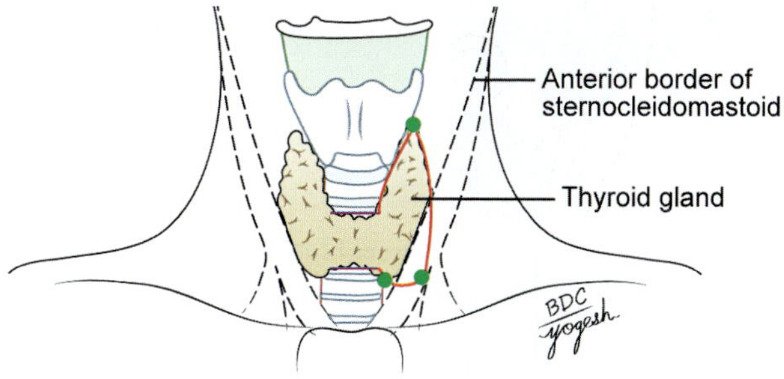


**Fig. 20.14:** Thyroid gland

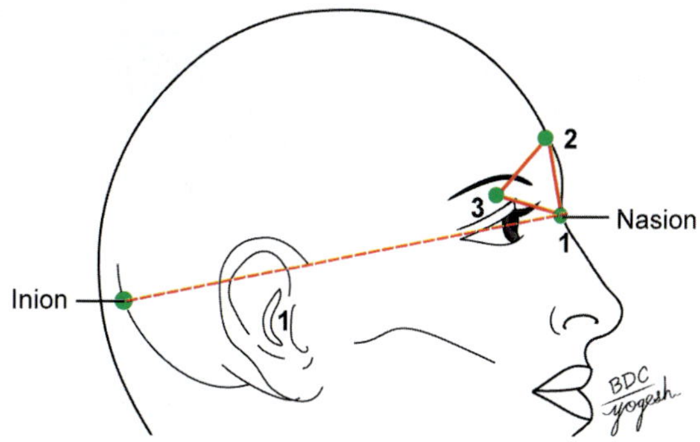


**Fig. 20.15:** Surface marking of frontal air sinus

## PARANASAL SINUSES

### Frontal Sinus

Frontal sinus is marked by a triangular area formed by joining these three points (Fig. 20.15):

- Point 1: At the nasion.
- Point 2: 2.5 cm above the nasion.
- Point 3: At the junction of medial one-third and lateral two-thirds of the supraorbital margin, i.e. at the supraorbital notch.

### Maxillary Sinus

The roof of maxillary sinus is represented by the inferior orbital margin; the floor, by the alveolus of the maxilla; the base, by the lateral wall of the nose. The apex lies on the zygomatic process of the maxilla.

*Competency:*
**AN43.7** Identify the anatomical structures in: (1) Plain X-ray skull; (2) AP view and lateral view, (3) Plain X-ray cervical spine—AP and lateral view, (4) Plain X-ray of paranasal sinuses.

## RADIOLOGICAL ANATOMY

In routine clinical practice, the following X-ray pictures of the skull are commonly used.

1. Lateral view for general survey of the skull including cervical vertebrae.
2. A special posteroanterior view (in Water's position) to study the paranasal sinuses.

## LATERAL VIEW OF SKULL (PLAIN SKIAGRAM)

In the lateral view of skull, one side of the head faces toward the radiographic film and other side to the X-ray tube.

For radiological examination, the skull should be observed for the features of (Fig. 20.16):

1. Cranial vault
2. Base of the skull.

### Cranial Vault

***Shape and size:*** It is important to be familiar with the normal shape and size of the skull so that abnormalities, like oxycephaly (a type of cranio-stenosis), hydrocephalus, microcephaly, etc. may be diagnosed.

***Structure of cranial bones:*** The bones are unilamellar during the first three years of life. Two tables separated by diploe appear during the fourth year, and the differentiation reaches its maximum by about 35 years when diploic veins produce characteristic markings in radiograms. The sites of the external occipital protuberance and frontal bone are normally thicker than the rest of the skull. The squamous temporal and the upper part of the occipital bone are thin.

Generalized thickened bones are found in Paget's disease. Thalassaemia, a congenital haemolytic anaemia, is associated with thickening and a characteristic sunray appearance of the skull bones. A localised hyperostosis may be seen over a meningioma. In multiple myeloma and secondary carcinomatous deposits, the skull presents large punched out areas Fractures are more extensive in the inner table than in the outer table.

***Sutures:*** The coronal and lambdoid sutures are usually visible clearly. The coronal suture runs downwards and forwards in front of the central sulcus of the brain. The lambdoid suture traverses the posteriormost part of the skull.

Obliteration of sutures begins first on the inner surface (between 30 and 40 years) and then on the outer surface (between 40 and 50 years). Usually, the lower part of the coronal suture is obliterated first, followed by the posterior part of the sagittal suture. Premature closure of sutures occurs in craniostenosis, a hereditary disease. Sutures are opened up in children by an increase in intracranial pressure.

***Vascular markings***

a. *Middle meningeal vessels:* The anterior branch runs about 1 cm behind the coronal suture. The posterior branch runs backwards and upwards at a lower level across the upper part of the shadow of the auricle.
b. The *transverse sinus* may be seen as a curved dark shadow, convex upwards, extending from the internal occipital protuberance to the petrous temporal.
c. The *diploic venous markings* are seen as irregularly anastomosing, worm-like shadows produced by the frontal, anterior temporal, posterior temporal and occipital diploic veins. These markings become more prominent in raised intracranial pressure.

***Cerebral moulding:*** Indicating normal impressions of cerebral gyri, can be seen. In raised intracranial tension,

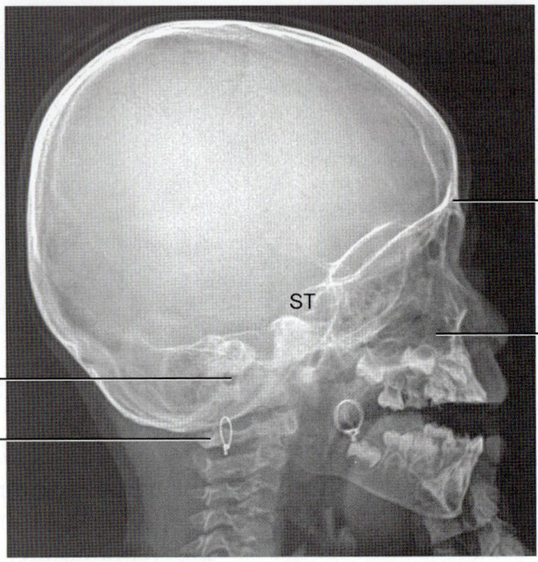


**Fig. 20.16:** Plane radiograph of skull: Lateral view (*Image courtesy*: Dr Janani Baradwaj)

the impressions become more pronounced and produce a characteristic *silver beaten* (or *copper beaten*) *appearance* of the skull.

***Arachnoid granulations:*** They may indent the parasagittal area of the skull to such an extent as to simulate erosion by a meningioma.

### *Normal intracranial calcifications*

a. Pineal concretions (brain sand) appear by the age of 17 years. The pineal body is located 2.5 cm above and 1.2 cm behind the external acoustic meatus. When visible it serves as an important radiological landmark.
b. Other structures which may become calcified include the choroid plexuses, arachnoid granulations, falx cerebri, and other dural folds.

***Auricle:*** The curved margin of the auricle is seen above the petrous temporal.

***Frontal sinus:*** It produces a dark shadow in the antero-inferior part of the skull vault.

### Base of Skull

1. ***Floor of the anterior cranial fossa*** slopes backwards and downwards. The shadows of the two sides are often seen situated one above the other. The surface is irregular due to gyral markings. It also forms the roof of the orbit.
2. ***Hypophyseal fossa*** represents the middle cranial fossa in this view. It is overhung anteriorly by the anterior clinoid process (directed posteriorly), and posteriorly by the posterior clinoid process. It measures 8 mm vertically and 14 mm anteroposteriorly. The interclinoid distance is not more than 4 mm. The fossa is enlarged in cases of pituitary tumours, arising particularly from acidophil or chromophobe cells.
3. ***Sphenoidal air sinus*** lies anteroinferior to the hypophyseal fossa. The shadows of the orbit, the nasal cavities, and the ethmoidal and maxillary sinuses lie superimposed on one another, below the anterior cranial fossa.
4. ***Petrous part of the temporal bone*** produces a dense irregular shadow posteroinferior to the hypophyseal fossa. Within this shadow, there are two dark areas representing the external acoustic meatuses of the two sides; each shadow lies immediately behind the head of the mandible of that side. Similar dark shadows of the internal acoustic meatuses may also be seen. The posterior part of the dense shadow merges with the mastoid air cells producing a honeycomb appearance.
5. In addition to the features mentioned above, the *mandible* lies anteriorly forming the lower part of the facial skeleton. The *upper cervical vertebrae* lie posteriorly and are seen as a pillar supporting the skull.

## ANTEROPOSTERIOR VIEW OF SKULL (PLAIN SKIAGRAM)

The skull anteroposterior (AP) view is a nonangled radiograph of the skull. This view provides an overview of the entire skull. In AP view, the back of patient's head is placed against the X-ray film.

*Advantages of AP view*: It gives overview of skull.

*The disadvantages of AP view* include:

- Overlap of bone makes it harder to evaluate the sinuses.
- Higher exposure of eyes to radiation than PA view.
- Higher magnification of the facial bones compared with the PA view.

### *Radiological features*

The following features can be seen in the plain skiagram of skull in AP view:

1. Structure of cranial bones
2. Sutures: Lambdoid, metopic (if present)
3. Arachnoid granulations
4. Calcifications of pineal body, arachnoid granulations and so on
5. Shadow of auricle

6. Air sinuses: Frontal, other sinuses are overlapped by bones
7. Shadows of orbit and nasal cavities
8. Nasal septum
9. Mandible
10. Denture.

## CERVICAL SPINE – ANTEROPOSTERIOR AND LATERAL VIEWS

The cervical vertebrae can be visualised better in lateral view with extended neck than in AP view.

### *Radiological features of the cervical spine*

The following features of the cervical vertebrae are observed radiologically (Fig. 20.17):

1. Body of cervical vertebrae
2. Intervertebral space (discs)
3. Pedicles
4. Shadow of spines
5. Articular processes – superior and inferior
6. Intervertebral foramen.

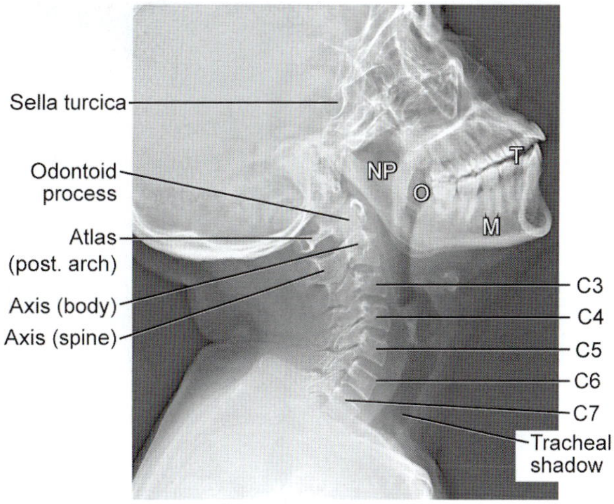


**Fig. 20.17:** Lateral view of plain radiograph of cervical spine in extended neck position (M: Mandible, T: Teeth, O: Air shadow in oropharynx, NP: Air shadow in nasopharynx, *Image courtesy*: Dr Janani Baradwaj)

## WATER'S VIEW FOR PARANASAL SINUSES

The radiography for visualisation of paranasal air sinuses: Water's view is useful for radiological visualization of paranasal air sinuses.

***Procedure:*** It is a special PA view of the skull taken with the head extended in such a way that the chin rests against the film with open mouth and the nose is raised from it (Water's position).

***Features*** (Fig. 20.18)

1. *Frontal sinuses*: These are seen clearly. They are located immediately above the nose and medial parts of the orbits.
2. *Maxillary sinuses*: These are also seen clearly below the orbit, on each side of nasal cavity.
3. Ethmoid and sphenoid sinuses are also visible.
4. *Sinusitis*: If a sinus is infected, the shadow is either hazy or radio-opaque.

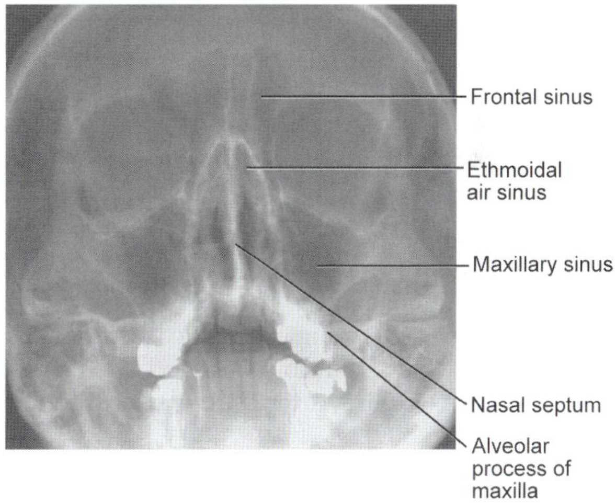


**Fig. 20.18:** X-ray of skull showing paranasal sinuses (Water's view/occipitomental view)

**Competencies:**

**AN43.8** Describe the anatomical route used for carotid angiogram and vertebral angiogram.

**AN43.9** Identify anatomical structures in carotid angiogram and vertebral angiogram.

### Carotid Angiogram

Carotid angiogram lateral view. A radio-opaque dye was injected into the carotid artery just before the radiograph was taken (Fig. 20.19). Internal carotid artery is seen to give an ophthalmic branch and then ends by dividing into a smaller anterior cerebral and a larger middle cerebral arteries.

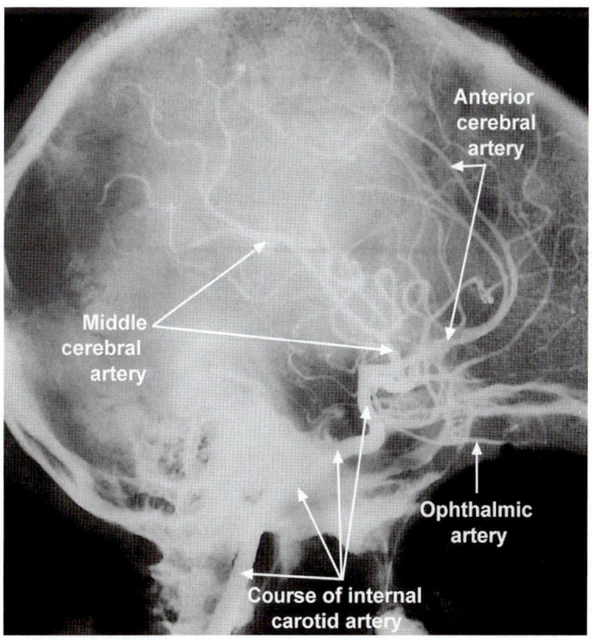


**Fig. 20.19:** Carotid angiogram

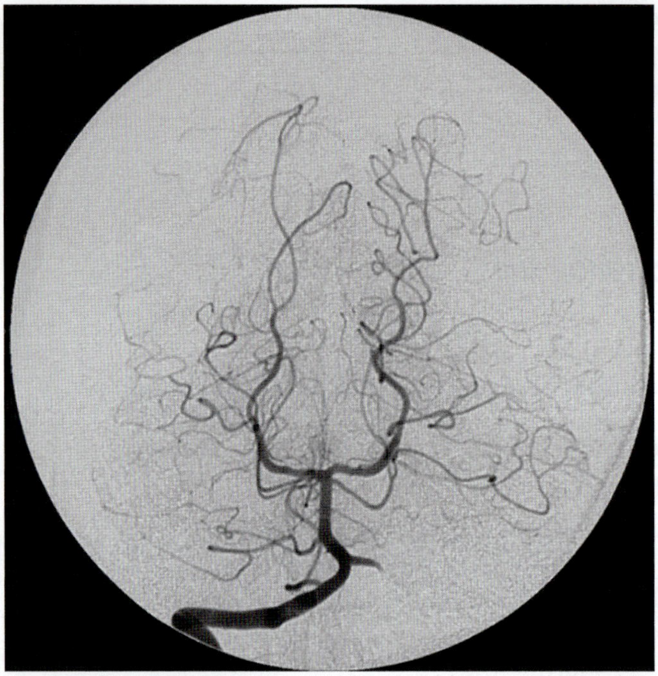

Fig. 20.20: Vertebral angiogram

### Vertebral Angiogram

A vertebral angiogram or vertebral artery angiography is used to visualize the vertebral arteries (Fig. 20.20). For the vertebral angiogram, a contrast dye is injected through the catheter, making the blood vessels visible on X-ray images. X-ray images or fluoroscopy images are captured to assess the flow of blood with injected dye through the vertebral arteries. It is useful to detect abnormalities like blockages, aneurysms, arteriovenous malformations, or other vascular disorders affecting the vertebral arteries.

BDC's Anatomy *e*-book

1. Further reading

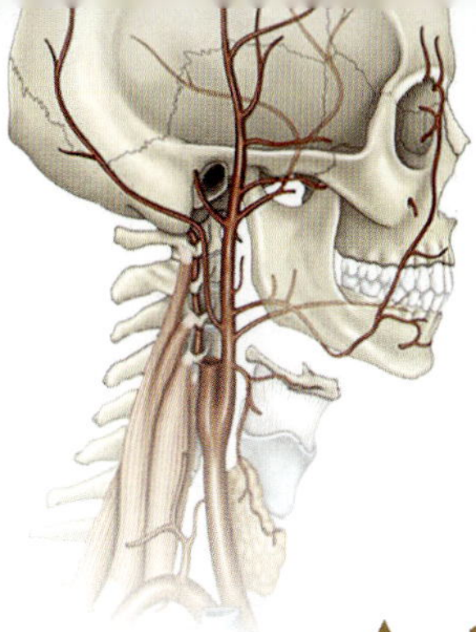

Appendix

# Parasympathetic Ganglia, Arteries and Pharyngeal Arches

## CERVICAL PLEXUS

Ventral rami of C1–C4 form the cervical plexus. C1 runs along hypoglossal and supplies geniohyoid and thyrohyoid. It also gives superior limb of ansa cervicalis, which supplies superior belly of omohyoid and joins with inferior limb to form ansa. Inferior limb of ansa cervicalis is formed by ventral rami of C2, C3. Branches from ansa supply sternohyoid, sternothyroid, and inferior belly of omohyoid. Cervical plexus also gives four cutaneous branches—lesser occipital (C2), great auricular (C2, C3), supraclavicular (C3, C4) and transverse or anterior nerve of neck (C2, C3).

### PHRENIC NERVE

Phrenic nerve arises primarily from ventral rami of C4 with small contributions from C3 and C5 nerve roots or through nerve to subclavius.

It is the only motor supply to its own half of diaphragm and sensory to mediastinal pleura, peritoneum and fibrous pericardium. Inflammation of peritoneum under diaphragm causes referred pain in the area of supraclavicular nerves supply, especially tip of the shoulders as their root value is also ventral rami of C3 and C4 (*see* Fig. 9.11).

## SYMPATHETIC TRUNK

Branches of cervical sympathetic ganglia of sympathetic trunk are given in Table A.1 (For details, *see* Chapter 8).

## PARASYMPATHETIC GANGLIA (Table A.2)

### SUBMANDIBULAR GANGLION

#### Location

The submandibular ganglion lies superficial to hyoglossus muscle in the submandibular region. Functionally, submandibular ganglion is connected to facial nerve, while topographically it is connected to lingual branch of mandibular nerve (*see* Fig. 7.14).

#### Roots

The ganglion has sensory, sympathetic and secretomotor or parasympathetic roots.

1. Sensory root is from the lingual nerve. It is suspended by two roots of lingual nerve.
2. Sympathetic root is from the sympathetic plexus around the facial artery. This plexus contains postganglionic fibres from the superior cervical ganglion of sympathetic trunk. These fibres pass through the ganglion and are vasomotor to the gland.

**TABLE A.1: Branches of cervical sympathetic ganglia**

| | *Superior cervical ganglion* | *Middle cervical ganglion* | *Inferior cervical ganglion* |
|---|---|---|---|
| Arterial branches | i. Along internal carotid artery as internal carotid nerve which gives deep petrosal, nerve to Muller's muscle, to dilator pupillae, to pineal gland<br>ii. Along common carotid and external carotid arteries for all 3 salivary glands | Along inferior thyroid artery | Along subclavian and vertebral arteries |
| Grey rami communicantes | Along 1–4 cervical nerves | Along 5 and 6 cervical nerves | Along 7 and 8 cervical nerves |
| Along cranial nerves | Along cranial nerves IX, X, XI and XII | — | — |
| Visceral branches | Pharynx, cardiac | Thyroid, cardiac | Cardiac |

**TABLE A.2: Connections of parasympathetic ganglia**

[*Note*: The sympathetic fibres arises from T1 spinal segment → Superior cervical ganglion → relay → postganglionic fibres form plexus around arteries]

| *Ganglia* | *Sensory root* | *Sympathetic root* | *Secretomotor root/ parasympathetic root* | *Motor root* | *Distribution* |
|---|---|---|---|---|---|
| Submandibular | Two branches from lingual nerve | Branch from plexus around facial artery | Superior salivatory nucleus → facial nerve → chorda tympani (joins the lingual nerve) → relay in ganglion | — <br> — | a. Submandibular <br> b. Sublingual <br> c. Anterior lingual glands |
| Pterygopalatine | Two branches from maxillary nerve | Deep petrosal from plexus around internal carotid artery | Superior salivatory nucleus, and lacrimatory nucleus → nervus intermedius → facial nerve → geniculate ganglion → greater petrosal nerve + deep petrosal nerve = nerve pterygoid canal | — | a. Mucous glands of nose, paranasal sinuses, palate, nasopharynx <br> b. Some fibres pass through zygomatic nerve → zygomaticotemporal nerve → communicating branch to lacrimal nerve → lacrimal gland and tensor tympani |
| Otic | Branch from auriculotemporal nerve | Plexus along middle meningeal artery | Inferior salivatory nucleus → glossopharyngeal nerve → tympanic branch → nerve tympanic plexus → lesser petrosal nerve. | Branch from nerve to medial pterygoid | a. Secretomotor to parotid gland via auriculotemporal nerve <br> b. Tensor veli palatini via nerve to med. pterygoid (unrelayed) |
| Ciliary | From nasociliary nerve | Plexus along ophthalmic artery | Edinger-Westphal nucleus → oculomotor nerve → nerve to inferior oblique | — | a. Ciliaris muscles <br> b. Sphincter pupillae |

3. Secretomotor root is from superior salivatory nucleus through nervus intermedius via chorda tympani which is a branch of cranial nerve VII. Chorda tympani joins lingual nerve. The parasympathetic fibres get relayed in the submandibular ganglion.

### Branches

The ganglion gives direct branches to the submandibular salivary gland.

Some postganglionic fibres reach the lingual nerve to be distributed to sublingual salivary gland and glands in the oral cavity.

## PTERYGOPALATINE GANGLION

### Location

Pterygopalatine or sphenopalatine is the largest parasympathetic ganglion, suspended by two roots of maxillary nerve. Functionally, it is related to cranial nerve VII. It is called the ganglion of 'hay fever'.

### Roots

The ganglion has sensory, sympathetic and secretomotor or parasympathetic roots.

1. Sensory root is from maxillary nerve. The ganglion is suspended by 2 roots of maxillary nerve.
2. Sympathetic root is from postganglionic plexus around internal carotid artery. The nerve is called deep petrosal. It unites with greater petrosal to form the nerve of pterygoid canal. The fibres of deep petrosal do not relay in the ganglion.
3. Secretomotor or parasympathetic root is from greater petrosal nerve which arises from geniculate ganglion of cranial nerve VII. These fibres relay in the ganglion.

### Branches

The ganglion gives number of branches. These are:

1. *For lacrimal gland:* The postganglionic fibres pass through zygomatic branch of maxillary nerve. These fibres hitch hike through zygomaticotemporal nerve into the communicating branch between zygomaticotemporal and lacrimal nerves, then to the lacrimal nerve for supplying the lacrimal gland.
2. *Nasopalatine nerve:* This nerve runs on the nasal septum and ends in the anterior part of hard palate. It supplies secretomotor fibres to both nasal and palatal glands.
3. *Nasal branches:* These are medial posterior superior branches for the supply of glands and mucous membrane of nasal septum; the largest is named nasopalatine; and lateral posterior superior branches for the supply of glands and mucous membrane of lateral wall of nasal cavity.
4. *Palatine branches:* These are one greater/anterior palatine and 2–3 lesser/posterior palatine branches. These pass through the respective foramina to supply sensory and secretomotor fibres to mucous membrane and glands of soft palate and hard palate.

5. *Orbital branches* for the orbital periosteum.
6. *Pharyngeal branches* for the glands of pharynx.

## OTIC GANGLION

### Location

The otic ganglion lies deep to the trunk of mandibular nerve, between the nerve and the tensor veli palatini muscle in the infratemporal fossa, just distal to the foramen ovale. Topographically, it is connected to mandibular nerve, while functionally it is related to cranial nerve IX.

### Roots

This ganglion has sensory, sympathetic, parasympathetic or secretomotor and motor roots (*see* Fig. 6.21).

1. Sensory root is by the auriculotemporal nerve.
2. Sympathetic root is by the sympathetic plexus around middle meningeal artery.
3. Secretomotor root is by the lesser petrosal nerve from the tympanic plexus formed by tympanic branch of cranial nerve IX. Fibres of lesser petrosal nerve relay in the otic ganglion. Postganglionic fibres reach the parotid gland through auriculotemporal nerve.
4. Motor root is by a branch from nerve to medial pterygoid. This branch passes unrelayed through the ganglion and divides into two branches to supply tensor veli palatini and tensor tympani

### Branches

The postganglionic branches of the ganglion pass through auriculotemporal nerve to supply the parotid gland.

The motor branches supply the two muscles—tensor veli palatini and tensor tympani.

## CILIARY GANGLION

### Location

The ciliary ganglion is very small ganglion present in the orbit. Topographically, the ganglion is related to nasociliary nerve, branch of ophthalmic division of trigeminal nerve, but functionally it is related to oculomotor nerve. This ganglion gets parasympathetic fibres.

### Roots

It has three roots—the sensory, sympathetic and parasympathetic. Only the parasympathetic root fibres relay to supply the intraocular muscles.

1. Sensory root is from the long ciliary nerve.
2. Sympathetic root is by the long ciliary nerve from plexus around ophthalmic artery.
3. Parasympathetic root is from a branch to inferior oblique muscle. These fibres arise from Edinger-Westphal nucleus, join oculomotor nerve and leave it via the nerve to inferior oblique, to be relayed in the ciliary ganglion.

### Branches

The ganglion gives 10–12 short ciliary nerves. These contain postganglionic fibres for the supply of constrictor or sphincter pupillae for narrowing the size of pupil and ciliaris muscle for increasing the curvature of anterior surface of lens. These are required during accommodation of the eye.

## ARTERIES OF HEAD AND NECK (Table A.3)

**TABLE A.3: Common carotid artery**

| *Artery* | *Beginning, course and termination* | *Branches* |
|---|---|---|
| Common carotid (Table A.3) | It is a branch of brachiocephalic trunk on right side and a direct branch of arch of aorta on the left side. The artery runs upwards along medial border of sternocleidomastoid muscle enclosed within the carotid sheath. The artery ends by dividing into internal carotid and external carotid at the upper border of thyroid cartilage (*see* Fig. 4.13) | Two terminal branches: Internal carotid and external carotid |
| Internal carotid | It is a terminal branch of common carotid artery. It first runs through the neck (cervical part), then passes through the petrous bone (petrous part), then courses through the sinus (cavernous part) and lastly lies in relation to the brain (cerebral part) | ***Cervical part:*** No branch<br>***Petrous part***<br>1. Caroticotympanic branches<br>2. Pterygoid branch<br>***Cavernous part***<br>1. Cavernous branches<br>2. Superior and inferior hypophyseal arteries.<br>***Cerebral part***<br>1. Ophthalmic artery<br>2. Anterior choroidal artery<br>3. Posterior communicating artery<br>4. Anterior cerebral artery<br>5. Middle cerebral artery |

*(Contd.)*

**TABLE A.3: Common carotid artery** *(Contd.)*

| *Artery* | *Beginning, course and termination* | *Branches* |
|---|---|---|
| External carotid | It is one of the terminal branches of common carotid artery and lies anterior to internal carotid artery. External carotid artery starts at the level of upper border of thyroid cartilage, runs upwards and laterally to terminate behind the neck of mandible by dividing into larger maxillary and smaller superficial temporal branches | 1. Ascending pharyngeal artery<br>2. Superior thyroid artery<br>3. Lingual artery<br>4. Facial artery<br>5. Occipital artery<br>6. Posterior auricular artery<br>7. Superficial temporal artery<br>8. Maxillary artery |
| Superior thyroid | It arises from anterior aspect of external carotid artery close to its origin. It runs downwards and forwards deep to the infrahyoid muscles to the upper pole of thyroid gland | 1. Infrahyoid branch<br>2. Superior laryngeal artery<br>3. Cricothyroid branch<br>4. Sternocleidomastoid branch<br>5. Anterior and posterior branches |
| Lingual | It arises from anterior aspect of external carotid artery forms a typical loop which is crossed by XII nerve. Its 2nd part lies deep to the hyoglossus. The 3rd part runs along the anterior border of hyoglossus and 4th part runs forwards on the under surface of tongue | 1. Suprahyoid artery<br>2. Dorsal lingual artery (3–4 in number)<br>3. Sublingual artery |
| Facial | This tortuous artery from anterior side also arises a little higher than lingual artery. It runs in the neck as cervical part and in the face as facial artery | 1. Ascending palatine artery<br>2. Tonsillar artery<br>3. Glandular branches for submandibular gland<br>4. Submental artery<br>5. Inferior labial artery<br>6. Superior labial artery<br>7. Lateral nasal artery |
| Occipital | It arises from the posterior aspect of external carotid artery and runs upwards along the lower border of posterior belly of digastric muscle. Then it runs deep to mastoid process and the muscles attached to it. The artery then crosses the apex of suboccipital triangle and then it pierces trapezius 2.5 cm from midline to supply the layers of scalp (*see* Fig. 4.13) | 1. Sternomastoid branches: Upper and lower<br>2. Mastoid branch<br>3. Meningeal branches<br>4. Muscular branches<br>5. Descending branch: Superficial and deep<br>6. Occipital branches |
| Posterior auricular | It arises from posterior aspect of external carotid artery, it runs along the upper border of posterior belly of digastric muscle to reach the back of auricle | 1. Stylomastoid branch<br>2. Auricular branch<br>3. Occipital branch |
| Ascending pharyngeal | It arises from the medial side of external carotid artery, close to its origin. It runs upwards and between pharynx and tonsil on medial side and medial wall of middle ear on the lateral side (*see* Fig. 4.13) | 1. Pharyngeal branches<br>2. Inferior tympanic branch<br>3. Meningeal branches |
| Superficial temporal | It is the smaller terminal branch of external carotid artery. It begins behind the neck of the mandible, runs upwards and crosses the preauricular point, where its pulsations can be felt. 5 cm above the preauricular point it ends by dividing into anterior and posterior branches (*see* Fig. 2.7) | 1. Transverse facial artery<br>2. Anterior auricular branch<br>3. Zygomatico-orbital branch<br>4. Middle temporal artery<br>5. Anterior and posterior divisions |
| Maxillary | It is the larger terminal branch of external carotid artery. It is given off behind the neck of the mandible. Its course is divided into 1st, 2nd and 3rd parts according to its relations with lateral pterygoid muscle. 1st part lies below the lateral pterygoid, 2nd part lies on the lower head of lateral pterygoid and 3rd part lies between the two heads | ***From the first part***<br>1. Deep auricular<br>2. Anterior tympanic<br>3. Middle meningeal<br>4. Accessory meningeal<br>5. Inferior alveolar<br>***From the second part***<br>1. Masseteric<br>2. Deep temporal<br>3. Pterygoid<br>4. Buccal |

*(Contd.)*

**TABLE A.3: Common carotid artery** *(Contd.)*

| *Artery* | *Beginning, course and termination* | *Branches* |
|---|---|---|
| | | ***From third part***<br>1. Posterior superior alveolar<br>2. Infraorbital<br>3. Greater palatine<br>4. Pharyngeal<br>5. Artery to pterygoid canal<br>6. Sphenopalatine |
| **Subclavian artery** | It is the chief artery of the upper limb. It also supplies part of neck and brain. On the right side, subclavian artery is a branch of the brachiocephalic trunk. On the left side, it is a direct branch of arch of aorta. The artery on either side ascends and enters the neck posterior to the sternoclavicular joint. The arteries of two sides have similar course. The artery arches from the sternoclavicular joint to the outer border of the first rib where it continues as the axillary artery. It is divided into three parts by the crossing of scalenus anterior muscle (*see* Figs 8.20 and 8.21) | ***From 1st part***<br>1. Vertebral artery<br>2. Internal thoracic artery<br>3. Thyrocervical trunk<br>a. Inferior thyroid artery<br>b. Transverse cervical artery<br>c. Suprascapular artery<br>4. Costocervical trunk (only on the left side)<br>a. Superior intercostal artery<br>b. Deep cervical artery<br>***From 2nd part***<br>Costocervical trunk only on the right side<br>***From 3rd part***<br>Dorsal scapular artery (occasional branch; if present, it replaces the deep branch of transverse cervical artery) |

## PHARYNGEAL APPARATUS (Table A.4 to A.6)

**TABLE A.4: Structures derived from skeletal and muscular components of pharyngeal arches** (*Source*: Textbook of Human Embryology, Yogesh Sontakke, 2e, CBS Publishers)

| *Pharyngeal arch* | *Muscles* | *Nerve* | *Skeletal elements* | *Ligament* |
|---|---|---|---|---|
| First arch (Meckel's cartilage) | Muscles of mastication (temporalis, masseter, medial and lateral pterygoid)<br>Tensor veli palatini<br>Tensor tympani<br>Anterior belly of digastric<br>Mylohyoid | Pretrematic: Chorda tympani<br>Post-trematic: Mandibular nerve | Premaxilla<br>Maxilla<br>Zygomatic bone Temporal bone<br>Incus Malleus | Anterior ligament of malleus<br>Sphenomandibular ligament |
| Second arch (Reichert's cartilage) | Muscles of facial expression<br>Posterior belly of digastric<br>Stylohyoid<br>Stapedius | Facial nerve | Stapes<br>Styloid process<br>Short (lesser) cornua of hyoid bone<br>Superior part of body of hyoid bone | Stylohyoid ligament |
| Third arch | Stylopharyngeus | Glossopharyngeal nerve | Greater cornua of hyoid bone<br>Lower part of body of hyoid bone | — |
| Fourth arch | Cricothyroid, constrictors of pharynx, muscles of palate except tensor veli palatini | Superior laryngeal nerve | Laryngeal cartilages except epiglottis | — |
| Sixth arch | Intrinsic muscles of larynx except cricothyroid | Recurrent laryngeal nerve | — | — |

**TABLE A.5: Derivatives of ectodermal clefts**

| *Pharyngeal cleft* | *Derivatives* |
|---|---|
| Dorsal part of first ectodermal cleft | Epithelium of external auditory meatus |
| Auricle | Six auricular hillocks; three from first arch and three from II arch |
| Rest of ectodermal clefts | Obliterated by the overgrowth of second pharyngeal arch. The closing membrane of the first cleft is the tympanic membrane |

| TABLE A.6: Derivatives of endodermal pouches | |
|---|---|
| ***Pharyngeal pouch*** | ***Derivatives*** |
| Dorsal ends of first and second pouches form tubotympanic recess | Proximal part of tubotympanic recess gives rise to auditory tube<br>Distal part gives rise to tympanic cavity and mastoid antrum<br>Mastoid cells develop at about 2 years of age |
| Ventral part of second pouch | Epithelium covering the palatine tonsil and tonsillar crypts<br>Lymphoid tissue is mesodermal in origin |
| Third pouch | Thymus and inferior parathyroid gland or parathyroid III<br>Thymic epithelial reticular cells and Hassall's corpuscles are endodermal<br>Lymphocytes are derived from haemopoietic stem cells during 12th week |
| Fourth pouch | Superior parathyroid or parathyroid IV |
| Caudal pharyngeal complex | Thymic element – part of thymus Lateral thyroid element – part of thyroid gland<br>Ultimobranchial body – parafollicular |

BDC's Anatomy *e*-book

1. Molecular regulation of pharyngeal arches
2. Clinical terms

# Index